Cardiovascular MRI

*Physical Principles
to Practical Protocols*

Cardiovascular MRI

*Physical Principles
to Practical Protocols*

VIVIAN S. LEE, MD, PhD

Professor
Departments of Radiology and of Physiology and Neuroscience
Vice Chair of Research
Department of Radiology
New York University School of Medicine
New York, NY

ILLUSTRATED BY

MARTHA HELMERS

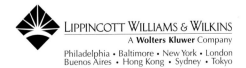

LIPPINCOTT WILLIAMS & WILKINS
A **Wolters Kluwer** Company
Philadelphia • Baltimore • New York • London
Buenos Aires • Hong Kong • Sydney • Tokyo

Acquisitions Editor: Lisa McAllister
Developmental Editor: Rebecca Barroso
Marketing Manager: Angela Panetta
Manufacturing Manager: Ben Rivera
Production Editor: David Murphy
Compositor: Publication Services, Inc.
Printer: The Maple-Vail Book Manufacturing Group

© 2006 by LIPPINCOTT WILLIAMS & WILKINS
530 Walnut Street
Philadelphia, PA 19106 USA
LWW.com

Printed in the USA

Library of Congress Cataloging-in-Publication Data

Lee, Vivian S., 1966-
    Cardiovascular MRI : physical principles to practical
protocols / Vivian
S. Lee ; illustrated by Martha Helmers.
        p. ; cm.
    Includes index.
    ISBN-13: 978-0-7817-7996-8 (alk. paper)
    1. Cardiovascular system—Magnetic resonance imaging. 2. Magnetic
resonance imaging. 3. Medical physics.   I. Title.
    [DNLM: 1. Cardiovascular Diseases—radiography. 2. Magnetic
Resonance Angiography—methods. 3. Magnetic Resonance Imaging
—methods.   WG 141.5.M2 L481c 2005]
    RC670.5.M33L44 2005
    616.1'07548—dc22

2005033038

This book is dedicated to my parents,
Samuel and Elisa Lee, and
my sister, Jennifer Lee,
for their love and inspiration;
and to my husband, Benedict Kingsbury,
and to my children,
Annelisa and Mira-Rose Kingsbury Lee,
for bringing me such joy in life.

CONTENTS

PREFACE

The world of magnetic resonance (MR) imaging is evolving at a pace that is at the same time awe-inspiring and overwhelming. In part, these developments can be attributed to the revolution in computer technology. More importantly, however, credit must be given to the remarkable ingenuity of MR physicists and engineers who, through the development of new tools and techniques, have made MR indispensable in the clinical setting. As a consequence of the extensive technical advances, a serious understanding of MR physics may seem beyond the grasp of most physicians. Experience teaching physics to physicians shows that this is not so!

From a practical perspective, users who have a working knowledge about the physics underlying the generation of MR images have considerable advantage over passive interpreters of imaging studies. Active participation in developing protocols and acquiring images helps to optimize performance and diagnostic quality. Artifacts and pitfalls can be recognized and, when possible, minimized or avoided. Moreover, a firm understanding of present-day techniques is vital to the adoption of new advances, which will continue for the foreseeable future.

The aim of this book is to provide clinicians in practice or in training with a firm foundation in the physical principles of how MR images are generated. Scientists new to MRI may also find this book a useful introduction; its practical perspective may be of particular interest to researchers seeking to have an impact on medical practice. The book is divided into three sections. Section I covers basic principles of MR physics, particularly those relevant to an understanding of cardiovascular MR imaging. Included also is a chapter that concentrates on safety issues (Chapter I-10). Section II focuses on the principles as applied to vascular imaging and emphasizes gadolinium-enhanced MR angiography in Chapter II-4. Section III turns to cardiac MR imaging, reviewing different categories of techniques and applications.

The foundational principles covered in the first part of the book are applicable across all of MRI. The concepts presented use classical-physics models of proton behavior so that only a high-school level of mathematics and physics is required. To refresh the reader's memory of this material, reviews of basic math and physics concepts are incorporated in the text. MR applications are focused on cardiovascular imaging, where the demands for fast and artifact-free images have created fertile ground for some of the most exciting innovations in MRI. From this book, students should be able to apply lessons learned in MR physics to customize and optimize current state-of-the-art cardiovascular MR imaging sequences and protocols.

Key Concepts are summarized at the beginning of each chapter. In the first few chapters, Background Reading sections are included to help the reader review basic mathematical and physics principles. These concepts are not optional. For the reader to follow the development of ideas in this book, an understanding of these sections is vital. Throughout the text, the take-home points are highlighted as Important Concepts. Additionally, Challenge Questions scattered throughout each chapter are intended to engage the reader in the learning process. At the end of each chapter, Review Questions provide an opportunity to apply lessons learned and to think beyond the material provided in the text. Many of the chapters in Sections II and III conclude with sample clinical Protocols for the reader to implement in his/her own practice. A glossary of terms is included at the end of the book.

ACKNOWLEDGMENTS

My parents, Professors Samuel and Elisa Lee, have devoted their professional lives to scientific research and to education. Their unquenchable spirit of inquiry instilled in me and in my sister Jennifer Lee, also now a physician-scientist, a fascination with the application of science and engineering to medicine. As devoted and loving parents, they created a family life that was committed to equality, hard work, and the flourishing of all. They have worked unceasingly to enable us to be what we are.

My career in Radiology was made possible by Carl Ravin, Chair of the Department of Radiology at Duke University, where I trained as a resident and where I discovered a passion for MRI. I received much encouragement from our residency program director, James Bowie, who assigned me to teach basic MR physics early in my training. My appreciation of the elegance of MR physics was kindled by the teachers at the Stanford-Duke MR physics course, especially Dwight Nishimura and his superb tutorial on k-space. He kindly agreed to use of some of this material in Chapter I-6 of this book, including the Review Questions. The world of MR science is warmly collegial—my education has come from very many physicists, engineers, and expert physician-scientists who have patiently answered my innumerable questions about MR physics over many years. Many have been very welcoming colleagues in the International Society of Magnetic Resonance in Medicine (ISMRM). I am indebted to them all.

The marvelous opportunity to do my MRI fellowship, then directed by Jeffrey Weinreb, Neil Rofsky, and Glenn Krinsky, at NYU meant an incomparable immersion in the fast-evolving practice of clinical body and cardiovascular MRI. In the last few years, our new Chair of Radiology at NYU, Dr. Robert Grossman, has made remarkable progress toward realizing his vision of our department as leading one of the top in the country. One of his achievements has been the development of a top-notch group of MR researchers, many of whom I have the pleasure to learn from and to collaborate with in research. The combination of outstanding MR scientists, superb fellows and residents, and a dedicated team of clinical faculty, technologists, nurses, and staff have made NYU a place in which I feel fortunate to work.

The material for this book has evolved from a series of MR physics lectures I have given at NYU over the years, having been challenged, critiqued, and improved by the participants. I thank them for inspiring preparation of this book. For cheerfully helping me to organize and juggle multiple responsibilities at work while preparing the manuscript, I am grateful to Lois Mannon, Carol Nazzaro, and Polina Khodora; to my research assistants Ambrose Huang, Manmeen Kaur, and Ting Song; and to my excellent colleagues in body and cardiovascular MRI: Elizabeth Hecht, Bachir Taouli, Michael Macari, Barbara Srichai, and Leon Axel.

For making this book possible, I am profoundly indebted to Martha Helmers. She created and edited over 400 illustrations and figures for this project. Martha is a photoradiologist extraordinaire as well as a self-taught master of software programs such as Photoshop and Illustrator. She has contributed her time, energy, and remarkable creativity with an admirable steadiness and selflessness. I am thankful for her talent, for her encouragement, and for her never-failing enthusiasm despite the daunting volume of work this project proved to involve.

Several friends and colleagues have devoted much time and meticulous attention to reading drafts of parts or all of this book. Henry Rusinek sharpened phrasing and clarified concepts throughout the book. For innumerable further invaluable and diverse suggestions for its improvement, I warmly thank: Louisa Bokacheva, Qun Chen, Robert Edelman, Sandra Moore, Niels Oesingmann, and Lon Simonetti. My thanks also to colleagues from other institutions—Debiao Li, Martin Prince and Hajime Sakuma for generously providing MR images for this text.

Above all, I wish to thank my husband, Benedict Kingsbury, for his love, generosity, strength of spirit, and boundless support of all my endeavors, and our beloved children, Annelisa and Mira-Rose Kingsbury Lee, for filling our lives with immeasurable happiness.

ABBREVIATIONS AND SYMBOLS

SYMBOLS

α = flip angle

α_E = Ernst angle

B_0 = B naught, strength of static magnetic field

B_1 = Strength of RF excitation magnetic field

f = precessional frequency, Larmor frequency, in units Hz or MHz

γ = gyromagnetic ratio

g = geometric factor

Δk = k-space voxel dimension

k_{total} = overall size of k-space

μ = magnetic moment

M = magnetization vector

N_{acq} = number of signal averages

N_{ex} = number of excitations

N_{PE} = number of phase-encoding steps

P = pressure gradient

ϕ = angle in transverse plane with respect to transverse axes

Q_p = pulmonary blood flow

Q_s = systemic blood flow

R1 = spin-lattice relaxivity

R2 = spin-spin relaxivity

SV = stroke volume

T1 = spin-lattice relaxation time

T2 = spin-spin relaxation time

TD = trigger delay

TE = echo time

TE_{eff} = effective echo time

TI = inversion time

TR = repetition time

V = velocity

Venc = encoding velocity

V_{maxFRE} = maximum flow-related enhancement velocity

ω = precessional frequency, Larmor frequency, in units rad/sec

ABBREVIATIONS

ADC = analog-to-digital converter

CI = cardiac index

cm = centimeter

CO = cardiac output

ECG = electrocardiographic

EDV = end diastolic volume

EF = ejection fraction

EPI = echo planar imaging

ESV = end systolic volume

Fast SPGR = fast spoiled gradient echo imaging

FID = free induction decay

FIESTA = fast imaging excitation with steady state acquisition

FFE = fast field echo

FLASH = fast low angle shot imaging

FRE = flow related enhancement

FSE = fast spin echo

FISP = fast imaging with steady state precession

FOV = field of view

G = gauss, 1/10,000 tesla

GRE = gradient recalled echo

HASTE = half-Fourier acquisition single-shot turbo spin echo

HLA = horizontal long axis

Hz = hertz, cycle per second

IR = inversion recovery

LVOT = left ventricular outflow tract

m = meter

MIP = maximum intensity projection

MOTSA = multiple overlapping thin-slab acquisition

MPR = multiplanar reconstruction

MP-RAGE = magnetization preparation rapid acquisition gradient echo

MR = magnetic resonance

MRA = magnetic resonance angiography

MRI = magnetic resonance imaging

msec = millisecond

PD = proton density

PE = phase-encoding

PSV = peak systolic velocity

recFOV = rectangular field of view

rad = radian

RARE = rapid acquisition with relaxation enhancement

RF = radiofrequency

ROI = region of interest

R-R interval = R wave – to – R wave interval

SAR = specific absorption rate

sec = second

SENSE = sensitivity encoding

SMASH = simultaneous acquisition of spatial harmonics

SPAMM = spatial modulation of magnetization

SPGR = spoiled gradient recalled echo

SSD = surface-shaded display

SSFP = steady state free precession

STIR = short tau inversion recovery

T = tesla

TFE = turbo field echo

TOF = time of flight

True FISP = fast imaging with steady state precession

TSE = turbo spin echo

turboFLASH = turbo fast low angle shot imaging

TW = trigger window

VCG = vectorelectrocardiogram

VLA = vertical long axis

VR = volume rendering

MR Physics

Overview of MRI and Basic Principles

The target audience for this book consists of radiologists, technologists, and others interested in medical imaging who want to understand how magnetic resonance (MR) images are made. The goals are to provide enough of a background in MR physics for the reader to use and optimize protocols for MR imaging (MRI), particularly cardiovascular MRI. Keeping in mind the rapid rate of innovation in the field of MRI, this book also aims to equip the reader with a sufficient foundation in MR physics to understand and incorporate future technological advances.

Section I of this book (Chapters I-1 through I-10) describes the general principles of MR physics. Section II puts these principles to practice in vascular imaging applications. Section III is devoted to cardiac imaging.

Section I is meant to be comprehensible to readers of all backgrounds. Although many theoretical principles are reviewed, the emphasis is always on their practical implications. Key mathematical and engineering ideas necessary to understand MRI are reviewed in Background Reading sections. Throughout the text, Challenge Questions are intended to engage the reader in the learning process. Take-home messages each section are summarized in "Important Concepts." *New terms* are italicized and defined in the Glossary at the end of this book. The main ideas of each chapter are summarized in "**Key Concepts**."

This first chapter introduces foundational principles of MRI. The topics of this chapter are: the behavior of hydrogen protons as tiny oscillating magnets in an external magnetic field, the hardware components of an MR system, an overview of image formation, the characteristics of an image that define its quality, and an introduction to pulse sequence diagrams—the recipes for making MR images.

KEY CONCEPTS

▶ Human bodies are made of 95% water. Each water molecule consists of two hydrogen atoms and one oxygen atom.

▶ Hydrogen protons have a special property—they behave like tiny magnets.

▶ Magnetic properties of a single proton (its magnetic moment) or of an aggregate of protons (net magnetization) can be depicted as a vector that may change size and orientation over time.

▶ When placed in a steady magnetic field, the magnetization of protons will align with the field, and their magnetic moments will precess around the axis of the field at the Larmor frequency.

▶ Precessing protons can be depicted as spinning vectors whose frequencies can be expressed in units of hertz (Hz, cycles per second, denoted by f) or of radians per second (as denoted by ω), where $\omega = 2\pi f$.

▶ Hydrogen protons in water molecules precess at different frequencies from those in fat molecules because of their different molecular environments.

▶ Radiofrequency excitation temporarily deflects magnetization from the direction of the external magnetic field. Afterward, magnetization will return to its initial direction via a process called relaxation.

▶ Radiofrequency excitation leads to the generation of MR signals, which are used to produce images; tissues have different appearances on MR images based, in part, on differences in their relaxation properties.

▶ To generate MR images, the positions of protons in the body are localized to specific parts of an image by means of magnetic field gradients and data processing using Fourier transformations.

▶ Defining characteristics of an image include its spatial resolution, signal-to-noise ratio, and contrast-to-noise ratio.

▶ Basic components of an MRI system include a superconducting magnet, transmitter and receiver coils, and gradient coils.

▶ A pulse sequence diagram is a recipe for generating an MR image. It describes the temporal coordination of radiofrequency excitation pulses, gradients, and signal measurements.

HUMANS AS PROTONS AND PROTONS AS MAGNETS

Each hydrogen nucleus consists of a single proton that can be considered as a simple magnet with a tiny magnetic field (Figure I1-1), referred to as its *magnetic moment*.

> **IMPORTANT CONCEPT:** Protons that constitute hydrogen nuclei behave like tiny magnets.

Although the magnetic field of a single proton is minuscule, the aggregate effect of hydrogen protons in the body is measurable. This is because approximately 95% of the body's mass is water (H_2O). Every mole (18 grams) of water contains 6.023×10^{23} oxygen atoms and twice as many hydrogen atoms. Thus, the body of an average 60 kg woman contains about 3.8×10^{27} hydrogen protons in water molecules, not including the protons in her fat!

While the nuclei of elements other than hydrogen, such as phosphorus, sodium, and fluorine, can also be used to generate MR images, the natural abundance of hydrogen in the body makes it particularly suitable for clinical imaging applications.

The generation of clinical MR images can be understood in terms of manipulations of the magnetization of hydrogen protons. Important concepts that will be discussed include the effects of large external fields on the magnetic moments of protons, the consequences of temporarily deflecting magnetic moments away from the direction of the large external field, and the magnetic moments' return to an equilibrium state following the deflection. Each of these concepts requires an understanding of some of the principles of electromagnetism and electromagnetic induction, which are reviewed in the following Background Reading.

BACKGROUND READING: Electromagnetism and Electromagnetic Induction

A magnetic field can be generated in different ways. The most familiar form of a magnet is a bar magnet. It is usually made of iron, and one end of the magnet acts as the north pole while the other is the south pole. Alternatively, a magnetic field can be generated by passing an electrical current through a wire. Current flowing through a loop of wire generates a magnetic field perpendicular to its plane. If the wire is configured as a solenoid—that is, it is coiled tightly in a cylinder (Figure I1-2)—then the magnetic field induced along each loop of the solenoid is added to the fields induced along the other loops, and consequently a substantial magnetic field can be generated along the length of the cylinder. If the current passing through the solenoid is steady, then the magnetic field will be steady, with a north pole at one end of the coil and a south pole at the other end. The strength of the magnetic field is directly proportional to the amount of current passing through the wire and is referred to at B_0 ("B zero" or "B naught"), typically measured in units of tesla or gauss, where 1 tesla (T) = 10,000 gauss (G).

Electromagnetic Induction

Another important concept in electromagnetism is *electromagnetic induction*, which describes the effect of a magnetic field on a nearby wire. A magnetic field changing over time will induce current to flow through the wire (Figure I1-3). The pattern of current flowing through the wire will reflect the pattern of fluctuation of the magnetic field. For example, if the field changes at a particular frequency f, then the current induced in the wire will also alternate with frequency f. A steady magnetic field does not induce any current in the nearby wire.

> **IMPORTANT CONCEPTS:** Current flowing through a loop of wire or through a solenoid will generate a magnetic field. A changing magnetic field will induce current in a nearby wire.

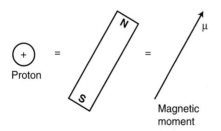

FIGURE I1-1. Protons as magnets. The proton that constitutes the nucleus of a hydrogen atom behaves like a tiny bar magnet. The magnetic field associated with the magnet, its magnetic moment, is expressed as a vector, **μ**.

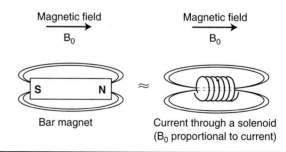

FIGURE I1-2. Electromagnetism. A magnetic field, B_0, can be created using a bar magnet or by applying current through a coil of wire (solenoid). Note that the lines of flux representing the magnetic field of the solenoid are oriented along the bore of the coil (dashed lines). The magnetic field also extends around the solenoid, creating what is referred to as the *fringe field*.

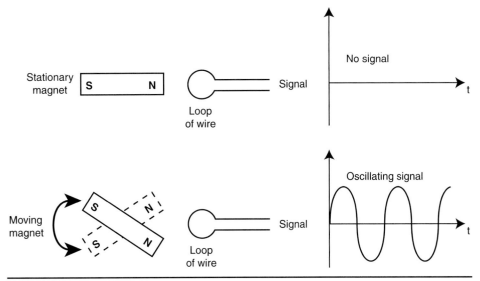

FIGURE I1-3. Electromagnetic induction. A static magnetic field (top) will not induce any current in a nearby loop of wire. However, a magnetic field changing over time (bottom) will induce a current in the loop of wire. The current will have the same frequency of oscillation as the magnetic field.

MAGNETIZATION AS VECTORS

The magnetic properties of a single proton or a population of protons can be depicted as a *vector*, with a certain magnitude and direction. The magnetic moment of a single proton is often denoted as μ (mu) (Figure I1-1), whereas the cumulative effect of a population of protons is given by the net magnetization, **M**. The lengths of the vectors μ and **M** are referred to as their magnitudes, and their directions are usually defined as their angles with respect to some fixed set of reference axes. Before the behavior of magnetic moments in an external magnetic field is described, a review of vectors and sines and cosines is provided in the next Background Reading section.

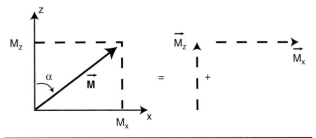

FIGURE I1-4. 2D magnetization vector in the xz plane. The vector **M** can be expressed as the sum of its z component, $\mathbf{M_z}$, and its x component, $\mathbf{M_x}$.

BACKGROUND READING: Vectors and Sines and Cosines

A vector is depicted as an arrow with a magnitude (or length) and angle (or orientation) with respect to some set of reference axes. Vectors can be constrained to lie within a plane (in which case they are called 2D) or they can point in any direction in space (in which case they are then called 3D). Any vector can be expressed as the sum of its x and y (for 2D) or x, y, and z components (for 3D). For example, a vector M in the xz plane with a magnitude **M** and angle α (alpha) relative to the z axis can be thought of as the sum of the x component, $\mathbf{M_x}$, and the z component, $\mathbf{M_z}$ (Figure I1-4).

Similarly, a 3D vector **M** can be expressed as the sum of its x, y, and z components: $\mathbf{M} = \mathbf{M_x} + \mathbf{M_y} + \mathbf{M_z}$.

In MR physics, the sum of $\mathbf{M_x} = \mathbf{M_y}$ can be denoted as $\mathbf{M_{xy}}$. Thus, **M** can be expressed as the sum of its z and xy components, $\mathbf{M} = \mathbf{M_z} + \mathbf{M_{xy}}$ (Figure I1-5). The angle that **M** makes with the z axis is usually referred to as α, while a second angle, ϕ (phi), describes the angle between $\mathbf{M_{xy}}$ and the x axis.

To determine the relationship between the magnitude M, lengths of the components $\mathbf{M_x}$ and $\mathbf{M_z}$ or $\mathbf{M_{xy}}$ and $\mathbf{M_z}$, and the angles α and ϕ, a review of sine and cosine functions is needed.

Definition of Sines and Cosines

A right triangle is defined as a triangle that has one 90° angle. Opposite the 90° angle is called the hypotenuse. Right triangles have useful properties that define the lengths of its sides relative to the angles formed by the sides and the length of the hypotenuse.

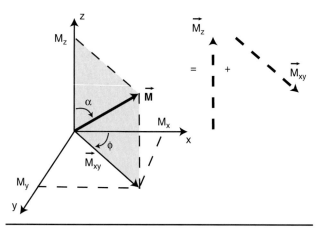

FIGURE I1-5. 3D magnetization vector. A 3D vector **M** can be represented as the sum of two components, **M**$_z$ and **M**$_{xy}$, where **M**$_z$ is considered the longitudinal magnetization, while **M**$_{xy}$ is the transverse magnetization.

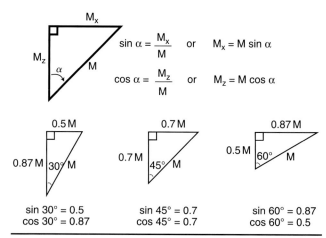

FIGURE I1-6. Sine and cosine definitions for a right triangle, with sample values for three examples of α.

For a right triangle (Figure I1-6), the sine (abbreviated as sin) of one of the non-90° angles is defined as the ratio of the length of the side opposite the angle divided by the length of the hypotenuse. The cosine (abbreviated as cos) of an angle is the ratio of the length of the adjacent side divided by the length of the hypotenuse. In other words, for the triangle in Figure I1-6,

$$\sin \alpha = M_x/M$$
$$\cos \alpha = M_z/M$$

These relationships are the same for all right triangles, regardless of size. Sine and cosine values for the entire range of angles have known values. These values can be used to determine the lengths of the sides of a triangle relative to the hypotenuse. Three sample α values are illustrated in Figure I1-6.

CHALLENGE QUESTION: What is sin 0? What is cos 0?

Answer: As the angle α approaches zero, then M_x approaches zero, so sin 0 = 0. M_z approaches M, so cos 0 = 1.

From these definitions, it follows that for the 2D vector shown in Figure I1-4, the x and z components have magnitudes or lengths that can be predicted knowing the length of M and the angle a:

$$M_x = M \sin \alpha$$
$$M_z = M \cos \alpha$$

CHALLENGE QUESTION: For the 3D vector shown in Figure I1-5, what are the magnitudes of the two components M_{xy} and M_z in terms of the magnitude M and the angle α?

Answer: $M_{xy} = M \sin \alpha$ and $M_z = M \cos \alpha$ (Figure I1-5).

MRI Reference Axes and Standard Terminology

Most MRI uses a magnet field formed by a large coil of superconducting wire, within which the subject is placed. The magnetic field directed along the main axis, or bore, of the magnet usually defines the z axis (Figure I1-7). Magnetization along the bore is referred to as *longitudinal magnetization*, while that perpendicular to the bore is called *transverse magnetization*. Because of the symmetry of magnetization in the transverse plane, the x and y directions are interchangeable. By convention, 3D magnetization vectors **M** are therefore considered in terms of their z (longitudinal) and xy (transverse) components: **M**$_{xy}$ + **M**$_z$. The angle of the vector **M** with respect to the z axis, α, is referred to as the *flip angle*.

> **IMPORTANT CONCEPT:** Magnetization along the direction of the bore of the magnet is referred to as longitudinal magnetization, while magnetization perpendicular to the bore is called transverse magnetization.

For clarification, although most MRI units are positioned so that the the bore of the magnet, the z axis, is horizontal, most textbook drawings of magnetization vectors depict the z axis pointing vertically (Figure I1-7).

> **IMPORTANT CONCEPT:** In most MR physics books, including this one, magnetization vector diagrams are illustrated with the z axis pointed vertically, but in MRI applications in real life the bore of the magnet (the z direction) is in fact usually horizontal.

Net Magnetization

In MRI, the protons across the imaging region do not usually have identical magnetic moments. Their lengths and

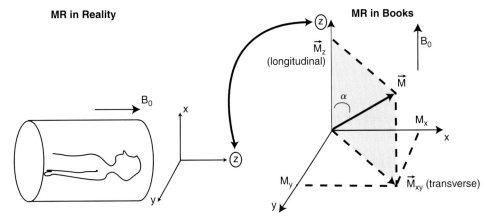

FIGURE I1-7. Orientation of magnetization in reality and in books.

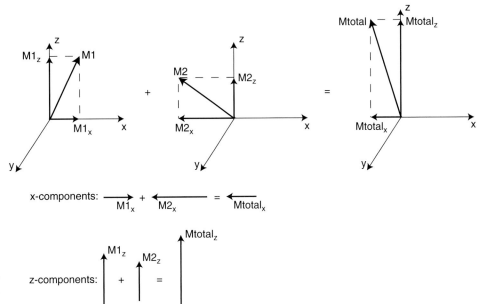

FIGURE I1-8. Vector addition in the xz plane can be accomplished by summing x and z components.

orientations are frequently different, depending on factors such as where they are in the magnetic field and in what types of tissues they are found. To determine the net magnetization of the entire population of protons, different subpopulations must be considered separately and their contributions to net magnetization summed. To determine net magnetization, the reader should feel comfortable with vector addition, which is reviewed in the following Background Reading.

BACKGROUND READING: Vector Addition

There are at least two different ways to perform vector addition. One is to overlay each vector from head to tail (Figures I1-4 and I1-5). For example, as shown in Figure I1-4, the vector M can be formed by the sum of

M_x and M_z, laid from head to tail. Similarly, in three dimensions, the magnetization vector is the sum of M_{xy} and M_z (Figure I1-5).

Alternatively, vectors can be summed by adding each of their orthogonal components, M_x, M_y, and M_z (Figure I1-8). For example, consider two vectors in the xz plane, M1 and M2. To add these two vectors, first break each vector down into its x and z components, $M1_x$, $M1_z$, $M2_x$, $M2_z$. Then sum the x components and z components separately: $Mtotal_x = M1_x + M2_x$. $Mtotal_z = M1_z + M2_z$. The resulting vector **Mtotal** is simply the sum of the component totals, **Mtotal** = $Mtotal_x$ + $Mtotal_z$.

Because vector addition is best understood by examples, the reader is referred to Figure I1-9. As illustrated in the figure, one key concept in vector addition is that vectors pointing in opposite directions cancel each other

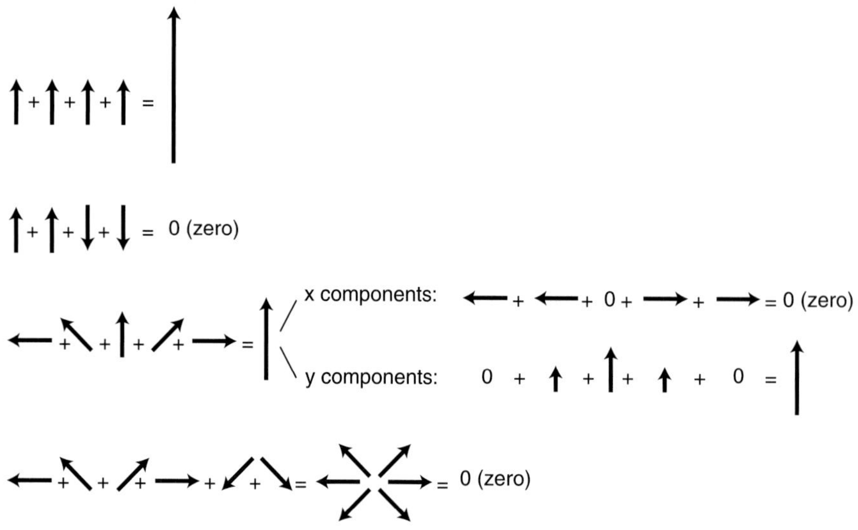

$\uparrow + \uparrow + \uparrow + \uparrow = \Big|$

$\uparrow + \uparrow + \downarrow + \downarrow = 0$ (zero)

$\leftarrow + \diagdown + \uparrow + \diagup + \rightarrow = \Big|$

x components: $\leftarrow + \leftarrow + 0 + \rightarrow + \rightarrow = 0$ (zero)

y components: $0 + \uparrow + \uparrow + \uparrow + 0 = \uparrow$

$\leftarrow + \diagdown + \diagup + \rightarrow + \diagup + \diagdown = 0$ (zero)

FIGURE I1-9. Examples of vector addition. In the third example, each vector is expressed in terms of its x or horizonal components ($\mathbf{M_x}$) as well as its y or vertical components ($\mathbf{M_y}$). A perfectly vertical vector has no x component; a horizontal vector has no y component. When components point in opposite directions, they cancel each other out.

out. Therefore, a large population of vectors that are randomly oriented, pointing in all directions, tends to sum to zero. Because for every vector, there will likely be a vector pointed in the opposite direction.

IMPORTANT CONCEPT: When vectors are added, the components that point in opposite directions cancel each other out.

UNDERSTANDING PRECESSION AND THE LARMOR EQUATION

Precession: The Spinning Gyroscope Analogy

Outside of the MR environment, the magnetic moments of protons in the body are oriented in a completely random fashion, and therefore net magnetization is zero.

What happens when these protons are placed in a strong external magnetic field?

Two aspects of the behavior of the magnetic moments can be observed. First, the magnetic moments tend to align with the external magnetic field. They behave like tiny bar magnets exposed to a strong magnetic field and are inclined to align with it. This creates a net magnetization.

Second, a magnetic moment placed in an external field is induced to rotate around the axis of the magnetic field. To understand this movement, known as *precession*, consider the analogy of a wobbling gyroscope (Figure I1-10). A spinning gyroscope oriented vertically spins without any wobbling. However, once tipped off axis, gravity causes the spinning gyroscope to start to wobble. The wobbling has its own frequency (f in Figure I1-10), which can be

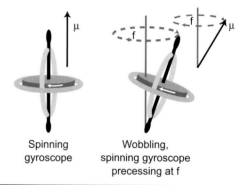

Spinning gyroscope

Wobbling, spinning gyroscope precessing at f

FIGURE I1-10. The wobbling, spinning gyroscope analogy for a precessing proton with magnetic moment **μ**.

considered independent of the frequency of spinning. The precession of protons' magnetic moments is akin to this wobbling. In the case of the gyroscope, the wobbling frequency depends on gravity, while for protons the precessional frequency depends on the strength of the external magnetic field, B_0. The *precessional frequency* is measured either in hertz (cycles per second, in which case it is denoted by f) or in radians per second (in which case it is denoted by ω, omega), where $\omega = 2\pi f$ and π (pi) is approximately 3.14.

When exposed to the B_0 magnetic field, all magnetic moments precess (or wobble) around the axis of the magnetic field. Although the magnetic moments precess at about the same frequency, they do not precess together (Figure I1-11), that is, they lack *phase coherence*. As a result, the transverse or M_{xz} components are randomly oriented. Based on the concepts of vector addition (Figure I1-9) and the very large number of protons in the tissue, transverse magnetization cancels out and is zero. Consequently, the net magnetization, **M**, is entirely longitudinal in the direction of B_0 and stationary.

Magnetic Moments with No Phase Coherence

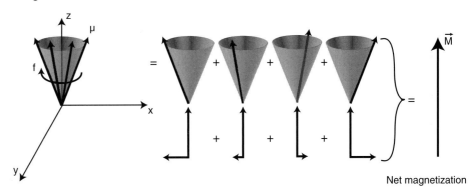

Net magnetization

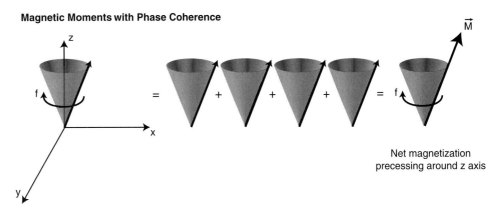

Magnetic Moments with Phase Coherence

Net magnetization
precessing around z axis

FIGURE I1-11. Precessing magnetic moments without (above) and with (below) phase coherence. When magnetic moments lack phase coherence, despite precessing at the same frequency, the transverse components in the xy plane cancel out (x components illustrated in figure), leaving only a net magnetization in the z direction. With phase coherence, the net magnetization also precesses around the z axis.

If the magnetic moments gain phase coherence, then the net magnetization precesses around the z axis at a frequency f (Figure I1-11). In other words, net magnetization acquires a transverse component that rotates in the xy plane with a frequency f.

While vectors are useful for showing the state of magnetization at a given point in time, other tools are better for depicting the behavior of magnetization vectors over time, such as precessing magnetic moments. Sinusoidal curves can illustrate the behavior of a single magnetic moment, populations of coherent moments, as well as populations of magnetic moments that are gradually losing phase coherence. The relationship between precessing vectors and their depiction as sinusoidal curves is detailed in the following Background Reading on precessing vectors, angular frequency, and sinusoidal curves.

BACKGROUND READING: Precessing Vectors, Angular Frequency, and Sinusoidal Curves

Precessing Vectors
When placed in an external magnetic field, the magnetic moments of protons precess around the axis of that field. Because it is difficult to depict a moving magnetization vector on paper, the precessing vector is instead represented by plotting one component of the vector (usually M_x or M_y) against time (Figure I1-12).

CHALLENGE QUESTION: What is the value of M_x at any point in time, if $\phi(t)$ is defined as the angle between M_{xy} and the x axis that changes over time? What about M_y?

Answer: The x component M_x changes over time and can be expressed using the cosine function (Figure I1-6 and Figure I1-13):

$$M_x(t) = M_{xy} \cos \phi(t)$$

where the angle of M_{xy} with respect to the x axis, ϕ, changes over time, as denoted $\phi(t)$. Similarly, the y component $M_y(t) = M_{xy} \sin \phi(t)$.

With precessing vectors, ϕ is changing constantly over time. As ϕ changes from zero to 90° ($\pi/2$) to 180° (π) to 360° (2π) and back around the circle again, the value of M_x will also change—from M_{xy} to 0 to $-M_{xy}$ and back to M_{xy} again (recall that cos 0° = 1, cos 90° = 0, cos 180° = −1, and cos 0° = cos 360° = 1).

The rate of change of ϕ per unit time is defined as an *angular frequency*, which is simply the precessional frequency. This frequency describes how fast

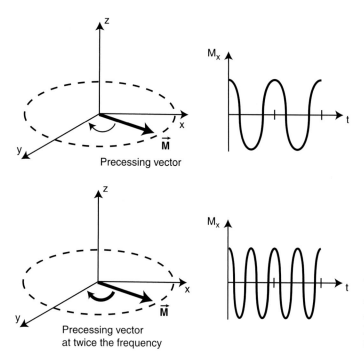

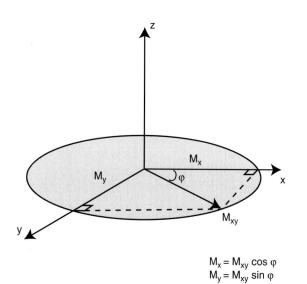

$$M_x = M_{xy} \cos \varphi$$
$$M_y = M_{xy} \sin \varphi$$

FIGURE I1-13. The x component of $\mathbf{M_{xy}}$ varies over time depending on its angle with respect to the x axis, ϕ.

the precessing magnetic moments spin around in the xy plane, and it can be expressed using different units. The use of different units can be confusing and merits a brief discussion and explanation.

Angular Frequencies

A common way to express the frequency of precessing vectors is in terms of cycles per second, or the number of full 360° rotations per second. The units of hertz (Hz) are used, where 1 Hz equals one cycle per second.

FIGURE I1-12. Precessing vectors. A precessing vector in the xy plane can be depicted in terms of its x component, $\mathbf{M_x}$, over time. The frequency of precession is twice as high in the lower example, resulting in a more "compressed"-appearing sinusoidal function for $\mathbf{M_x}$.

When frequency is expressed in these units, the symbol f is usually used for angular frequency.

Alternatively, angular frequency can be expressed in units of radians per second, where one full cycle (360°) is equal to 2π (two pi, or about 6.28) radians. This means that one cycle per second equals 2π radians per second. When angular frequency is expressed in radians per second, the symbol ω (omega) is usually used.

Both expressions of angular frequency, f and ω, are useful in MRI. In particular, ω is useful for relating frequency to the angle ϕ that a magnetic moment makes with the x axis. After precessing for time t, ϕ, in units of radians, simply equal to the product of ω and t (ωt). Therefore, the precessional behavior of magnetization over time can be expressed in terms of M_x using the equation

$$M_x(t) = M_{xy} \cos \phi(t) = M_{xy} \cos \omega t$$

The faster the vector spins, the higher the frequency ω, and the more sinusoidal oscillations will occur per unit time. Figure I1-12 illustrates two precessing moments, one at twice the frequency of the other.

CHALLENGE QUESTION: What is the relationship between frequencies expressed in f and ω?

Answer: The two are related simply by:

$$\omega = 2\pi f \quad \text{or} \quad f = \omega/2\pi$$

For example, if f = 64,000,000 Hz (or 64 MHz), then
ω = 64,000,000 cycles/sec × 6.28 rad/cycle
   = 402,112,859 rad/sec.

Sinusoidal Functions

There are certain properties of cosine and sine functions that are useful to understand for MR imaging. One concept is that of symmetric and asymmetric functions. Cosine is a *symmetric* function (Figure I1-14). This means that the cosine curve is a mirror image of itself around time = 0. In other words, $\cos(-\omega t) = \cos \omega t$. In contrast, sine curves are *asymmetric functions*: $\sin(-\omega t) = -\sin(\omega t)$.

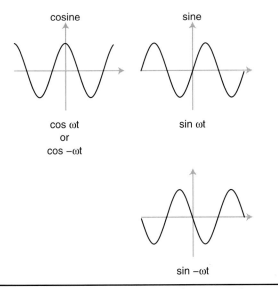

FIGURE I1-14. Symmetry of the cosine function and asymmetry of the sine function.

Precessing Vectors with and without Phase Coherence

Instead of just one magnetic moment, consider what happens when there is a collection of many precessing magnetic moments.

If all the vectors precess together, then they have phase coherence. The overall amplitude of the net magnetization will be equal to the sum of the individual components, and the net magnetization will have a frequency equal to that of any individual magnetic moment (Figure I1-15, top).

What happens if the frequencies of the individual components are slightly different? They lose phase coherence and no longer precess together. Then the net magnetization curve will resemble that shown in the lower two parts of Figure I1-15. As the magnetic moments drift in frequency, the sinusoidal functions no longer sum in a straightforward way. At a reference time point (the midpoint of the curves plotted in Figure I1-15), the magnetization adds. However, away from this point, signal from magnetization vectors precessing at different frequencies cancels partly, resulting in attenuation of the signal away from the midpoint.

The resulting magnetization sinusoidal curve begins to take on the shape of a *sinc function*. Mathematically, a sinc function can be expressed as

$$\text{sinc } x = (\sin x)/x \qquad (\text{and sinc} = 1 \text{ for } x = 0)$$

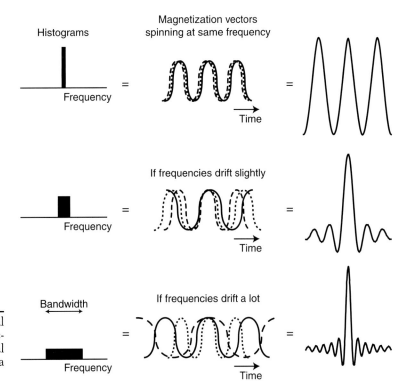

FIGURE I1-15. Transverse magnetization signal over time from many precessing magnetization vectors. With greater drifts in frequency, the net signal looks less like a sinusoidal function and more like a sinc function.

As illustrated in the figure, there is a relationship between the range of frequencies and the appearance of the resulting signal. Specifically, the greater the drift in the frequencies or the wider the range of frequencies used to form the sinc function, the more "compressed" the curve appears (Figure I1-15). The extreme frequency contributions result in the narrowing of the summed signal and its side ripples.

In MR terms, the range of frequencies is referred to as the *bandwidth* and is defined as the highest frequency minus the lowest frequency.

The Larmor Frequency and the Larmor Equation

One of the most important concepts of MR physics is the *Larmor equation*, which describes the relationship between the precessional frequency and the external magnetic field to which the protons are exposed.

The Larmor equation says that the angular frequency at which the magnetic moments precess around the axis of the magnetic field, called the *Larmor frequency*, is proportional to the strength of the magnetic field. The higher the field strength, the faster the precession,

$$f = \gamma B$$

where f = precessional frequency, B is the magnetic field strength, and γ (gamma) is the *gyromagnetic ratio*. γ depends on the type of nucleus being imaged. For hydrogen protons, $\gamma \cong 42.6$ megahertz per tesla (MHz/T; recall that a frequency denoted f is measured in cycles per second, or hertz, and 1 MHz = 1 million cycles per second). Compared to other nuclei, hydrogen protons have a large gyromagnetic ratio. This, in addition to their natural abundance, makes hydrogen ideal for MR imaging because small changes in the magnetic field cause large, and readily measurable, changes in signal. For a 1.5 T magnet, the Larmor frequency is

$$f = 42.6 \text{ MHz/T} \times 1.5 \text{ T} = 63.9 \text{ MHz} \approx 64 \text{ MHz}$$

or about 64 million cycles per second. If the magnetic field were uniformly and perfectly 1.5 T throughout, then all protons in the magnet's bore would precess around the z axis at the same frequency of about 64 MHz.

IMPORTANT CONCEPT: The Larmor equation states that the frequency of precession of magnetic moments around the axis of an external magnetic field, called the Larmor frequency, is proportional to the strength of the magnetic field.

As will be discussed later, no MRI system has a perfectly homogeneous magnetic field, B_0, throughout its bore. What then is the effect of heterogeneity in the magnetic field? The answer lies simply in understanding the Larmor equation: Protons that are exposed to slightly different magnetic fields will precess at slightly different frequencies. More specifically, protons that are exposed to fields less than 1.5 T will precess slightly more slowly than those exposed to 1.5 T, while those exposed to fields greater than 1.5 T will precess more quickly.

Frequency and Phase

In MRI, the effects of magnetic field differences on the precessing of protons are characterized in terms of *frequency* and *phase*. Frequency is the rate of change of phase. It is described simply as the number of cycles (or millions of cycles) per second. By the Larmor equation, frequency changes directly in proportion to the strength of the magnetic field.

What about phase? Phase refers to the orientation of one magnetization vector relative to some reference. It can be thought of as the angle between two vectors or between a vector and a reference axis, for example the angle ϕ between a vector M_{xy} and the x axis (Figure I1-13). If two protons start in the same position but precess at different frequencies, then with time the protons will be out of phase; that is, there will be a phase difference between them. The greater the frequency difference between two protons, the greater the phase difference over a given time. For a given difference in frequencies, the more time elapsed, the greater the phase difference separating the two protons. However, phase shift is uniquely defined only across a range of 360°. When a phase shift exceeds 360° (say, 370°), it becomes indistinguishable from a phase shift 360° less (say, 10°). Nevertheless, the cumulative phase difference between two protons precessing at two frequencies is proportional to the difference in frequencies and to the duration of time that has passed (Figure I1-16).

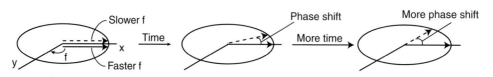

FIGURE I1-16. Frequency and phase are directly related. Protons with higher frequencies (solid vector) will become out of phase with those precessing at lower frequency (dashed vector). The phase shifts increase over time.

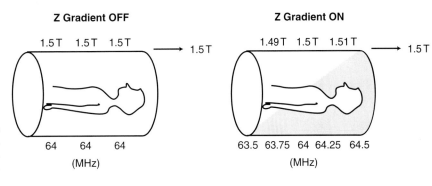

FIGURE I1-17. Varying the magnetic field with a z gradient alters the precessional frequencies of protons along the z direction.

> **IMPORTANT CONCEPT:** Protons exposed to different magnetic fields will precess at different frequencies. Consequently, phase differences will progressively accumulate between their magnetic moments.

Gradients

Precessional frequencies can be deliberately made to vary with position in the magnetic field by applying a magnetic field *gradient* along a given direction. A magnetic field gradient refers to a magnetic field that varies in a certain direction (Figure I1-17). In the setting of a gradient, the precessional frequencies of protons vary spatially in a predictable fashion. For example, with a linear magnetic field gradient in the z direction (Figure I1-17), the field toward the subject's feet is slightly weaker than 1.5 T, while the field toward the head is slightly stronger. The protons at the feet therefore precess more slowly than the middle of the body, and those in the head precess more quickly. For a given linear magnetic field gradient, the range of precessional frequencies across the field of view, Δf, or the bandwidth, can be predicted using the Larmor equation,

$$\Delta f = \gamma \Delta B$$

where ΔB is the range of magnetic field strengths across relevant region.

> **IMPORTANT CONCEPT:** Magnetic field gradients cause precessional frequencies to vary spatially in a predictable fashion, according to the Larmor equation.

Spatial variation of the external magnetic field causes a corresponding variation in Larmor frequencies for the magnetic moments exposed to the gradient. What would the effect of deliberately varying precessional frequencies to vary have on the net magnetization? Based on the previous Background Reading (Figure I1-15), the cumulative signal from protons exposed to a linear magnetic field gradient will resemble a sinc function (Figure I1-18).

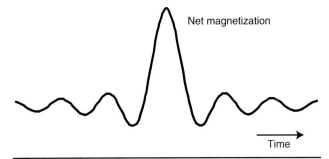

FIGURE I1-18. The composite signal from protons exposed to a magnetic field gradient resembles a sinc function.

Fat versus Water

So far, the discussion about the Larmor frequency has assumed that all hydrogen nuclei are alike, but they are not. The molecular environment experienced by a given hydrogen proton is not exactly equal to B_0, but depends on the nature of its surrounding electron cloud, which tends to shield it from the external magnetic field. In water, hydrogen atoms are bound to oxygen; in fat, hydrogen atoms are bound to carbon. Oxygen attracts the electron cloud away from the hydrogen atoms more strongly than carbon does (that is, the oxygen-hydrogen bond is said to be more polar than the carbon-hydrogen bond). Less shielded by their electron clouds, the protons in water "see" a stronger magnetic field than the protons in fat do. As a result, the precessional frequency of water protons is slightly faster than that of fat protons. At 1.5 T, the difference is about 220 Hz. For example, if water protons are precessing at 63,864,220 Hz (approximately 64 MHz) at 1.5 T, then the fat protons experiencing the same magnetic field will precess at 63,864,000 Hz or 220 Hz slower (Figure I1-19). The frequency difference is proportional to the B_0 magnetic field strength. At 3 T, the frequency difference is about 440 Hz.

> **IMPORTANT CONCEPT:** At 1.5 T, fat protons precess 220 Hz slower than water protons. The difference is proportional to B_0.

This difference can be advantageous in certain situations, such as when selective imaging of fat or water is desired (as discussed in Chapter I-9). This difference can also

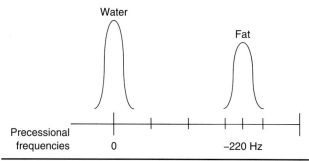

FIGURE I1-19. Precessional frequencies of protons in fat and water at 1.5 T.

create certain artifacts, such as chemical shift artifacts, which are reviewed in Chapter I-5 (Figure I5-22) and Chapter I-9 (Figure I9-3).

THE "MAGNET"

To produce MR images, the magnetic properties of hydrogen protons are manipulated, measured, and imaged in an MR system, which consists of a complex collection of hardware and software. A clinical MR imaging unit, often referred to colloquially as the "magnet," actually consists of several different components that are necessary for imaging. Before delving into the specific steps needed to make an MR image, it is important to understand and to differentiate these components (Figure I1-20):

1. Superconducting magnet and shim coils
2. Transmitting coil
3. Receiving coil
4. Gradient coils

These components are described below.

(1) Superconducting Magnet

One of the requirements for making MR images is that the protons of the body must be exposed to a relatively large external magnetic field. Although low-field permanent (ferromagnetic) magnets are sometimes used for this purpose in specialized extremity imaging, for cardiovascular MR imaging a magnetic field strength of 1 to 3 T is needed. To generate such a field, a superconducting magnet is used.

The superconducting magnet consists of a solenoid of wire, typically made of niobium-titanium, tightly wound to form a solenoid or cylinder around the bore of the magnet. When a constant current flows through the wire, a static, relatively uniform magnetic field is generated within the bore of the magnet, aligned in the direction of the bore. At room temperature, niobium-titanium has normal resistance. However, when niobium-titanium is cooled to less than 9.5 kelvins (recall that zero kelvin, or

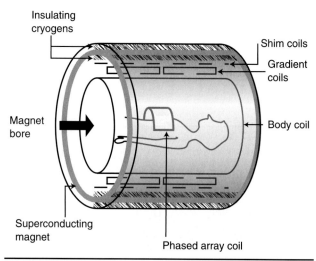

FIGURE I1-20. The main components of a superconducting MR imaging system.

0 K, is absolute zero, the lowest temperature possible), it becomes superconducting. The term *superconducting* means that there is no resistance to current flowing through the wires, so the magnet stays on with no energy added. This has important practical implications. Once a superconducting magnet is ramped up and fully installed, it is always on, regardless of whether the computer console appears to be on or not. As a result, all safety guidelines (as discussed in Chapter I-10) must be followed, even after hours when the lights are out!

> **IMPORTANT CONCEPT:** A superconducting magnet, once ramped up and fully installed, is always on. Safety precautions must be taken around the clock with all MR systems.

The operating expenses of a superconducting magnet come from maintenance of the cooling agents, or cryogens. Older systems use liquid helium (4.2 K) around the wires and an additional insulating layer of liquid nitrogen (77 K) around the helium (Figure I1-21). Newer systems use only the liquid helium and a cold-head compressor instead of the liquid nitrogen.

A magnet *quench* refers to the loss of superconductivity of the main magnet. Quenching is dangerous for several reasons. Once superconductivity is lost, the resistance of the niobium-titanium wire generates considerable heat, which causes rapid evaporation of the cryogens. Helium gas escapes from the cryogen bath (making a loud, hissing noise), and its large volume can displace the oxygen from the room. This is dangerous for the subject and for personnel. Also, in a closed room the helium release can cause a drop in pressure, or a vacuum, in the room. Therefore for safety reasons, all MR scanner rooms must have both ventilation equipment that removes the helium to an outside environment and an oxygen monitor that

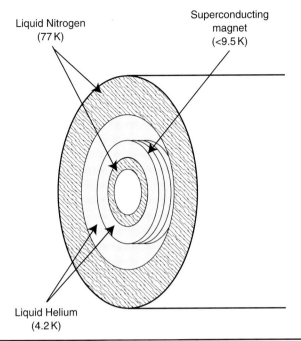

Liquid Nitrogen (77 K)

Superconducting magnet (<9.5 K)

Liquid Helium (4.2 K)

FIGURE I1-21. Cryogens maintain superconductivity. In older systems a combination of liquid nitrogen and helium is used. New machines use liquid helium and cold-head compressors to cool the helium.

sounds in case the oxygen level drops. Quenching can also cause serious damage to the superconducting coils.

Just how strong is a magnetic field of 1.5 T or 3 T? For comparison, the magnetic field at the earth's equator is approximately 0.3 G or 0.00003 T, while at the North Pole it is approximately 0.7 G. A typical refrigerator magnet is about 500 G or 0.05 T.

The main magnetic field, B_0, is always on, but it is not perfectly homogeneous. That is, the field is not exactly 1.5 T throughout the bore. The inhomogeneity of a field is typically described in parts per million (ppm). A 1% degree of inhomogeneity would translate into 10,000 ppm. Manufacturers of MRI systems provide specifications on field homogeneity over a specified field of view. A high-end system has inhomogeneity of less than 1 ppm across a 40–50 cm spherical field of view. *Shimming* refers to the use of additional coils (known as shim coils, shown in Figure I1-20) to improve the field homogeneity over the area of imaging. Shimming is particularly important after a subject is introduced into the magnet bore because the presence of the body distorts the magnetic field.

One consequence of maintaining a high field in the bore of the magnet is the resulting fringe field outside of the magnet (see Figure I1-2). The fringe field can cause unwanted effects on people and equipment outside of the magnet and even outside of the imaging room. *Shielding* is required to reduce the fringe field and can be achieved actively with compensatory coils built into the magnet design and passively with steel lining in the walls of the

room. The field strength outside the magnet decreases with the cube of the distance. Safety lines around the magnet for electrical equipment are usually defined by the distance from the magnet (perimeter) at which the magnetic field is 5 G or less. Additional safety considerations for clinical MRI are provided in Chapter I-10.

(2) Transmitting Coil

As will be discussed subsequently, making an MR image requires excitation of the protons whereby their orientations are deflected from the axis of the B_0 field by a second magnetic field, called B_1, that is temporarily applied. The radiofrequency pulses that generate the B_1 field are emitted by the *transmitting coil*. Typically the B_1 magnetic field strengths generated by the transmitting coil are on the order of 10–20 microtesla (μT), much weaker than the B_0 magnetic field. Radiofrequency excitation can be performed by a set of coils, referred to as the body coil, within the main structure of the magnet (Figure I1-20) or by a separate coil positioned directly over the regions of imaging interest, such as a transmit/receive head coil.

(3) Receiving Coil

Signal reception in MRI is based on electromagnetic induction. As the magnetic moments of hydrogen protons precess, they generate a fluctuating magnetic field. Placing a loop of wire, the *receiving coil*, in the vicinity of this changing magnetization causes current to be induced in the wire. The induced current has a frequency identical to the rate of oscillation of the magnetic field. The strength of the current reflects the amplitude of the magnetization. Therefore, the current from the receiving coil can be used to measure proton magnetization and its behavior on time.

A variety of coils can be used to receive signals. Even the body coil can be used as a receiving coil. For better cardiovascular images, however, surface coils that are positioned closer to the body, such as a *phased-array coil*, are usually preferred over volume coils such as the body coil. A phased-array coil consists of several small coils (known as elements), which can each receive signal simultaneously and independently. Typical cardiovascular phased-array coils have 4 to 8 elements per array, and two arrays, one positioned anteriorly over the chest and the other posteriorly under the back, are used for imaging. Peripheral phased-array coils for lower-extremity imaging may have up to 36 or more elements.

CHALLENGE QUESTION: When would it be necessary to use a body coil for receiving signal?

Answer: Subjects who are large and who barely fit into the bore of the magnet must be imaged with the body coil because additional surface coils do not fit.

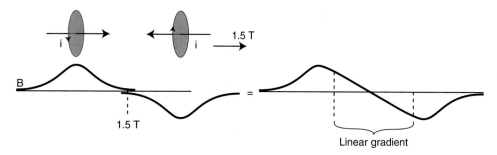

FIGURE I1-22. Gradient coils. Application of current in opposite directions in a pair of gradient coils causes local magnetic field changes centered around each coil. The cumulative effect of both coils is to cause a change in the magnetic field strength that varies approximately linearly with distance.

Receiver coils are connected to the MR computer console via hardware that includes *receiver channels*. Each receiver channel relays a separate MR signal into the computer for analysis. Most commercial cardiovascular MR systems presently have between 4 and 32 receiver channels. In an ideal situation, each element of a phased-array coil is connected to its own receiver channel. However, with a limited number of receiver channels signals from several coils must typically be combined, or multiplexed, to each receiver channel.

(4) Gradient Coils

While the body coil, transmitter coils, and receiver coils are used to generate MR signals, the gradient coils are used primarily for spatial localization of the signal, as will be discussed in Chapter I-5. The gradient coils are three pairs of coils, used to generate magnetic field gradients in the x, y, or z directions (a gradient in the z direction is illustrated in Figure I1-17). In combination, they can be used to create oblique gradients for off-axis imaging. How a pair of gradient coils generates a magnetic field gradient is illustrated and explained in Figure I1-22.

The amplitude of a magnetic field created by a pair of gradient coils depends on the amount of current passing through each coil (Figure I1-23). When the current through each coil is equal, the gradient is centered between the two coils, and the magnetic field halfway between the two coils remains at 1.5 T. The stronger the current in each gradient coil, the greater the resulting magnetic field gradient. If the current directions are reversed in the two gradient coils, then the gradient will change to the opposite direction. The activity of the gradient coils is typically plotted showing the strength of the gradient over time (Figure I1-23). As illustrated in Figure I1-23, the gradient coils generate a linear gradient across a limited segment of the magnet bore. The useful imaging field of view is determined by the range of gradient linearity.

It is important to emphasize that the magnetic fields of gradient coils are superimposed on the main magnetic field, B_0. That is, they add to or take away from the 1.5 T field. Whereas B_0 is always aligned in the z direction, the gradients can be oriented in any direction. For example, a gradient in the x direction, G_x, causes a *change* in B_0 along

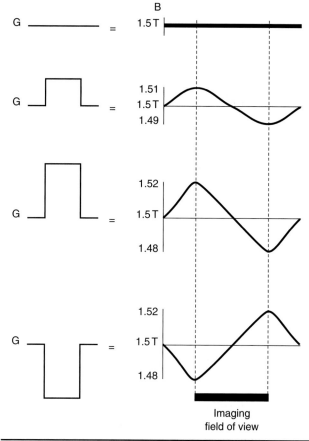

FIGURE I1-23. Different gradient strengths and polarity result from different current strengths in the gradient coils. The conventional representation for gradients is shown on the left, where the height of the bars reflects the amplitude of the gradient, while the horizontal axis reflects time. Positive (above the horizontal axis) and negative (below the horizontal axis) gradient strengths lead to gradients with opposite polarity.

the x direction, although B_0 remains oriented in the z direction (Figure I1-24).

Gradient performance measures are described using the terms *peak amplitude, rise time*, and *slew rate*, and these terms are frequently cited as a measure of the potency of a particular MR unit (Figure I1-25). The peak amplitude, expressed in millitesla per meter (such as 40 mT/m), describes the maximum gradient strength across the imaging field of view. Peak amplitudes for cardiovascular MR

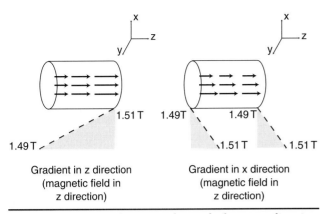

FIGURE I1-24. Gradients can be applied in any direction. Compare the effects of a gradient in the z direction (left) with a gradient in the x direction (right). In both cases, the main magnetic field is aligned in the z direction.

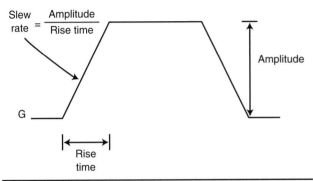

FIGURE I1-25. Definitions of gradient amplitude (or strength), slew rate, and rise time.

systems range from 20 to 45 mT/m. As illustrated in Figures I1-22 and I1-23, the gradient is not truly linear throughout the entire magnet bore. Nonlinearities in the gradients at the ends of the field of view can lead to image distortion. The range across which the maximum gradient strength is expected to apply with near linearity is provided by manufacturers of MR systems and is usually about 35 cm to 50 cm.

Rise time (microseconds or μsec) refers to the time for a gradient to reach its maximum amplitude starting from zero. Slew rate (mT/m/msec or T/m/sec) describes the slope of the rise (Figure I1-25). In general, the relationship between the variables can be expressed as

$$\text{Slew rate (T/m/sec)} = \frac{\text{amplitude (mT/m)}}{\text{rise time (}\mu\text{sec)}/1000}$$

although in some cases, the highest slew rate may be sustainable only for a short time—not long enough to reach the desired amplitude.

CHALLENGE QUESTION: What is the slew rate for a gradient that has a rise time of 200 microseconds (μsec) and a maximum gradient strength of 30 mT/m?

Answer: Using the preceding equation, the slew rate is 30 mT/m divided by 200 μsec (0.2 msec), or 150 mT/m/msec or 150 T/m/sec.

Slew rates on commercial cardiovascular MR systems are commonly about 100 to 200 mT/m/msec.

MRI IN A NUTSHELL

Having reviewed the basic properties of protons in a magnetic field and having introduced some of the core hardware components that constitute an MR system, the stage is set now for an overview of how MR images are actually generated.

The five basic steps can be summarized as follows and are depicted schematically in Figure I1-26:

1. By placing a subject into the bore of the magnet and exposing tissue magnetic moments to an external magnetic field, the magnetic moments are made to align with the field and net magnetization is generated.
2. The magnetization is perturbed by brief application of a radiofrequency pulse from the transmitting coil. This is referred to as *radiofrequency excitation*.
3. The magnetization is then allowed to return to its equilibrium state. This is referred to as *relaxation*. Signals emitted by the relaxing protons are collected using the receiver coil.

To localize signal from different regions in the body, magnetic field gradients are applied during Steps 2 and 3 using the gradient coils.

4. The process is then repeated many times, typically between 128 and 256 times.
5. All the signals are collected in a data space referred to as *k-space*, which is then transformed into an image by a mathematical process called a *Fourier transformation*.

This section provides the reader with a framework for a deeper understanding to be gained in subsequent chapters in Section I. More Background Reading on k-space and Fourier transformations follows.

Step 1: Magnetization Is Created

Outside of the MRI unit, the magnetic moments of the protons in the body are randomly aligned. Because of their random orientation, there is no net magnetization, and **M** = 0 (no matter how magnetic the personality!).

When the subject is placed inside the bore of the MRI unit, he or she becomes exposed to the static magnetic field, B_0. The magnetic moments tend to line up along the axis of the bore. As a result, a net magnetization of the subject is created.

MRI in a Nutshell

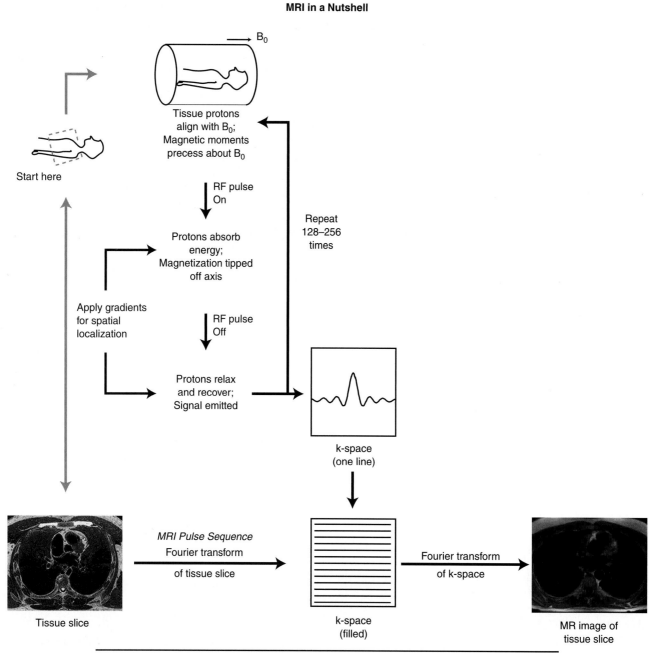

FIGURE I1-26. MRI in a nutshell (see text).

How "magnetic" does the subject become? Not very magnetic. Because of thermal fluctuations, net magnetization is only about 0.3 to 5 protons/million. That is, for every two million protons in the body, the 1.5 T field causes about 1,000,001 to point north for every 1,000,000 pointing south. Although the magnetization effect is small, the natural abundance of protons makes the cumulative magnetization sufficiently large to be measurable.

When a person is placed in the magnet, the process of alignment of the magnetic moments of the protons is not instantaneous. It takes about 1 to 10 seconds, depending on the tissue type. As will be discussed in more depth later, the time constant that expresses this rate of alignment is referred to as the T1 ("tee one") relaxation.

Step 2: Magnetization Is Perturbed (Chapter I-2)

Once the protons become aligned with the main magnetic field and a net magnetization, **M**, is created, the MR imaging process can begin. First, a radiofrequency (RF) pulse is applied by the transmitting coil. The RF pulse represents a weak magnetic field, called B_1, oriented perpendicular to B_0, that tilts the net magnetization away from the direction of the bore of the magnet. The angle of the tilt is called the flip angle. This process is referred to as *RF excitation*.

Step 3: Magnetization Relaxes Back to Equilibrium State (Chapters I-3 and I-4)

Once the RF pulse has excited the protons, tipping their magnetization toward the transverse plane, the transmitting coil is turned off. The rotating transverse component of net magnetization induces current in the receiver coil. This current is amplified and measured as MR signal. The signal has a sinusoidal pattern that typically looks like the functions shown in Figure I1-18. Each signal is digitized and stored as one line of the data space, called k-space.

Once the RF pulse ends, the magnetic moments are exposed again only to the static B_0 magnetic field and will tend to relax back to their ground state, becoming realigned with B_0.

Spatial Localization (Chapter I-5)

A fundamental feature of MR imaging is its ability to achieve *spatial localization*. The term spatial localization refers to the ability to differentiate signal from protons in the body based on their location. If protons in a tumor emit a distinct signal, it is important not only to know that a tumor is present but also to determine where the tumor lies. Is it in the left side of the chest or the right side of the chest? Is it in the heart or in the spine? MR imaging achieves spatial localization by application of magnetic field gradients using gradient coils during Steps 2 and 3.

Step 4: Repetition of the Process

To make an MR image, Steps 2 and 3 are repeated again and again, typically 128 to 256 to 512 times. Each repetition adds another piece of data to k-space, until it is completed or filled. The number of repetitions depends on the type of image desired. In general, the higher the spatial resolution of the image, the greater the number of repetitions.

Step 5: Fourier Transformation of the Raw k-Space Data to an MR Image (Chapters I-6, I-7)

To make the MR image, the k-space data are subjected to a mathematical process called a *Fourier transformation*, or Fourier transform for short, which is performed by the MR computer. The Fourier transform of k-space is the MR image that provides an anatomic depiction of tissue in the body. The relative brightness and darkness of different tissues in the image, referred to as image contrast, depend on the tissue properties that are accentuated by the MR imaging process. As will be discussed later in this section, factors that can affect image contrast include the timing and shapes of RF and gradient pulses and the flip angle, among others.

> **IMPORTANT CONCEPT:** MR images are made by repeatedly exciting protons in the body and then recording the signals received during their relaxation.

THE FOURIER TRANSFORMATION AND TEMPORALLY AND SPATIALLY VARYING SIGNALS

The Fourier transformation is a mathematical tool that permeates all of MRI physics. This section is intended to give the reader an intuitive feel for it. One-dimensional Fourier transformations are used to to analyze MR signals detected by the receiving coil, whereas two- and three-dimensional Fourier transformations are applied to k-space to generate MR images. In all cases, the fundamental principles and properties of the Fourier transformation are the same. One important difference between MR signals and MR images is the domain over which signals vary. For example, MR receiver signals vary over time. In contrast, MR images represent signals that vary over distance or space. Before discussing the Fourier transformation, it is important to distinguish these two types of signals: temporally varying and spatially varying signals (Figure I1-27). Temporally and spatially varying signals are reviewed in the following Background Reading.

BACKGROUND READING: Temporally and Spatially Varying Signals

In MRI there are two categories of signals: those that vary over time and those that vary over space or distance. When plotted graphically, the amplitude of time-varying signals varies with time while spatially varying signals vary with distance or space (Figure I1-27). The meaning of signal frequency in each context is discussed below.

First, frequency can be understood in terms of temporal frequency: the variation of a signal over time. For example, sounds represent signals that vary over time. The higher the frequency, the faster the waves vary in amplitude over time. This is detected by our ears in terms of a higher pitch. Time-varying signals are central to MR physics because protons in an external magnetic field precess. Their precessing behavior gives rise

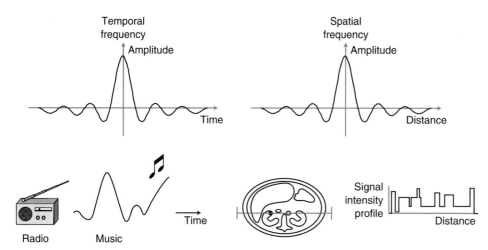

FIGURE I1-27. Temporally varying (left) and spatially varying (right) signals. Sounds, such as music emanating from a radio, are time-varying signals, where the amplitude of sound can be plotted over time. An MR image is representative of a spatially varying signal. A signal intensity profile through one horizontal row of the image is a signal that varies with distance.

to signals that have sinusoidal patterns that can be described in terms of temporal frequencies (cycles per unit time), such as the Larmor frequency.

Second, frequency can be understood in terms of spatial frequency; that is, the variation of a signal across space rather than time. Unlike temporal frequency, which is measured in units of cycles per unit time (such as Hz), the units of spatial frequency are in cycles per unit distance. For example, a uniform image has no spatial variation and therefore has a spatial frequency of zero. An image with alternating black and white vertical bars has a dominant spatial frequency that is inversely proportional to the spacing of the bars. An image with thick, widely spaced bars has a low spatial frequency, whereas one with thin, finely spaced bars has a high spatial frequency. Although it may not be obvious at first, the information contained in any cross-sectional slice of tissue can also be described in terms of spatial frequency components.

> **IMPORTANT CONCEPTS:** Signals can be temporally varying or spatially varying, and analyses of both can be performed using Fourier transformations.

The Fourier Transformation: Definition

To understand how MR images are generated, it is imperative that the reader become familiar and comfortable with some of the basic properties of the Fourier transformation. The introduction to the Fourier transformation provided here is supplemented in Chapter I-6, which focuses on k-space and its properties.

The Fourier transformation, or Fourier transform (FT), provides a means of understanding and analyzing signals of different frequencies. The FT is based on an important theorem that states that a function or curve can be expressed as the sum of a combination of sine and cosine components of different frequencies. The FT of a function is the mathematical process by which the sine and cosine components, their different frequencies and amplitudes, are determined. The FT can be presented as a histogram of the amplitudes of each component frequency. The sum of these components recreates the function.

Another way is to consider the FT as the recipe for how to make a function. The ingredients are sine and cosine functions of different frequencies. The FT defines the amounts or amplitudes of each of the sines and cosines needed to generate the function.

In MR applications, FTs can be one-, two-, or three-dimensional. (The exact mathematical expression for the FT is given in Chapter I-6.) Two important properties of FTs are discussed in the next subsection. Then, illustrated in subsequent subsections are some examples of FTs. For simplicity, FTs are expressed in terms of cosine functions (and not sine functions) in the following discussion. Chapter I-7 explores in more detail the relationship between sine and cosine components of the FT.

Properties of the Fourier Transformation

There are two properties of the Fourier transformation that are important to understand: the duality property and the linearity property.

Duality Property

Consider a function f whose Fourier transform, FT(f), is equal to g. The *duality property* means that the FT of g, FT(g) will be equal to f. In fact, Fourier transforms are not exactly governed by the duality property (some mathematical corrections are needed). However, conceptually, the duality property does apply and is used in qualitative explanations of MR physics in this book.

Linearity Property

The FT also has the property of linearity, which, in mathematical terms, means that

$$FT(f_a + f_b) = FT(f_a) + FT(f_b)$$

that is, the FT of the sum of two functions is equal to the sum of the FTs of each function. It follows then that $FT(2f) = 2\,FT(f)$. That is, if the original function is doubled in amplitude, the FT of the function will also be doubled in amplitude.

One-Dimensional FT

The one-dimensional (1D) FT is applied to functions of a single variable, such as the time-varying signal measured by the receiving coil. Any such function can be expressed as the sum of sines and cosines of different temporal frequencies. The 1D FT of a function provides a histogram of how much of each of those sines and cosines are needed to recreate the function. Examples are shown in Figure I1-28, where for simplicity, only cosine contributions are illustrated.

> **IMPORTANT CONCEPT:** The Fourier transform of a function can be thought of as a histogram of the frequencies of sinusoidal functions that, when summed together, generate the original function.

CHALLENGE QUESTION: Why is the Fourier transformation of a simple sinusoidal function with frequency ω (such as parts a through c, Figure I1-28) depicted as two spikes rather than one?

Answer: Cosine is a symmetric function, and therefore cos ωt is indistinguishable from cos −ωt. Because they are indistinguishable, whenever a spike appears for ω, the same spike will appear at −ω. Consequently, all the cosine components of the Fourier transformation illustrated in Figure I1-28 are symmetric about the value, ω = 0.

Consider part d in Figure I1-28, where the function is constant over time. The only frequency represented in this function is a frequency of zero. (Recall that cos 0 = 1.) Therefore, the FT of the constant function is a spike at frequency zero. By the duality property, the FT of a function that consists of a spike at zero is then simply a constant function.

CHALLENGE QUESTION: Intuitively, why is the FT of a spike a constant function? (Hint: Review Figure I1-15.)

Answer: From Figure I1-15, the function that results when a narrow range of frequencies are summed together is a broad sinc function. As more frequencies are summed, the central peak of the

sinc function gets narrower and taller, while the side lobes diminish. If the range of frequencies were to get even wider, the sinc function would get even narrower. Taken to the extreme, a bandwidth that includes all frequencies (a constant function) will result in a curve that looks like a single spike with no sidelobes. In other words, the FT of the spike is a constant.

In MR physics, the 1D FT is useful for understanding such concepts as RF excitation and signal reception. Typically the 1D FTs are applied to time-varying signals, so the frequencies are expressed in Hz (or MHz or kHz).

Two-Dimensional FT

In MR physics, applications of 2D FTs are usually used for spatially varying functions. Rather than one axis of frequencies, the 2D FT has two axes of frequencies, which define spatial variations in each of two directions. With a view toward understanding k-space, the frequency values in the 2D FT will be named k_x and k_y, to describe the spatial frequency components of a 2D image in the x and y directions, respectively.

This concept of a 2D FT is best understood by a review of examples, shown in Figure I1-29, which are discussed in more detail next.

Examples of 2D FT

Uniform Gray Levels

In parts A and B of Figure I1-29, images that contain only a uniform gray level can be plotted as constant functions in both x and y directions. A constant function has no variation, and therefore its FT is a spike at zero (see Figure I1-28). Therefore, the 2D FT of a uniform shade of gray has a value only at its center point, where k_x and k_y are zero. The brighter the gray level (B), the higher the amplitude of the value in the center of the 2D FT map.

Vertical and Horizontal Ripples

Figure I1-29C illustrates an image that consists of vertically oriented ripples which have no spatial variation in the y direction. The lack of spatial variation in the y direction corresponds to a sinusoidal function with a frequency of zero ($k_y = 0$). The spatial frequency for the variations in x have a frequency k_x (and also $−k_x$).

The pattern is similar in part D, although the ripples are oriented horizontally, so that the Fourier transform has spikes at positive and negative values of k_y, whereas $k_x = 0$.

Waffle Pattern

A sum of horizontal and vertical ripples, resembling a waffle, is shown in Figure I1-29E. The waffle is an excellent example of the property of linearity. The FT of the

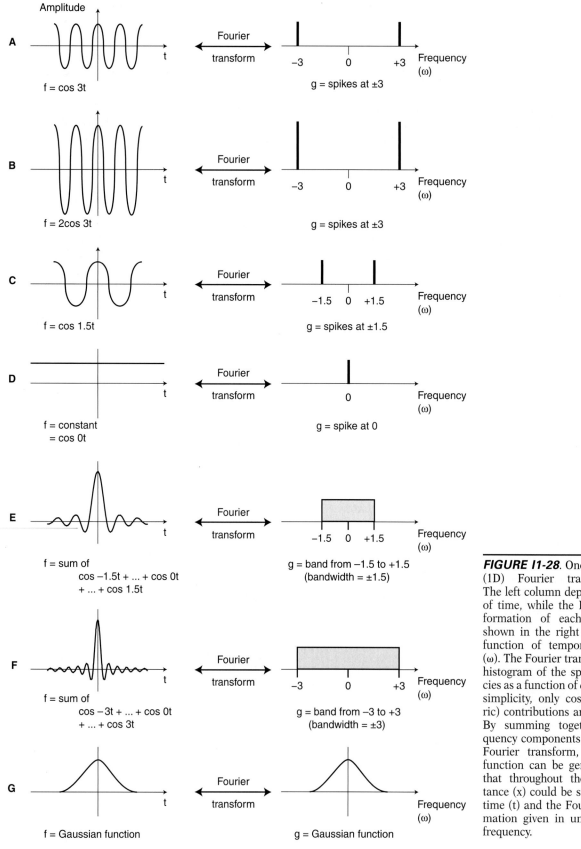

FIGURE I1-28. One-dimensional (1D) Fourier transformations. The left column depicts functions of time, while the Fourier transformation of each function is shown in the right column as a function of temporal frequency (ω). The Fourier transform plots a histogram of the spatial frequencies as a function of ω (cos ωt). For simplicity, only cosine (symmetric) contributions are considered. By summing together the frequency components shown in the Fourier transform, the original function can be generated. Note that throughout the figure, distance (x) could be substituted for time (t) and the Fourier transformation given in units of spatial frequency.

2D Fourier Transforms

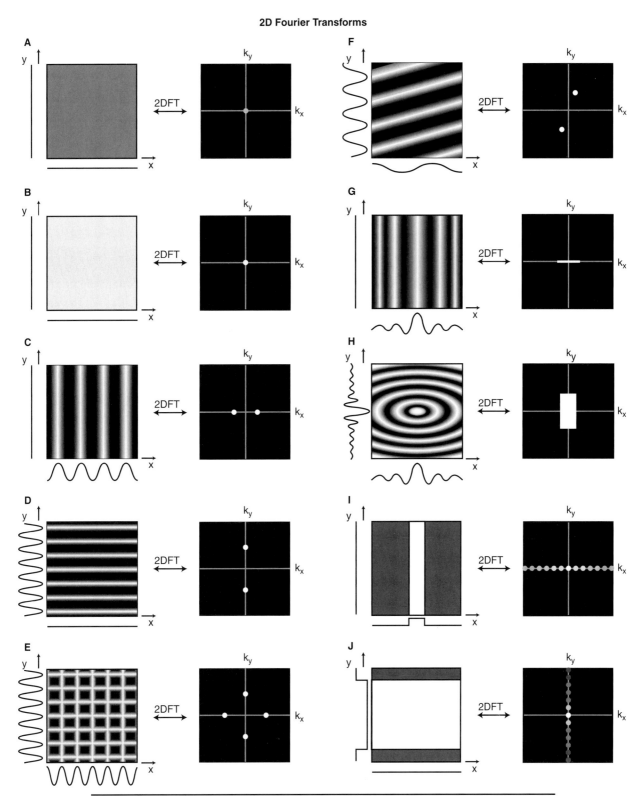

FIGURE I1-29. Two-dimensional (2D) Fourier transformations (2DFT). Examples A through J illustrate how spatial variations in an image (left columns) can be considered in terms of their spatial variations in the y and x directions (drawn to the left and below each figure, respectively). Spatial variations are expressed in terms of spatial frequencies on the 2D Fourier transform histogram (right columns). k_x corresponds to x-direction spatial frequency, $\cos k_x x$, while k_y corresponds to y-direction spatial frequency, $\cos k_y y$. The relative amplitudes of different frequency components are indicated by the brightness of the dots in 2D FT map. Summing the spatial frequency components defined in the Fourier transform will return the original 2D image.

waffle is simply the FT of the horizontal ripples plus the FT of the vertical ripples. In this example, the spatial frequency in the x direction is slightly higher than the example shown in Figure I1-29C, hence the spikes are located at higher values of k_x.

Oblique Ripples

Oblique ripples are depicted in Figure I1-29F. The asymmetric pattern shown has spatial variation in both x and y simultaneously. The variation has a higher frequency along the y direction than along the x direction. The Fourier transform consists of spikes at positions with nonzero k_x and k_y values, where k_y is higher in value than k_x.

Sinc Function

Analogous to the 1D sinc function (Figure I1-28E), a 2D version of the sinc function is illustrated in Figure I1-29G. The Fourier transform of a sinc function is a band of frequencies. In this case, the spatial variation is only across the x direction, so that the Fourier transform has nonzero values only for k_x across a narrow range, while $k_y = 0$ because there is no spatial variation in the y direction. A function with sinc-type spatial variation in both x and y is shown in Figure I1-29H.

Although the duality property applies in all the examples shown in Figure I1-29, just to make the point explicitly, the converse of parts G and H is shown in parts I and J. The 2D FT of a vertical or horizontal bar of high intensity in an image is simply a sinc function in the 2D Fourier transform.

> **IMPORTANT CONCEPT:** The 2D Fourier transform represents the 2D spatial frequency histogram that can be used to describe completely any 2D image.

MR Images and 2D FT

Clearly, most of the images that are generated by MRI systems are more complex than rippled potato chips and Belgian waffles. Nonetheless, the concept of the Fourier transform can be easily extended once the basics are understood. Each point in the 2D FT map corresponds to a particular pattern of ripples. For example, the points along the k_x axis describe vertical ripples of varying widths. Points along k_y describe horizontal ripples. Off-axis points in the 2D FT map reflect the contributions of oblique ripples (Figure I1-29F). Points nearer the center of k-space correspond to widely spaced ripples, while those near the edges relate to tightly spaced ripples.

According to the Fourier transformation theorem, any image can be described in terms of the different patterns of ripples that constitute the image. Based on the linearity property, the resulting FT is the sum of all of the different

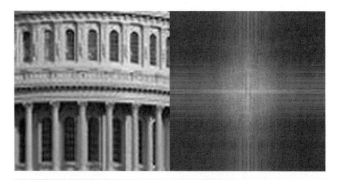

FIGURE I1-30. Image of part of a building (left) and its 2D FT (right).

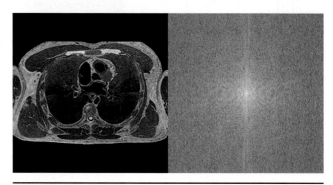

FIGURE I1-31. Tissue slice (left) and its 2D FT (right).

frequency components of the image. With information contained in the Fourier transform, the original image can be reconstructed by summing up all the spatial frequency components represented in the FT (white dots in the FT map). Using the recipe analogy, the 2D FT describes how much of each frequency (combinations of k_x and k_y) is needed to produce the image.

Consider, for example, the more complex 2D image shown in Figure I1-30, which depicts a building with prominent horizontal and vertical components. The 2D FT is shown alongside the image. Not surprisingly, the FT has significant contributions along the k_x and k_y axes.

What about a less geometric image? Figure I1-31 shows an image of a tissue slice of the body alongside its 2D FT. In contrast to the building, the distribution of spatial frequencies in the 2D FT map is more dispersed across the range of frequencies. Nonetheless, the information in the 2D FT still represents the spatial frequency map for the original tissue slice. It turns out that the 2D FT of a tissue slice is a ubiquitous feature of MR imaging. Another name for the 2D FT of the tissue slice is *k-space*! As will be discussed in great detail in Chapter I-6, the process of generating an MR signal results in the FT of the original tissue slice.

CHALLENGE QUESTION: If k-space is the 2D FT of the original tissue slice, what function should be applied to k-space to produce an image that depicts the tissue anatomy and why?

Answer: The Fourier transform! By the duality property, the FT of k-space should return an image that is nearly identical to the original tissue slice.

With an understanding of the 2D Fourier transform, some properties of k-space become clear. The center of k-space contains the low-spatial-frequency information (overall shades of white or gray), which defines image contrast, while the peripheral parts of k-space contain the high-spatial-frequency components, which affect spatial resolution (fine ripples). A more thorough discussion of k-space is provided in Chapter I-6.

> **IMPORTANT CONCEPT:** The 2D Fourier transformation of an image depicts the spatial frequency components of the image that, when summed together, will generate the image. The central portions of the 2D Fourier transformation map contain the lower-spatial-frequency information, while the periphery contains the higher-frequency components.

IMAGES AND THEIR DEFINING CHARACTERISTICS

To make an MR image, k-space data are subjected to the process of a Fourier transformation. What is the nature of the k-space data and the resulting MR image? Both are simply *arrays* or grids of numbers (Figure I1-32). When the values of the numbers are converted to a gray scale of *signal intensities*, the array becomes an image. Each box in the array or grid corresponds to a *voxel* in the image. Depictions of k-space as an image are shown in Figures I1-30 and I1-31. MR images are also arrays of numbers. Before discussing the MR images themselves, a brief Background Reading on the relationship between arrays and images is provided next.

BACKGROUND READING: Arrays and Images

A digital image, such as an MR image, is simply an array, or grid, of numbers. To display the numbers as an image, the computer converts the numbers into a gray scale of brightnesses, referred to as signal intensities, according to the convention that the higher the number, the brighter the voxel, and the lower the number, the darker the voxel (Figure I1-32).

MR signal intensities (with arbitrary units) are scaled by the MR system in an arbitrary fashion to ensure a reasonable use of the range of gray-scale intensities on the computer monitor. The signal intensity values, while proportional to tissue properties such as T1 and others, are not comparable from study to study, much less from system to system. (Note that

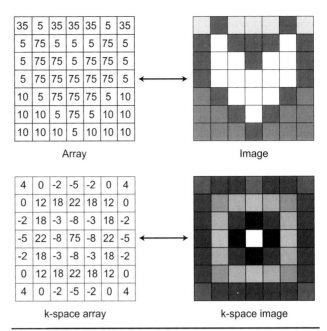

FIGURE I1-32. Arrays and images. A sample 2D image (above) and sample 2D k-space (below) are expressed as arrays of numbers (left) and as gray-scale images (right). To make the image, the numbers in the array are translated into signal intensities, where lower numbers appear darker and higher numbers brighter.

this is an important difference between MRI and computed tomography (CT) imaging, where the attenuation measurements, in Hounsfield units, reflect tissue density and are scaled in a standard fashion from CT system to CT system.)

k-space also consists of an array of numbers. Sometimes, k-space is also depicted as an image (Figure I1-30 and I1-31) where the brightness of the voxels in the image reflects the amplitude of each spatial frequency component.

MR images are used to "see" inside the body. They are intended to be faithful representations of the anatomic structures in the body. However, the reproductions are not perfect. How accurate the images are depends on several of their characteristics, which are collectively referred to as image quality and are usually considered to indicate their diagnostic usefulness. The most commonly used parameters to describe an image are its basic features—number of dimensions, size, and matrix size—and measures of its quality—spatial resolution, signal-to-noise ratio, image contrast, and presence of artifacts. Each of these parameters is described in the following subsections.

Dimensions, Field of View, and Matrix

Most MR images are either two-dimensional (2D) or three-dimensional (3D). 2D MR images are representations of tissues slices of the body. These slices have a defined thickness, typically 3 to 10 mm. The anatomic structures may not be perfectly homogeneous across the thickness of the slice, so the 2D MR image should be thought of as an average of the information. For reasons that will become evident in later chapters (Chapters I-4 and I-5), with 2D imaging, the two dimensions have different properties and different names, usually referred to as *frequency-encoding* and *phase-encoding* directions.

With 3D MR imaging, the image reflects a volume rather than a slice. The third dimension is usually referred to as the *partition dimension*, while the other two retain their typical nomenclature of frequency and phase. Advantages of 3D imaging include a more complete representation of all the tissue in a given region and the ability to postprocess and reformat images into any slice plane for a better representation of tissue geometry and relationships between structures. Because acquisition times increase substantially with 3D imaging, fast imaging methods are usually implemented for 3D techniques.

Sometimes, the term "4D" MR imaging is used. This usually refers to the acquisition of multiple 3D datasets over time, so that the fourth dimension is time.

The *field of view (FOV)* defines the size of the anatomic region being imaged. FOV is measured in centimeters (cm) or millimeters (mm) and is defined for each dimension. For example, a typical FOV for an axial image of the chest might be 400 mm × 300 mm. On most commercial systems, the maximum FOV in any direction is 50 cm or 500 mm. On some systems the maximum FOV may be only 35 cm or 350 mm.

The imaging *matrix* describes the number of pixels or voxels that are comprised in the image and is expressed as the product of the number of voxels along each dimension. For a 2D image, a typical matrix is 256 × 256. The imaging matrix need not be symmetric. For example, a 2D matrix might be 256 × 128. The default values for imaging matrix sizes are typically powers of 2, such as 128, 256, or 512, or at least multiples of 8, because the Fourier transformation is simpler to compute with such numbers. A 3D image might have a matrix of three unequal numbers such as 256 × 128 × 96. If a matrix is given by two or three unequal numbers, the larger is usually the number of voxels in the frequency-encoding direction, while the smaller correspond to the phase-encoding direction(s). This is because additional phase-encoding lines directly add to image acquisition times. In terms of image quality, for a given FOV, the larger the matrix size, the less pixelated and sharper the image usually appears.

Image Spatial Resolution

The spatial resolution of an image is usually defined as the ratio of the field of view (FOV) and the number of voxels in the image or matrix:

$$\text{Spatial resolution}_x = \text{FOV}_x/\text{number of voxels in image in x direction,}$$

$$\text{Spatial resolution}_y = \text{FOV}_y/\text{number of voxels in image in y direction,}$$

$$\text{Spatial resolution}_z = \text{Slice thickness.}$$

For example, if an image FOV is 250 mm and the imaging matrix is 256 × 256, then the spatial resolution will be approximately 1 mm. If the image is larger, say a FOV of 500 mm, then the same imaging matrix would result in voxels that are about 2 mm in size, and the image resolution would be 2 mm. Conversely, for a 250 mm image with a matrix of 512 × 512, the resolution and voxel size would be 0.5 mm. Spatial resolution need not be the same in all directions. For a matrix of 256 × 512 and a 500 mm image, the spatial resolution would be 2 mm × 1 mm; that is, 2 mm in one direction and 1 mm in the other. Voxels that have the same size in all three dimensions are referred to as *isotropic voxels*. As will be discussed in Chapter I-8, voxel dimensions and spatial resolution are not necessarily interchangeable.

The spatial resolution roughly defines the size of the smallest features that may be detected in the image, such as small lesions or tiny vessels. The better the spatial resolution, the smaller the abnormality that can be resolved, or, alternatively, the sharper the appearance of all objects in the image (Figure I1-33). Spatial resolution is only one parameter that determines the conspicuity or detectability of pathology. Other factors include image contrast, noise, and presence of artifacts.

> **IMPORTANT CONCEPT:** Spatial resolution is a parameter of image quality that reflects the size of the smallest features that may be detected and the sharpness of object edges.

Signal-to-Noise Ratio

Signal refers to what is received by the receiver coils and used to make images. It is typically measured in terms of the signal intensity of the voxels in an image. The term

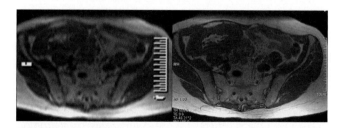

FIGURE I1-33. Images with lower (left) and higher (right) spatial resolution.

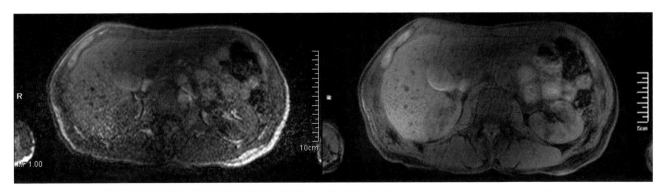

FIGURE I1-34. Images with lower (left) and higher (right) SNR.

noise does not refer to the banging sounds of the system but rather the *image noise*, which is composed of the random, undesirable perturbations of signal that arise from the body, instrument electronics, and computer calculations. Noise contributes to the graininess or mottled appearance of images. All images contain noise. The goal of MR images is to maximize the signal relative to noise. The parameter that measures this relationship is the *signal-to-noise ratio (SNR)*, which is defined as

$$SNR = \frac{Signal}{Noise}$$

Among the factors that contribute to the SNR of an image are the time taken to acquire the data for the image and the amount of magnetization within each voxel that contributes to the signal. The relationship is approximately:

$$SNR \approx C \times Magnetization \times \sqrt{time}$$

where the constant C includes many other factors, most notably the receiver coil's sensitivity to the signal.

The amount of magnetization within a voxel depends on three main factors: (1) the way in which the RF pulse and gradients are applied and the signal sampled, (2) intrinsic characteristics of the tissue magnetization, and (3) the volume of the voxel. The first two factors are the subjects of other chapters in Section I. The volume of a voxel is important because, with larger voxels, more protons contribute to signal, and therefore more signal is generated.

CHALLENGE QUESTION: What is the relationship between SNR and spatial resolution?

Answer: SNR and spatial resolution are inversely related. The higher the spatial resolution, the smaller the voxel, and the lower the SNR.

IMPORTANT CONCEPT: SNR and spatial resolution are inversely related. Small voxels have lower SNR.

The SNR is proportional to the square root of time. That is, if the acquisition time is doubled, the SNR will increase by a factor of about 40% (since $\sqrt{2} = 1.4$) (Figure I1-34).

IMPORTANT CONCEPT: SNR is proportional to the square root of time.

Although throughout this book the strength of the external magnetic field is assumed to be 1.5 T, it is worth noting that SNR increases linearly with field strength. All other things being equal, a 3 T MRI system should theoretically provide twice the SNR of a 1.5 T system.

Measurements of SNR are frequently used to compare different imaging techniques. In practical terms, signal is simply defined as the average or mean signal intensity in the region of interest. The noise corresponds to the standard deviation of signal intensity values. In most MRI, noise does not vary across the image. For simplicity, noise is estimated in air that is included in the imaging field:

$$SNR \text{ of tissue} = \frac{Average \ signal \ intensity \ of \ tissue}{Standard \ deviation \ of \ air}$$

This formula does not apply when parallel imaging techniques are used; parallel imaging techniques are introduced in Chapter I-8.

Contrast-to-Noise Ratio

The contrast-to-noise ratio (CNR) is a parameter that reflects the visibility or conspicuity of findings in an image, for example, the detectability of a tumor or the demarcation between myocardium and blood pool (Figure I1-35). It also takes into account the effects of noise on conspicuity:

$$CNR \text{ for tissues A and B} = \frac{Signal \ A - Signal \ B}{Noise}$$

For a given degree of contrast, the greater the image noise, the more difficult it is to distinguish a tissue A from its background, B.

As with SNR, noise is measured by the standard deviation of signal in air:

CNR for tissues A and B

$$= \frac{\text{Avg signal intensity A} - \text{Avg signal intensity B}}{\text{Standard deviation of air}}$$

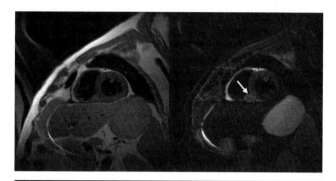

FIGURE I1-35. Image contrast. By changing the parameters for an MR acquisition, many types of image contrast can be generated. In this subject with melanoma metastases, the right ventricular mass (arrow) is best seen on the "fat-suppressed T2-weighted" image (right) because it has greater contrast compared with the normal myocardium. The "T1-weighted" image on the left shows little contrast between the lesion and myocardium.

Artifacts

Even with high spatial resolution, high SNR and high CNR, an image can still be ruined by artifacts (Figure I1-36). Imaging artifacts can arise from a variety of sources. Many artifacts are ubiquitous, such as physiologically based artifacts arising from respiratory or bowel motion and blood flow. Others may be intrinsic to the way MR images are acquired. Some arise because of technical problems such as hardware or software malfunctions. The identification and diagnosis of image artifacts are some of the greatest challenges of MRI. Throughout this book, specific artifacts will be discussed in the sections that describe the underlying physics leading to these artifacts. Additionally, artifacts that lead to pitfalls in interpretation of gadolinium-enhanced MR angiography are considered in Chapter II-4, and those involved in cine gradient echo cardiac MRI in Chapter III-4.

PULSE SEQUENCE DIAGRAM: AN INTRODUCTION

To make an MR image, the transmitting coil, the three gradient coils, and the receiver coil must be turned on and off in a precisely coordinated fashion to produce an image with desired characteristics and quality. The orchestration of these actions is referred to as a *pulse sequence*. Pulse sequences are depicted in *pulse sequence diagrams*, which provide instructions for how to make an MR image. The

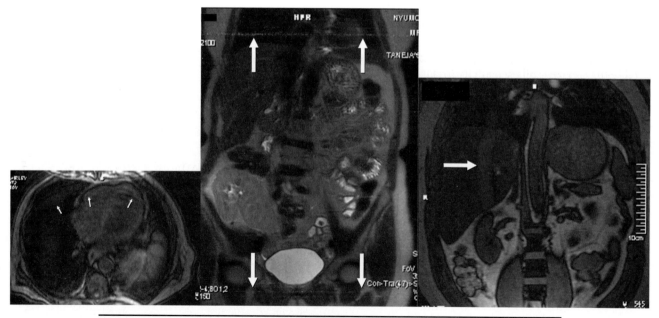

FIGURE I1-36. Examples of MRI artifacts. Motion artifacts (arrows) caused by breathing (left), zipper artifacts (horizontal pale lines at top and bottom of image, arrows) caused by scanning with the room door open (middle), and ghosting artifact (arrow) of the aorta projecting over the liver (right) are some causes of artifacts that degrade image quality.

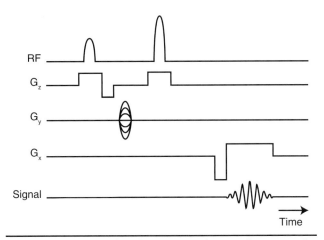

FIGURE I1-37. Sample pulse sequence diagram for a spin echo sequence. The diagram shows when each of the gradients is applied—their strength and duration—in order to generate a desired signal (echo). The horizontal axis is time.

pulse sequence diagram plots the activity of the transmitting coil (RF), three gradient coils (G_x, G_y, G_z), and receiver coil (Signal) over time (the horizontal axis). The heights of the RF pulse and gradient coil plots reflect the strength or amplitude of each. A typical pulse sequence diagram is shown in Figure I1-37.

In most cases, the pulse sequence diagram shows how a single line of k-space is collected, and the reader infers that to generate an image, what happens in the diagram is repeated a number of times to collect the full dataset for k-space, with slight variations as demarcated (as in G_y, in this example, where the varying amplitude G_y gradient pulses from one excitation to the next are superimposed in one symbol). Using the convention where z represents the craniocaudal direction, most pulse sequence diagrams depict the imaging of an axial slice of the body. If other imaging planes are desired, the gradient components need to be relabeled accordingly.

REVIEW QUESTIONS

1. The Larmor frequency at 1.5 T is about 64 MHz. Assuming a gyromagnetic ratio $\gamma = 42.6$ MHz/T,
   a. What is the precessional frequency or Larmor frequency at 1 T?
   b. What is the precessional frequency or Larmor frequency at 3 T?

2. Protons precess at slightly different frequencies in fat and water because of the slightly different local environments of the protons in each. At 1.5 T, a proton precesses 220 Hz more slowly in fat than in water.
   a. What is the difference in precessional frequencies at 1 T?
   b. What is the difference in precessional frequencies at 3 T?

3. Ideally all protons in the magnet bore should experience the same magnetic field, for example 1.5 T. But this does not occur, especially once a person is placed into the bore of the magnet. The process of shimming the magnet can help improve the homogeneity of the field, but only to a point. Consider the implications of a field that is uniform to within 6 ppm. This means that the field will have an error of

   $\pm 6/1,000,000 \times 1.5$ T $= 9/1,000,000$ T $\sim 1/100,000$ T so that the range of the magnetic field strengths will be 1.49999 T to 1.50001 T. With a magnet of this specification, what will be the range of precessional frequencies of the protons in the magnet when no gradients are on? (Assume $\gamma = 42.6$ MHz/T.)

4. If a maximum gradient strength is 25 mT/m at 1.5 T and the field of view is 50 cm, then what is the range of magnetic field strengths across the field of view when the maximum gradients are applied? What is the range of precessional frequencies in this state? (Assume $\gamma = 42.6$ MHz/T.)

5. The signal received from a receiver coil during application of a magnetic field gradient has the appearance shown in Figure I1-18. How would it be possible to determine how many protons are precessing across the range of frequencies induced by the magnetic field gradient?

6. The image shown in Figure I1-Q6 was generated using a field of view of 50 cm. What is the likely cause of the warping at the ends of the image?

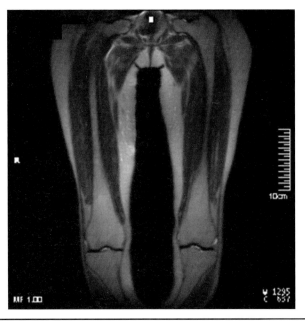

FIGURE I1-Q6A. Image with warping at ends.

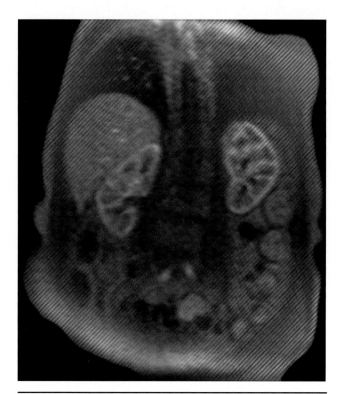

FIGURE I1-7A. Image with corduroy artifact. (Courtesy of N. Oesingmann, Ph. D.)

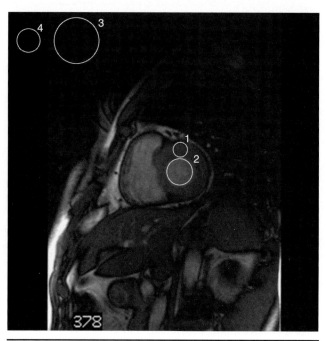

FIGURE I1-Q8. Image showing different regions of interest.

7. The image depicted in Figure I1-Q7 shows a corduroy artifact across the image. What change in k-space would give rise to an artifact with this appearance?

8. You are asked to determine the signal-to-noise ratio for myocardium in the image in Figure I1-Q8, which has the following regions of interest defined for you. What is the myocardial signal-to-noise ratio? What is the myocardium-to-blood contrast-to-noise ratio? (SD = standard deviation)

Regions of Interest (ROIs):
1. Mean = 85, SD = 16
2. Mean = 195, SD = 29
3. Mean = 11, SD = 5
4. Mean = 0, SD = 0

RF Excitation and Signal Generation

This chapter introduces the processes by which protons in the body interact with RF excitation pulses, generate signals, and then recover to their equilibrium state. An understanding of the general principles is needed before specifics can be discussed in more detail, such as the differences in properties of various tissues (Chapter I-3), the types of signals that can be generated for MR imaging (Chapter I-4), and the collection of data in k-space to produce MR images (Chapters I-5 and I-6).

KEY CONCEPTS

▶ Longitudinal magnetization is stationary and does not contribute to signal measured by a receiver coil.

▶ Transverse magnetization, by precessing in the transverse plane, can generate measurable signal.

▶ Longitudinal magnetization must be tipped into the transverse plane by a radiofrequency (RF) pulse to produce measurable signal.

▶ RF pulses are weak magnetic fields, B_1, that must rotate at the same frequency at which protons precess in order to achieve resonance and excitation.

▶ With an RF pulse, protons are tipped to a given flip angle at a rate dependent on the strength of the B_1 magnetic field.

▶ B_0 magnetic field inhomogeneities cause heterogeneous RF excitation, whereas B_1 heterogeneity may result in failure to attain the desired flip angle of excitation.

▶ At equilibrium, precessing magnetic moments have no phase coherence and therefore no net transverse magnetization; RF excitation induces phase coherence.

▶ When RF excitation ends, magnetic moments return to their equilibrium state aligned with B_0; this process can be described in terms of the decay of the transverse magnetization (T2, T2′, and T2*) and the recovery of longitudinal magnetization (T1).

▶ T1 recovery and T2 decay curves are exponential curves with time constants T1 and T2, respectively.

TRANSVERSE VERSUS LONGITUDINAL MAGNETIZATION

The net magnetization, **M**, represents the sum of the magnetic moments of all of a subject's individual protons within the magnet bore. Before launching into details about how to manipulate and measure **M**, it is important to explain first why the behavior of **M** is usually analyzed in terms of its two components: transverse magnetization, or M_{xy}, and longitudinal magnetization, or M_z. As discussed in Chapter I-1, the longitudinal magnetization, M_z, is static. Since a static magnetic field induces no current in the receiver coil, M_z is not directly measured. In contrast, the transverse component of magnetization, M_{xy}, precesses about the z axis in the xy plane. Provided there is phase coherence, the precessing magnetization can induce a current in the receiver coil, which can be recorded as signal.

IMPORTANT CONCEPT: Net magnetization is best analyzed in terms of its longitudinal (M_z) and transverse (M_{xy}) components separately. M_{xy} generates measurable signal, while M_z, because it is static, does not.

RADIOFREQUENCY (RF) EXCITATION

RF Excitation: The Concept

When a person is placed into the bore of the magnet, his or her protons will align in the direction of the main magnetic field. Magnetic moments are not stationary; they precess about the z axis. But because the protons lack phase coherence, the transverse component of their magnetic moments are completely random and sum to zero. Therefore, the net magnetization is completely longitudinal. Longitudinal magnetization is static, and therefore no signal is measurable.

CHALLENGE QUESTION: How can the net magnetization be made measurable?

Answer: To make the signal detectable by a receiver coil, the alignment or orientation of the magnetization vectors must be

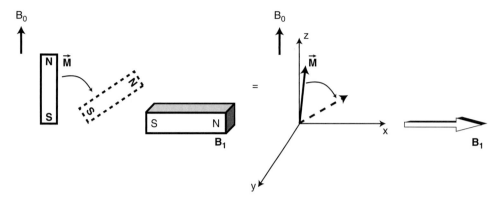

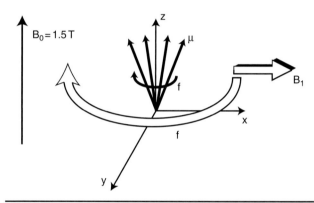

FIGURE I2-1. RF excitation. A B_1 magnetic field in the xy plane tips **M** away from the longitudinal axis.

changed from longitudinal to transverse, and the tranverse magnetization must have phase coherence. The RF excitation pulse achieves both requirements.

The orientation of any magnet can be influenced simply by exposure to a magnetic field oriented in a different direction (Figure I2-1). Radiofrequency (RF) excitation operates on this principle. An RF pulse is a relatively weak magnetic field oriented in the xy plane that pulls the magnetic moments away from the longitudinal direction toward the transverse plane. Distinct from B_0, the magnetic field of the RF pulse is referred to as B_1 ("B one").

In addition to tipping the magnetization into the transverse plane, the RF pulse also achieves phase coherence. This means that with RF excitation, all the magnetic moments of the protons precess together around the z axis at 64 MHz (Figure I1-11). Because of the properties of electromagnetic induction, a coherent M_{xy} can induce an oscillating current in a nearby receiver coil. Hence, an RF pulse creates MR signal by converting static longitudinal magnetization into coherently precessing transverse magnetization.

> **IMPORTANT CONCEPT:** By tipping the net magnetization away from the longitudinal axis into the transverse plane and by inducing phase coherence, the RF excitation pulse generates measurable MR signal.

RF Excitation: Requiring Resonance

There is one additional condition necessary for RF excitation. In the superconducting magnet, even though the net magnetization, **M**, is a stationary vector aligned with the z axis, the individual magnetic moments (μ) precess around the z axis at the Larmor frequency, or about 64 MHz at 1.5 T. For the RF pulse to have any effect on these protons, B_1 must also spin around the z axis at the same 64 MHz frequency. In other words, B_1 must *resonate* with the protons, as in "Magnetic <u>Resonance</u> Imaging." As long as the B_1 magnetic field rotates around the xy plane at the same

FIGURE I2-2. Resonance. To achieve resonance, B_1 must rotate about the z axis at the same frequency as the magnetic moments of the protons, that is, at the Larmor frequency (f).

frequency as the protons are precessing, it will be able to engage and pull the magnetization vector down toward the xy plane (Figure I2-2).

> **IMPORTANT CONCEPT:** For excitation to occur, RF excitation pulses must resonate with the protons; that is, the RF pulse frequency must match precisely the precessional (Larmor) frequency of the protons.

When B_1 resonates with the precessing protons, it causes **M** to be tipped away from the z axis and into the xy plane. Protons that are not precessing at the same frequency as B_1 will not be affected. This observation has important implications. To excite all the protons in the field of view with an RF pulse at 64 MHz, all the protons must precess at 64 MHz. For this to occur, the magnetic field must be exactly 1.5 T throughout the field of view. Magnetic field inhomogeneity, either intentional (created by the use of gradient coils) or unintentional (created by metal in the subject's body, for example), will cause protons to deviate from the expected Larmor frequency. Then, only the subset of the protons that still precess at 64 MHz will be excited. Consequently, B_0 inhomogeneity can be a substantial source of image artifacts (Figure I2-3). However, under certain circumstances, the necessity for resonance can also be used to advantage, for example, in the selective excitation of single slices of tissue (Chapter I-5).

RF Excitation: Flip Angle

The flip angle, α (alpha), is defined as the angle the magnetization vector is tipped away from the z axis by the RF pulse (Figure I2-4). For example, if the the flip angle is 10 or 15°, the magnetization vector is tipped only slightly away from the z axis. A flip angle of 90° tips the vector completely into the xy plane. Once tipped, the magnetization vector precesses around the z axis at the Larmor frequency (Figure I2-4).

The amount of measurable signal resulting from an RF excitation pulse is equal to the transverse component of **M**, M_{xy}. The longitudinal component, M_z, reflects the signal that is available for measurement following the next RF pulse. From Chapter I-1, Figure I1-5,

$$M_{xy} = M \sin \alpha$$
$$M_z = M \cos \alpha$$

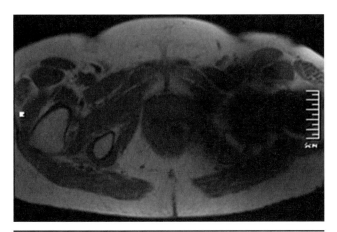

FIGURE I2-3. B_0 heterogeneity caused by a hip prosthesis, resulting in imperfect resonance and excitation around the region of the metal implant.

CHALLENGE QUESTION: What are the measurable (M_{xy}) and stored (M_z) magnetization components following a flip angle of 90°?

Answer: All of the magnetization is moved into the xy plane following a 90° pulse, and none is left in the z direction. Therefore, $M_{xy} = M$, while $M_z = 0$, since sin 90° = 1 and cos 0° = 0.

The magnetization vector can also be tipped beyond the xy plane to angles greater than 90°. For example, if tipped 180°, **M** is longitudinal but points in the opposite direction along the z axis (Figure I2-4). How a rotating magnetic field in the xy plane can cause protons to flip 180° will be explained in the next section.

It is also worth noting that repeatedly tipping the magnetization with several RF pulses in rapid succession causes a cumulative increase in the flip angle that is the sum of each individual RF pulse's effect. For example, if three identical 15° RF pulses are applied back-to-back, then the net effect would be a 45° flip angle. Similarly, if the vector is tipped 180° and then tipped another 180°, for a total of 360°, the magnetization vector will again be at 0° or back where it started.

Sometimes it is useful to consider the flip angle in terms of its fraction of a full 360° cycle. For example, a 90° flip angle represents one-quarter of a cycle, while 45° is one-eighth of a cycle.

> **IMPORTANT CONCEPT:** The flip angle is a measure of the energy of an RF pulse used to tip a magnetization vector. The flip angle determines the relationship between the measured signal and the amount of magnetization available to generate signal following the next RF excitation.

RF Excitation: The Implementation

To understand how to achieve a desired flip angle, a more thorough explanation of the RF pulse is needed.

RF excitation can be thought of as a magnetic field, B_1, rotating in the xy plane at the Larmor frequency. To simplify

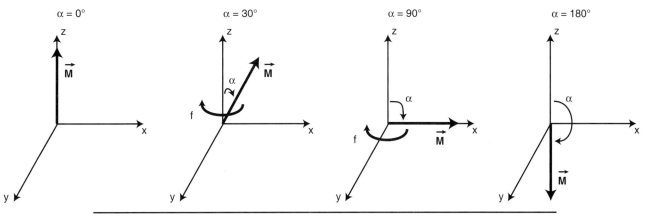

FIGURE I2-4. Examples of different flip angles from 0° to 180°.

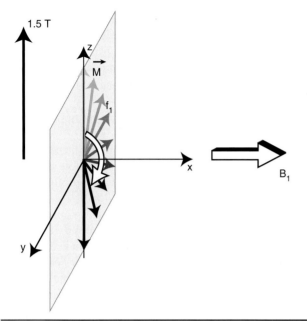

FIGURE I2-5. B_1 induces precession about its axis at a frequency f_1. Using a rotating frame of reference where B_1 is aligned with the x axis, the precession of the magnetization vector about the B_1 magnetic field is expressed as an oscillation about the x axis in the yz plane. The frequency f_1 is proportional to strength of B_1.

matters, it can be helpful to ignore the rotational behavior of B_1 and simply consider it to be a stationary magnetic field, say along the x axis (Figure I2-5). (This is sometimes referred to as a "rotating frame of reference.") As soon as B_1 is turned on, the net magnetization will be inclined to align in the same direction as B_1. The main magnetic field, B_0, is still on, of course, and so the protons remain primarily aligned in the z-axis direction. Nevertheless, B_1 will have a real, albeit small, effect on magnetization.

CHALLENGE QUESTION: Other than orientation and phase coherence, what other effect does B_1 have on the magnetic moments?

Answer: Just as B_0 causes the magnetic moments to precess about the z axis, B_1 will cause the magnetic moments to precess about the axis of B_1.

How can magnetic moments precess around the axis of B_1? The behavior of the magnetization vector during an RF pulse is illustrated in Figure I2-5, where B_1 is assumed to be aligned with the x axis. Its effect is analogous to the effect of B_0 making protons precess about the z axis in the xy plane. A magnetic field oriented in the x direction will cause the magnetization to precess in the yz plane. In other words, the magnetization will tip down toward the xy plane, swing beyond it to the opposite end of the z axis, and then swing back again toward z.

CHALLENGE QUESTION: What is the rate of oscillation of M about B_1?

Answer: The precessional frequency of protons in response to B_1 can be computed using the Larmor equation.

This rate of oscillation or precession, f_1, will be proportional to the strength of B_1, according to the Larmor equation:

$$f_1 = \gamma B_1$$

and is independent of B_0.

How long the RF pulse must be kept on to achieve a desired flip angle depends on the precessional frequency, f_1, which in turn depends on B_1. The field strength of B_1, typically 10–25 microtesla or μT (0.00001–0.000025 T), is much lower than that of B_0. Therefore, the precessional frequency of magnetization around the B_1 axis, f_1, is much lower than f (64 MHz). For example, for $B_1 = 10\ \mu T$,

$$f_1 = 42.6\ \text{MHz/T} \times 10\ \mu T = 426\ \text{Hz}$$

A frequency of 426 Hz, or 426 cycles per second, means that the protons will precess around B_1 about once every 2 milliseconds, since

$$\frac{1\ \text{sec}}{426\ \text{cycles}} = \frac{1000\ \text{msec}}{426\ \text{cycles}} = \frac{2.34\ \text{msec}}{\text{cycle}}$$

A flip angle of 360° can be achieved in 2.34 msec, a flip angle of 180° would take half the time, or 1.17 msec, and a 90° flip angle would require a 0.587 msec pulse.

CHALLENGE QUESTION: How would a stronger B_1 affect the flip angle?

Answer: Based on the Larmor equation, the stronger the B_1, the faster the precession associated with B_1, and therefore the shorter the time needed to induce the desired flip angle.

For a B_1 of 20 μT, the precessional frequency associated with B_1 would be twice as fast, or 852 Hz. Each cycle would therefore take half as long. That is, the magnetization vector would precess around B_1 once every 1.17 msec. Hence, a flip angle of 180° would be achieved in only 0.587 msec, while a 90° flip angle would require 0.294 msec.

So far, the rotating behavior of B_1 at 64 MHz has been ignored. Reintroducing it now does not change any of the flip angle calculations described above. Rather than a simple trajectory, the path taken by the net magnetization vector as it is tipped away from the z axis toward the xy plane takes the course of a spiral down to the transverse plane and beyond (Figure I2-6). The stronger the B_1 field, the faster the spiral and the more quickly the magnetization will tip into the transverse plane.

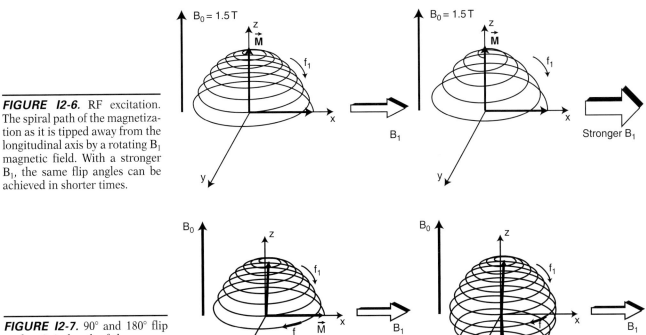

FIGURE I2-6. RF excitation. The spiral path of the magnetization as it is tipped away from the longitudinal axis by a rotating B_1 magnetic field. With a stronger B_1, the same flip angles can be achieved in shorter times.

FIGURE I2-7. 90° and 180° flip angles. Spiral path of the magnetization vector during an RF pulse. For a given B_1, a 180° excitation requires twice as long as a 90° excitation.

Flip angles greater than 90° can be achieved by leaving the RF pulse on after the magnetization vector has reached the transverse plane. As shown in Figure I2-7, the magnetization vector continues to spiral toward the negative z axis. A flip angle of 180° is achieved with a pulse twice as long as a 90° pulse. If the RF pulse is left on even longer, the magnetization vector will spiral back up to the transverse plane (270° flip angle), returning to its original orientation aligned with the z axis (360° flip angle).

Magnetic Field Inhomogeneities and B_0 and B_1

When the B_0 magnetic field is not perfectly homogeneous, some protons will precess at frequencies other than the expected Larmor frequency. At 1.5 T, an RF pulse that has a frequency of 64 MHz will excite only protons precessing at 64 MHz. All others will *not* be excited by the RF pulse. To compensate for some degree of B_0 inhomogeneity, RF pulses are designed to include a range of frequencies around the Larmor frequency.

CHALLENGE QUESTION: What form would an RF pulse have that contained a range of frequencies?

Answer: A sinc function (Figure I1-15).

The B_1 field is assumed to affect all protons to the same degree, but this is only true if the B_1 field is homoge-

neous across the entire area of interest. B_1 inhomogeneities affect the flip angle achieved by the RF excitation pulse. For example, if B_1 is 20 μT throughout most of the body but only 10 μT in one region, then the RF pulse used to create a 90° flip angle in most of the body will cause a only 45° flip angle around this area. Consequently, the strength of signal will decrease substantially in this region. This problem can be particularly challenging at 3 T, where B_1 heterogeneities and the so-called dielectric effect can cause significant imaging artifacts (Figure I2-8).

> **IMPORTANT CONCEPT:** Magnetic field inhomogeneities can lead to heterogeneous RF excitation. Some protons may not be excited by the RF pulse (B_0 heterogeneity), while others may not achieve the desired flip angle (B_1 heterogeneity).

Phase of the RF Pulse

An important feature of the RF pulse is its phase. *RF phase* refers to the orientation of the transverse component, M_{xy}, following an RF pulse. For example, two RF pulses with a phase difference of 90° are shown in Figure I2-9.

In a repetition of a pulse sequence, the phase of the RF pulse can be deliberately varied from one RF pulse to another in order to ensure that the phase of the resulting M_{xy} signal differs from one repetition to another. This option is exploited in spoiled gradient echo imaging, discussed in Chapter I-4.

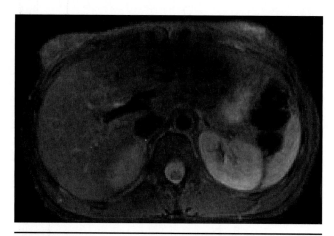

FIGURE I2-8. B_1 heterogeneity and dielectric effect cause lower signal in the region of the left lobe of the liver at 3 T.

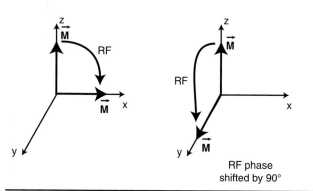

FIGURE I2-9. RF phase. Two 90° RF pulses that differ in phase by 90°.

The Decay and the Recovery: Transverse (T2) and Longitudinal (T1) Relaxation

What happens after B_1 is turned off? Exposed only to the B_0 magnetic field, the net magnetization **M** will return to its original, pre-RF pulse, equilibrium state. This process can be viewed in two independent parts:

1. The loss of phase coherence (T2 relaxation or *T2 decay*)*
2. The recovery of longitudinal magnetization (T1 relaxation or *T1 recovery*)

Although there is some interdependence between the T1 and T2 relaxations, it is easiest to consider these properties as independent. The rates of T2 decay and T1 recovery vary across different tissues, giving rise to one means of characterizing and distinguishing between tissues and pathology. Additionally, most MR contrast agents work by causing changes in these rates, as will be discussed in Chapter I-3.

The Decay: Transverse (T2) Relaxation

Immediately after B_1 is turned off, what kind of signal would be expected from the receiver coil? The transverse magnetization, M_{xy}, will be precessing in the xy plane. As an oscillating magnetic field, M_{xy} induces a current in a nearby receiver coil.

CHALLENGE QUESTION: What is the frequency of the signal measured by the receiver coil?

Answer: The Larmor frequency.

The measured signal (*echo*) is a simple sinusoidal signal, oscillating at about 64 MHz at 1.5 T (Figure I2-10). Its initial amplitude is proportional to the magnitude of M_{xy}.

However, in reality, once B_1 is turned off, phase coherence is lost quickly (Figure I2-11). Two factors contribute to the loss of phase coherence: *intrinsic relaxation*, due to tissue-specific properties (T2), and *extrinsic relaxation*, due to magnetic field inhomogeneities (*T2′ relaxation*). *T2 relaxation* occurs because of the variability in the exchange of energy between adjacent protons and is an intrinsic tissue property. Many pathologic states have different T2 relaxation properties from normal tissues (Chapter I-3). T2′ decay happens because of B_0 magnetic field inhomogeneities. According to the Larmor equation, protons exposed to different magnetic fields will precess at slightly different frequencies and therefore lose phase coherence. The cumulative effects of T2 and T2′ relaxation are referred to as *T2* relaxation* or T2* decay.

With the rapid loss of phase coherence, the measured signal rapidly declines. When the individual magnetic moments become randomly distributed around the xy plane, M_{xy} becomes negligible (Figure I2-11).

> **IMPORTANT CONCEPT:** The loss of phase coherence can be attributed to an intrinsic tissue charateristic (T2) and magnetic field inhomogeneities (T2′). Collectively, these factors result in a decay of the measured signal, referred to as T2* relaxation or T2* decay.

The term *free induction decay (FID)* is used to describe the behavior of the transverse magnetization immediately after applying the RF pulse (Figure I2-12). "Free" refers to the freely precessing protons no longer forced to be coherent by the RF pulse, "induction" refers to the current induced by the oscillating magnetization across the receiver coil, and "decay" refers to the loss in signal over time.

The rate at which the overall transverse magnetization decreases is described by a time constant called T2*, which includes contributions from T2 and T2′. Note that

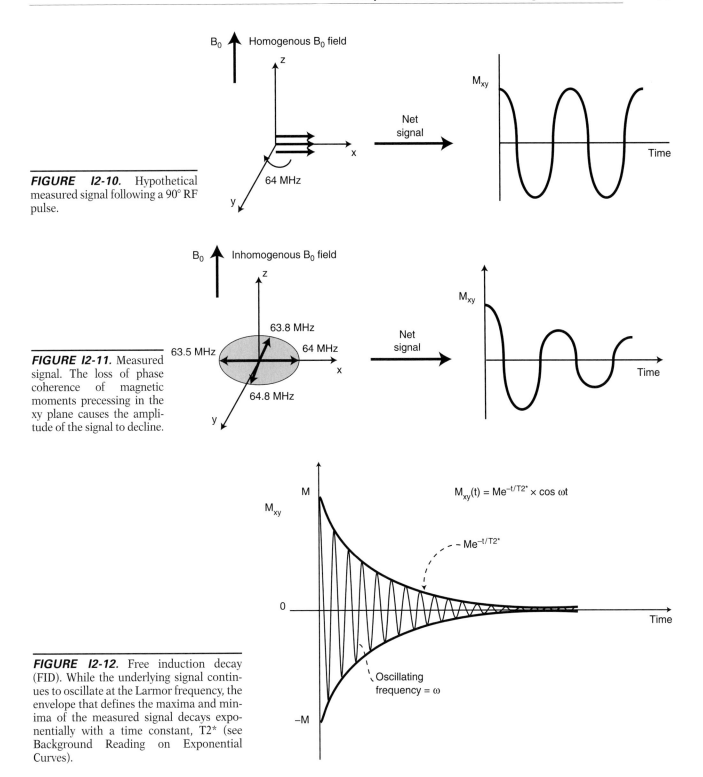

FIGURE I2-10. Hypothetical measured signal following a 90° RF pulse.

FIGURE I2-11. Measured signal. The loss of phase coherence of magnetic moments precessing in the xy plane causes the amplitude of the signal to decline.

$$M_{xy}(t) = Me^{-t/T2^*} \times \cos \omega t$$

FIGURE I2-12. Free induction decay (FID). While the underlying signal continues to oscillate at the Larmor frequency, the envelope that defines the maxima and minima of the measured signal decays exponentially with a time constant, T2* (see Background Reading on Exponential Curves).

the terms T2, T2*, and T2′ refer both to the types of signal decay themselves and to the numerical time constants of the exponential decay curves. By definition, the T2, T2*, and T2′ values define the time after which the maximum transverse signal has decayed by 63%. For most tissues other than fluids, T2 times are less than 100 msec. For a review of exponential curves, the following Background Reading is provided.

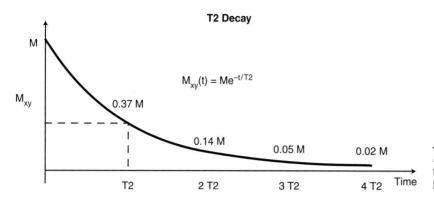

T2 Decay

$M_{xy}(t) = Me^{-t/T2}$

M

M_{xy}

0.37 M

0.14 M

0.05 M

0.02 M

T2   2 T2   3 T2   4 T2   Time

FIGURE I2-13. Exponential T2 decay. The time constant, T2, represents how long it takes for the signal to have decayed by 63%.

Background Reading: Exponential Curves

Both the decay of the transverse magnetization (T2 relaxation) and the recovery of longitudinal magnetization (T1 relaxation) can be described by exponential curves. Each will be discussed in turn using their respective exponential equations.

Exponential Decay (T2)

Many effects observed in nature can be described by *exponential decay* curves. This situation occurs when the amount of something (such as a radioactive element) that decays per unit of time is a fixed fraction of the amount that is present. As the amount of the element decreases, the amount of decay per unit time decreases in proportion. The exponential decay of transverse magnetization can be expressed in the same way. The basic equation is

$$M_{xy}(t) = Me^{-t/\tau}$$

where M is the value of transverse magnetization immediately following the RF pulse, and therefore also its maximum value. The time constant, τ (tau), is the parameter that describes the rate of decay. For T2 or T2* decay, the time constant τ = T2 or T2*, respectively. Like the number π, e is an irrational number, 2.71828 . . ., with natural significance.

The best way to understand the exponential decay equation is to examine the value of M at different time points t (Figure I2-13). For example, at t = 0, immediately after the RF pulse has finished,

$$M_{xy}(t = 0) = Me^0 = M$$

recalling that any number to the 0th power = 1. The values for M_{xy} at times t = τ (or t = T2), t = 2τ, t = 3τ, and t = 4τ are listed in Table I2-1. Note that over time the overall signal decays to a small fraction of its original value (5% and 2% at t = 3τ and 4τ, respectively).

▶ **TABLE I2-1 Exponential Decay Values for**
$M_{xy}(t) = Me^{-t/\tau}$, where τ = T2 or T2*

Time	Magnetization, M_{xy}
0	M
τ	0.37 M
2τ	0.14 M
3τ	0.05 M
4τ	0.02 M

To get a better feeling for typical T2 decay, consider a representative value of T2 = 20 msec. At 20 msec after the RF pulse, the measured signal diminishes to 37% of its original value. After 40 msec, the measured signal is 14%, while after 60 msec it is only 5% of its original value. The fast rate of T2 decay places strict constraints on the window of opportunity for signal measurement. If signal is measured too late after the RF pulse (where "too late" might be only 60 msec!), then there will be virtually no signal left.

A tissue with longer T2, say 40 msec, will demonstrate a slower decay of signal. That is, all things being equal, tissues with longer T2 times will have more signal at any given time than those with short T2 times.

> **IMPORTANT CONCEPT:** The longer the T2, the slower the decay; the shorter the T2, the faster the decay.

Exponential Decay of a Sinusoidal Function

For an exponentially decaying curve that is also oscillating or sinusoidal (like the FID in Figure I2-12), the equation that describes the process is

$$M_{xy}(t) = Me^{-t/\tau}\cos \omega t$$

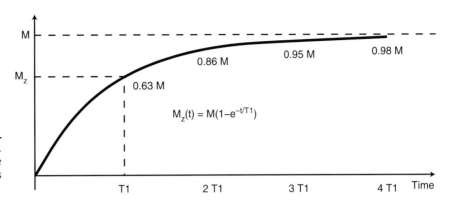

T1 Recovery

$M_z(t) = M(1-e^{-t/T1})$

FIGURE I2-14. Exponential T1 recovery. The time constant, T1, represents the time needed for the signal to recover 63% of its maximum value.

the product of the sinusoidal function (cos ωt, where ω is the frequency of oscillation) and the exponential function, $Me^{-t/\tau}$, that describes the decay.

CHALLENGE QUESTION: In the case where M_{xy} describes the FID, what is the value of ω?

ANSWER: ω is the Larmor frequency. (As discussed in Section I, Chapter 1, to convert the Larmor frequency, f, from units of Hz into ω, in radians per second, use the relation ω = 2πf.)

Exponential Recovery

A companion to exponential decay is *exponential recovery* (Figure I2-14). The equation used to describe this curve is

$$M_z(t) = M(1 - e^{-t/\tau})$$

In this case, M represents the maximum value of the longitudinal magnetization after full recovery, while τ (tau) again is a time constant, this time referred to as the T1 relaxation time. This time τ describes a time constant for recovery rather than decay.

Again, it is easiest to understand the recovery equation by looking at values of M(t) at different time points. Initially, at t = 0,

$$M_z(t = 0) = M(1 - e^0) = M(1 - 1) = 0$$

The values for M_z at times t = τ (or t = T1, in the case of T1 recovery), t = 2τ, t = 3τ, and t = 4τ are listed in Table I2-2. Note that for exponential recovery, after a time equaling 3 or 4 time constants, the overall signal has recovered almost completely to its maximum value (95% or 98%, respectively).

To get a better feel for typical T1 recovery curves, consider a representative value of T1 = 500 msec. At 500 msec after the RF pulse, the measured signal will have recovered to about 63% of its original value. After

TABLE I2-2 Exponential Recovery Values for $M_z(t) = M(1 - e^{-t/\tau})$, where τ = T1

Time τ	Magnetization, M_z
0	0
τ	0.63 M
2τ	0.86 M
3τ	0.95 M
4τ	0.98 M

1000 msec, the longitudinal magnetization will have reached 86% of its original value, while by 1500 msec it will be nearly its full value (95%). A tissue with a longer T1 time, say 800 msec, will recover more slowly. That is, all things being equal, tissues with long T1 times will have less magnetization than tissues with short T1 times.

Note that unlike the exponential decay of transverse magnetization, the exponential recovery of longitudinal magnetization recovers without oscillation. It is therefore always depicted as a simple recovery curve, without a sinusoidal component.

IMPORTANT CONCEPT: The longer the T1, the slower the recovery; the shorter the T1, the faster the recovery.

TABLE I2-3 Magnetization at T1 and T2 times

Time τ	M_z, T1 Recovery	M_{xy}, T2 Decay
0	0	M
τ	0.63 M	0.37 M
2τ	0.86 M	0.14 M
3τ	0.95 M	0.05 M
4τ	0.98 M	0.02 M
5τ	0.994 M	0.006 M

The expected decays (from M to 0) and recoveries (from 0 to M), expressed in terms of T1 and T2 values, are given in Table I2-3. Note the complementary nature of these two phenomena.

> **IMPORTANT CONCEPT:** M_z just before a 90° pulse will equal the measured M_{xy} just after the pulse. Hence, although M_z is not measurable, it is just one RF pulse away from being measurable.

The Recovery: Longitudinal (T1) Relaxation

Longitudinal magnetization recovers on a slower time scale than the loss of phase coherence. Typical values for T1 relaxation times are on the order of 500–1500 msec for tissues other than water. The concept of T1 is complementary of T2. Where T2 describes decay and loss of transverse signal, T1 describes recovery of longitudinal magnetization and regrowth of potential signal.

With MR imaging, the application of RF pulses and measurement of signal is a repetitive process. Longitudinal recovery attained before application of the RF pulse will determine the amount of transverse magnetization or signal available for the measurement. *A 90° RF pulse transforms any given M_z into an equal M_{xy} just after the pulse.* The more complete the longitudinal recovery, M_z, the greater the measured signal resulting from a 90° pulse.

PUTTING T1 AND T2 TOGETHER

The processes of T2 decay and T1 recovery are plotted together in Figure I2-15. The exponential decay of the transverse component of magnetization is described as T2 or T2* relaxation or decay, while the recovery of longitudinal magnetization is referred to as T1 relaxation or recovery. Figure I2-15 depicts the temporal relationship between the fast T2 decay (T2 = 10–100 msec) and the slower T1 recovery (T1 = 500–1500 msec). By the time longitudinal signal has recovered to any significant degree, there is no measurable transverse component, because there is complete loss of phase coherence. Consequently, the exponential recovery of longitudinal magnetization is depicted without the oscillations associated with transverse magnetization.

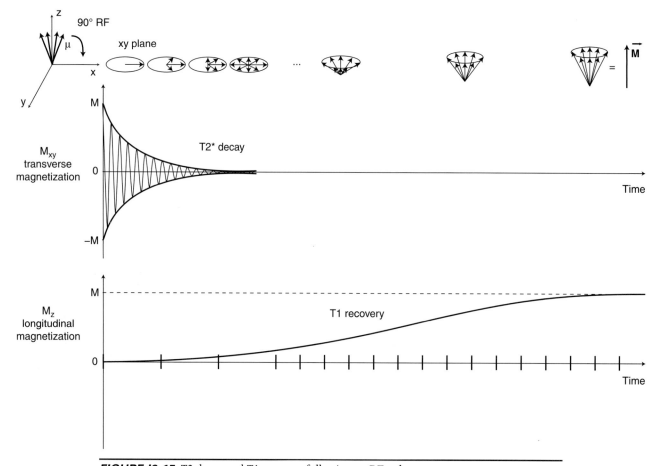

FIGURE I2-15. T2 decay and T1 recovery following an RF pulse.

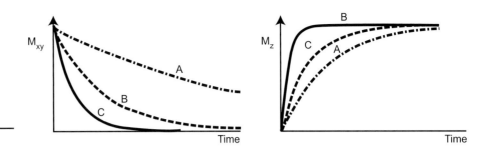

FIGURE I2-Q4.

REVIEW QUESTIONS

1. To review:
   a. What is the Larmor equation?
   b. What is the value of the gyromagnetic ratio for protons (give units)?
   c. What is the precessional frequency or Larmor frequency (in MHz) for protons at 1.5 T?
   d. What is the field strength corresponding to a Larmor frequency of 128 MHz?

2. Assume that at 1.5 T a 10 μT magnetic field, B_1, rotating in the xy plane at 64 MHz, induces a 90° flip angle in 0.6 msec.
   a. How long should the RF pulse be left on to achieve a 45° flip angle?
   b. Compute B_1 needed to be to achieve a 90° flip angle in 0.2 msec?
   c. What key property of the RF system would have to be changed to be useful for imaging at 3 T?
   d. Once resonance is ensured, how long would it take for the 10 μT B_1 RF pulse to achieve 90° flip angle at 3 T?

3. For a magnetization vector, **M**, in the z direction with magnitude M, how much transverse magnetization would result from a 30° flip angle RF pulse? How much longitudinal magnetization would remain? (Hint: sin 30° = 0.5 and cos 30° = 0.87.)

4. Longitudinal magnetization recovery curves and FID curves, for three tissues A, B, and C, are shown in Figure I2-Q4. The T1 and T2 values for the tissues are given in the following table. Match the tissues with the labels A, B, and C.

Tissues	Curve Label
Myocardium: T1 = 800 msec and T2 = 30 msec	____
Blood: T1 = 1200 msec and T2 = 250 msec	____
Fat: T1 = 250 msec and T2 = 60 msec	____

5. The three tissues in Question 4 are subjected to a 60° flip angle RF pulse. Which tissue will have the most signal following a second RF pulse 100 msec after the first?

Chapter 3

Tissue Characteristics and Contrast Agents: PD, T1, and T2

The brightness of the voxels in an MR image is directly proportional to the amount of signal measured by the receiver coils. MR pulse sequences can be designed to emphasize different tissue properties, such as proton density (PD), T1 relaxation time, T2 relaxation time, motion, vascularity, and oxygenation, among others. The basic properties of PD, T1, and T2 are reflected in all MR images to a greater or lesser extent depending on the pulse sequence design. These three properties are briefly introduced in this chapter. Most exogenous contrast agents are designed to alter the T1 or T2 relaxation times of tissues. Some of the contrast agents commonly used in cardiovascular MR imaging are reviewed.

KEY CONCEPTS

▶ T1 relaxation times reflect spin-lattice interactions. T1 times are shortest when molecular motion approaches the Larmor frequency.

▶ Gadolinium chelates are contrast agents used predominantly to shorten T1 relaxation times of surrounding protons.

▶ The relationship between the concentration of gadolinium contrast material and signal intensity is neither linear nor monotonic.

▶ T2 relaxation times reflect spin-spin interactions. T2 times are shortest for slow rates of molecular motion.

▶ Relaxivity is the inverse of the relaxation time, and relaxivity of multiple tissues or components is additive.

PROTON DENSITY

Proton density reflects the number or percentage of "MR visible" protons per unit volume. It does not refer to the number of hydrogen nuclei in a tissue. The majority of protons are generally not visible by MR because they are associated with large macromolecules and have very short T2 times (0.1 msec or less). As a percentage of total protons, MR visible protons make up about about 10% to 11% of all protons for most tissues. For example, for muscle, MR visible protons comprise 9.3% of all protons, while for cerebrospinal fluid (CSF) the value is about 10.8%. Sequences that have image contrast based on differences in proton density (called "proton density-weighted") are useful in musculoskeletal applications to help visualize low-signal structures such as bone and ligaments, but they are not commonly used in cardiovascular MR applications.

T1 RELAXATION: SPIN-LATTICE OR LONGITUDINAL RELAXATION

The goal of this and the following section is to give the reader an intuitive understanding about why some tissues have long T1 and T2 relaxation times and others have short relaxation times. To gain this insight, it is important to appreciate differences in the molecular motion of protons in different tissues, because the local field fluctuations associated with molecular motion can promote or delay T1 and T2 relaxation.

The T1 relaxation time depends on the net transfer of energy to (or absorption from) the environment, or "lattice." This transfer occurs only when a proton encounters a magnetic field fluctuating close to its Larmor frequency, which in turn depends on the magnetic field, B_0, to which it is exposed (Figure I3-1). Th field fluctuations depend on rates of molecular motion.

All molecules are in a constant state of random motion. Rates of molecular motion vary for different tissues. Water molecules in pure water are relatively small and move very quickly, so the protons in them experience field fluctuations at a frequency much higher than the Larmor frequency at 1.5 T. Proteins and other macromolecules are larger and

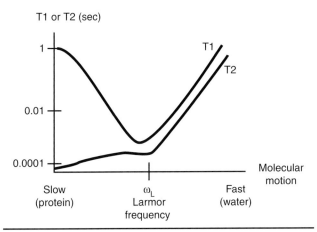

FIGURE I3-1. T1 and T2 times associated with different types of molecules are plotted according to rates of molecular motion relative to the Larmor frequency (assuming $B_0 = 1.5$ T).

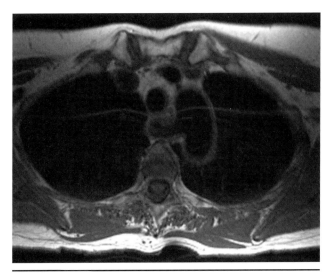

FIGURE I3-2. Effects of differences in T1 relaxation times on image signal intensity in a subject with aberrant right subclavian artery. Tissues such as fat and bone marrow have short T1 relaxation times and therefore have greater signal than tissues such as muscle. The technique used to acquire this image caused signal loss in flowing blood, hence the absence of signal in all vessels.

relatively slow-moving, so protons in them experience a field that changes much more slowly than the Larmor frequency at 1.5 T. It turns out that protons in fat have a natural frequency of motion that is close to the Larmor frequency at 1.5 T, and therefore the longitudinal relaxation of fat is fast, and its T1 time is very short. Water molecules that interact with proteins and macromolecules are slowed by their attraction to them, so protein-containing fluids also have short T1 times. Protons in the majority of tissues other than free water are at the slower end of the spectrum, slower than the Larmor frequency.

CHALLENGE QUESTION: Do tissues with short T1 times tend to be higher or lower in signal intensity on MR images compared with tissues with long T1 times?

Answer: Tissues with shorter T1 usually have higher signal intensity (Figure I3-2).

> **IMPORTANT CONCEPT:** T1 relaxation is fastest when the frequency of molecular motion is close to the Larmor frequency.

Short T1 times mean faster recovery of longitudinal magnetization and therefore more measurable signal following each RF excitation pulse (Figure I3-2).

T1 Contrast Agents: Gadolinium Chelates

Although the intrinsic T1, T2, and proton-density differences of tissues can be a useful basis for diagnosing disease with MRI, frequently exogenous contrast agents are administered to improve the detection and characterization of pathology. In cardiovascular MRI, intravenous

contrast agents are widely used for a number of reasons, including imaging vascular anatomy and pathology, assessing blood supply to normal and pathologic tissues, and evaluating myocardial viability. Contrast agents that shorten T1 relaxation times are desirable because they result in increased signal on T1-weighted images. The most commonly used agents are chelates of gadolinium (Gd^{3+}), a heavy metal ion that alters the T1 relaxation of adjacent protons as a result of its strong paramagnetic properties. Manganese chelates (Mn^{2+}) are less commonly used.

Gadolinium is a lanthanide element in the family of rare earth metals. It has seven unpaired electrons. Each unpaired electron contributes to a strong magnetic moment, and therefore the gadolinium atom is paramagnetic; that is, it adds to the external magnetic field. The magnetic moment (μ) of each unpaired electron is 657 times as great as the magnetic moment of a proton. Because the rate of longitudinal relaxation is proportional to the square of the moment (μ^2), gadolinium contrast agents cause nearby protons to relax a million times faster than usual. Note that the gadolinium is not directly imaged. Rather, its effect on longitudinal relaxation of protons is responsible for the measured signal change.

> **IMPORTANT CONCEPT:** Gadolinium chelates are effective contrast agents because they cause nearby protons to relax much faster than usual.

The Gd^{3+} ion has nine sites to which water molecules can bind, but for that very reason the free gadolinium ion, like other heavy metals, is toxic, because those binding sites may attach to chemical groups on the body's proteins that normally bind to other ions such as calcium. Therefore, chelating agents are used to bind most of the sites, reducing the toxicity of the agent. The nature of the chelate determines the biodistribution and clearance of the gadolinium contrast agent. Several different gadolinium chelates are available commercially (Figure I3-3). One of the most widely used agents, gadopentetate dimeglumine, uses a diethylenetriamine pentaacetic acid (DTPA) chelate to bind eight of the nine binding sites, leaving the ninth site for water to approach the paramagnetic center of the molecule.

Properties of several commonly used commercially available gadolinium chelates are described in the following list, and their chemical structures are shown in Figure I3-3.

(1) Gadopentetate dimeglumine (Gd DTPA) [Magnevist, Berlex/Schering]

- 0.5 mol/L concentration
- Linear structure
- Ionic agent: Gd-DTPA dissociates into gadopentetate^{2-} and 2 meglumine^{1+}
- Osmolarity: 1960 mOsm/kg (each molecule dissociates into 3 ions)
- 15 mL = 35 mOsm (recall that normal osmolarity of serum is 285 mOsm/L)
- Dose: 0.1 mmol/kg body weight
- In Europe, doses up to 0.3 mmol/kg have been approved

- Biological elimination half-life: 1.6 hr (91% excreted by 24 hr)
- Excretion: renal (glomerular filtration)
- T1 relaxivity (r1): ~4–5 L/mmol-s

(2) Gadodiamide (Gd DTPA-BMA) [Omniscan, GE Healthcare]

- 0.5 mol/L concentration
- Linear structure
- Nonionic agent
- Osmolarity: 789 mOsm/kg
- Dose: 0.1–0.3 mmol/kg body weight
- Biological elimination half-life: 1.2 hr (95–98% excreted by 24 hr)
- Excretion: renal (glomerular filtration)
- T1 relaxivity (r1): 4–5 L/mmol-s

(3) Gadoteridol (Gd HP-DO3A) [Prohance, Bracco]

- 0.5 mol/L concentration
- Macrocyclic (ring) ligand
- Nonionic agent
- Osmolarity: 630 mOsm/kg
- Dose: 0.1–0.3 mmol/kg body weight
- Biological elimination half-life: 1.6 hr (94% excreted by 24 hr)
- Excretion: renal (glomerular filtration)
- T1 relaxivity (r1): 4–5 L/mmol-s

(4) Gadobenate dimeglumine (Gd-BOPTA) [MultiHance, Bracco]

- 0.5 mol/L concentration
- Linear structure

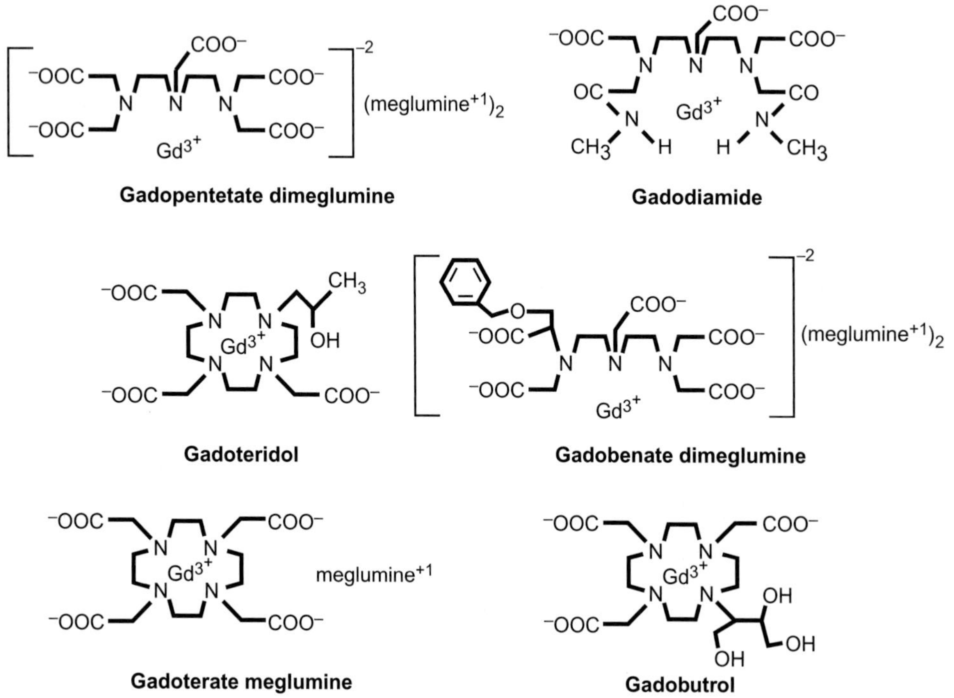

FIGURE I3-3. The most commonly used commercially available gadolinium contrast agents.

- Ionic agent
- Osmolarity: 1970 mOsm/kg
- Dose: 0.1 mmol/kg body weight
- Biological elimination half-life: 1.2–2.0 hr
- Excretion: renal (glomerular filtration), 0.6–4% excreted via biliary route
- T1 relaxivity (r1): ~9–10 L/mmol-s

(5) Gadoterate meglumine (Gd-DOTA) [Dotarem, Guerbet] (not available in the United States)

- 0.5 mol/L concentration
- Macrocyclic (ring) ligand
- Ionic agent
- Osmolarity: 1400 mOsm/kg
- Dose: 0.1–0.3 mmol/kg body weight
- Excretion: renal (glomerular filtration)
- T1 relaxivity (r1): ~4–5 L/mmol-s

(6) Gadobutrol [Gadovist, Schering] (not available in the United States)

- 1 mol/L concentration
- Macrocyclic (ring) ligand
- Ionic agent
- Osmolarity: 1603 mOsm/kg
- Dose: 0.1–0.3 mmol/kg body weight
- Excretion: renal (glomerular filtration)
- T1 relaxivity (r1): ~4–5 L/mmol-s

Dose of Gadolinium Chelates

Doses of gadolinium contrast agents are scaled to subject weight. Most of the gadolinium chelates are administered at doses of 0.1–0.3 mmol/kg body weight. The term *single dose* refers to 0.1 mmol/kg; a *double dose* means 0.2 mmol/kg. For commercial preparations that are 0.5 mol/L, a single dose corresponds to about 12–15 mL for an average-sized (60–75 kg) individual.

In terms of subject body weight in kilograms (kg) or pounds (lb), the dose calculation can be estimated as

$$0.1 \text{ mmol/kg} = 0.2 \text{ mL/kg subject body weight}$$
$$0.1 \text{ mmol/kg} \approx 0.1 \text{ mL/lb subject body weight}$$

A table of doses for commercial preparations that are 0.5 mol/L is provided (Table I3-1).

CHALLENGE QUESTION: How many mL of gadolinium contrast material would be required to administer a single dose to a 75 kg person? What about a 100 kg person?

Answer: A single dose equals 0.1 mmol/kg or approximately 0.2 mL/kg. Thus, a single dose equals 15 mL for a 75 kg person and 20 mL for a 100 kg person.

Safety of Gadolinium Chelates

One measure of the safety of gadolinium chelates is their stability in vivo, which in large part depends on the how tightly the gadolinium ion is bound to its chelate. On this basis, gadoteridol (Prohance) is the most stable, while gadodiamide (Omniscan) is the least. However, to date, no harmful effects have been reported in humans due to release of free gadolinium ions with these agents. Moreover, there has been no correlation between the release of gadolinium ion and adverse events.

Large numbers of clinical safety studies have shown all agents to be safe and well tolerated. The total incidence of adverse events is generally less than 5%, and the incidence of any single adverse event is 1% or less. The most common reactions are nausea, emesis, hives, and headache. Anaphylactoid reactions have been reported with use of each of the agents. The true incidence is unclear, but is likely betweeen 1 : 100,000 and 1 : 500,000. Allergy to one agent is not associated with allergies to the others.

Certain side effects have been reported for specific agents. With gadopentetate dimeglumine (Magnevist), asymptomatic transient increases in serum iron have been measured in 15–30% of subjects. With both gadopentetate dimeglumine (Magnevist) and gadodiamide (Omniscan), serum bilirubin levels increase slightly in 3–4%, but generally return to baseline within 24 to 48 hours. The higher osmolarity of gadopentetate dimeglumine (Magnevist) compared to the other agents is particularly important in the setting of extravasation from the injection site. Recently, gadodiamide (Omniscan) has been shown to interfere with some laboratory measurements of serum calcium, leading to spuriously low concentrations of serum calcium, particularly in patients with renal insufficiency (1).

Because of concerns of accumulation of free gadolinium, the safety of administering gadolinium chelates in patients with renal failure has been studied intensively. The data show that these agents are safe in renal insufficiency and that no additional precautions are needed in this population. Additionally, deoxygenated sickle erythrocytes have been shown in vitro to align perpendicular to a magnetic field. Consequently, the package insert warns about the potential risk of vaso-occlusive complications in

▶ **TABLE I3-1 Standard Doses for Gadolinium Contrast Agents**

Patient weight (lb)	Single dose (0.1 mmol/kg)	Double dose (0.2 mmol/kg)
100 lb (45.5 kg)	10 mL	20 mL
150 lb (68.2 kg)	15 mL	30 mL
200 lb (90.9 kg)	20 mL	40 mL
250 lb (113.6 kg)	25 mL	50 mL
300 lb (136.4 kg)	30 mL	60 mL

subjects with sickle cell anemia. However, there is no evidence to support increased clinical concern in this patient population or those with other hemoglobinopathies.

Gadopentetate dimeglumine is known to cross the placenta freely, and it is assumed that the other MR contrast agents behave in a similar fashion. In general, administration of gadolinium chelates in pregnancy is considered contraindicated. Gadopentetate dimeglumine is excreted at concentrations of about 0.009% (range 0.001%–0.04%) of the total dose in human breast milk over the first day after injection, and the oral absorption of gadolinium from the gastrointestinal tract is extremely low (2). However, many centers still recommend that nursing mothers not breastfeed for 24–48 hrs after administration.

> **IMPORTANT CONCEPT:** Gadolinium chelates are among the safest diagnostic contrast agents administered in medicine, but they should not be administered to pregnant patients without careful consideration.

For additional details about safety, the reader is referred to recent review articles. General MR safety is discussed in Section I, Chapter 10.

Distribution of Gadolinium Chelates

The gadolinium chelates just described are considered extravascular agents. After intravenous injection, the agents rapidly equilibrate between the intravascular and extravascular/extracellular compartments. Therefore, for gadolinium-enhanced MR angiography, images are acquired during the first passage of the bolus through the arterial vessels and before there is substantial venous or interstitial enhancement.

These agents do not cross the intact blood-brain barrier. Their distribution and clearance are identical to those of other agents that are excreted by renal glomerular filtration.

Nonproportionality of MR Signal Intensities to Gadolinium Concentrations

Gadolinium chelates shorten T1 relaxation times and therefore lead to higher signal intensity on T1-weighted images. However, unlike CT, where the concentration of iodinated contrast material in tissues can be calculated directly from the voxel attenuation measurements, in MRI the signal intensities are not proportional to gadolinium concentrations. In fact, the relationship is not even monotonic. That is, beyond a certain concentration (depending on the pulse sequence), the signal intensity starts to *de*crease with increased gadolinium concentration (Figure I3-4).

The main reason for the unexpected relationship between gadolinium concentration and MR image signal

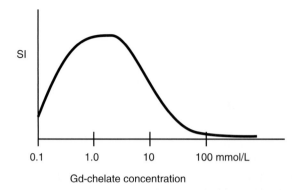

FIGURE I3-4. Schematic relationship between MR signal intensity (T1-weighted sequence) and gadolinium contrast concentrations plotted on a logarithmic scale. At low doses, where T1 effects dominate, the signal intensity increases nonlinearly with concentration. However, above a certain concentration (depending on the characteristics of the pulse sequence), the T2 effects become more important and lead to signal loss.

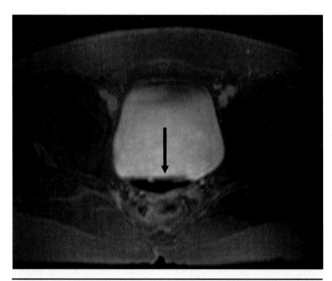

FIGURE I3-5. T2 effects of concentrated gadolinium contrast material in the bladder. Axial fat-suppressed T1-weighted image shows high signal intensity from gadolinium contrast excretion in the urine. However, in the dependent portion of the bladder (arrow), the signal intensity is markedly reduced because of the T2-shortening effects of the highly concentrated (and dense) gadolinium contrast.

intensity is that gadolinium contrast agents shorten not only T1 but also T2 relaxation times. At high concentrations of gadolinium chelate (Figure I3-5), T2 shortening is substantial enough to cause signal loss, overcoming the effect of T1 shortening.

> **IMPORTANT CONCEPT:** The relationship between gadolinium contrast concentration and MR signal intensity is not linear and not even monotonic. At high gadolinium concentrations, T2 effects dominate and cause signal loss.

The complex relationship between gadolinium concentration and image signal intensity has important consequences for cardiovascular MR imaging. First, where gadolinium chelates are highly concentrated, such as in veins draining the intravenous injection site and the renal calyces and bladder, the signal intensity may be paradoxically low and impair image interpretation. Second, for cardiac perfusion imaging, where gadolinium contrast agents are used as tracers for blood flow, image signal intensity cannot be used directly to quantify the amount of gadolinium in the blood pool or myocardium without more sophisticated tools (Section III, Chapter III-7).

Gadolinium Concentrations and T1 and T2 Relaxation Times

The effects of gadolinium on T1 and T2 relaxation times of adjacent protons can be readily calculated. The way in which gadolinium contrast material shortens T1 and T2 relaxation times of water can be understood best in terms of *relaxivity*, R1 or R2, which is the inverse of T1 or T2, respectively:

$$R1 = \frac{1}{T1} = r1 \times C$$
$$R2 = \frac{1}{T2} = r2 \times C$$

where r1 and r2 are the *relaxivity constants* specific for a given contrast agent and C is the concentration of gadolinium chelate (mmol/L). For gadopentetate dimeglumine,

r1 is approximately 4 L/mmol-sec, and r2 is approximately 5 L/mmol-sec.

As the concentration of gadolinium chelates increases, the T1 values shorten and therefore tissues appear brighter. The competing effects of T2 shortening are also evident from these equations because as the concentration of gadolinium increases T2 shortens as well. A short T2 means low signal intensity on all MR images including a T1-weighted image (Figure I3-6).

CHALLENGE QUESTION: What are the T1 and T2 relaxation times of gadopentetate dimeglumine straight out of the commercially prepared bottle (0.5 mol/L), and what are the implications of these values for MR imaging?

Answer: Gadopentetate dimeglumine has a concentration of 0.5 mol/L (or 500 mmol/L). Given that r1 = 4 L/mmol-sec while r2 = 5 L/mmol-sec,

$$T1 = \frac{1}{r1 \times C} = \frac{1}{4 \times 500} = 0.5 \text{ msec}$$
$$T2 = \frac{1}{r2 \times C} = \frac{1}{4 \times 500} = 0.4 \text{ msec}$$

A T2 of 0.4 msec means that the measured transverse magnetization decays almost instantaneously. Pure gadolinium will appear black on just about any MR image (Figure I3-6).

> **IMPORTANT CONCEPT:** T1 and T2 relaxation times are inversely proportional to gadolinium concentrations. Higher concentrations of gadolinium not only shorten T1 times but also shorten T2 times.

Gadolinium Concentrations in Tissues

The foregoing calculations apply to aqueous solutions of gadolinium. When gadolinium contrast material is in tissue, then the overall T1 and T2 relaxation times for the tissue will depend both on the T1 and T2 of the gadolinium contrast material and on the intrinsic T1 and T2 values of the tissue, according to the *additivity of relaxivity*.

$$R1_{tissue+Gd} = R1_{tissue} + R1_{Gd}$$
$$R2_{tissue+Gd} = R2_{tissue} + R2_{Gd}$$

Recall that relaxivity, R1,2, is the inverse of relaxation time, R1,2 = 1/T1,2.

$$\frac{1}{T1_{tissue+Gd}} = \frac{1}{T1_{tissue}} + \frac{1}{T1_{Gd}}$$
$$\frac{1}{T2_{tissue+Gd}} = \frac{1}{T2_{tissue}} + \frac{1}{T2_{Gd}}$$

> **IMPORTANT CONCEPT:** Relaxivity (the relaxation rate or inverse of T1 and T2 times) is additive.

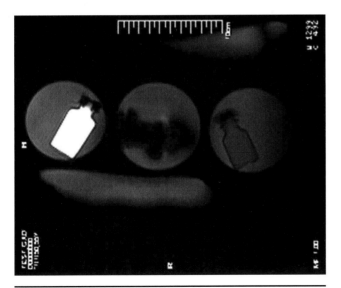

FIGURE I3-6. Three vials immersed in water and imaged with a T1-weighted gradient echo sequence. On the left, the vial contains diluted gadopentetate dimeglumine, in the center, an unopened commercial vial of gadopentetate dimeglumine, and on the right, a vial of saline. The T2 shortening effect of the concentrated gadolinium causes marked signal loss.

CHALLENGE QUESTION: For most solid organs such as the myocardium, gadolinium contrast material dominates the T1 relaxation of the gadolinium-enhanced tissue. To understand why, calculate the T1 time for a cardiac perfusion study in which the T1 of myocardium is 800 msec and the concentration of gadolinium in the heart is 1 mmol/L.

Answer: At a concentration of 1 mmol/L and assuming r1 = 4 L/mmol-sec, the T1 of the gadolinium component is

$$T1 = \frac{1}{r1 \times C} = \frac{1}{4 \times 1} = 0.25 \text{ msec} = 250 \text{ msec}$$

By the additivity of relaxivity,

$$T1 = \frac{1}{T1_{myocardium+Gd}} = \frac{1}{T1_{myocardium}} + \frac{1}{T1_{Gd}}$$

$$= \frac{1}{800} + \frac{1}{250} = 0.00125 + 0.004 = 0.00525$$

$$T1_{myocardium+Gd} = \frac{1}{0.00525} = 190 \text{ msec}$$

The combination of myocardium and gadolinium has a T1 of 190 msec, which is close to the T1 of gadolinium contrast material with its T1 of 250 msec, but very different from the myocardium with its longer T1 of 800 msec. The additivity of relaxivity means that the material with a much shorter T1 will dominate the cumulative T1 effects.

Dependence of T1 on Field Strength

T1 relaxation times vary with B_0 field strength. The Larmor frequency of protons increases directly with B_0 (Larmor equation), but intrinsic molecular motion patterns do not change. Most tissues have molecular motion on the slower end of the spectrum illustrated in Figure I3-1. Thus, at higher field strengths the molecular motion of most tissues is even further away from the Larmor frequency than at 1.5 T. T1 relaxation occurs less efficiently, resulting in longer T1 values for most tissues at higher fields. For example, gray matter of the brain has a T1 time of about 998 msec at 1.5 T, which increases to 1250 msec at 4 T, and the T1 of white matter increases from 718 msec at 1.5 T to 1070 msec at 4 T. Compared to other tissues, the T1 of fat does not increase as much. Therefore, on T1-weighted images at higher field strengths fat seems brighter relative to other tissues than at 1.5 T. This can create artifacts in the imaging, but it can also be addressed by application of fat saturation pulses (Section I, Chapter 9).

IMPORTANT CONCEPT: T1 relaxation times are longer for most tissues, except fat, at higher B_0 field strengths.

T2 RELAXATION: SPIN-SPIN OR TRANSVERSE RELAXATION

The T2 relaxation time reflects the rate of loss of phase coherence in transverse magnetization. Loss of coherence is caused by variability of local magnetic fields within a tissue. Fluctuations in the local magnetic field depend on the molecular motion of small magnetic moments. To produce dephasing, the local field variations must be relatively constant over several milliseconds. High-frequency fluctuations will average out and cause no net effect. Thus, the relationship between T2 relaxation time and rates of molecular motion is relatively straightforward (Figure I3-1)—the faster-moving protons (such as those in free water) have the least effect on the magnetic field and hence the longest T2 relaxation times, while slower-moving protons have shorter T2 times. At the Larmor frequency, T1 relaxation also leads to a loss of phase coherence. This is referred to as the "T1 contribution to T2" and can be seen in Figure I3-1 as a focal decrease in T2 at the Larmor frequency of molecular motion.

T2, T2′, and T2*

The loss of phase coherence measured after an RF pulse is referred to as T2*. T2* rates depend on two main factors: fluctuations in local magnetic fields resulting from intrinsic molecular motion and diffusion (T2) and magnetic field inhomogeneities that occur at the macroscopic level (T2′). Magnetic field inhomogeneities (T2′) usually dominate the T2* decay. The relationship between the loss of phase coherence contributed by different factors can be described by the principle of the additivity of relaxivity (the same as for longitudinal rates):

$$R2^* = R2 + R2'$$

or

$$\frac{1}{T2^*} = \frac{1}{T2} + \frac{1}{T2'}$$

where relaxivity, R2, is the inverse of T2 time. Analogous to T1 relaxivity, T2* will be determined by the fastest component of the dephasing process. For example, if T2 = 50 msec and T2′ = 5 msec, then T2* will be a bit shorter than the smaller of the values:

$$\frac{1}{T2^*} = \frac{1}{50} + \frac{1}{5} = 0.02 + 0.2 = 0.22$$

$$T2^* \cong 4.5 \text{ msec}$$

IMPORTANT CONCEPT: From the two factors, T2′ and T2, that contribute to phase coherence loss, the dominant factor is the one that causes the greatest dephasing (typically T2′ due to B_0 field inhomogeneities).

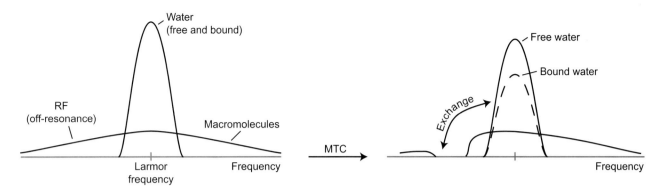

FIGURE I3-7. Magnetization transfer. Magnetization transfer contrast results from application of an off-resonance RF pulse, which saturates magnetization associated with macromolecular protons but not free water. The free exchange of this magnetization with water associated with the macromolecules results in saturation of signal in solid organs such as muscle and myocardium, thereby reducing their signal for angiographic applications.

Dependence of T2 on Field Strength

Unlike T1, there is very little dependence of T2 on B_0 field strength. At higher field strengths, intrinsic tissue T2 relaxation times shorten only slightly. However, T2* times are usually shorter because at higher B_0, because magnetic field homogeneity may be more difficult to achieve.

Free Water versus Bound Water: Magnetization Transfer

The relationship between molecular motion and T2 relaxation times is exploited in MR imaging using a technique called *magnetization transfer*, which is used in some angiographic applications to suppress signal from background tissues relative to blood in vessels.

Magnetization transfer relies on the difference in T2 relaxation times between free, unbound water protons and protons that are bound to macromolecules. Before going into the details of magnetization transfer, two concepts must be introduced. First is the inverse relationship between T2 relaxation times and the range of resonance frequencies of a tissue. In Chapter I-2, the Larmor frequency was defined for protons at 1.5 T as about 64 MHz. In reality, the resonance frequency is not one single frequency but a range of frequencies (Figure I3-7). This range can be relatively narrow or broad, depending on the T2 characteristics of the protons. Protons with long T2 times have narrow resonance, while protons with short T2 times have broader resonance. The second concept is that magnetization or energy freely exchanges between macromolecular protons and the water protons bound to the macromolecules.

As discussed previously, free water, because of its fast molecular motion, has a very long T2 time. Macromolecules and protons that are bound to them have much shorter T2 times. In most tissues other than

TABLE I3-2 Typical T1 and T2 Relaxation Times at 1.5 T

Tissue	T1 (msec)	T2 (msec)
Fat	250	60
Myocardium	800	30
Liver	575	50
Arterial Blood	1200	250
CSF	2000	1000

blood, a significant proportion of water protons are bound to macromolecules. A consequence of the differences in relaxation times is that free water has a very narrow resonance bandwidth around the Larmor frequency, while bound protons have a much broader resonance. To achieve magnetization transfer contrast, a special broad-bandwidth RF pulse is applied off resonance, several kHz away from the resonance frequency of water (Figure I3-7). The RF pulse saturates the signal from these bound protons. The saturated magnetization of the macromolecules exchanges with the bound water, causing signal loss. As a consequence, most tissues other than free water and fat are suppressed with magnetization transfer.

T1 AND T2 TIMES FOR NORMAL AND DISEASED TISSUES

In general, most normal tissues have relatively short T1 and T2 times (Table I3-2), while fluids, such as blood, cerebrospinal fluid, or cystic lesions, usually have relatively long T1 and T2 times. Additionally, many types of pathology, including many malignant tumors, generally have longer T1 and T2 times than normal tissues of their origins. As will be discussed in Chapter I-4, the distribution of T1 and T2 times has implications when considering how to modify image contrast for maximum conspicuity of pathology.

REVIEW QUESTIONS

1. Why is free gadolinium ion (Gd^{3+}) toxic?

2. What concentration of gadolinium contrast material would be needed in the aorta to achieve a T1 value of 50 msec? Assume the T1 of blood is 1200 msec, and r1 = 4 L/mmol-sec.

3. Direct injections of gadolinium contrast material.
   a. In some applications, contrast material is injected directly into the vessels of interest, bypassing the venous circulation. For example, direct injections into coronary arteries are being investigated in laboratories studying real-time MR coronary interventions. If gadopentetate dimeglumine is drawn up directly from the original vial and injected into the vessel, T1-weighted images show a signal void in the vessel. Why?

   b. To overcome the problem described in (a), a dose of gadolinium contrast can be diluted in normal saline solution. If 5 mL of contrast material is injected into a bag of 250 mL normal saline (dilution of 50:1), what will be the T1 and T2 values of the dilute mix? What will be the appearance of this mixture on MR images?

4. How many mL of gadolinium contrast material (at 0.5 mol/L) would make a single dose for a child who weighs 10 kg? What about a double dose?

REFERENCES

1. Prince MR, Erel HE, Lent RW, Blumenfeld J, Kent KC, Bush HL, Wang Y. Gadodiamide administration causes spurious hypocalcemia. Radiology 2003; 227:639–646.
2. Kubik-Huch RA, Gottstein-Aalame NM, Frenzel T, Seifert B, Puchert E, Wittek S, Debatin JF. Gadopentetate dimeglumine excretion into human breast milk during lactation. Radiology 2000; 216:555–558.
3. Shellock FG, Kanal E. Safety of magnetic resonance imaging contrast agents. J Magn Reson Imaging 1999; 10:477–484
4. Runge VM. Safety of approved MR contrast media for intravenous injection. J Magn Reson Imaging 2000; 12:205–213.

Chapter 4

Echoes

Most MR images can be characterized as either *spin echo* or *gradient echo* images. This chapter focuses on how each type of image is produced and their properties and explores the parameters that can be manipulated to alter image contrast with each approach. The techniques for reducing acquisition times for each type of sequence will be discussed. Finally, specific applications of spin echo and gradient echo sequences in cardiovascular MR imaging are introduced. More detailed explorations are covered in Sections II and III of this book.

KEY CONCEPTS

▶ Two main types of echoes are used for generating MR images: spin echoes and gradient echoes.

▶ Gradient echoes are generated following a single RF pulse that can have a flip angle of less than 90° and a pair of dephasing and rephasing gradients.

▶ Gradient echo images have T2* weighting; unlike spin echoes, the effects of magnetic field inhomogeneities are not eliminated with gradient echoes.

▶ Partial flip angle gradient echo imaging leaves residual longitudinal magnetization for subsequent repeated RF excitations to be performed in quick succession.

▶ With gradient echo images, the sequence parameters that affect image contrast are the repetition time (TR), echo time (TE), and flip angle.

▶ T1-weighted spoiled gradient echo images are generated with relatively long TR, short TE, and large flip angles, while T2*-weighted images rely on short TR, long TE, and small flip angles.

▶ Multiecho gradient echo acquisitions improve efficiency of gradient echo imaging.

▶ Steady-state free-precession gradient echo imaging using balanced gradients provides image contrast that is T2/T1 weighted and requires short TR (<5 msec) and homogeneous B_0 magnetic field.

▶ Spin echo images are generated following two RF pulses (typically a 90° and a 180° pulse) and a pair of dephasing and rephasing gradients.

▶ With spin echoes, the two sequence parameters that affect image contrast are the TR, which determines T1 contrast, and the TE, which determines T2 contrast.

▶ T1-weighted spin echo images are produced using short TR and short TE, while T2-weighted images rely on long TR and TE.

▶ Fast spin echo imaging improves the efficiency of spin echo imaging by a factor equal to the echo train length (ETL), but at the price of reduced image contrast.

▶ Half-Fourier single-shot fast spin echo sequences generate images as fast as one second per slice, but are limited by high specific absorption rate (SAR), decreased T2-weighted image contrast, and relatively low signal-to-noise ratio.

▶ Spin echo imaging reduces the effects of B_0 field inhomogeneities that cause T2' decay, allowing intrinsic T2 relaxation differences to be visualized.

GRADIENT ECHOES

Gradient Echoes: The Concept

A *gradient recalled echo (GRE)*, or gradient echo, is produced by the application of a pair of gradient pulses that serve to *dephase* and then partially *rephase* magnetic moments. The process of rephasing generates an echo within the free induction decay (FID) time; this echo is sampled or measured with the receiver coil and used to fill k-space. This chapter explains how gradient pulses generate echoes and affect image contrast. The methods for spatial encoding of gradient echoes will be discussed in Chapters I-5 and I-6.

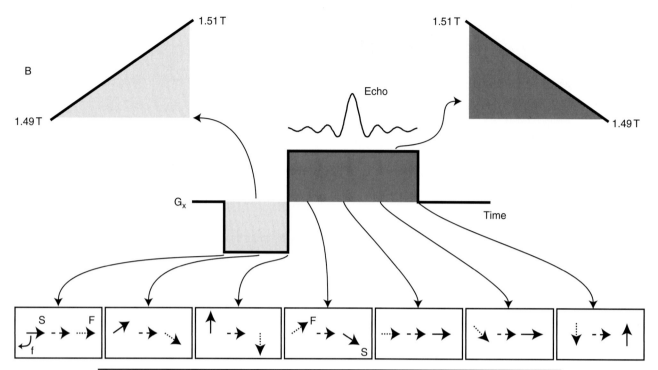

FIGURE I4-1. Gradient recalled echo. By first dephasing and then rephasing magnetic moments, the gradients produce a gradient echo. Protons that initially experience a magnetic field less than 1.5 T with the dephasing lobe (S, slow) will subsequently be exposed to a magnetic field greater than 1.5 T with the rephasing lobe (F, fast). In this example, maximum refocusing occurs at the midpoint of the rephasing lobe.

The process of controlled, intentional dephasing and then rephasing of the magnetic moments is illustrated in Figure I4-1.

Controlled Dephasing

As introduced in Chapter I-2, following an RF excitation pulse, the transverse component of magnetization precesses about the xy plane with phase coherence. However, once the RF pulse ends, the magnetic moments begin to dephase, and the measured signal decays. With gradient echo imaging, a gradient that is applied during this process causes accelerated dephasing (Figure I4-1). By convention, the gradient is applied in the x direction.

Controlled Rephasing

To generate a gradient echo, a second gradient pulse is then applied, with reversed polarity. Wherever the dephasing gradient caused the field to be greater than 1.5 T, the reversed gradient causes it to be less than 1.5 T, and vice versa. Hence, protons that had been precessing more slowly will now precess faster, whereas those that had been faster will now be slower. Consequently, the rephasing gradient reverses the dephasing caused by the first gradient and brings the magnetic moments back in phase.

At the moment of maximum phase coherence, the peak of the gradient echo is formed. If the reversed gradient is left on longer, accelerated dephasing will occur, and the echo will decay (Figure I4-2).

> **IMPORTANT CONCEPT:** Gradients always cause dephasing. Gradient echo imaging relies on controlled dephasing and then rephasing of magnetic moments.

The gradient echo is usually sampled during the entire duration of gradient reversal. The time between the peak of the RF pulse and the point of maximal refocusing (typically the midpoint of the gradient reversal) is called the *echo time (TE)* (Figure I4-2). The MR signals that are generated with gradient echo imaging are usually referred to as T2*-weighted because the amplitude of the echo is governed by T2* decay (FID) (Chapter I-2).

CHALLENGE QUESTION: If gradient echoes are affected by T2* decay, then is there truly perfect rephasing of the magnetic moments as illustrated in Figure I4-1?

Answer: No! There will be some residual dephasing of the magnetic moments as a result of T2* decay, even at the peak of the gradient echo formation.

> **IMPORTANT CONCEPT:** Gradient recalled echo images have T2* weighting, which includes the effects of both field inhomogeneities and intrinsic T2 differences of tissues. Field inhomogeneity effects are not eliminated with use of gradient refocusing.

Gradient-Induced Phase Shifts

The amplitudes and durations of the dephasing and rephasing gradients are two parameters that can be varied in MR imaging. The question of how they affect the gradient echo process is explored in this section.

Gradients cause dephasing by inducing protons to precess at different frequencies along the direction of the gradient at different locations. The gradient amplitude determines how fast this dephasing occurs. The stronger the gradient, the faster the dephasing. For example, if a gradient with a particular amplitude G is applied for a duration t and causes the faster protons to be 90° ahead of the slower protons, then a gradient twice as strong, 2G, will accomplish the same phase difference in half the time. Alternatively, if the original gradient amplitude G is applied for twice as long, 2t, the protons will have twice the phase difference, or 180°.

This observation can be generalized by stating that the phase shift is proportional to both the strength of the gradient and the duration of the gradient. In mathematical terms, the phase shift, $\Delta\phi$, for constant G_x, can be expressed as

$$\Delta\phi = 360° \times \Delta ft = 360° \times \gamma\Delta B_{gradient}t$$
$$= 360° \times \gamma x G_x t$$

That is, $\Delta\phi$ depends on the difference in precessional frequencies, Δf, and the length of time, t, during which the frequencies are different. The frequency difference can be related to the magnetic field strength difference, $\Delta B_{gradient}$, by the Larmor equation, where γ is the gyromagnetic ratio. The field strength difference is in turn related to the gradient strength, G_x, and distance between protons, x, along the direction of the gradient.

When drawn in the format of a typical pulse sequence diagram, where the strength of the gradient is plotted as the height of the pulse and the duration is its length, phase shift can be considered as proportional to the area under the gradient curve (Figure I4-3).

Depending on the degree of dephasing desired, different combinations of gradient strengths and durations can be used, as illustrated in Figure I4-4.

> **IMPORTANT CONCEPT:** Phase shift is proportional to the area under the gradient curve. For a constant gradient, the phase shift is related to gradient strength × gradient duration.

Partial Flip Angle Imaging: A Free Lunch

With gradient echo imaging, a flip angle α of less than 90°, called a *partial flip angle*, can be used to shorten the time intervals between RF pulses (TR) and therefore to shorten the acquisition time.

How much transverse and longitudinal magnetization results from a partial flip angle RF pulse? Recall the relationship reviewed in Chapter I-1 (Background Reading on Vectors and Sines and Cosines) and illustrated in Figure I1-5. The magnitude of the transverse magnetization is equal to the magnitude of the magnetization vector, **M**, multiplied by the sine of the flip angle, sin α, while the longitudinal component is the magnitude multiplied by the cosine of the flip angle, cos α.

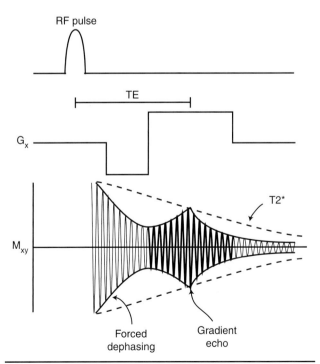

FIGURE I4-2. Formation of the gradient echo during T2* decay (free induction decay, or FID). The peak of the gradient echo occurs at a time called the echo time, TE, following the RF pulse.

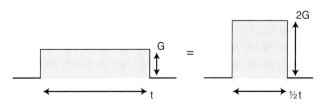

FIGURE I4-3. Phase shift is proportional to area under the gradient curve. The same phase shift can be achieved in half the time by doubling the amplitude of the gradient.

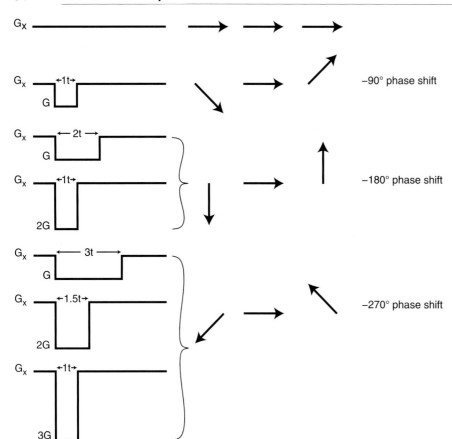

FIGURE I4-4. Relationship between gradient amplitude and duration and resulting degree of dephasing.

$-90°$ phase shift

$-180°$ phase shift

$-270°$ phase shift

IMPORTANT REVIEW POINT: Any magnetization vector, M, can be expressed in terms of its transverse component in the xy plane, M_{xy}, which reflects measurable signal, and its longitudinal component, M_z, which represents stored or potential signal. The magnitude of each component is related to the flip angle, α, by the following equations:

$$M_{xy} = M \sin \alpha$$
$$M_z = M \cos \alpha$$

A Free Lunch

The "magic" of gradient echo imaging is that the sum of the magnitudes of the transverse and longitudinal magnetization components is greater than the magnitude of the original magnetization vector. Another way of thinking about this is to say that the sum of the lengths of the two sides of a right triangle are always greater than the length of the hypotenuse. (Note that this is a property of the magnitudes of the sides only; the sum of the two vectors, $\mathbf{M_{xy}}$ and $\mathbf{M_z}$, exactly equals $\mathbf{M}$.)

To get a better feeling for this relationship, consider a few examples of flip angles and the resulting longitudinal and transverse magnetization values in Figure I4-5 and Table I4-1.

Why is the partial flip angle such a useful feature? Following a partial flip angle excitation, a considerable amount of transverse magnetization can be generated for measurable signal. Yet, immediately following this excitation, there can still be substantial residual longitudinal magnetization for a subsequent excitation. For example, consider a 30° RF excitation pulse. For a net magnetization of amplitude M, the measurable signal in the transverse plane immediately after the excitation will have amplitude 0.5 M, while 0.87 M remains in the longitudinal direction. This means that a 30° RF pulse generates only half has much signal as would a 90° pulse, but it leaves 87% of the magnetization for another 30° RF pulse.

IMPORTANT CONCEPT: Partial flip angle gradient echo imaging amounts to a "free lunch" because the sum of the magnitudes of the transverse and longitudinal magnetization components can exceed the magnitude of the original net magnetization. Following partial flip angle excitation, residual longitudinal magnetization (the amount depending on the flip angle, α) is available for a subsequent RF pulse.

Reaching Equilibrium with Gradient Echo Pulse Sequences

In many applications of gradient echo imaging, partial flip angle RF pulses are applied in quick succession without sufficient time for full T1 recovery between each pulse (Figure I4-6). The state of transverse and longitudinal

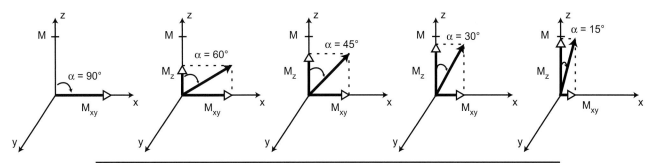

FIGURE I4-5. Longitudinal and transverse magnetization following RF pulses of 90°, 60°, 45°, 30°, and 15°.

▶ **TABLE I4-1**

		Flip Angle				
		90°	**60°**	**45°**	**30°**	**15°**
Measured Signal:	M_{xy} (transverse) = $M \sin \alpha$	M	0.87 M	0.7 M	0.5 M	0.26 M
Potential Signal:	M_z (longitudinal) = $M \cos \alpha$	0	0.5 M	0.7 M	0.87 M	0.97 M

magnetization evolves over the first several RF excitations, after which a steady-state equilibrium is reached. The magnetization at equilibrium depends on the balance between two factors: the decrease in longitudinal magnetization resulting from each RF excitation and the amount of recovery of longitudinal magnetization during the time between successive RF excitations, called the *repetition time* or TR (Figure I4-6). Recovery depends on the relationship between the T1 relaxation time of tissues and the TR. With larger flip angles, more of the longitudinal magnetization is lost with each RF pulse. With longer TRs, shorter T1 relaxation times, or both, more is recovered in each interval.

Figure I4-6 also shows how the flip angle affects the equilibrium that is reached. Immediately after each 30° pulse, M_z is 0.87 M, where M is the prepulse magnetization, while the magnitude of the transverse component, M_{xy}, is 0.5 M. In this example, some T1 recovery occurs during the TR interval, but it is not complete. Therefore, at the time of the second RF pulse, M_z has not fully recovered to M. If it has recovered to 0.94 M, then following the next 30° RF pulse, the transverse component will be half of 0.94 M, or 0.47 M, while the longitudinal component will be 0.87 × 0.94 M, or 0.82 M. After several RF pulses, a balance is achieved at which the recovery of M_z through T1 relaxation during the TR is equal to the amount by which it is decreased by each RF pulse.

In the same example, consider what happens if the flip angle is increased to 60°. Following each RF pulse, M_z is 0.5 M, while the magnitude of the transverse component, M_{xy}, is 0.87 M. That is, the fraction of the longitudinal

magnetization that is converted to measurable signal is considerably higher following a 60° pulse than following a 30° pulse. However, because the T1 relaxation of the tissue shown in this example is long relative to the TR, longitudinal recovery is modest in each repetition time. Therefore, the equilibrium is established at a much lower level of longitudinal magnetization. Consequently, the actual measured signal will be less with 60° RF pulses than with 30° pulses. The dampening of signal by repeated RF excitations in gradient echo imaging is commonly referred to as *saturation*. As shown in Figure I4-6, saturation is greater with higher flip angle excitations.

> **IMPORTANT CONCEPT:** After repeated partial flip angle excitations, a balance is achieved between the decrease in longitudinal magnetization resulting from each RF excitation and the longitudinal recovery that takes place during the interval between RF pulses.

Maximizing Signal in Gradient Echo Imaging

The maximum signal for a given tissue with known T1 value can be achieved when the following relationship between flip angle, α_E, TR, and T1 is fulfilled:

$$\cos \alpha_E = e^{-TR/T1}$$

The optimal flip angle, α_E, is known as the *Ernst angle*. When the TR is much larger than T1, then α_E approaches 90°. On the other hand, when the TR is much smaller than T1, then the optimal flip angle α_E is small and close to 0°.

Image Contrast: Balance between Flip Angle, TR, and T1

Figure I4-6 illustrates the effects of flip angle on *one* tissue. Parameters that are important for image contrast are TR, TE, and the T1 of tissues. To gain some insight into how TR, TE, and flip angle can be used to bring out differences due to tissue T1 and T2 relaxation times, consider the

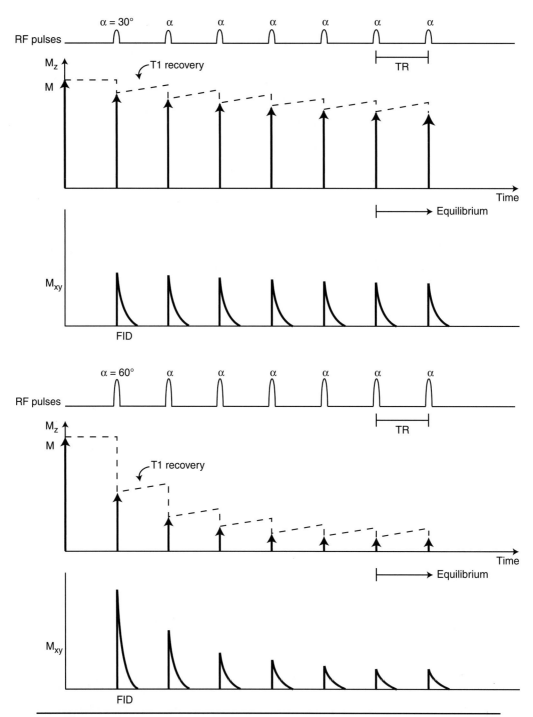

FIGURE I4-6. Longitudinal magnetization (M_z) and transverse magnetization (M_{xy}) after a series of RF pulses causing (a) 30° and (b) 60° flip angle.

following three commonly used versions of gradient echo sequences in cardiovascular MRI:

A. Long TR and Large Flip Angle

With gradient echo imaging, even a long TR is usually shorter than the T1 relaxation times of most tissues. Nevertheless, a long-TR sequence allows tissues with short T1 times to recover a substantial amount of longitudinal magnetization compared to tissues with long T1 times. If enough time is available for longitudinal recovery, then higher flip angles can be used without saturating the signal. Figure I4-7 illustrates the effect of long TR and large flip angle on tissues with short and long T1 values.

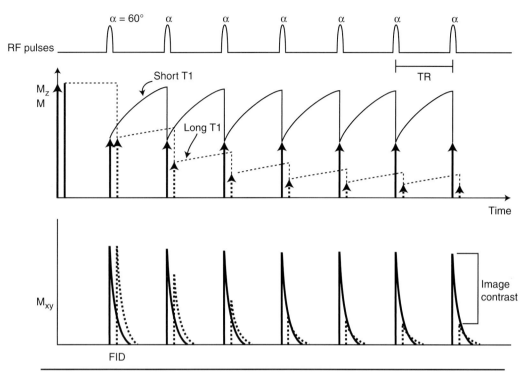

FIGURE I4-7. Gradient echo sequence with long TR and large flip angle results in image contrast for tissues with differing T1 relaxation times (short T1, solid line; long T1, dashed line).

With long TR times, differences in T1 times are brought out because there is enough time for differences in longitudinal recovery to become apparent. The longer the TR times relative to the T1 recovery times, the higher the flip angle that can be used without saturating signal.

B. Short TR and Small Flip Angle

If TR is much shorter than T1, then there will be no significant recovery between each RF pulse. This means that the signal will simply depend on the flip angle, and there will be very little contrast based on differences in tissue T1 times. A high flip angle will lead to minimal residual longitudinal magnetization after each pulse and, consequently, very low signal (Figure I4-6). If TR is much less than T1, a small flip angle is usually used (Figure I4-8).

C. Gadolinium-Enhanced Imaging

Gadolinium-enhanced MR imaging provides a third option of generating contrast. The T1-shortening effects of gadolinium contrast material are dramatic. For gadolinium-enhanced MR angiography, the T1 of blood can become as short as 20 msec. As illustrated in Figure I4-9, because the recovery of longitudinal magnetization is so fast with gadolinium contrast material, short TR times and higher flip angles can be used.

CHALLENGE QUESTION: How can the contrast between gadolinium-enhanced tissues and background unenhanced tissues be further increased?

Answer: By increasing the flip angle. Recall that gadolinium contrast material acts by shortening T1 relaxation times of the protons around it. If T1 is sufficiently short, then longitudinal magnetization of gadolinium-containing tissues will recover sufficiently even with high flip angles. However, with larger flip angles, the background tissues will become almost completely saturated and generate minimal signal. As a consequence, the contrast between gadolinium-enhanced tissues and background tissues will be even greater than the contrast at low flip angle.

> **IMPORTANT CONCEPT:** A long TR and a larger flip angle bring out differences in T1 relaxation times with gradient echo imaging. Conversely, shorter TR and a smaller flip angle minimize T1 weighting. Gadolinium-enhanced imaging favors a short TR and a larger flip angle to maximize contrast between gadolinium-enhanced vessels and other tissues.

Acquisition Times for Gradient Echo Imaging

How long does it take to make a gradient echo image? Following each RF excitation, a gradient echo is used to

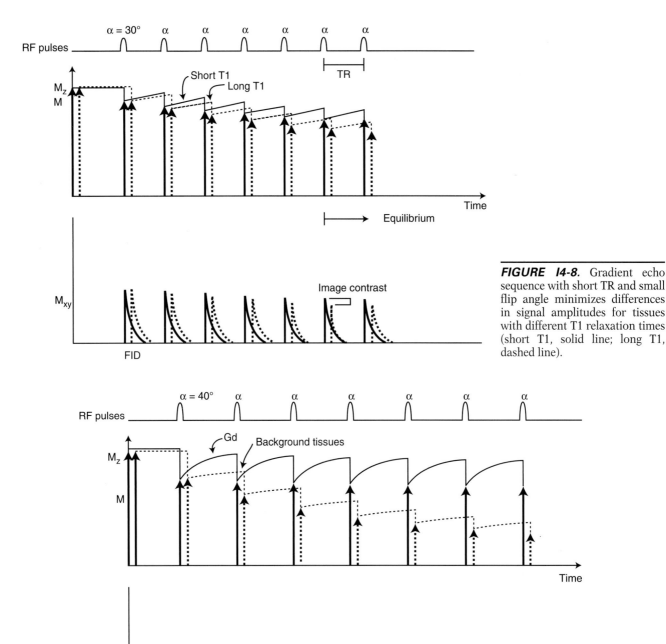

FIGURE I4-8. Gradient echo sequence with short TR and small flip angle minimizes differences in signal amplitudes for tissues with different T1 relaxation times (short T1, solid line; long T1, dashed line).

FIGURE I4-9. Gadolinium enhanced gradient echo imaging. The short T1 relaxation time of tissue containing gadolinium ensures that its signal is significantly higher than that of tissues with longer T1 times, despite high flip angles.

fill a single line of k-space. For 2D imaging, to fill an entire 2D k-space, many echoes—typically 128 to 256—need to be collected. For reasons that will be more apparent in the next chapter, the number of echoes is referred to as the *number of phase-encoding steps*, N_{PE}. The total time needed to acquire enough data to make an image, the *acquisition time* or T_{acq}, depends on N_{PE} and on the repetition time TR. That is,

$$T_{acq} = N_{PE} \times TR$$

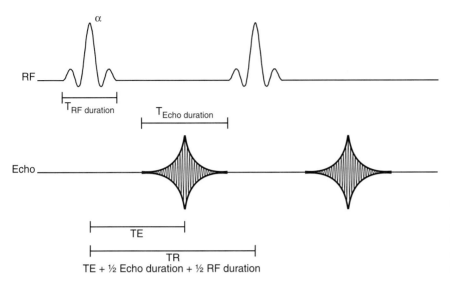

TE + ½ Echo duration + ½ RF duration

FIGURE I4-10. With fast gradient echo imaging, the TR is only slightly longer than the TE. Consequently, methods that reduce the TE will in turn reduce the TR and shorten acquisition times.

for 2D gradient echo imaging. Therefore, short TR times are necessary for fast gradient echo imaging.

What are the factors that contribute to the TR for a gradient echo sequence? As illustrated in Figure I4-10, the TR is related to the duration of the RF pulse, the duration of the echo, and the TE.

Fast Imaging with Gradient Echoes

How short can the TR of a gradient echo sequence be? Because residual longitudinal magnetization after a partial flip angle RF pulse may be sufficient to allow a repeat excitation almost immediately after an echo is sampled, the TR does not need to be much longer than the TE (Figure I4-10). The TE for gradient echo imaging can be as short as 1 msec or less with MR systems that have strong gradients and fast slew rates. Corresponding TR times can be as little as 2 msec or even less.

Very short TRs mean fast imaging, because the acquisition time for an MR image is directly proportional to TR. With a short TR, acquisition times can be a fraction of a second for 2D imaging and less than 10 seconds for 3D imaging.

As will be more fully explored in Section I Chapter 8, these very short TR and TE times are achieved by minimizing the duration of each component of the pulse sequence that contributes to TR. In this section, the technique of shortening the TE by reducing the duration of the dephasing lobe of the gradient echo is illustrated.

> **IMPORTANT CONCEPT:** With gradient echo imaging, especially 3D gradient echo sequences, the TR need only be slightly longer than the TE. Therefore, methods that shorten TE will also shorten TR and hence reduce acquisition times.

Shortening the Dephasing Lobe

For gradient echo sequences, the echo is sampled only during application of the rephasing gradient. For reasons that will be discussed in subsequent chapters, the duration of this sampling period must be adequate to achieve desired signal-to-noise ratios and spatial resolution. Since no signal is measured during the dephasing lobe of the gradient, dephasing can be made as short as possible.

CHALLENGE QUESTION: How is it possible to have a shorter dephasing duration?

Answer: Make the dephasing gradient amplitude stronger than that of the rephasing gradient (Figure I4-11).

The duration of the dephasing lobe is dependent on the maximum gradient strength of the system. The stronger the gradients, the shorter the dephasing duration. Why is this helpful? From Figure I4-2, the shorter the dephasing lobe, the shorter the echo time. As illustrated in Figure I4-11, shorter echo times can directly translate into faster repetitions of the gradient echo process, thereby leading to shorter acquisition times for MR imaging.

> **IMPORTANT CONCEPT:** For faster imaging, stronger gradients are advantageous because the same degree of dephasing can be achieved in shorter times, leading to shorter TE. With some gradient echo sequences, a shorter TE translates into shorter TR and consequently, shorter acquisition times.

Spoiled versus Steady-State Gradient Echo Imaging

With gradient echo imaging, the TR times can be shorter than the T2* of most tissues. This means that the transverse magnetization may not have fully decayed before

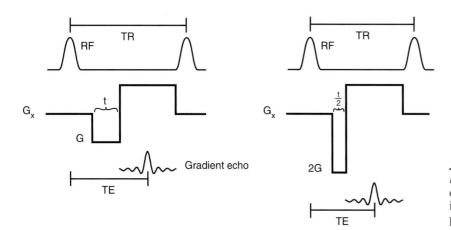

FIGURE I4-11. Stronger dephasing gradients lead to shorter TE and TR. The dephasing lobe is shortened by using the strongest possible gradients.

the next RF pulse occurs. Residual transverse magnetization can be troublesome because, after the next RF pulse, it is tipped away from the xy plane and contributes to longitudinal magnetization. Subsequent RF pulses may tip it into the transverse plane again. If this process is not well controlled, the contribution of the transverse magnetization to the measured signal can easily corrupt the image contrast and cause the so-called *band artifact* (Figure I4-12). The easiest way to solve this problem is to eliminate all the transverse magnetization before the subsequent RF pulse, a process called *spoiling*. These sequences are referred to as *spoiled gradient echo* sequences. So far, the discussion in this chapter has assumed spoiled gradient echo imaging. However, it is important to differentiate between spoiled gradient echo and another type of gradient echo imaging commonly used in cardiovascular MR imaging, known as *steady-state gradient echo* imaging. (Manufacturers have different terminology for each, as summarized in Table I4-2.) The distinction between the two types of gradient echo sequences is based on what happens to the transverse signal that has not fully decayed before the next RF pulse.

The concept behind steady-state gradient echo imaging is that under certain circumstances, the residual transverse magnetization can actually be used to increase the measured signal. Recent advances in technology have enabled the application of steady-state gradient echo imaging to body and cardiovascular MRI, with major improvements in image signal-to-noise and contrast-to-noise ratios in shorter imaging times.

More specifics about each type of gradient echo sequence are provided in the following two sections.

Spoiled Gradient Echo Imaging

The three most commonly used ways to spoil a gradient echo sequence are as follows:

1. *Long TR:* If TR is more than 3 to 4 times the T2 relaxation times—preferably greater than 500 msec, or at

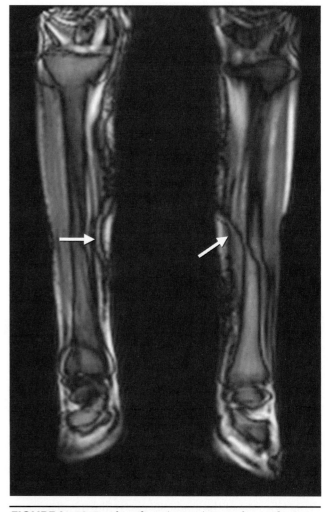

FIGURE I4-12. Band artifacts (arrows) in gradient echo imaging resulting from undesired contributions of transverse magnetization to measured signal.

least greater than 200 msec—then the transverse magnetization will be spoiled by dephasing.

2. *RF spoiling:* If a phase offset is added to each successive RF pulse (see Chapter I-2, Figure I2-9), then the

TABLE I4-2

Spoiled Gradient Echo	Steady-State Gradient Echo*
FLASH (fast low angle shot)	True FISP (fast imaging with steady-state precession)
SPGR (spoiled GRASS)	FIESTA (fast imaging employing steady-state acquisition)
FFE (fast field echo)	Balanced FFE (fast field echo)

* Steady-state gradient echo sequences listed are confined to balanced steady-state free precession sequences used in cardiovascular imaging (1).

phases of the residual transverse magnetization vectors will cancel each other out because of their reduced coherence or wide distribution of orientations.

3. *Spoiler gradients:* The third approach to spoiling is to extend the duration of the readout gradient beyond the sampling of the echo and before the next RF pulse. The prolonged application of the gradient causes accelerated dephasing of the residual transverse magnetization (Figure I4-13). These extra gradient pulse durations are referred to as *spoiler gradients* or *crusher gradients*.

Out of these three, the spoiler gradient method is most commonly used.

Image Contrast in Spoiled Gradient Echo Imaging

In spoiled gradient echo imaging, the three main parameters that affect image contrast are the TR, the TE, and the flip angle. How these are used to achieve desired image contrast is described next.

Spoiled gradient echo images are usually either T1 or T2* weighted. With spoiled gradient echo imaging, true *T2-weighted imaging* is difficult to achieve because gradients, unlike 180° refocusing pulses in spin echo imaging (discussed later in this chapter), do not eliminate the loss of transverse magnetization caused by field inhomogeneities (T2*). The image contrasts that can be achieved by manipulating TR, TE, and flip angle are given in Table I4-3.

The longer the TR and the higher the flip angle, the more *T1-weighted* the image becomes. The longer the TE, the more T2*-weighted the image is (Figure I4-14).

> **IMPORTANT CONCEPT:** For spoiled gradient echo imaging, longer TR results in more T1 weighting, while longer TE causes more T2* weighting.

TABLE I4-3 Spoiled Gradient Echo Imaging Parameters

Image Contrast	TR	Flip Angle	TE
T1 weighting	**long**	**large**	short
T2* weighting	shorter	smaller	**long**
PD weighting	short	**small**	short

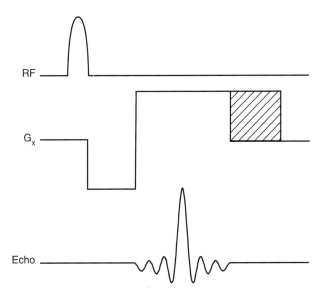

FIGURE I4-13. Spoiler or crusher gradient in a spoiled gradient echo sequence extends the rephasing lobe (dashed area) to "crush" residual transverse magnetization before subsequent RF excitation.

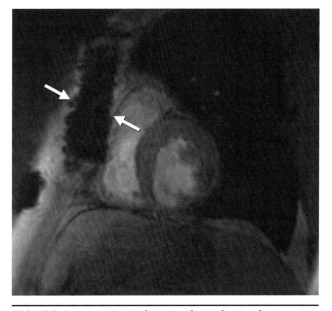

FIGURE I4-14. T2* weighting with gradient echo imaging. Metallic sternal wires accelerate T2* decay and cause the low signal of the wires to be exaggerated on this image. With the *blooming artifact*, the extent of signal loss (arrows) exceeds the region of the metal wires because the sequence used a long TE (9 msec). See also Figure I4-18.

Signal intensity, SI, detected using gradient echo sequences can be expressed as the product of three factors that reflect the contribution of proton density, longitudinal recovery, and transverse decay. Recall from Chapter I-2 that the exponential recovery of longitudinal magnetization can be described as a function, $1 - e^{-t/T1}$, whereas the expression for exponential decay of transverse magnetization is $e^{-t/T2^*}$. The equation for SI for a spoiled gradient echo sequence is given in terms of TR and TE times and reflects dependence on the flip angle, α:

$$SI = \frac{N(H)\sin \alpha \left\{1 - e^{(-TR/T1)}\right\}\left\{e^{(-TE/T2^*)}\right\}}{\left\{1 - (\cos \alpha)(e^{(-TR/T1)})\right\}}$$

The factor N(H) refers to proton density and reflects the total net magnetization available to produce an MR signal.

Before analyzing the patterns of image contrast resulting from different combinations of TR, TE, and α, one important question to be addressed is why MR images have to be either T1 weighted or T2 (or T2*) weighted. If tissues have different T1 and T2 relaxation times, why not use both to create differences in image intensity and to enhance the conspicuity of pathology? The reason for this is that, as discussed in Chapter I-3, for most tissues, T1 and T2 times tend to be correlated. Tissues have either relatively short T1 and T2 times (normal tissues) or relatively long T1 and T2 times (water, pathology). Consider a tissue with short T1 and short T2. The short T1 will give large signal intensity because of faster T1 recovery, yet the short T2 will decrease signal because of more T2 decay. Conversely, for a tissue with long T1 and T2, the long T1 will decrease signal, but the long T2 will increase signal.

The competing effects of T1 and T2 values on signal intensity mean that parameters of the sequence must be chosen to favor either a T1 or T2* basis for visualizing tissue with spoiled gradient echo imaging. To achieve T1 weighting, a long TR and large flip angle will emphasize T1 differences, while short TE will minimize T2* contrast. Conversely, for T2* weighting, a long TE will bring out T2* differences, while a short TR and low flip angle will minimize T1 contrast. To minimize both T1 and T2* weighting and achieve proton density weighting, a small flip angle and short TR and TE should be used (Table I4-3).

> **IMPORTANT CONCEPTS:** Most tissues have either long T1 and long T2 or short T1 and short T2. Consequently, parameters for imaging usually must be selected to favor either T1-weighted imaging or T2(*)-weighted imaging while minimizing the other.

Extensions of Spoiled Gradient Echo Imaging

Multislice Gradient Echo Imaging
When TR times are much longer than TE, then multiple slices can be imaged during the time after each echo and before the next RF pulse. The number of slices that can be imaged depends on how many RF-echo units can fit into one TR. Since TE is defined as the time from the center of the RF pulse to the center of the echo, the full time from the start of the RF pulse to the end of the echo is at least equal to 1/2 RF + TE + 1/2 echo duration (Figure I4-10). Consequently, the number of slices that can be measured for a given TR is

$$\text{Number of slices} \approx \frac{TR}{\frac{1}{2} RF \text{ duration} + TE + \frac{1}{2} \text{Echo duration}}$$

as depicted in Figure I4-15.

For example, if the TR is 180 msec, TE 4.4 msec, and the total time from start of RF to end of echo is 8 msec, about 20 slices could be imaged in the time conventional gradient echo imaging takes to acquire one slice.

CHALLENGE QUESTION: How long would the acquisition time be for a spoiled gradient echo acquisition with TR = 180 msec, TE = 4.4 msec, 128 phase-encoding steps, and coverage of 20 slices?

Answer: The acquisition time for a 2D gradient echo sequence is given by

$$T_{acq} = TR \times N_{PE}$$

So, for the parameters given,

$$T_{acq} = 180 \text{ msec} \times 128 = 23 \text{ sec}$$

As discussed above, all 20 slices can be acquired in this 23 sec acquisition. Because the duration is within the breath-holding capacity of most people, the pulse sequence could be performed during suspended respiration to minimize motion artifacts in thoracic or abdominal imaging.

Multiecho Gradient Echo Imaging
Multiple gradient echoes can be sampled with each RF pulse to improve imaging efficiency. A series of gradient reversals is applied to generate multiple gradient echoes following a single RF pulse (Figure I4-16). The multiple echoes must be sampled in a short time before the FID has decayed completely. The number of echoes that can be generated before T2* decay depends on how rapidly gradient switching occurs and how fast each echo can be sampled. The sampling of multiple echoes reduces the time available for multislice imaging. Consequently, the use of these two techniques must be balanced depending on the imaging needs.

If all 64 to 128 lines of k-space for a single image can be generated with a single RF excitation, then the sequence is referred to as a *single-shot* gradient echo sequence. One commonly used single-shot sequence is echo planar

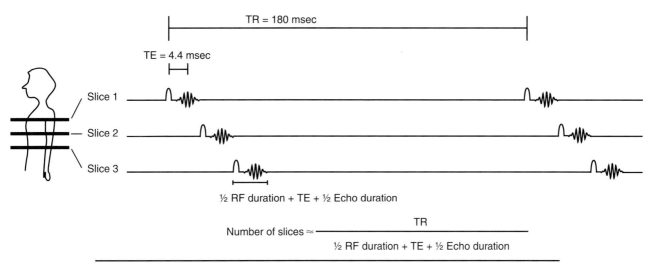

FIGURE I4-15. Multislice gradient echo imaging.

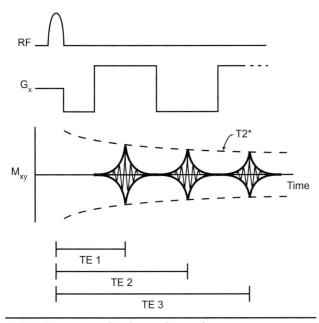

FIGURE I4-16. Multiecho gradient echo imaging. Repeating the gradient reversal results in a series of echoes that can each be used to fill k-space.

imaging (see Chapter I-6 for more details). Because the echoes are acquired during T2* decay, the single-shot sequences are typically heavily T2* weighted.

> **IMPORTANT CONCEPT:** Fast gradient echo imaging options include the acquisition of imaging data from multiple slices and multiple echoes within a single TR.

TurboFLASH

For some applications, such as gadolinium-enhanced myocardial perfusion, fast T1-weighted gradient echo

imaging is desired. To improve T1 weighting in the setting of very short TR and TE, an inversion prepulse (180°) or saturation prepulse (90°) is applied before a series of gradient echoes are acquired (Figure I4-17). A prepulse is an RF excitation pulse applied before the conventional imaging RF pulse to manipulate image contrast; prepulses are discussed further in Chapter I-9. In one implementation, referred to as *turboFLASH* (turbo fast low angle shot imaging), single-shot T1-weighted images can be produced using an inversion or saturation prepulse. Other terms for this sequence include magnetization-prepared rapid acquired gradient echo (MP-RAGE).

CHALLENGE QUESTION: What would be the image contrast resulting from a very short TR and TE, low flip angle, and no prepulse?

Answer: The images would be proton density-weighted. The short TR and low flip angle would minimize T1 weighting, while the short TE would minimize T2* weighting.

An inversion recovery turboFLASH sequence is illustrated in Figure I4-17. Following a 180° inversion pulse and a short delay known as the *inversion time* (TI), a series of gradient echoes are generated in quick succession during a portion of longitudinal recovery. The inversion pulse accentuates differences between tissues with different T1 times. The RF excitation pulses have low flip angles so as not to perturb longitudinal recovery. TR and TE are minimum, because image contrast does not depend on recovery of longitudinal signal between RF pulses. If a full set of echoes (say, 128) is collected with each inversion prepulse, then the sequence is considered to be analogous to a single-shot sequence. The actual image contrast for this method is complex because the acquisition of the echoes occurs during T1 relaxation. As will be discussed in Chapter III-7, turboFLASH sequences are commonly used in cardiac applications, particularly perfusion imaging (Figure I4-18).

Steady-State Gradient Echo Imaging

Unlike spoiled gradient echo imaging, where residual transverse magnetization is considered a nuisance and all efforts are made to eliminate it, steady-state gradient echo imaging seeks to harness the signal from residual magnetization. In cardiovascular imaging, the most common implementation of steady-state imaging is referred to as *True FISP*, *balanced FFE*, or *FIESTA* (Table I4-2, Figure I4-19). For reasons discussed subsequently, the image intensity depends directly on T2 and inversely on T1 relaxation times. This is often expressed as T2/T1 image contrast.

Steady-state gradient echo imaging results in a complex behavior of magnetization. Figure I4-20 illustrates

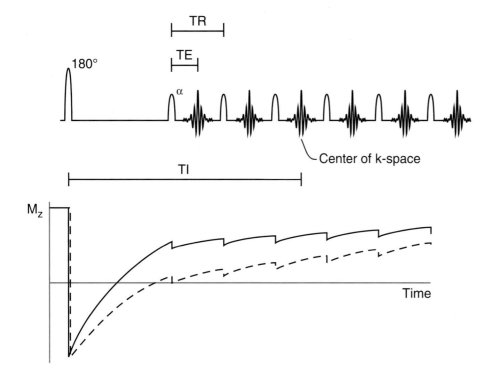

FIGURE I4-17. The turboFLASH gradient echo sequence generates fast T1-weighted images with a magnetization preparation prepulse, a series of low flip angle RF pulses, and short TR and TE. The inversion time, TI, may be defined as the time from the inversion pulse to the acquisition of the echo filling the center of k-space (as shown here). An alternative definition of TI is the time from the inversion pulse to the acquisition of the first echo.

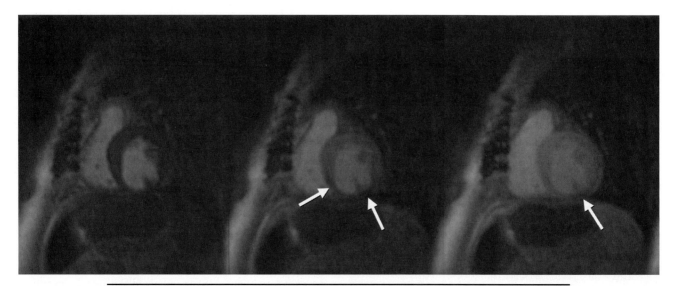

FIGURE I4-18. Perfusion images using a turboFLASH sequence at three different time points following intravenous injection of gadolinium contrast material. Each image is acquired in less than 0.4 sec. Hypoperfusion of inferior wall infarct is illustrated (arrows). This is the same patient as shown in Figure I4-14; note that the blooming artifact from the sternal wires is considerably less with use of a TE of 1 msec.

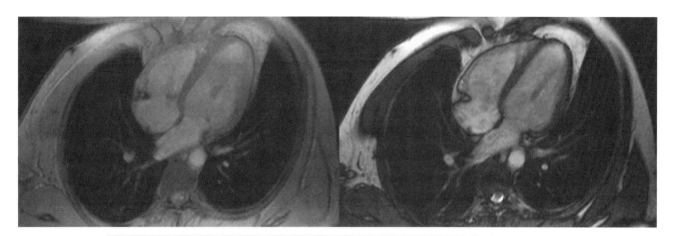

FIGURE I4-19. Cardiac MR images acquired using spoiled gradient echo on left and steady-state gradient echo imaging on right. Whereas spoiled gradient echo relies on inflow of unsaturated protons for high signal intensity of the blood pool, steady-state gradient echo relies on T2 differences to generate excellent blood-myocardium contrast.

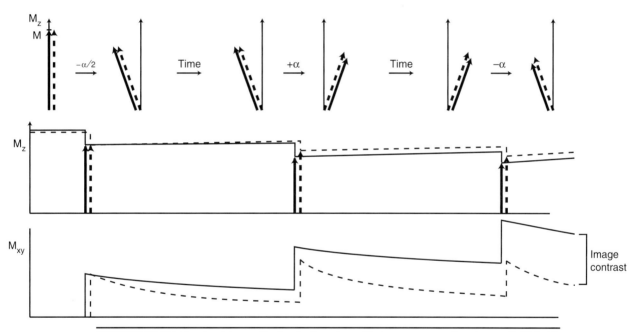

FIGURE I4-20. Steady-state gradient echo imaging with two representative tissues, fluid (with T2 close to T1, solid line) and muscle (T2 shorter than T1, dotted line). Most soft tissue will behave like muscle. Fat, even though its T1 is short, also has a relatively short T2 and behaves like fluid.

how a steady-state gradient echo sequence can achieve T2/T1 contrast. An initial $-\alpha/2$ pulse is followed by a series of $+\alpha$, $-\alpha$, $+\alpha$ RF pulses of alternating sign. After each RF pulse, an echo is sampled. If TR is much shorter than T2, the residual transverse magnetization will be substantial. Tissues with longer T2 times will have more residual magnetization left from one excitation to another. This contributes to the T2 weighting of these images.

With steady-state gradient echo sequences, T1 differences will also influence image contrast. The shorter the

T1, the more longitudinal relaxation and signal will be measured. Hence, the signal intensity will be inversely related to T1.

The image contrast for steady-state gradient echo imaging depends on the T2/T1 ratio and is different from most of the imaging methods described so far. In general, the images appear T2 weighted. Water and blood have long T2 and long T1 times. Most other tissues, other than fat, have much shorter T2 times than T1. Fat has not only a short T2 but also a relatively short T1. Therefore, on steady-state gradient echo imaging, blood and other fluids

IMPORTANT CONCEPT: With steady-state gradient echo imaging, image contrast depends not on T1 or T2 alone but on their ratio, T2/T1. Fluid-containing structures (vessels and blood) and fat produce high signal intensity compared with other tissues.

as well as fat have higher signal intensity than background tissues (Figure I4-19).

The implementation of steady-state gradient echo pulse sequences requires a high-performance MR system. Fast gradients are required to ensure short enough times to preserve transverse magnetization. Typically TR must be on the order of 5 msec or less.

Other requirements for the steady-state gradient echo sequences are related to the need to control the transverse magnetization from one excitation to the next. Recall that the transverse magnetization is directly dependent on maintaining phase coherence of protons. What can disrupt the phase coherence? Field inhomogeneities and unbalanced gradients are the two main factors. Field inhomogeneities cause protons to precess at different frequencies, leading to loss of the transverse magnetization and to flash band artifacts (Figure I4-12). To compensate for the dephasing effects of gradients, steady-state gradient echo sequences have balanced gradients to ensure equal amounts of dephasing and rephasing, a concept illustrated in Figure I4-21.

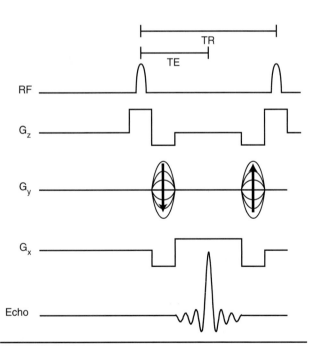

FIGURE I4-21. Pulse sequence diagram for steady-state gradient echo imaging with balanced gradients. The net areas under the gradient curves equal zero. Balanced gradients minimize gradient-induced dephasing from one echo to the next and ensure that steady state is maintained.

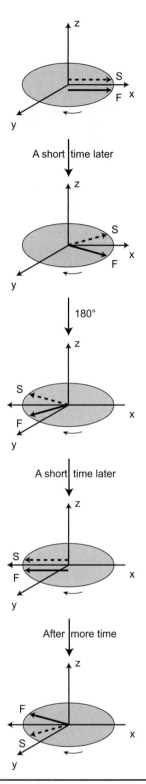

FIGURE I4-22. Spin echo. With a 90° RF pulse, longitudinal magnetization is tipped into the transverse plane. After a short time, slight differences in precessional frequencies manifest as a phase shift between protons. Following a 180° refocusing RF pulse, the relationship of the protons is reversed, with the slower protons moving ahead of the faster protons. When the faster protons catch up with the slower protons, a spin echo is formed. Over time, phase shift reaccumulates.

IMPORTANT CONCEPT: Steady-state gradient echo imaging requires short TRs and TEs, field homogeneity, and balanced gradients.

SPIN ECHOES

Many commonly used MR pulse sequences rely on spin echoes to generate MR images. How spin echoes are produced is discussed in this section.

Following an RF excitation pulse with a 90° flip angle, the transverse magnetization decays rapidly, governed by the T2* relaxation time (FID). The decay is rapid in part because of intrinsic T2 effects, which vary across tissues, but mostly because of inhomogeneities in the B_0 magnetic field. To make a spin echo, a second RF pulse is applied after the 90° pulse. The second RF pulse is called a *refocusing pulse* because it has the effect of refocusing the dephased magnetic moments; it typically requires a *refocusing angle* of 180°. With refocusing, net transverse magnetization grows to form a measurable echo of the original FID (Figure I4-22).

How does the 180° refocusing pulse reverse dephasing (Figure I4-22)? Immediately after the initial 90° RF pulse, dephasing occurs because of B_0 heterogeneity and intrinsic T2 decay. The B_0 heterogeneity means that some protons are exposed to slightly stronger local magnetic fields and therefore, according to the Larmor equation, precess slightly *faster*, while others are exposed to slightly weaker fields and therefore precess slightly *slower*. It is easiest to understand the 180° pulse as flipping the magnetic moments within the transverse plane, so that the relationship of the protons is reversed (Figure I4-22). The faster protons are moved behind the slower protons. Over time, the fast protons catch up, and with this rephasing, a spin echo is formed. The spin echo decays following dephasing of the protons again.

Spin Echo Minimization of T2′ Effects

There are several observations that can be made about the spin echo. First, the time at which the echo occurs can be predicted relative to the time when the 180° refocusing pulse is applied. The echo time or TE, is defined as the time between the 90° RF pulse and the peak of the echo. Because the time that it takes to rephase protons equals the time it takes to dephase, the 180° pulse occurs, by definition, at time TE/2 (Figure I4-23). This means that it is possible to manipulate exactly when the echo occurs by applying the 180° RF pulse at half the desired echo time after the 90° pulse.

Second, the maximum amplitude of the spin echo is lower than the maximum amplitude of the original FID echo (Figure I4-23). While the 180° pulse does eliminate the dephasing effects that result from variations in magnetic fields or B_0 inhomogeneity (T2′), fluctuations due to spin-spin interactions (true T2) cannot be eliminated

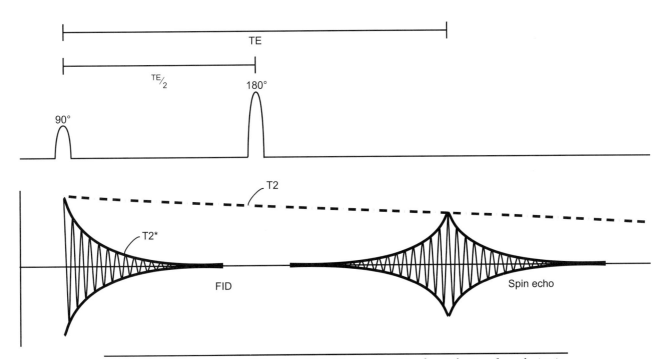

FIGURE I4-23. Spin echo and T2 effects. T2* of the FID consists of contributions from the intrinsic T2 relaxation of the tissue (T2) and other effects (T2′) such as B_0 inhomogeneity. The 180° flip angle eliminates the effects of field inhomogeneity (T2′) but not T2. The peak amplitude of the spin echo is slightly less than that of the FID, according to an exponential decay governed by T2.

(Chapter I-3). Therefore, the decrease in maximum amplitude of the spin echo reflects the intrinsic tissue T2 relaxation alone. The echo time influences the amount of T2 decay. The longer the echo time, the lower the amplitude of the echo.

> **IMPORTANT CONCEPT:** Spin echo imaging eliminates the effects of B_0 field inhomogeneities but not the intrinsic T2 relaxation effects.

MR imaging that uses a single 90° pulse followed by a single 180° pulse to generate a single echo is referred to as *conventional spin echo imaging*. Figure I4-24 illustrates what happens to M_{xy} and M_z, the transverse and longitudinal components, during the 90°–180° echo process.

Image Contrast Using Spin Echoes

The two main parameters that can be controlled in spin echo imaging are the repetition time (TR) and the echo time (TE). How these are used to achieve T1-weighted images and T2-weighted images is described next (Figure I4-25).

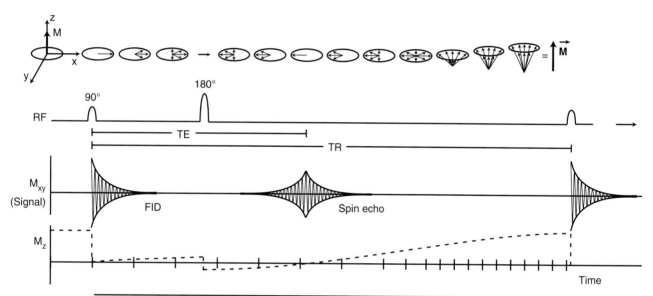

FIGURE I4-24. Behavior of transverse (M_{xy}, signal) and longitudinal (M_z) magnetization during a spin echo. With spin echo imaging, only the spin echo, and not the FID, is recorded.

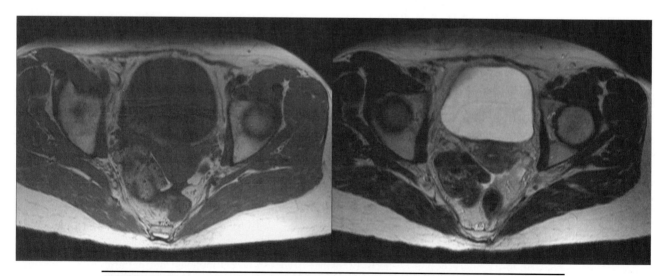

FIGURE I4-25. Fast spin echo images that demonstrate T1 weighting (TR 500 msec, TE 9 msec) and T2 weighting (TR 8700 msec, TE 116 msec). Fat is high in signal on T2-weighted images because of the echo train imaging.

Use of TR to Determine T1 Contrast

The term "T1-weighted" refers to images with intensity differences that are based on T1 relaxation time differences. Careful selection of the repetition time, TR, can bring out these differences. The TR is important because it defines the amount of time following each 90° RF pulse for the longitudinal magnetization to recover before the next 90° pulse. Tissues with different T1 times will recover at different rates, and these affect the amount of longitudinal magnetization available to generate an echo following the subsequent RF excitation. Tissues with longer T1 times have less signal than tissues with shorter T1 times. Selection of an appropriate TR for image contrast depends on the T1 values of the different tissues.

For example, consider two tissues, such as fat and muscle, with T1 values of 300 msec and 700 msec. The effects of different TR times on image contrast between these two tissues are illustrated in Figure I4-26.

For maximum T1 contrast, the TR should have an intermediate value between the T1 values of the tissues with the shortest and longest T1 times. In the example in

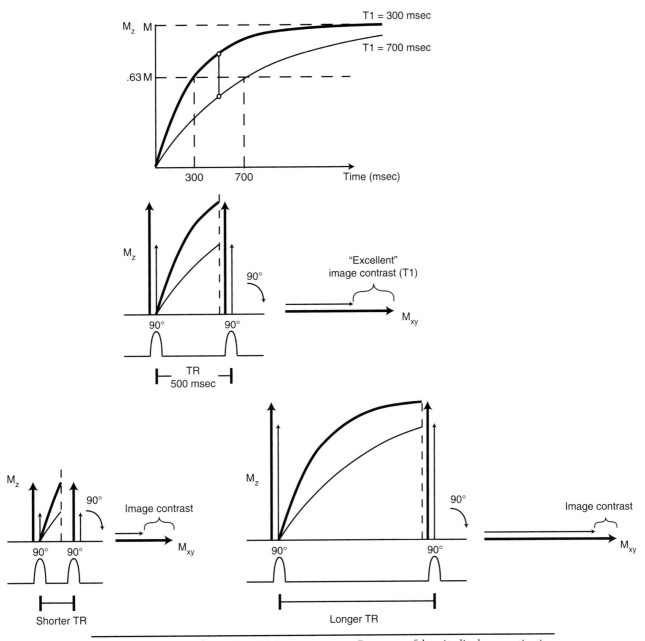

FIGURE I4-26. TR determines T1 image contrast. Recovery of longitudinal magnetization between RF (90° in this example) pulses determines the amount of image contrast. To maximize contrast between two tissues, the TR should have an intermediate value between their T1 times.

Figure I4-26, a TR of about 500 msec produces a large difference in signal intensity between the tissues with T1 times of 300 msec and 700 msec. (The TR for optimal contrast between two tissues with T1 values T1$_a$ and T1$_b$ is actually given by

$$TR = \frac{[\ln(T1_a/T1_b)]T1_aT1_b}{T1_a - T1_b}$$

where ln is the natural logarithm. In this example, the optimal TR is actually 445 msec.) Because the resulting difference in signal intensity is due primarily to differences in T1 times, the images are considered T1 weighted.

If the TR is very short (say, 200 msec), then the overall signal amplitude will be low for both tissues, because neither recovers much longitudinal magnetization between RF excitations. If the TR is greater than 1000 msec, the image contrast between the two tissues will be low because both will have recovered most of their longitudinal magnetization. Spin echo sequences with TR times on the order of 2–3 times as large as the T1 relaxation times of the tissues of interest will show very little T1 weighting or T1 contrast.

> **IMPORTANT CONCEPTS:** For optimal T1 contrast, the TR should have an intermediate value between the T1 relaxation times of the tissues of interest. To minimize T1 contrast, the TR should be at least 2–3 times as long as the T1 times of most tissues.

Because most tissues have T1 times of between 200 and 1200 msec, T1-weighted spin echo sequences have a TR between 500 and 800 msec, referred to as "short TR" sequences. Conversely, to minimize T1 differences across tissues, "long TR" sequences are used, where TR is typically about 1500–2000 msec. Because, a long TR means a longer acquisition time, typically TR does not exceed 2000 msec.

Use of TE to Determine T2 Contrast

The term "T2-weighted" refers to images with intensity differences that are based on T2 relaxation time differences. Careful selection of the echo time, TE, can bring out these differences. At longer echo times, signal amplitude decreases for all tissues, but those with longer T2 times have more signal than those with shorter T2 times. Selection of an appropriate TE depends on the T2 times of the tissues to be imaged.

For example, consider two tissues with T2 values of 70 msec and 130 msec (Figure I4-27). A very short TE, say 30 msec, will result in minimal image contrast, because magnetization will not have decayed substantially in either tissue. A very long TE, say 300 msec, will generate negligible signal, because magnetization from both tissues will have decayed considerably. It turns out that optimal T2 contrast occurs at a TE that is intermediate between the T2 times of the tissues of interest. So for the example, a TE of about 100 msec (intermediate between 70 msec and

130 msec) would generate images with considerable T2 contrast. (The TE for optimal contrast for two tissues with T2 values equal to T2$_a$ and T2$_b$ is actually given by

$$TE = \frac{[\ln(T2_a/T2_b)]T2_aT2_b}{T2_a - T2_b}$$

where ln is the natural logarithm. In this example, the optimal TE is actually 94 msec.)

In general, because most tissues have T2 times between 20 and 250 msec, T2-weighted spin echo sequences have TE times of at least 80–100 msec. These are generally referred to as "long TE" sequences. Conversely, for sequences with relatively little T2 weighting, "short" TE times, generally less than 50 msec, are used to minimize T2 differences while maximizing the amount of signal.

> **IMPORTANT CONCEPTS:** For optimal T2 contrast, the TE should have an intermediate value between the T2 relaxation times of the tissues of interest. To minimize T2 contrast, the TE should be short relative to T2 relaxation times.

Putting TR and TE Together

The signal intensity (SI) produced by a spin echo sequence depends on the relationhip between sequence TR and tissue T1 as well as between sequence TE and tissue T2. Recall from Chapter I-2 that the exponential recovery of longitudinal magnetization can be described as a function, $1 - e^{-t/T1}$, while the expression for exponential decay of transverse magnetization is $e^{-t/T2}$. Put in terms of TR and TE times, SI for a spin echo sequence is given by

$$SI = N(H) \times (1 - e^{-TR/T1}) \times (e^{-TE/T2})$$
$$= PD \text{ effect} \times T1 \text{ effect} \times T2 \text{ effect}$$

N(H) again refers to proton density and reflects the total magnetization available to generate signal.

The opposing effects of T1 and T2 on signal intensity suggest that the parameters of a spin echo sequence, TR and TE, must be chosen to favor T1 or T2. To obtain T1-weighted images, it is imperative that T2 weighting be minimized, while for T2-weighted images, T1 weighting must be minimized. Chapter I-9 presents strategies that make T1 and T2 contrast additive, such as short inversion time inversion recovery sequences.

> **IMPORTANT CONCEPT:** With spin echo imaging, the effects of T1 and T2 times on signal intensity are conflicting. Hence, for T1-weighted images, T2 weighting must be minimized, while for T2-weighted images, T1 weighting must be minimized.

Figure I4-28 depicts the effects of different combinations of TR and TE times in a spin echo sequence for tissues

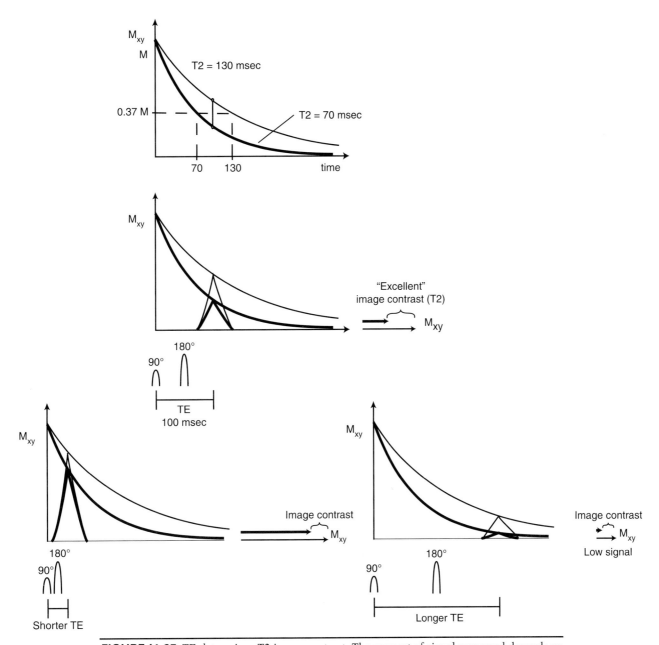

FIGURE I4-27. TE determines T2 image contrast. The amount of signal measured depends on differences in T2 decay at the selected TE time. Differences in amplitudes of the echoes are plotted for three TEs. If the goal is to maximize contrast between two tissues, then the TE should have an intermediate value between their T2 times.

with different T1 and T2 times. These strategies are considered in the following paragraphs.

(a) Short TR and short TE: T1-weighted imaging. A short TR emphasizes T1 contrast, and a short TE minimizes T2 contrast. This combination is perfect for T1-weighted imaging.

(b) Long TR and long TE: T2-weighted imaging. A long TR minimizes T1 contrast, while a long TE brings out T2 contrast. This combination is perfect for T2-weighted images.

(c) Long TR and short TE: Proton density-weighted imaging. With a long TR and short TE, there is neither much

T1 weighting nor much T2 weighting. The image is then mainly *proton density (PD)-weighted.*

(d) Short TR and long TE: Not recommended. This combination of parameters is bad and should not be used. With a short TR and long TE, T1 and T2 effects cancel each other out. Pathologic tissues or fluid-filled structures will have signal intensities that may be either brighter, darker, or the same as normal tissue, making images difficult to interpret.

Typical parameters for spin echo sequences with different types of image contrast are summarized in Table I4-4.

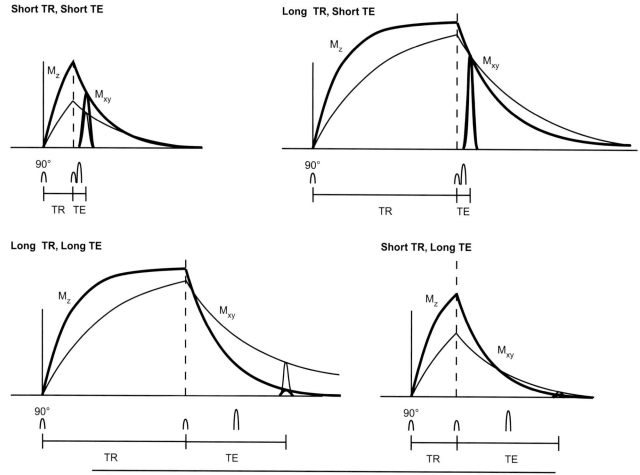

FIGURE I4-28. The combination of long and short TR and TE on M_z (shown to the left of the vertical dashed lines) and M_{xy} (to the right of the dashed lines) for "normal" tissues, shown as a thick line (shorter T1 and T2 times) versus "pathology" and fluid-filled structures, shown as a thin line (longer T1 and T2 times).

▶ **TABLE I4-4 Spin Echo Parameters**

	Short TR (500–800 msec)	**Long TR (≥1200 msec)**
Short TE (<50 msec)	T1	PD
Long TE (≥80 msec)	Not used	T2

IMPORTANT CONCEPTS: T1-weighted spin echo images are generated using short TR and short TE, while T2-weighted images rely on long TR and long TE.

Spin Echoes and Acquisition Times

As with gradient echo sequences, the acquisition time for an MR spin echo image depends on the TR and the number of phase-encoding steps:

$$T_{acq} = N_{PE} \times TR$$

As with gradient echoes, because the process of making an image requires multiple repetitions of the spin echo process, it is important to consider how one 90°–180° echo sequence affects subsequent echoes. For example, it may seem desirable to shorten TR as much as possible in order to reduce acquisition times, but a short TR will have a substantial impact on the echo from the second excitation. If TR is too short, little longitudinal magnetization will have recovered and therefore, following the next 90°, there will be very little measurable FID or echo. Thus for spin echo imaging, TR times are typically at least as long as one T1 time of relevant tissue, say 500–2000 msec.

CHALLENGE QUESTION: What is the acquisition time needed to generate a 128 × 128 image (N_{PE} = 128) with a TR of 500 msec? What if the matrix is 512 × 512? What about for T2-weighted imaging with TR equal to 2000 msec?

Answers: Based on the formula for acquisition time,

$$T_{acq} = N_{PE} \times TR = 128 \times 0.5 \text{ sec} = 64 \text{ sec} \sim 1 \text{ min}$$

For a 512 × 512 matrix,

$$T_{acq} = N_{PE} \times TR = 512 \times 0.5 \text{ sec} = 256 \text{ sec} \sim 4 \text{ min}$$

For a longer TR,

$$T_{acq} = 128 \times 2 \text{ sec} = 256 \text{ sec} \sim 4 \text{ min}$$

$$T_{acq} = 512 \times 2 \text{ sec} = 1024 \text{ sec} = 16.7 \text{ min}$$

For imaging in the brain, where there is minimal motion, acquisition times such as those just computed would be acceptable. In the chest or abdomen, where respiratory motion can degrade images, a single acquisition would result in poor image quality. The artifacts can be made less apparent by performing repeated acquisitions and averaging their results to generate one image. This process is called *signal averaging*. When multiple signals need to be averaged, the acquisition times increase proportionally to the *number of acquisitions*, N_{acq}, so that the formula for acquisition time becomes

$$T_{acq} = TR \times N_{PE} \times N_{acq}$$

With 4 acquisitions, a single 128 × 128 matrix spin echo image through the heart would then take

$$\begin{aligned} T_{acq} &= TR \times N_{PE} \times N_{acq} \\ &= 2000 \text{ msec} \times 128 \times 4 = 1024 \text{ sec} \end{aligned}$$

or about 16.7 min. In the world of clinical MRI, where subjects are scheduled in 30 minutes to 1 hour appointment intervals, these conventional spin echo sequences would be considered too *slow* and impractical. As will be discussed next, several methods are employed to speed up spin echo imaging.

Multislice Spin Echo Imaging

The acquisition schemes described so far produce only one image in acquisition times of several minutes. As with gradient echo imaging, one strategy for improving efficiency is to generate images from multiple slices in the same acquisition time.

To allow M_z to recover after each 90° RF pulse, the repetition times are typically much longer than the echo times, and therefore the time following the echo can be usefully spent collecting imaging data from other slices (Figure I4-29). The number of slices or images that can be acquired in this case depends roughly on how many 90°–180° echo units can fit into a TR. The number of slices that can be measured in a TR is approximately

$$\text{Number of slices} \approx \frac{TR}{\frac{1}{2}\text{RF duration} + TE + \frac{1}{2}\text{Echo duration}}$$

With a T2-weighted sequence with TR = 2000 msec and TE = 100 msec, just under 20 slices can be imaged in the same time it would take to image a single slice. Similarly, with a T1-weighted sequence with TR = 500 msec and TE = 20 msec, almost 25 slices can be imaged.

Fast Spin Echo

The efficiency of spin echo imaging is vastly improved with the generation of more than one echo after each 90° RF pulse. The technique is referred to as *fast spin echo (FSE), turbo spin echo (TSE), rapid acquisition with relaxation enhancement (RARE),* or *echo train imaging.* After the first spin echo peaks, the transverse components of the magnetic moments continue to precess at slightly

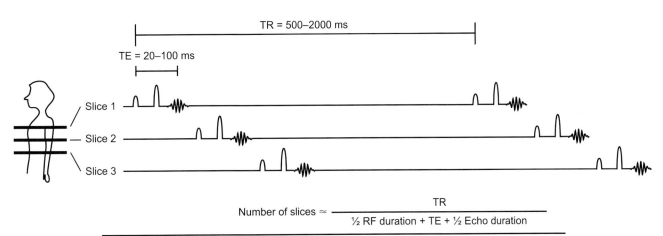

FIGURE I4-29. Multislice spin echo imaging. During the time between the spin echo and the subsequent 90° RF pulse, additional echoes can be acquired from other imaging slices. The total number of slices that can be imaged in the same time as a single slice depends on the number of times the 90°–180° echo (which takes about ½ RF duration + TE + ½ Echo duration) can fit into the TR interval.

different frequencies and dephase (Figure I4-30). This dephasing can be reversed again by the application of a second 180° pulse, leading to formation of a second echo. The maximum amplitude of the second echo will be less than that of the FID and slightly less than that of the first echo, according to the T2 decay properties of the tissue.

The number of echoes generated for every 90° RF excitation pulse is called the *echo train length (ETL)*. ETL measures the improvement in efficiency of the fast spin echo pulse sequence compared with conventional spin echo imaging. The higher the ETL, the shorter the acquisition time:

$$T_{acq} = \frac{TR \times N_{PE} \times N_{acq}}{ETL}$$

CHALLENGE QUESTION: A T2-weighted image is to be obtained of the chest with matrix 128 × 128 and TR = 2000 msec. Compare acquisition times for (a) conventional spin echo imaging and (b) fast spin echo with echo train length of 16.

Answer: With conventional spin echo imaging, 128 TRs are required. The acquisition time would be 256 sec or about 4 min with one acquisition. Because this time is too long for a breath hold, multiple signals would be needed to reduce respiratory

artifacts in the image. For N_{acq} = 2–4, acquisition times would be 8–16 min. However, fast spin echo imaging with ETL = 16 requires only 8 TRs to generate the image. The acquisition time is reduced to 16 sec, which is within the time frame of a single breath hold, so signal averaging is no longer needed.

Fast spin imaging can also be implemented in a multislice mode (Figure I4-31). Multislice echo train imaging works well with T2-weighted sequences, where TR is much longer than the duration of the echo train, so that echo trains from multiple slices can fit into each TR.

> **IMPORTANT CONCEPT:** Fast spin echo imaging improves the efficiency of spin echo imaging by a factor equal to the echo train length (ETL).

Considerations for Echo Train Imaging

Limits on How Many Echoes Can Be Obtained after Each 90° RF Pulse

The ETL depends on the balance between T2 decay and *interecho spacing*, defined as the time between consecutive echoes in an echo train (Figure I4-32).

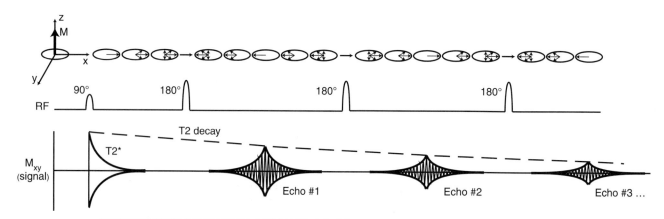

FIGURE I4-30. Fast spin echo or turbo spin echo imaging. Transverse magnetization is repeatedly refocused with a series of 180° RF pulses. The number of echoes acquired after each 90° RF excitation is referred to as the echo train length.

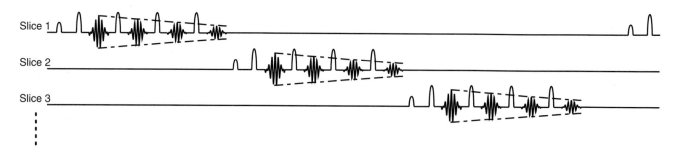

FIGURE I4-31. Multislice fast spin echo imaging with echo train length of four. For ease of viewing, RF pulses and echoes for a given slice are illustrated together.

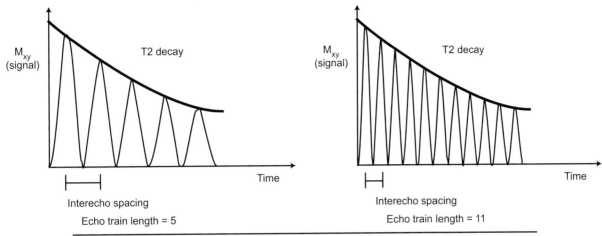

FIGURE I4-32. Interecho spacing in fast spin echo imaging. Shorter interecho spacing enables more echoes to be collected over a given time.

Because the maximum amplitude of spin echoes declines with time according to T2, the number of echoes depends on the rate of decay and on how fast each echo can be generated and sampled. Recall from Chapter I-2 that by the time four T2 times have elapsed, only 2% of the magnetization remains. The shorter the interecho spacing, the more echoes can be acquired during this window. Interecho spacing depends on how much time is needed to apply the 180° RF pulses and how long it takes to sample the echo. New MR systems with fast gradient slew rates and high sampling frequencies can generate and sample echoes in less than 5 msec. This means that within a decay of 4 T2 times—say about 300 msec—more than 60 echoes can be collected!

Impact of Sampling Echoes at Multiple TEs on Image Contrast

MR echoes are used to fill k-space, which in turn is subjected to a Fourier transformation to generate an image. As will be discussed in more detail in Chapter I-6, the central portions of k-space define image contrast, while the periphery of k-space encodes high-spatial-resolution details of an image. With conventional spin echo imaging, all echoes are collected at the same TE. When multiple echoes are sampled at different TEs, it becomes important to specify the placement of the echoes in k-space, especially those that fill the center of k-space. The image contrast for a fast spin echo image is defined by the *effective TE* or TE_{eff} (Figures I4-33 and I4-34), which is the TE corresponding to the echo that is used to fill the center of k-space. TE_{eff} can be thought of as approximately equivalent to TE for conventional spin echo sequences.

IMPORTANT CONCEPT: The central lines of k-space determine image contrast. The TE of the echo that fills the center line of k-space is referred to as the effective TE or TE_{eff}.

Because the image is generated using data acquired from a range of echo times, the actual T2 weighting of a fast spin echo image is inferior to that of a single-echo technique, where all the echoes in k-space are acquired at the same TE. For example, in Figure I4-34, even though TE_{eff} = 80 msec, many lines of k-space have much shorter TE times, which results in less T2 weighting. This means that when imaging tissues with only slightly different T2 relaxation times, differences that may be clear on conventional T2-weighted spin echo images may be less perceptible on echo train images. Longer ETLs tend to reduce T2 contrast.

IMPORTANT CONCEPT: The image contrast in fast spin echo imaging is inferior to that of conventional spin echo imaging, because the echoes used to fill k-space have a range of echo times.

Impact of Sampling Echoes at Multiple TEs on Sharpness of the Image

One important consequence of fast spin echo imaging is that objects in the image, particularly small objects, become blurred in the phase-encoding direction (2). This blurring is worse for long echo train sequences, particularly when the central lines of k-space are collected early in the echo train and the peripheral lines collected late. Blurring is less apparent for tissues with long T2 times. To minimize blurring, echo trains should be kept relatively short, using short interecho spacing, and long effective TEs favored.

Fat on Echo Train Imaging

Fat has a short T2 relaxation time and should be low in signal intensity on T2-weighted images compared to most tissues. However, on all echo train spin echo images, whether T1- or T2-weighted, fat is bright. This is attributed to the phenomenon of J-decoupling. The interested reader is referred to a separate publication (3).

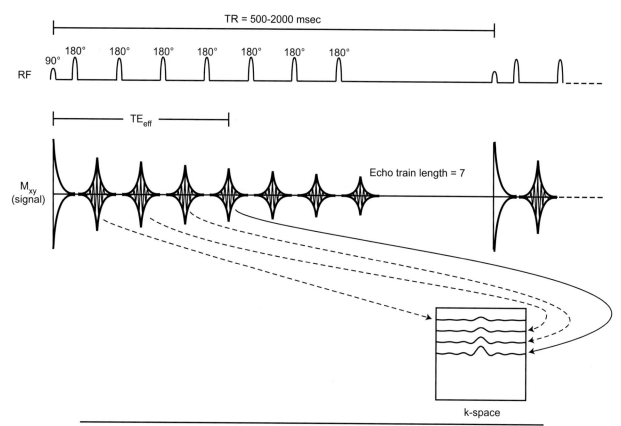

FIGURE I4-33. Image contrast with fast spin echo imaging. Selection of the echo (the fourth in this example) that is used to fill the center of k-space determines the TE$_{eff}$, which, in turn, defines the degree of T2 image contrast.

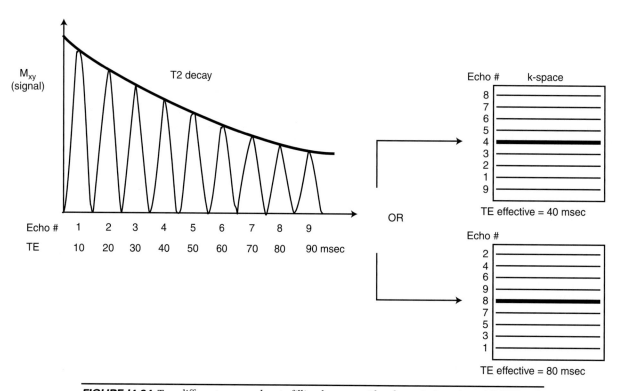

FIGURE I4-34. Two different approaches to filling k-space with echo train imaging with ETL = 9. In the top example the fourth echo (TE$_{eff}$ = 40 msec) fills the center, while in the bottom example the eighth (TE$_{eff}$ = 80 msec) is used. In the bottom example, the images would be more T2 weighted.

The high signal from fat on fast spin echo images can be beneficial or detrimental in cardiovascular MR imaging applications. For example, the high signal intensity of fat that surrounds structures such as the pericardium or aorta improves the definition of these structures. However, the high signal intensity of epicardial fat surrounding coronary arteries reduces contrast between the bright vessels and their surroundings. As will be discussed in Chapter I-9, several strategies for suppressing the signal from fat are available and are widely used.

> **IMPORTANT POINT:** Although fat does not have a long T2 time, it is bright on T2-weighted fast spin echo imaging.

Half-Fourier Single-Shot Echo Train Spin Echo Imaging

Taken to the extreme, fast spin echo imaging can be used to perform ultrafast imaging using half-Fourier single-shot methods. Single-shot fast spin echo imaging can be achieved by filling just over half of k-space (Chapter I-7). For example, for an image with 128 phase-encoding steps, about 68 echoes must be measured and the remaining 60 filled in by computation. Even so, the single-shot approach is possible only with very short interecho spacing. For an interecho spacing of 5 msec, the time to the last of 68 echoes will be about 340 msec. After 340 msec most signal has decayed, but by placing the later echoes far away from the center of k-space, the half-Fourier single-shot approach can produce an image in less than 400 msec! *Half-Fourier acquisition single-shot turbo spin echo (HASTE)* imaging is widely used in cardiac and body imaging because, as an ultrafast sequence, it is much less sensitive to artifacts resulting from cardiac and respiratory motion.

What determines the image contrast in single-shot spin echo imaging? As in other fast spin echo approaches, image contrast depends on the echoes that are used to fill the central portions of k-space. For example, if the echo that occurs at 63 msec after the 90° RF pulse is the one used to fill the central line of k-space, then the TE_{eff} is 63 msec (Figure I4-35). The adjacent echoes (at 58 msec and 68 msec) are used to fill the lines just around the central line, while the echoes that occur much earlier and later are used to fill the peripheral lines.

CHALLENGE QUESTION: What is the TR of a single-shot echo train spin echo sequence?

ANSWER: TR is defined as the repetition time between RF excitation pulses that are used to generate a given image. With single-shot echo train imaging, only one RF excitation is used for each pulse. Therefore, because there is no second RF excitation, the time between RF pulses is infinite (∞). The pulse sequence parameters for such a sequence can be expressed as $TR/TE_{eff}/\text{refocusing angle} = \infty/63\ \text{msec}/180°$. Some manufacturers use the parameter TR in this sequence to describe the time between imaging consecutive slices.

Special Considerations for HASTE

Specific Absorption Rate (SAR)

As discussed with other safety issues in Chapter I-10, one important safety consideration with MR pulse sequences is the amount of energy transferred to a subject by application of RF pulses. This energy is converted into heat, which is usually rapidly dissipated by the body through blood circulation and other mechanisms. The deposition of energy is quantified as *specific absorption rate (SAR)*. SAR limits are set by regulatory agencies such as the U.S. Food and Drug Administration (FDA) to minimize the risk of unsafe heating of patients during clinical imaging.

Half-Fourier single-shot echo train sequences require application of numerous 180° pulses in quick succession. Compared to conventional and fast spin echo sequences, single-shot methods have high SAR. Therefore, although in theory the single-shot sequence could be repeated

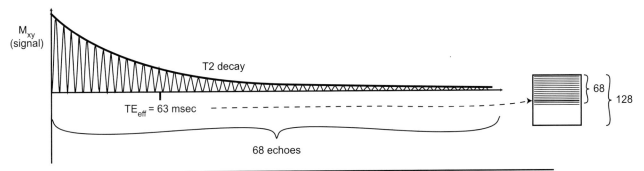

FIGURE I4-35. Half-Fourier single-shot echo train imaging. Following a single 90° RF pulse, an echo train of 68 echoes is collected and used to fill 68 of the 128 lines of k-space. The remainder of k-space is computed based on the symmetry of k-space (which is discussed in greater detail in Chapter I-7). In this example, the echo sampled at 63 msec after the RF pulse is used to fill the central line of k-space for an effective TE of 63 msec.

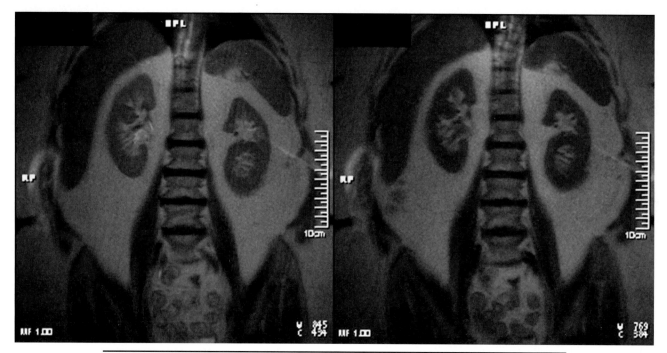

FIGURE 14-36. Example of half-Fourier single-shot fast spin echo images obtained with a refocusing pulse of 180° (left) and 150° (right). Note the reduced image quality with the smaller refocusing angle, particularly in detailing the renal calyces.

as often as every 400 msec, in practice each image is acquired less frequently, such as once per second. This allows 600 msec between acquisitions to keep the average energy deposition below SAR limits.

Another strategy for reducing SAR is to decrease the refocusing flip angle below 180°. Depending on the patient body habitus, the flip angle may need to be reduced to as low as 150° to meet SAR limits. The incomplete focusing decreases the amplitude of the echo and degrades image quality (Figure 14-36). In general, reducing the refocusing flip angle to much less than 150° is not desirable; it may be better to reduce SAR by increasing the time between RF pulses instead.

Signal-to-Noise Ratio

Although the HASTE sequence is extremely fast and therefore carries with it the advantages of minimizing respiratory and cardiac motion artifacts, it generates relatively low signal. Many of the echoes used to fill k-space occur after long echo times and after significant decay of transverse magnetization. To make matters worse, only about half of the data is truly collected. Consequently, the resulting image has an inferior signal-to-noise ratio compared to one in which all of k-space is filled with measured signal (Figure 14-37). This sequence generally does not do well in combination with other manipulations that lower signal further, such as frequency-selective fat saturation pulses or the use of the body coil rather than surface or phased-array coils for signal reception.

Image Contrast and Sharpness

As with echo train imaging in general, single-shot echo train sequences have T2 weighting that is inferior to conventional spin echo imaging at a TE equal to TE_{eff}. Detection of differences between tissues with only slightly different T2 relaxation times may be more difficult or impossible with these sequences when compared with conventional single-echo spin echo sequences or fast spin echo images with shorter echo trains. Additionally, because of the long echo train length, small objects may appear blurred, especially when a short TE_{eff} is used.

IMPORTANT CONCEPTS: Half-Fourier single-shot fast spin echo sequences are useful in cardiovascular MR imaging because they are fast, with acquisition times on the order of one second per slice. Limitations of the sequence include high energy deposition due to repeated 180° refocusing pulses, decreased T2-weighted image contrast, and relatively low signal-to-noise ratio.

GRADIENT ECHO VERSUS SPIN ECHO: SUMMARY

In summary, clinical MR pulse sequences can be classified as either gradient echo or spin echo. Each has its specific advantages.

Gradient echo imaging is typically faster, but it results in lower signal-to-noise ratios than spin echo imaging.

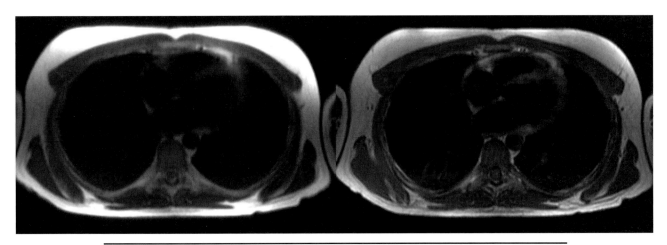

FIGURE I4-37. HASTE (left) vs. fast spin echo (right) images in the same subject, illustrating the lower signal-to-noise ratio (and lower spatial resolution) of the single-shot sequence.

Because smaller flip angles are used, there is usually less energy deposition (SAR) with gradient echo images. However, spoiled gradient echo methods are quite sensitive to undesirable T2* effects caused by field inhomogeneities and other susceptibility-inducing factors such as metal and air-tissue interfaces. Spoiled gradient echo images are usually either T1 weighted or T2* weighted. Steady-state gradient echo sequences, unlike their spoiled counterparts, have image contrast that is based on differences in T2/T1. They require short TRs and excellent magnetic field homogeneity.

Spin echo images minimize susceptibility or T2* effects by use of multiple 180° refocusing pulses, and therefore true T2-weighted images can be obtained. However, the 90° and 180° pulses with spin echo sequences require longer acquisition times. Both T1- and T2-weighted images can be obtained with spin echo sequences.

In clinical practice, gradient echo images are used for 2D or 3D T1-weighted imaging with and without gadolinium contrast agents, such as for MR angiography or contrast-enhanced cardiac imaging, and for flow-sensitive imaging and cardiac contractility studies. Spin echo images are usually reserved for T2-weighted imaging and for the assessment of anatomic structures, including the heart and vessel wall.

IMPORTANT CONCEPTS: Spin echo images are typically used for T2-weighted sequences and high resolution anatomic imaging, whereas gradient echo images are used for fast T1-weighted imaging, including flow-sensitive imaging as well as assessment of cardiac function. New steady-state gradient echo methods produce fast images of the heart with predominantly T2-weighted image contrast between blood and myocardium.

REVIEW QUESTIONS

1. Characterize the predominant image contrast for spin echo sequences with the following parameters:

	TR	TE or TE_{eff}	ETL	Weighting? (T1, PD, T2)
a.	500	20	1	
b.	1200	40	1	
c.	1500	80	1	
d.	1500	80 (effective)	32	
e.	1500	120	1	

Rank these sequences from that with the most T2 weighting to that with the least T2 weighting:
Most ____ ____ ____ ____ ____ Least

2. Characterize the predominant image contrast for gradient echo sequences with the following parameters:

	TR	TE	Flip Angle	Spoiling?	Weighting?
a.	200	2	80	Yes	
b.	200	4	80	Yes	
c.	25	10	25	Yes	
d.	25	4	15	Yes	
e.	4	1.5	60	No*	

*Balanced gradients

3. Consider a T1-weighted spin echo sequence with TR = 700 msec, T2 = 30 msec, and 100 phase-encoding steps.
   a. For a conventional spin echo sequence, what is the acquisition time for this sequence using a single acquisition?

Consider the following ways in which the sequence can be modified to provide images of the heart:

b. How many slices can be acquired in the same acquisition time if the total time from 90° RF excitation to the end of the echo is 35 msec?

c. A fast spin echo version of this sequence can be performed with spin echoes at TEs of 20, 30, 40, 50, 60 msec. How can one obtain image contrast that is similar to the conventional spin echo sequence described above? How will the image contrast for this sequence compare with that of the conventional spin echo sequence? What is the acquisition time for this sequence? How many slices can be imaged if the total time from 90°–180°–5 echoes is now 70 msec?

4. Match the sequences to the right that can be used to generate the following kinds of image contrast:

a. T1-weighted imaging: _____

b. T2-weighted imaging: _____

c. T2*-weighted imaging: _____

(1) Conventional spin echo

(2) Fast spin echo

(3) Half-Fourier single-shot fast spin echo

(4) Spoiled gradient echo

(5) True FISP steady-state gradient echo

5. Why are not there spoiled and steady-state spin echo imaging sequences?

REFERENCES

1. Duerk JL, Lewin JS, Wendt M, Petersilge C. Remember true FISP? A high SNR, near 1-second imaging method for T2-like contrast in interventional MRI at .2 T. J Magn Reson Imaging 1998; 8:203–208.

2. Constable RT, Gore JC. The loss of small objects in variable TE imaging: implications for FSE, RARE, and EPI. Magn Reson Med 1992; 28:9–24.

3. Henkelman RM, Hardy PA, Bishop JE, Poon CS, Plewes DB. Why fat is bright in RARE and fast spin-echo imaging. J Magn Reson Imaging 1992; 2:533–540.

Chapter 5

Spatial Localization and Introduction to k-Space

If a subject were placed into the magnet bore and subjected to an RF pulse at the Larmor frequency, then all the protons in the bore would become excited. Without the use of gradients, the protons would generate one collective signal measurable by the receiver coils (Figure I5-1). This signal would include contributions from the entire body, without any differentiation based on location. Such a signal could not be used to make an MR image, because to make an MR image, spatial localization is required.

Spatial localization is the essential process of any imaging test. Signal must be differentiated based on location so that a spatial map of the signal can be presented as a diagnostic image. In MRI, this is achieved primarily with magnetic field gradients, which are applied in clever ways and at strategic times during the MR pulse sequence. For 2D imaging, spatial localization can be considered in three steps. First, *slice-select gradients* are used so that only a thin slice of tissue is excited and emits signal. Then, to localize signal within a given slice, two sets of gradients are applied: *frequency-encoding gradients* during the echo, and *phase-encoding gradients* at some time between the RF pulse and the echo. Standard descriptions of a 2D pulse sequence assume a transverse slice orientation. Slice-selective excitation is therefore performed using gradients in the z direction, frequency encoding with x gradients, and phase encoding with y gradients (Figure I5-2). But in real applications, these three orthogonal directions are freely interchangeable. For 3D imaging, excitation can be performed using slab-selective excitation or nonselective excitation. Then spatial localization is performed using one frequency-encoding gradient and two sets of phase-encoding gradients.

This chapter uses conventional explanations to describe spatial localization. Imaging artifacts that are associated with each step in spatial localization are also reviewed. In the next chapter, spatial localization will be revisited, with a view toward a deeper understanding of the wonders of k-space.

KEY CONCEPTS

▶ The goal of spatial localization is to identify the origins of signal on a voxel-by-voxel basis to generate a spatial map of signal intensity.

▶ Signal intensity values are determined for each voxel with coordinates x, y, and z, by using magnetic field gradients in the x, y, and z directions.

▶ Linear gradients cause Larmor frequencies to change linearly with distance along the direction of the gradient.

▶ For 2D imaging, localization in the z direction is achieved by slice-selective excitation. A slice-select gradient is applied during RF excitation; the thickness of the slice and its profile depend on the slice-select gradient strength, the transmitter bandwidth, and the nature of the RF excitation pulse.

▶ Localization in the x direction is accomplished using a frequency-encoding gradient, while localization in the y direction requires a phase-encoding gradient.

▶ The echo is sampled during the frequency-encoding gradient; for accurate signal measurement, the sampling frequency must be at least twice as high as the largest frequency measured (the Nyquist theorem).

▶ Phase-encoding gradients are applied at times other than RF excitation and signal sampling.

▶ The dephasing caused by gradients can be reversed with rephasing lobes.

▶ Although the carrier frequency of the Larmor frequency (64 MHz) is used for MR imaging, MR RF pulses and signals are low frequency (Hz or kHz), subject to modulation and demodulation.

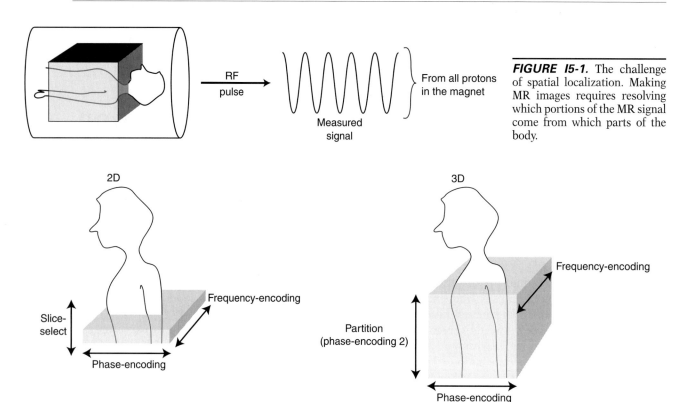

FIGURE I5-1. The challenge of spatial localization. Making MR images requires resolving which portions of the MR signal come from which parts of the body.

FIGURE I5-2. Standard nomenclature for 2D and 3D spatial localization, assuming an axial imaging 2D slice or axial 3D slab.

Before beginning the discussion of spatial localization, it is necessary to review the concepts of *modulation* and *demodulation*. Although the Larmor frequency is about 64 MHz, most of the signals used to make MR images—the RF excitation pulses and the echoes or signals recorded—are actually much lower in frequency, on the order of kilohertz (kHz) rather than megahertz (MHz). (Recall that 1 kHz = 1000 Hz, while 1 MHz = 1,000,000 Hz.) Low-frequency RF pulses are modulated with the high Larmor frequency to achieve RF excitation, while the high-frequency echoes are demodulated back to lower frequencies for signal processing. The following Background Reading provides an introduction to the concepts of modulation and demodulation.

BACKGROUND READING: Modulation and Demodulation

The concept of modulation and demodulation is the key behind the function of a familiar household appliance, the AM/FM radio. AM stands for *amplitude modulated* signal, while FM is *frequency modulated*. Radios transmit sounds originating far away. The range of frequencies that comprise the human voice and music is approximately 1–2 kHz. How can these sounds be transmitted miles away? To transmit sound waves far distances, frequencies much higher than 1–2 kHz must

be used. Think about the effect of standing atop a sky-scraper (alongside a transmitter) and yelling at the top of your lungs. The total audience for your broadcast would be rather limited, and the competition with other broadcasters would be pretty fierce. On the other hand, higher frequencies, such as in the hundreds of kHz or tens of MHz range (AM 820 kHz or FM 93.9 MHz, for example) can travel miles and penetrate buildings, with minimal interference from other carrier frequencies. But the human ear cannot hear these frequencies.

Radios work because the lower frequencies of voice and music can be superimposed onto a high-frequency carrier wave. The radio transmitter achieves this by a process called modulation, which can be performed by amplitude modulation (Figure I5-3) or, as in the case of MRI, frequency modulation. The radio receiver removes the high carrier frequency and recovers the music by demodulation (Figure I5-3).

MR operates in a similar way. The RF pulse has a bandwidth of a few kHz, while the 64 MHz Larmor frequency is the carrier frequency. When transmitted, the RF pulse is modulated to a 64 MHz carrier frequency to achieve resonance. In terms of the echo produced, the high-frequency signal received is centered around 64 MHz, but for analysis the MR computer demodulates the signal into its low-frequency (kHz) components.

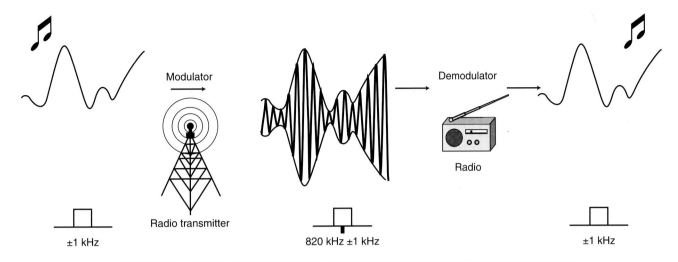

FIGURE I5-3. Radio transmission. Low-frequency music is modulated by a high carrier frequency required for transmission over long distances. The radio receives the signal and demodulates it back to the original low-frequency, audible, signal that is heard as music. The bandwidths of frequencies are depicted beneath each signal. (Note that in this example the signal is amplitude modulated. With MR, the signal is frequency modulated, which is harder to depict graphically, but conceptually rather similar.)

> **IMPORTANT CONCEPT:** MR transmitter and receiver signals are low-frequency (kHz), modulated to and demodulated from the 64 MHz Larmor carrier frequency.

Z-AXIS LOCALIZATION: SLICE-SELECT GRADIENTS AND CROSS-TALK ARTIFACTS

For 2D imaging, RF excitation is performed during application of a slice-select gradient so that only tissue within a thin slice is excited and will subsequently generate signal. Slice-select gradients ensure that all of the measured signal will originate from the same position in the z direction (assuming a transverse slice). With slice-select gradients, the z coordinate for spatial localization is predetermined, and protons outside the desired coordinates do not contribute to signal intensity.

Slice-selective excitation takes advantage of the requirement for resonance. A linear magnetic field gradient in the z direction causes the magnetic field strength to vary along the z axis (Figure I5-4). If the RF pulse consists of a pure 64 MHz signal, then only a very thin slice of tissue at 1.5 T will be excited. All other protons will be oblivious to the RF excitation pulse because they do not fulfill resonance conditions.

CHALLENGE QUESTION: Why would this scenario of a perfect 64 MHz RF excitation pulse not be a desirable way to achieve slice-selective excitation?

Answer: This scenario would not be desirable because the slice that would be excited by a pure 64 MHz pulse would be infinitesimally thin and contain too few protons to generate measurable signal for imaging.

A real RF pulse has a finite width and includes a range of frequencies. For example, the range might be from 63.998 to 64.002 MHz. The 0.004 MHz, or 4 kHz, range of frequencies is referred to as the *transmitter bandwidth* (Figure I5-4). (Note that this bandwidth is different from the more commonly encountered *receiver bandwidth*, which will be discussed later with frequency encoding.) Bandwidths in MRI are usually expressed as $\pm f_{max}$ kHz, where f_{max} is the maximum frequency in the range, so that a 4 kHz transmitter bandwidth could also be written as ± 2 kHz.

Slice Thickness

The relationship between slice-select gradient strength, transmitter bandwidth, and slice thickness is explored in this section (Figure I5-5).

The gradient strength is the ratio of the change in magnetic field, ΔB_0, over a given distance, Δd. For the slice-select gradient, G_z (mT/m),

$$G_z = \frac{\Delta B_0}{\Delta d}$$

To relate ΔB_0 to transmitter bandwidth, Δf, use the Larmor equation, $f = \gamma B$, to yield $\Delta f = \gamma \Delta B$. Substitute $\Delta B_0 = \Delta f / \gamma$,

$$G_z = \frac{\Delta f}{\gamma \Delta d}$$

Expressed in terms of slice thickness,

$$\Delta d = \frac{\Delta f}{G_z \gamma}$$

This equation says that to get thinner slices (smaller Δd), a lower transmitter bandwidth (Δf) and/or higher gradient strength (G_z) are necessary.

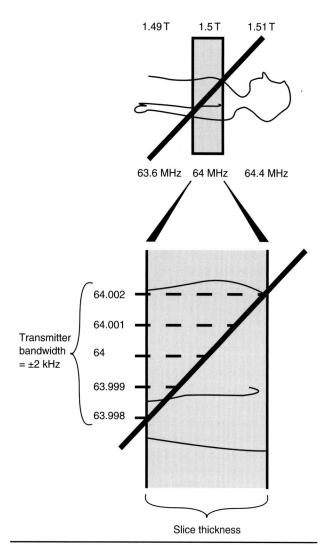

1.49 T   1.5 T   1.51 T

63.6 MHz   64 MHz   64.4 MHz

64.002

64.001

Transmitter
bandwidth
= ±2 kHz

64

63.999

63.998

Slice thickness

FIGURE I5-4. Slice-select gradient. A gradient is applied in the z direction so that protons are exposed to different magnetic fields along the length of the body and therefore precess at different frequencies. For a transmitter bandwidth of ±2 kHz, the slice that will resonate with the RF pulse will include all protons precessing at 63.998–64.002 MHz. A narrower transmitter bandwidth gives rise to a thinner slice.

CHALLENGE QUESTION: Using a slice-select gradient of 20 mT/m to excite a slice with thickness 5 mm, what is the range of frequencies that should be included in the RF excitation pulse? What about a 10 mm slice?

Answer: Using the equation above and recalling that 5 mm = 0.005 m,

$$G_z = 20 \text{ mT/m} = (\Delta f/42.6 \text{ MHz/T})/0.005 \text{ m}$$

$$\Delta f = 20 \text{ mT/m} \times 0.005 \text{ m} \times 42.6 \text{ MHz/T}$$

$$= 4.26 \text{ kHz} = \pm 2.13 \text{ kHz}$$

For a slice of twice the thickness, the range of frequencies would have to be doubled to ±4.26 kHz.

RF Pulses, Fourier Transforms, and Slice Profiles

One important concept in slice-selective excitation is the *slice profile*. The slice profile describes the amount of excitation caused by a slice-selective RF excitation pulse, both within the desired imaging slice and beyond. An ideal slice profile for a 90° RF excitation pulse is depicted in Figure I5-6, where the tissues within the slice are tipped uniformly by 90°, while tissues outside the slice experience no excitation.

What is the relationship between the RF excitation pulse and the slice profile? It turns out that there is a one-to-one correspondence between the Fourier transform of the RF pulse and the slice profile (Figure I5-6, for example).

Recall from Chapter I-1 that the Fourier transform describes the relative amounts of signal at all the component frequencies of an RF pulse. During application of the slice-select gradient, these frequencies correspond to different locations along the slice-select direction. They define the boundaries of the slice to be imaged.

The amplitude component of the Fourier transform describes how much energy is contained in each frequency component of the RF signal. This in turn defines the extent of RF excitation achieved at each location within the slice.

If the contributions are uniform across the transmitter bandwidth, then the Fourier transform will be a perfect rectangle. The slice profile will also be "ideal."

CHALLENGE QUESTION: What is the appearance and duration of the RF pulse that will result in perfect slice excitation?

Answer: An infinitely long sinc function.

> **IMPORTANT CONCEPT:** The Fourier transform of the RF pulse determines the excitation profile of the imaged slice.
> A rectangular Fourier transform corresponds to an "ideal" slice profile, where the slice is uniformly excited to the desired flip angle, without any excitation of tissue outside the slice.
> To achieve such a perfect excitation, the RF pulse would have to be an infinitely long sinc function.

Faster and Truncated Sinc RF Pulses and Their Slice Profiles

Long RF pulses are usually detrimental to MR imaging efficiency, and infinitely long RF pulses are clearly not practical. One useful feature of the sinc functions is that most of the information in the curve is contained within the central peak and a few ripples to either side of the curve. Hence, the RF pulse can be truncated to reduce the time needed for RF excitation. RF pulse durations can be further reduced by the use of stronger slice-select gradients.

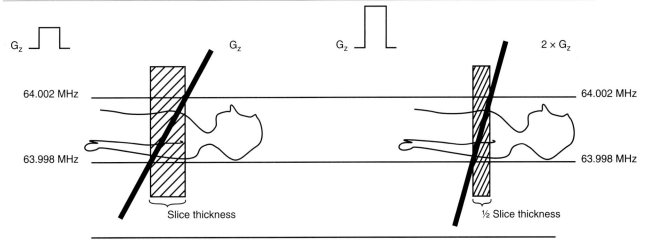

FIGURE I5-5. Slice thickness, transmitter bandwidth, and gradient strength. For a fixed transmitter bandwidth of ± 2 kHz, the slice thickness can be halved by doubling the amplitude of the slice-select gradient.

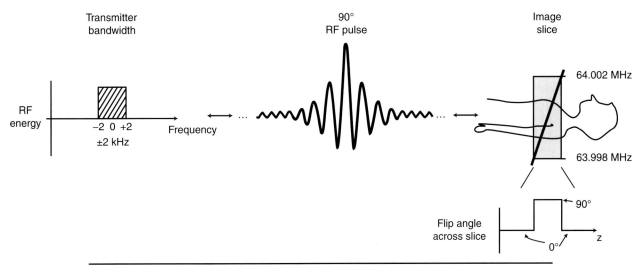

FIGURE I5-6. "Ideal" RF pulse for perfect slice profile. The ideal RF pulse for exciting a slice is a sinc pulse. All protons within the slice are excited to 90°, whereas none of the tissue outside the slice is excited (0° flip angle). The transmitter bandwidth profile (left) represents a one-dimensional Fourier transformation of the RF pulse, as does the slice profile (right).

To understand the effects of truncated RF pulses on slice profiles, more Background Reading is provided on sinc functions, truncated sinc functions, and their Fourier transforms. It is important to understand this section, because many of the themes will recur in the later section on receiver bandwidth and echo sampling.

BACKGROUND READING: Sinc Functions, Truncated Sinc Functions, and their Fourier Transforms

Sinc Functions
The sinc function is defined as $f(x) = (\sin x)/x$ (except at $x = 0$, where sinc $x = 1$). The sinc function plays a central role in MR imaging because MR signals and

RF pulses commonly represent the sum of sinusoidal functions across a relatively narrow range of frequencies. The Fourier transform (FT) of any function is a histogram of the amounts of different frequencies that, when summed, generate the function (Chapter I-1). The range of frequencies used to generate a sinc curve is referred to as the bandwidth. Bandwidth is usually centered around the zero frequency (demodulated) and expressed as $\pm f_{max}$ kHz or $2f_{max}$ kHz, where f_{max} is the maximum frequency in the range. For example, a ± 1 kHz bandwidth would mean that the range of frequencies includes -1 kHz through $+1$ kHz. This could also be expressed as a bandwidth of 2 kHz.

One useful property of sinc functions is worth reviewing. As shown in Figure I1-15 and Figure I5-7,

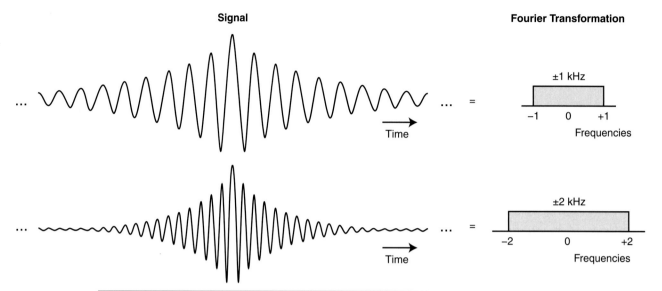

Signal   **Fourier Transformation**

FIGURE I5-7. Two sinc functions with different bandwidths. Note that these functions are infinitely long.

the wider the bandwidth comprised in the sinc function, the narrower the main peak of the sinc curve and the smaller the ripples. That is, at higher bandwidths the sinc function looks more and more "compressed." The "compressed" appearance results from the contributions of the higher frequencies (Figure I1-15). This concept is extremely important and recurs throughout many topics in MR physics!

> **IMPORTANT CONCEPT:** Higher bandwidths correspond to more "compressed" sinc functions.

Truncated Sinc Function and its Fourier Transform

In an ideal world, to generate an RF pulse that contains an equal representation of all frequencies across the desired transmitter bandwidth, the RF pulse would have to be infinitely long in duration (note the ". . ." symbols on both sides of the sinc functions shown in Figure I5-7). But in MR imaging, time is always of paramount concern, so a long RF pulse is out of the question. In fact, "sinc" functions in MR are actually truncated sinc curves. Typically, the degree of truncation is defined in terms of the numbers of *periods* (full oscillations from positive to negative to positive peak) that are included in the curve (Figure I5-8).

What happens to the Fourier transform of the sinc function when it is truncated? It no longer has the appearance of a perfect rectangle. Rather than a uniform contribution of all frequencies within the bandwidth, the truncated sinc function becomes a variable mix of different amounts of different frequencies in

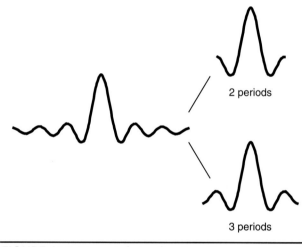

2 periods

3 periods

FIGURE I5-8. Truncated sinc function. Truncation of a sinc function is usually defined in terms of number of periods of oscillation, that is, the number of time the curve traverses one cycle of maximum-minimum-maximum.

the bandwidth and also starts to include some frequencies above and below the desired bandwidth (Figure I5-9).

> **IMPORTANT CONCEPTS:** The Fourier transform of a sinc function of infinite duration is a rectangular function. Truncation of a sinc function leads to distortion of the rectangular Fourier transform—the more severe the truncation, the larger the distortion. Truncation and its effects are determined by the number of periods included in the sinc function.

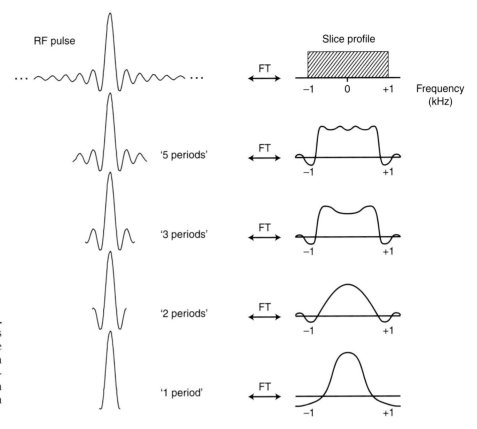

FIGURE I5-9. Fourier transforms of truncated sinc functions. The appearance of the Fourier transform depends only on the number of periods in the truncated sinc function within the pulse duration and *not* on the duration of the pulse.

What happens to the slice profile when a sinc RF pulse is truncated? A truncated RF pulse will cause some parts of the slice, such as the center, to be excited as desired, but other areas, such as the edges, will be excited either more or less than expected. In addition, there may be excitation outside the slice (Figure I5-10). Imperfect excitation means that an RF pulse intended to cause a 90° flip angle may cause a 100° flip angle at the edges of the slice. Outside the slice, where there should be no excitation, the truncated sinc RF pulse will cause small excitations (for example, ±15° flip angle). Although these effects may seem unimportant, they can dramatically affect image contrast and image quality.

The slice profile depends on the number of periods included in the truncated RF pulse and not necessarily on the actual duration of the RF pulse. By using stronger slice-select gradients, the time needed to include, say, three periods in the RF pulse can be shortened.

CHALLENGE QUESTION: Why do stronger slice-select gradients shorten the RF pulse needed to achieve a given slice profile?

Answer: If slice-select gradients are stronger, then the transmitter bandwidth increases correspondingly for a given slice thickness. An RF pulse with higher transmitter bandwidth will be more "compressed" than that with a lower transmitter bandwidth. Since the slice profile is dependent only on the number of periods contained in the RF pulse, a higher-bandwidth RF pulse requires less time for the same number of periods or the same slice profile.

> **IMPORTANT CONCEPT:** Higher-bandwidth RF pulses are more "compressed" and therefore require a shorter time to include the same number of periods as a lower-bandwidth signal.

Two scenarios are illustrated in Figure I5-11. A certain slice-select gradient is applied across the body so that the transmitter bandwidth is ±1 kHz and excites a 5 mm thick slice with a 1 msec, two-period RF pulse. If the gradient strength is doubled, then the transmitter bandwidth for the same 5 mm thick slice would double to ±2 kHz. At this bandwidth, the RF pulse would look much more "compressed"; in fact, with double the frequencies, it would be twice as "compressed." Two periods would now require only half as long, or 0.5 msec. Alternatively, if the RF pulse duration was maintained at the same 1 msec duration, the RF pulse would include four periods instead of two, resulting in a much improved slice profile with the stronger slice-select gradient.

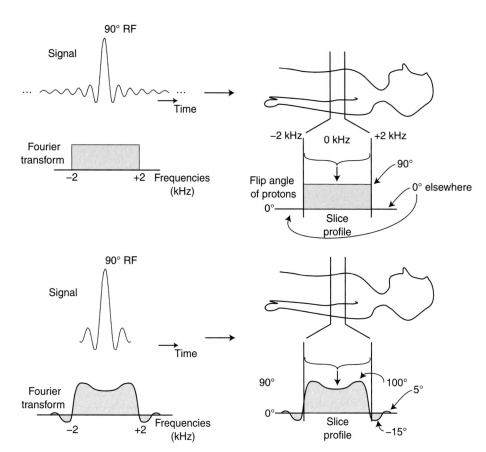

FIGURE I5-10. Truncation of a sinc RF pulse translates into imperfect slice excitation.

Stronger gradients can be used to advantage in one or a combination of the following three ways:

1. *To reduce the RF pulse time:* With double the slice-select gradient strength, the RF pulse duration in the example can be halved without sacrificing the quality of the slice profile.
2. *To improve the slice profile:* With double the gradient strength, the same RF pulse time of 1 msec will include four periods instead of two periods, resulting in a more rectangular slice profile.
3. *To reduce the slice thickness:* With double the gradient strength, if the original RF pulse transmitter bandwidth is maintained, then the excited slice will be half as thick at 2.5 mm. The quality of the slice profile will be identical to that of the original 5 mm slice.

> **IMPORTANT CONCEPT:** Strong slice-select gradients can be used to (1) reduce the duration of the RF pulse, (2) improve the slice profile of the same slice thickness, and/or (3) reduce the slice thickness.

Cross-Talk

Cross-talk artifacts are the effects of imperfect slice profiles on the imaging of neighboring slices. For 2D imaging, to ensure that small lesions are not missed, imaging would ideally be performed using a series of contiguous thin slices. With MR imaging, this would require that each 2D slice be excited uniformly, one at a time, without any stray excitation outside the desired slice (Figure I5-12). In fact, imperfect slice profiles caused by routine truncation of the RF pulses result in imperfect excitation of all slices, particularly at their edges, as well as unintentional excitation of tissue just outside the slice. The consequence is imperfect representation of tissues in the images.

Reducing Cross-Talk

As shown in Figure I5-12 at the bottom, there are two main approaches to reducing cross-talk.

Interslice Gaps

Most 2D imaging is described in terms of a given slice thickness and an *interslice gap*, such as "8 mm thick slices with 2 mm thick gaps." The gap is a portion of tissue between slices that is deliberately excluded to avoid the partial excitation caused by imperfect slice profiles.

How much interslice gap is reasonable? The gap depends on the slice profile, which in turn depends on the

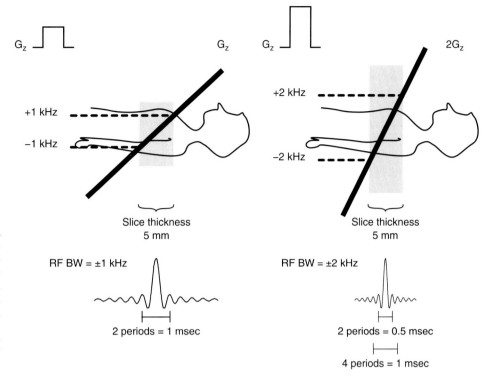

FIGURE I5-11. Slice-select gradients. The stronger slice-select gradient (right) increases the transmitter bandwidth for a given slice thickness, resulting in a more "compressed" sinc function for the RF pulse and consequently shorter time for the same number of periods in the RF pulse.

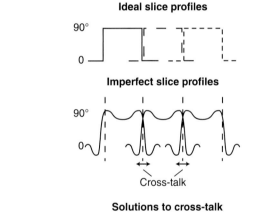

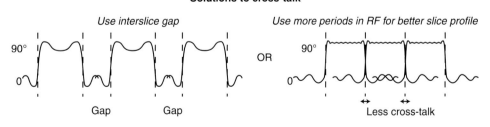

FIGURE I5-12. Cross-talk. Top: Ideal slice profile, where each slice-select RF pulse achieves a uniform 90° excitation across each slice and 0° outside. Middle: Typical nonideal slice profile demonstrating the imperfect excitation at the edges of slices, which is referred to as cross-talk and results from a truncated RF pulse. Bottom: Two solutions to cross-talk: (1) separate the slices with an interslice gap (left) or (2) improve the slice profile by adding lobes to the RF pulse (right).

number of periods in the RF pulse. It can be shown that, given the slice profile associated with a two-period RF pulse (Figure I5-9), the corresponding *slice thickness to gap ratio* should be about 5:1. This means that using a two-period RF pulse, 5 mm slices should be acquired with 1 mm gaps or 10 mm slices with 2 mm gaps. For a four-

period RF pulse, the required gap is less, because the slice profile is better; the slice thickness to gap ratio can be about 10:1.

Note that, whereas some manufacturers of MRI equipment describe slice thicknesses and gaps in terms of actual distances (e.g., 5 mm slices with 1 mm gaps), others use the term *distance factor*, which expresses the gap as a fraction of the slice thickness. For example, in the setting of a two-period RF pulse with slice thickness–to–gap ratio of 5:1, the distance factor would be 1/5 or 0.2. Similarly, for a four-period RF pulse, the distance factor would be 1/10 or 0.1.

> **IMPORTANT POINT:** The optimal slice–to–interslice gap ratio for a two-period RF pulse is 5:1 (distance factor 0.2), while for a four-period RF pulse, the ideal ratio is 10:1 (distance factor 0.1).

Increasing the Number of Periods in the RF Pulse

By using more periods of the sinc curve to better approximate the ideal shape of the RF pulse, slice profiles will improve and there will be less cross-talk. This comes at the expense of time, unless stronger gradients are used.

Dephasing Caused By Slice-Select Gradients

As discussed in Chapter I-4, application of a gradient always causes dephasing. What kind of dephasing is caused by the slice-select gradient and what are its consequences?

The slice-select gradient is applied during the RF pulse to ensure that only a thin slice of tissue is excited. The gradient is in the slice-select direction. For example, for an axial slice, the gradient will be along the bore of the magnet (z axis). This means that along the z axis, within each slice, the protons will be precessing at slightly different frequencies. What happens if the protons within a slice precess at different frequencies? They dephase, and their signals cancel out. If this dephasing is severe, there will be no signal to measure, causing a serious problem!

To minimize the effects of the slice-select gradient, a compensatory gradient lobe can be applied after the slice-select gradient (Figure I5-13).

> **IMPORTANT CONCEPT:** All gradients cause dephasing and require application of gradients of opposite polarity to rephase the magnetic moments.

As illustrated in Figure I5-13, the area under the rephasing lobe is only half the area under the main portion of the slice-select gradient because the dephasing effect occurs only for the protons that are precessing coherently in the transverse plane. At the start of the RF pulse, the magnetic moments are fully longitudinal. Because they are precessing incoherently, they are not affected by magnetic field gradients. The transition from incoherent longitudinal to coherent transverse magnetization occurs over the course of the RF excitation. As an approximation, the protons precess incoherently for the first half of the RF pulse and coherently during the latter half. Hence, the rephasing lobe needs only to be half as large as the dephasing lobe.

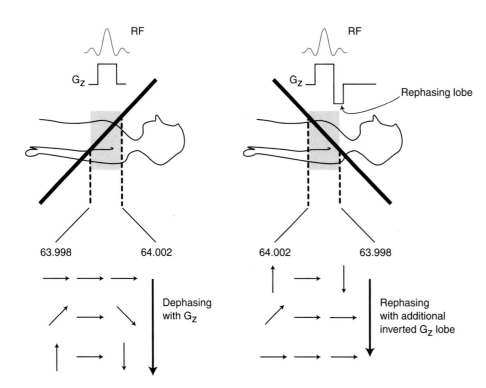

FIGURE I5-13. Compensatory rephasing lobe of the slice-select gradient. To reverse the intraslice dephasing caused by the slice-select gradient, a rephasing lobe is used. In this example, the rephasing lobe is half the duration of the slice-select gradient.

Slice Selection in Spin Echo and Gradient Echo Imaging

For gradient echo imaging, the slice-select gradient is applied during the RF excitation only. For spin echo imaging, the gradient is always applied during the 90° RF pulse and is usually also applied during the 180° pulse. No additional gradient lobes are needed to correct the dephasing effects of the slice-select gradient during the 180° pulse. This is because for the 180° pulse, the dephasing and rephasing occur during the first and second halves of the pulse, respectively. The complete pulse sequence diagrams for a conventional spin echo and a gradient echo sequence are given in Figure I5-14, illustrating the RF pulse and slice-select gradient (G_z) portions discussed so far.

X AXIS LOCALIZATION: FREQUENCY-ENCODING GRADIENTS AND CHEMICAL SHIFT ARTIFACT

Just as in the slice-select process, gradients are also used to localize the source of signal along the x direction using the process of frequency encoding. For this step of spatial localization, the gradient is applied during the sampling of the echo. With application of the frequency-encoding gradient, protons are made to emit signals of different frequencies depending on their location along the x direction. The gradient effectively encodes the location of a proton along the x axis by the frequency of its signal. For example, the frequency-encoding gradient shown in Figure I5-15 (left) causes protons in the right arm to precess at 63.95 MHz, while those in the spine precess at 64 MHz and those in the left arm at 64.05 MHz.

> **IMPORTANT DISTINCTION:** Whereas slice-select gradients are applied during the RF pulse, frequency-encoding gradients are applied during the sampling of the echo to encode spatial location based on the frequency of signal measured.

For reasons that will become apparent later, the frequency-encoding direction is usually defined as the direction which has the broadest span. For a conventional axial slice of the chest or abdomen, the frequency-encoding gradient is usually applied along the x direction from left to right. For brain imaging, on the other hand, frequency encoding is typically anterior to posterior. Because the signal is sampled during the frequency-encoding gradient, this gradient is also referred to as the *readout gradient*.

Three major effects of the frequency-encoding gradient on the actual signal measured should be considered. First,

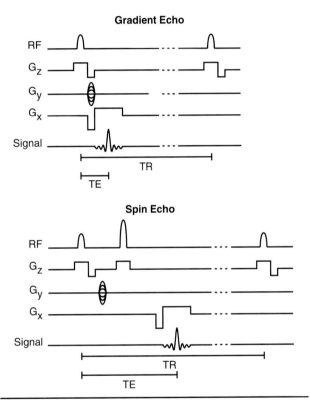

FIGURE I5-14. Pulse sequence diagram for gradient echo and spin echo sequences.

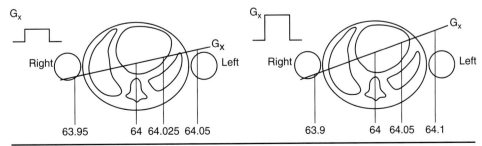

FIGURE I5-15. Frequency-encoding gradient in the x-direction, G_x, causes the precessional frequencies of protons to vary linearly with position in that direction. A gradient twice as strong, shown on the right, causes the spread of precessional frequencies to be twice as great.

how the gradient changes the appearance of the echo will be discussed.

CHALLENGE QUESTION: What will be the appearance of the echo that represents the composite of signals across a range of frequencies?

Answer: The echo will resemble a sinc function. The wider the range of frequencies, the more "compressed" the sinc function (Figure I5-7).

> **IMPORTANT CONCEPT:** With a frequency-encoding gradient, the echo will comprise signals from across a range of frequencies and have the appearance of a sinc function.

Second, consider how the application of a frequency-encoding gradient can help spatial localization.

CHALLENGE QUESTION: How can position along the x axis be extracted from the echo that is measured during application of a frequency-encoding gradient?

Answer: Apply a Fourier transform to the measured echo!

The Fourier transform of a function gives a histogram of the different frequency components that make up that function (Figure I5-16). If frequencies are linearly distributed along the x direction, then the Fourier transform of the resulting signal will provide a a map of the total amount of signal being generated at each location along the x axis. Each frequency component will include signal from the entire column of tissue that shares the same position along x. As discussed in Chapter I-4, the amount of signal measured at each location will depend on properties of the tissue (proton density, T1 and T2 relaxation time) and parameters of the pulse sequence such as TR, TE, and (for gradient echo imaging) flip angle. Sample results for T1-weighted and T2-weighted images are shown in Figure I5-16.

> **IMPORTANT CONCEPT:** The Fourier transform of an echo sampled during application of a frequency-encoding gradient provides the sum of the signals for each column of tissue along the frequency-encoding direction.

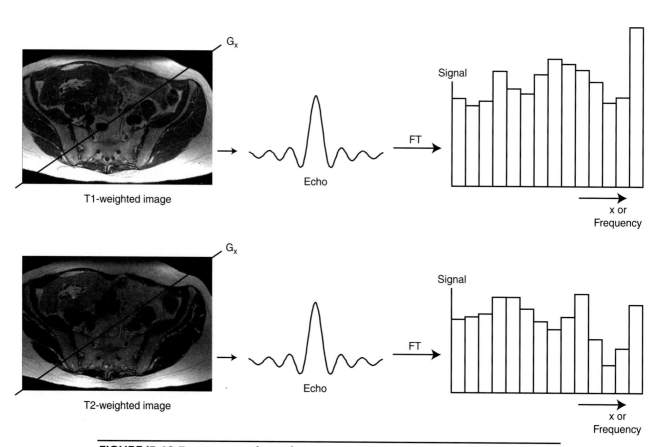

FIGURE I5-16. Frequency encoding. A frequency-encoding gradient causes the echo to have the appearance of a sinc function. When subjected to a Fourier transform, the echo is decomposed into a frequency histogram that describes the amount of signal at each frequency. Each frequency "encodes" a specific location along the x axis.

The third consequence of the frequency-encoding gradient is dephasing. Gradients always cause dephasing. A rephasing gradient is necessary to compensate for the dephasing (Figure I5-17).

With frequency encoding gradients, the compensation lobe always happens first, so that the reverse gradient first causes dephasing, and then the frequency-encoding gradient causes rephasing. The amount of dephasing or rephasing is proportional to the area under the gradient curve. Hence, the area under the dephasing lobe is equal to half the area under the rephasing lobe. This way, rephasing is greatest during the midpoint of the rephasing lobe. If this seems reminiscent of the discussion of how gradient echoes are made, then you are thinking along the right lines! The frequency-encoding gradient is used in gradient echo imaging to make the echo. In spin echo imaging, the frequency-encoding gradient is also used and adds a gradient echo component to the spin echo.

> **IMPORTANT CONCEPT:** The frequency-encoding gradient creates a gradient echo by use of a dephasing and a rephasing gradient. This gradient echo is the sole source of echo formation for gradient echo imaging, whereas in spin echo imaging the echo comprises spin echo and gradient echo contributions.

Receiver Bandwidth and Sampling Frequency

The receiver bandwidth is the range of frequencies sampled by the receiver during application of the frequency-encoding gradient. For a given field of view, the stronger the frequency-encoding gradient, the wider the receiver bandwidth. For example, if the gradient is very strong and causes the magnetic field to vary from 1.497 T to 1.503 T from one end of the image to the other, then the corresponding range of Larmor frequencies will be relatively large. Using the Larmor equation, this gradient can be computed and corresponds to a bandwidth of ±128 kHz or 256 kHz.

If, on the other hand, the gradient is weak and the field varies only from 1.4998 T to 1.5002 T, then the range of frequencies will be smaller, ± 8 kHz or 16 kHz (Figure I5-15).

The receiver bandwidth is different from transmitter bandwidth in that the receiver bandwidth applies to the range of frequencies contained within the echo, while the transmitter bandwidth refers to the range of frequencies contained within the RF excitation pulse. However, conceptually, the two share many things in common. The measured signal is demodulated from the 64 MHz carrier frequency to a center frequency of 0 Hz. Receiver bandwidths are typically described in the Hz or kHz range. Also the stronger the frequency-encoding gradient, the wider the range of frequencies; that is, the higher the receiver bandwidth for a given distance in the x direction.

One important new concepts is that the receiver bandwidth is constrained by the *sampling frequency*, which is defined as the rate at which the echo is sampled and digitized. When an MR signal is generated, it has the appearance of a sinc function. This signal must be collected by the receiver coil and digitized into a series of numbers to be stored in k-space. This process is performed by an *analog-to-digital converter (ADC)*. The sampling frequency is the rate at which the analog-to-digital conversion occurs. For example, for a sampling frequency of 500 kHz, 500,000 samples can be taken per second, while for a sampling frequency of 1 MHz, 1,000,000 samples can be measured per second. The total number of samples taken is determined by the number of voxels desired in the frequency-encoding direction. For example, if the image matrix is 256 × 256, then at least 256 samples of each echo are needed (Figure I5-18).

CHALLENGE QUESTION: How long would it take to sample the echo 256 times if the sampling frequency is 256 kHz?

Answer: 256 kHz corresponds to 256,000 samples per second. Therefore 256 samples would take 1/1000 of a second, or 1 msec.

Because the sampling frequency is finite, the recorded version of the sinc function may not be a perfect representation of the actual echo (Figure I5-18). How well the echo is represented depends on the relationship between

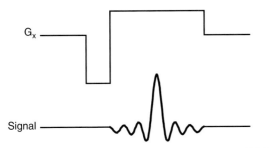

FIGURE I5-17. Dephasing lobe of frequency-encoding gradient. To correct for the phase dispersion caused by the presence of the rephasing lobe, this gradient is preceded by a dephasing lobe. The area under the dephasing lobe is equal to half the area under the rephasing lobe.

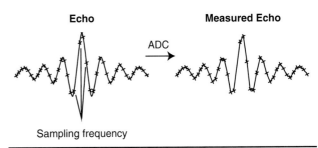

FIGURE I5-18. Sampling frequency and analog-to-digital conversion. Example of the effects of the ADC on the measured echo compared with the actual echo. Digitization of the signal results in some loss of information contained the original signal.

the sampling frequency and the highest-frequency components of the signal. This relationship is described by the *Nyquist theorem of sampling*, which states that to detect a signal of a frequency f accurately, the signal must be sampled at a frequency of at least twice the frequency, 2f. Background Reading is provided next to explain the Nyquist theorem in more detail.

BACKGROUND READING: Nyquist Theorem

The Nyquist theorem is best understood by looking at a sinusoidal signal and understanding how a computer must sample the signal to represent it correctly. The analog signal is emitted continuously, but the computer must take discrete measurements and therefore can only sample short segments of the signal at fixed intervals. The frequency at which the computer can measure the signal is the sampling frequency. If the sinusoidal signal has a frequency f, consider what happens with different sampling frequencies . For example, if the signal is sampled at that very same frequency f, what kind of representation of the signal would be collected by the MR system? The answer is that the measured signal will have the same value at every sample, leading to a contant signal that in no way reflects the original sinusoidal signal!

What if the sampling occurs more often than f, but still less than 2f? The data points sampled by the

computer will trace out a sinusoidal curve, but not one that represents the original signal—rather, one with a much lower frequency. This is called *undersampling*. This can be seen in old Western movies where stagecoach wheels appear to turn slowly backwards as the stagecoach rolls forward—the spokes of the wheels are undersampled in the movies with low frame rates.

The Nyquist theorem states that the sampling must be at least twice as frequent as f (2f) for the frequency to be represented accurately. At a minimum sampling frequency of 2f, both the maxima and minima can be detected, as shown at the bottom in Figure I5-19, and therefore the original signal can be more accurately represented. Of course, it is desirable to sample at more than 2f to ensure better representation of the original signal.

It follows from the Nyquist theorem that if the signal contains a range of frequencies, then, to ensure that the highest frequency, f_{max}, is adequately preserved, the sampling frequency must be at least $2f_{max}$.

> **IMPORTANT CONCEPT:** When a range of frequencies is represented in a signal, such as in an MR echo, then the sampling frequency must be at least twice that of the highest frequency to ensure that all frequencies are properly represented. If the highest frequency is adequately sampled, then all the lower frequencies will also be sufficiently sampled for representation.

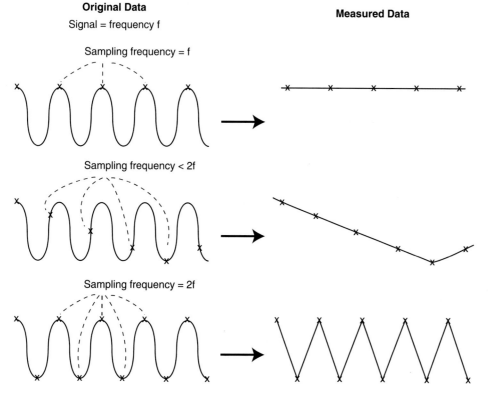

Original Data
Signal = frequency f

Measured Data

Sampling frequency = f

Sampling frequency < 2f

Sampling frequency = 2f

FIGURE I5-19. Effect of sampling frequencies on representation of sinusoidal functions. Undersampling results in inaccurate representations of the original data. The minimum sampling frequency for a signal with frequency f, according to the Nyquist theorem, is two times f (2f).

With application of a frequency-encoding gradient, the receiver bandwidth defines the range of frequencies to be sampled. A typical receiver bandwidth (demodulated) might be ±128 kHz across the entire field of view. In other words, the signal will include all frequency components between -128 kHz and 128 kHz.

CHALLENGE QUESTION: What must be the sampling frequency to sample accurately all frequency components of a signal with receiver bandwidth of ±128 kHz?

Answer: Based on the Nyquist theorem, the sampling frequency must be at least twice the highest frequency of 128 kHz, that is, 256 kHz.

For a receiver bandwidth of ±128 kHz or 256 kHz, the sampling frequency must be at two times the highest frequency, that is, 2×128 kHz or at least 256 kHz. Similarly, for a receiver bandwidth of ±16 kHz or 32 kHz, the sampling frequency must be 2×16 kHz or 32 kHz. Hence, it turns out that the receiver bandwidth and sampling frequency are practically interchangeable numbers. For most purposes, they can be thought of as identical. A receiver bandwidth of 256 kHz (±128 kHz) means a sampling frequency of 256 kHz.

> **IMPORTANT CONCEPT:** In MR jargon, the receiver bandwidth and the sampling frequency are almost interchangeable. If a system is described as having a high receiver bandwidth, this means that the sampling frequency is sufficiently high to sample the highest frequency in the receiver bandwidth.

Receiver Bandwidth Terminology

Different manufacturers use different systems for describing receiver bandwidths. One approach is more intuitive but less specific—receiver bandwidth is described as the range of frequencies represented across the image in the direction of the frequency-encoding gradient. The receiver bandwidth is expressed in $\pm$kHz, where the 0 kHz position is assumed to be the center of the field of view.

Another approach is to express the receiver bandwidth in terms of the range of frequencies across each voxel in the frequency-encoding direction. For example, for an image that contains 256 voxels in the frequency-encoding direction (x axis), then a ±128 kHz (or 256 kHz total) total receiver bandwidth would translate into a 1 kHz/voxel bandwidth. Frequently the units of receiver bandwidth on a per-voxel basis are in Hz/voxel, so a 1 kHz/voxel bandwidth might be expressed instead as 1000 Hz/voxel. For ease in comparing the bandwidth for different manufacturers, Table I5-1 shows a typical range of receiver bandwidth values for images with 256 and 512 voxels in the frequency-encoding direction.

Faster Imaging with Stronger Gradients and Higher Receiver Bandwidths

It is important to understand a manufacturer's specifications for sampling frequencies or receiver bandwidths because they relate directly to the speed at which the MR unit can produce images. To understand this concept, it is necessary to realize that the sampling frequency directly determines how long it takes for the full echo to be sampled.

For example, a sampling frequency or receiver bandwidth of 256 kHz means that the signal or echo is sampled 256,000 times per second. Sampling a signal 256 times would take 1/1000 of a second, or 1 msec. In contrast, if a receiver bandwidth or sampling frequency is 64 kHz, it would take four times as long, or 4 msec, to sample a signal 256 times. The length of sampling time can be important in determining acquisition time. For most gradient echo imaging, especially 3D gradient echo imaging, where the total TR can be on the order of only a few msec, an extra millisecond or two to sample the echo can have a dramatic effect on the TR and TE and, consequently, the acquisition times (Figure I5-20). As with RF excitation pulses, stronger frequency-encoding gradients can also be used to shorten the echo duration and consequently shorten TR and TE. For spin echo imaging, the time needed to sample the echo usually does not affect the imaging time. One exception to this rule is the case of long echo trains that require short interecho spacing. The longer the echo sampling time with fast spin echo imaging, the shorter the echo train length and the longer the acquisition time.

The drawback of faster imaging and higher receiver bandwidths is lower signal-to-noise ratios. The signal-to-

▶ **TABLE I5-1 Receiver Bandwidth Conversions**

256 Frequency-Encoding Voxels		512 Frequency-Encoding Voxels	
BW across Image	*BW per Voxel*	*BW across Image*	*BW per Voxel*
±16 kHz = 32 kHz	125 Hz/voxel	±16 kHz = 32 kHz	62 Hz/voxel
±32 kHz = 64 kHz	250 Hz/voxel	±32 kHz = 64 kHz	125 Hz/voxel
±64 kHz = 128 kHz	500 Hz/voxel	±64 kHz = 128 kHz	250 Hz/voxel
±128 kHz = 256 kHz	1000 Hz/voxel	±128 kHz = 256 kHz	500 Hz/voxel

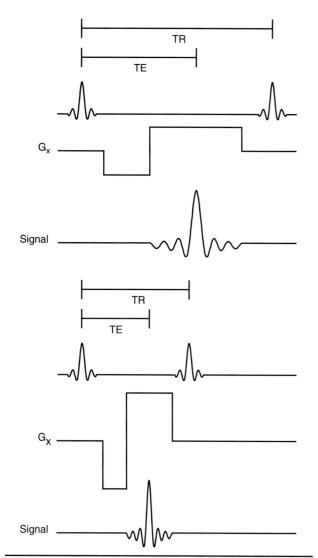

FIGURE I5-20. Higher gradient strengths and faster sampling frequencies mean shorter TR and faster imaging. Note the much shorter TR and TE for the lower example where a stronger G_x is used.

noise ratio that can be achieved depends on the time spent sampling the signal. Less sampling time results in a lower signal-to-noise-ratio. Therefore, careful selection of a receiver bandwidth must balance the opposing demands of shorter acquisition times and higher signal-to-noise ratios in MR imaging.

> **IMPORTANT CONCEPT:** Sampling frequency and receiver bandwidth directly determine the time used in sampling the echo. Shorter sampling times can translate into faster imaging but at the expense of lower signal-to-noise ratios.

Chemical Shift Artifact (of the First Kind)

The underlying assumption in frequency encoding is that differences in frequencies of signals from the body are solely due to differences in position along that axis. For example, if the center frequency is 0 Hz (demodulated signal), then any proton precessing at +200 Hz will be assumed to be located to one side of the center, say to the right (Figure I5-21), while a proton precessing at −200 Hz will be assumed to be to the left. This assumption works fine, provided that the magnetic field is perfectly uniform throughout (1.5 T) and provided that all the hydrogen protons are water protons with identical Larmor frequencies.

In Chapter I-1, however, it was stated that fat protons precess 220 Hz more slowly than water protons at 1.5 T because of their different molecular environment. This is known as *chemical shift*. What happens if fat is in the center of the field of view? The fat protons precess at a lower frequency, so the MR computer will localize the signal from the fat to the left side of the center, because by definition, anything precessing slower than 0 Hz must be coming from a location to the left. Therefore, fat will increase the total amount of signal from the areas to the left (causing higher signal intensity), while the region where the fat is actually positioned will have no signal. This creates a dark band in the center and a bright band to the left, the so-called *chemical shift artifact of the first kind*. (There is a second kind of chemical shift artifact, discussed in Chapter I-9.)

The nature and severity of the artifact depends on the receiver bandwidth and the relative location of fat and water in the frequency-encoding direction. As illustrated in Figure I5-21, a receiver bandwidth of 200 Hz/voxel results in a chemical shift equivalent to a displacement of one voxel at each fat-water interface. At a lower receiver bandwidth, the chemical shift artifact will be more apparent. For example, a receiver bandwidth of 120 Hz/voxel will result in an artifact that is about 2 voxels wide (Figure I5-22); a receiver bandwidth of 50 Hz/voxel will show an artifact that is 4 voxels wide.

CHALLENGE QUESTION: In Figure I5-22, in which direction is the frequency-encoding gradient increasing?

Answer: Since the dark band artifact is on the left edges of organs surrounded by fat, the frequency-encoding gradient must increase from the subject's left to right.

If the receiver bandwidth is higher than 220 Hz, as also depicted in Figure I5-21, then the chemical shift artifact will not be a problem. With a bandwidth of 560 Hz/voxel, for example, the shift is not visible because it causes misplacement that is less than one voxel. This is the case with most cardiovascular applications, where high receiver bandwidths are used to achieve faster imaging. Therefore, chemical shift artifacts of the first-kind are not commonly encountered. With conventional spin echo sequences, used in other MR applications, chemical shift artifacts may still be common because lower receiver bandwidth sequences are desired for their higher signal-to-noise ratios.

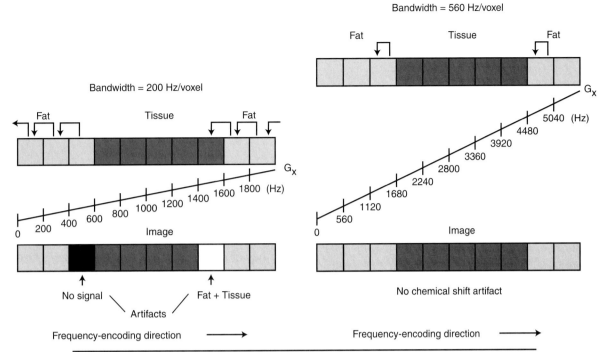

FIGURE I5-21. Chemical shift artifact depends on receiver bandwidth. On the left, with a bandwidth of 200 Hz/voxel, the more slowly precessing fat protons (light gray) are interpreted as arising from a lower (more leftward) point along the magnetic field gradient. The chemical shift artifact is one voxel wide at the interface of fat and water. On the right, there is no chemical shift artifact at higher receiver bandwidths, because differences in precessional frequencies between water and fat are contained within a single voxel.

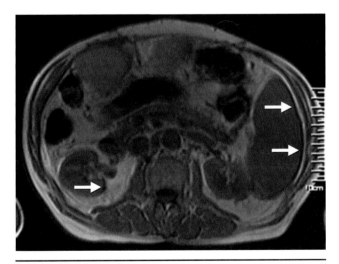

FIGURE I5-22. Chemical shift artifact. The loss of signal (arrows) along the left sides of interfaces between organs such as the kidneys or spleen and fat reflect chemical shift artifact of the first kind. The receiver bandwidth for this image was 120 Hz/voxel.

IMPORTANT CONCEPT: Chemical shift artifact results from mismapping of the more slowly precessing fat protons compared with water protons (about 220 Hz at 1.5 T). The mismapping becomes apparent as artifactual white or dark bands at fat-water interfaces in the frequency-encoding direction when the receiver bandwidth is less than about 220 Hz/voxel.

Frequency-Encoding Gradients and Spin Echo and Gradient Echo Imaging

Frequency-encoding gradients are used with both spin echo and gradient echo sequences. In both cases, they are balanced with a dephasing lobe. For gradient echo imaging, the frequency-encoding gradient generates the gradient echo itself. For spin echo imaging, the frequency-encoding gradient is applied during the spin echo. The measured spin echo represents the composite of the gradient echo and spin echo.

The relative timing of G_x compared with the rest of the pulse sequence diagram is depicted in Figure I5-14.

PHASE-ENCODING GRADIENTS

With slice-select gradients and frequency-encoding gradients, MR signal can be localized in two dimensions, z and x, to specific columns of tissue along the x direction. The third and final step of spatial localization requires phase-encoding gradients to determine the signal intensity values for each voxel along the y direction in every column. Unlike slice-select gradients and frequency-encoding gradients, which change the *frequencies* of protons, phase-encoding gradients change *phase*.

As reviewed in Chapter I-1, differences in precessional frequencies directly result in accumulated differences in phase. The stronger the gradient, the faster the dephasing; the longer a gradient is on, the greater the phase dispersion. Once the gradient is turned off, the protons will return to precessing together at the Larmor frequency, but they will maintain their phase dispersion. With a phase-encoding gradient in the y direction, the phase shift will depend on the duration and strength of the gradient and will linearly vary with position along the y axis (Figure I5-23).

In an MR pulse sequence, the phase-encoding gradient is applied for a short duration at some point other than during the RF excitation or echo. The phase-encoding step of spatial localization requires that the process of RF excitation through echo sampling be repeated numerous times using a different phase-encoding gradient to achieve different phase shifts each time. The number of repetitions usually equals to the number of voxels in the y direction. The number of voxels in the y direction is therefore typically referred to as the number of phase-encoding steps, or N_{PE}.

For each distinct application of the phase-encoding gradient, the echo measured will differ. For example, when no phase-encoding gradient is applied (expressed as a phase encoding gradient of zero, Figure I5-23), there will be maximal signal amplitude, because within each column the protons will be in phase and will sum to create a large signal. If strong phase-encoding gradients are applied, then within each column considerable dephasing of the protons will occur, and the net signal measured will be low because dephased magnetic moments cancel each other (Figure I5-23).

Phase-Encoding and Frequency-Encoding Example

The way in which phase-encoding and frequency-encoding gradients can be combined to solve the spatial localization challenge is best illustrated with a smaller image matrix. Consider an image with a matrix of 3×2 (Figure I5-24), where x = 3 in the frequency-encoding direction and y = 2 in the phase-encoding direction. After the frequency-encoding gradient and Fourier transform of the echo, signal is measured that contains three different frequencies, corresponding to the three columns. For each of the three positions along x, there are two unknown signal intensity values to be determined.

To accomplish spatial localization, two sets of echoes need to be collected, each with a different phase-encoding gradient. For simplicity, let one phase-encoding gradient be zero, and let the second cause a 180° phase shift between the two voxels of each column (Figure I5-24).

With no phase-encoding gradient, the Fourier transform of the signal will have three frequency components, one for each column. The amplitude aparture components equals the sum of the magnitudes of the magnetization vectors of both voxels in that column. In the example given, the sum of the magnitude of the components from the left column equals 5, from the middle column equals 42, and from the right equals 21.

This means that:

$$A = a_1 + a_2 = 5$$
$$B = b_1 + b_2 = 42$$
$$C = c_1 + c_2 = 21$$

For the second phase-encoding step, the phase-encoding gradient is applied with sufficient duration and strength to cause a 180° phase shift between the top and bottom rows of tissue. The resulting echo will be smaller in amplitude, because the signals in each of the two voxels in a column are completely out of phase. In fact, the resulting signal for each column will simply be the difference between the signal amplitudes of the two voxels. For this example, the amplitudes of the three frequency components are 1 for the left column, −4 for the middle column, and 7 for the right column.

Translated into equations,

$$A' = a_1 - a_2 = 1$$
$$B' = b_1 - b_2 = -4$$
$$C' = c_1 - c_2 = 7$$

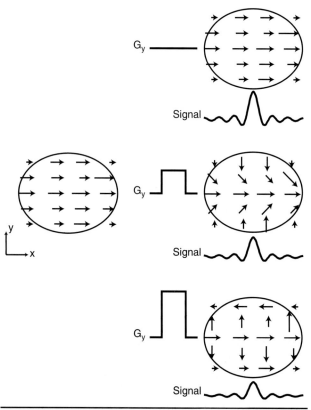

FIGURE I5-23. Phase-encoding gradient in the y direction with no phase-encoding gradient (top), a weak phase-encoding gradient (middle), and a strong phase-encoding gradient (bottom). The amplitude of each magnetic moment (arrows) will reflect the relationship between tissue properties and imaging parameters.

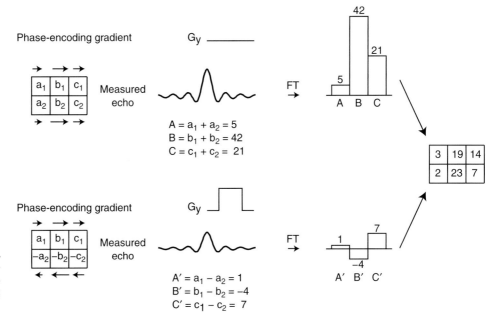

Phase-encoding gradient

G_y ─────

Measured echo

$A = a_1 + a_2 = 5$
$B = b_1 + b_2 = 42$
$C = c_1 + c_2 = 21$

FT →

Phase-encoding gradient

G_y

Measured echo

$A' = a_1 - a_2 = 1$
$B' = b_1 - b_2 = -4$
$C' = c_1 - c_2 = 7$

FT →

FIGURE I5-24. Spatial localization example. Example of phase-encoding gradients for a 3×2 matrix.

For each column, there are now two equations to solve for the two unknown signal intensity values. For example, to solve for a_1 and a_2, the following two equations must be solved using algebra:

$$a_1 + a_2 = 5$$
$$a_1 - a_2 = 1$$

The solution to the two unknowns is $a_1 = 3$ and $a_2 = 2$. The values for the other two columns can be similarly determined (Figure I5-24).

While this example of $N_{PE} = 2$ is simplistic, it illustrates the principle of using phase-encoding gradients to generate enough equations to solve for the unknown values of signal intensities along the y direction.

CHALLENGE QUESTION: For an imaging matrix with $N_{PE} = 128$, how many times does the phase-encoding gradient need to be applied and echoes sampled to solve the spatial localization problem?

Answer: 128 times. By the rules of algebra, to solve for an equation with 128 unknowns (the values of signal intensities in a given column of tissue), 128 different versions of the equation are necessary. Each phase-encoding step can be made to produce a different version of the equation with different coefficients for the unknowns.

N_{PE} Phase-Encoding Steps

The problem of the more typical case of a much larger number of phase-encoding voxels, say 128 or 256, is illustrated in Figure I5-25. Generalizing from the above example, for any given column of tissue, the only way to solve for the individual signal intensity components of each of the N_{PE} voxels in the column is to generate N_{PE} separate equations expressing different relationships between the voxel signals.

For example, with a zero phase-encoding gradient, all magnetization vectors in a given column remain in phase. Hence, the Fourier transformation of the resulting echo will equal the sum of signals from all voxels in each column (all coefficients = 1). For the first column, the amplitude of the frequency component corresponding to this location would be $A = a_1 + a_2 + a_3 + \cdots + a_{128}$. Whether most of the signal is coming from the front/anterior voxels (a_1, a_2, ...) or from the back/posterior (... a_{127}, a_{128}), is unknown thus far.

To solve for the 128 unknown values of any given column, such as a_1, a_2, a_3, ..., a_{128}, another 127 versions of the equations with these unknowns are needed, each of which must express some other combination of a_1, a_2, a_3, ..., a_{128} with different coefficients. Each different phase-encoding step accomplishes this goal. As illustrated in the 3×2 example, a strong phase-encoding gradient can be designed to induce a $180°$ phase shift from voxel to voxel in any given column, so that the resulting signal measured would be $a_1 - a_2 + a_3 - \cdots - a_{128}$ for column A (coefficients $+1$, -1, $+1$, etc).

Once all 128 phase-encoding steps have produced 128 distinct equations, all 128 unknowns for each column can be solved for, and spatial localization achieved! The array then can be converted to a gray-scale image, which is the MR image.

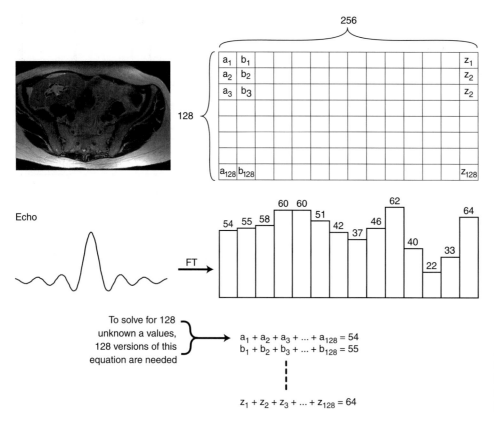

FIGURE I5-25. The phase-encoding challenge. The result applying a zero phase-encoding gradient is illustrated.

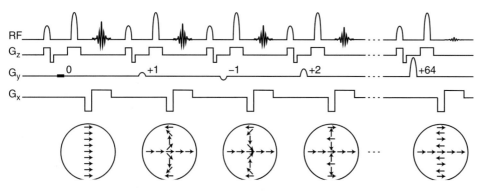

FIGURE I5-26. Phase-encoding steps. The effects of different phase-encoding steps on the phase difference across protons in the y direction are shown.

> **IMPORTANT CONCEPT:** The number of voxels in the phase-encoding direction, N_{PE}, determines the number of times different echoes must be generated in order to perform spatial localization in the phase-encoding direction.

Phase-Encoding Gradients and Phase Shifts

For a typical imaging matrix, say 128 or 256 voxels in the y direction, then 128 or 256 different phase-encoding steps are needed for spatial localization. How are the phase-encoding gradients varied from step to step?

A phase-encoding gradient of zero is always used for one step. Then each increment in phase-encoding is defined so that the gradient causes a relative phase shift of a multiple of 360° across the entire y direction of the image. That is, for a phase-encoding step of 1, the phase shift is +360° (from −180° to +180°) from one end of the image to the other in the y direction, while for a phase-encoding step of −1, the phase shift is −360° (from +180° to −180°) (Figure I5-26). A phase-encoding step of +2 causes a phase shift of +720° (from −360° to +360). A phase-encoding step of +3 causes a phase shift of +1080° (from −540° to +540°), and so on. For 128 phase-encoding steps, the phase-encoding steps typically range from −63 to +64. For the ultimate phase-encoding step of +64, the total phase shift of +64 × 360° across the 128 voxels in the y direction works out to a 180° phase shift between each two adjacent voxels. This highest phase-encoding step demands the maximum phase-encoding gradient strength.

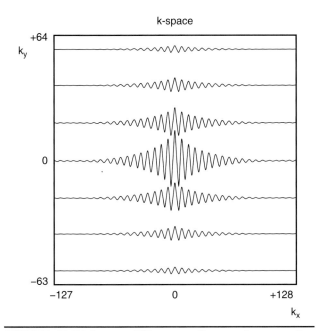

FIGURE I5-27. k-space filling according to phase-encoding step. Echoes with greatest amplitude, associated with minimal or no phase-encoding gradients, are used to fill the central lines of k-space, whereas the higher phase-encoding steps are used to fill the edges of k-space.

CHALLENGE QUESTION: Which phase-encoding step results in the maximum amplitude echo?

Answer: The phase-encoding step with no phase-encoding gradient generates the strongest echo, because with no phase-encoding gradient, there is no phase shift across voxels in the y direction. The echo equals the sum of all the signal amplitudes along y.

Phase-Encoding Steps and k-Space Filling

As described in Chapter I-1, each echo fills one line of the 2D data space called k-space. Depending on the phase-encoding gradient used, each echo differs from the next. For example, the echo with the greatest magnitude is usually that associated with zero phase-encoding gradient. The echoes associated with higher phase-encoding gradients are usually lower in amplitude because of the induced dephasing. As will be discussed in the next chapter, the order in which k-space is filled with each echo is specifically defined (Figure I5-27). The central line of k-space corresponds to zero phase-encoding gradient. Around the central lines are the echoes from phase-encoding steps 1 and −1 (weak gradients). Next the ±2 phase-encoding step echoes are stored, and so on, with the highest-order phase-encoding step echoes (−63 and +64) stored at the very edges of k-space. When filled in this way, the Fourier transform of k-space will produce the desired MR image.

Why Are Higher Phase-Encoding Gradient Steps Considered Important for Fine Image Detail?

With the highest phase-encoding gradients, the phase shift of adjacent voxels approaches 180°. If tissue in the column is homogeneous, that is, all protons have the same amplitude, then the net signal from the image will be negligible because magnetic moments oriented in opposite directions will cancel. Only at sharply defined edges or where there are fine variations in signal, such as small blood vessels, will there be signal at high phase-encoding steps. This is why the periphery of k-space is edge-determining and contains the information about fine details or edges.

> **IMPORTANT CONCEPT:** The signals with the highest amplitude are located in the center of k-space, while the periphery of k-space contains signal that is most sensitive to sharply defined edges and fine details.

Pulse Sequence Diagrams for Spin Echo and Gradient Echo MRI

For both spin echo and gradient echo imaging, the phase-encoding gradient is applied only briefly and not during the RF excitation or echo sampling. To indicate the changing G_y amplitudes for each RF excitation, a standard symbol is used for phase-encoding gradients, as illustrated in Figure I5-14.

THREE-DIMENSIONAL MRI SPATIAL LOCALIZATION

So far, the discussion of spatial localization has assumed that imaging is confined to a 2D slice. With 3D imaging, spatial localization is even more challenging.

RF excitation is performed using a nonselective or a slab-selective pulse. An axial slab can be selectively excited by applying a gradient applied in the z direction during the RF pulse. Alternatively, if no gradient is applied during the RF pulse, then an RF pulse at 64 MHz will excite the entire volume of tissue in the magnetic field.

CHALLENGE QUESTION: How will the characteristics of a slab-selective RF pulse will be different for a wide 3D slab compared with a thin 2D slice?

Answer: The RF pulse will have to excite a wider range of frequencies (higher or wider transmitter bandwidth). Therefore it will have a narrower, more compact appearance compared with a low-bandwidth 2D excitation pulse.

Because an entire volume of tissues is excited by the RF pulse, spatial localization requires determining the individual voxel contributions from the entire volume in all

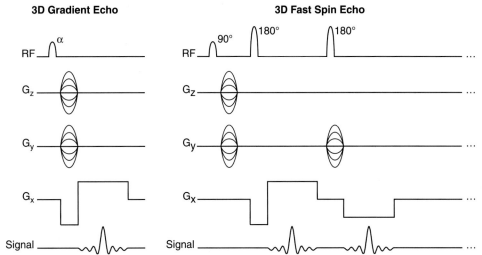

3D Gradient Echo   **3D Fast Spin Echo**

FIGURE I5-28. 3D Gradient echo and spin echo pulse sequence diagram, where both z and y gradients are used to achieve phase encoding.

three dimensions. Strategies employ frequency-encoding gradients during the echo for localization in one dimension and two sets of phase-encoding steps, N_{PE1} and N_{PE2}, for the other two. Because each phase-encoding step in one dimension requires a full set of phase-encoding steps in the other, the total acquisition times for 3D imaging are increased by a factor of N_{PE2} over 2D methods.

Typical pulse sequence diagrams for 3D gradient echo and spin echo sequences are shown in Figure I5-28. Because of time demands with spin echo sequences, 3D strategies usually use high-echo-train fast spin echo methods. As will be discussed in Chapter I-8, for both spin echo and gradient echo approaches, the goal is to minimize the number of phase-encoding steps to keep acquisition times feasible for routine clinical application.

REVIEW QUESTIONS

1. For detection of subtle atheromatous plaque in the aorta, thin-section ECG-gated spin echo imaging is desired. Consider the effect of gradient strength on transmitter bandwidth, RF excitation, and slice profile.

   a. Using a 1.5 T system with a 10 mT/m maximum gradient strength, the RF pulse uses a 2.13 kHz (or ±1.07 kHz) transmitter bandwidth to generate a 5 mm slice. A two-period RF pulse is used, which takes 1 msec. What is a reasonable interslice gap to minimize the effects of cross-talk?

   b. With a hardware upgrade, the maximum gradient strength is now increased to 20 mT/m. You decide that the benefits of this improved gradient strength

should be focused on reducing the slice thickness. What is the minimum slice thickness you can obtain with the same transmitter bandwidth with this stronger gradient strength? Draw the appearance of the RF pulse at the higher gradient strength? What interslice gap should you use? Use Figure I5-Q1A.

   c. Images with the slice thickness used in part b do not have sufficient signal-to-noise ratios to be interpretable. You increase the slice thickness back to 5 mm, keeping the gradient strength of 20 mT/m. You notice that the minimum interslice gap (distance factor) recommended by the system has decreased. Why is this?

   d. In most cases, the interslice gap is small compared to the imaging slice and can be ignored. However, in some settings, complete imaging coverage of the entire region is desired (for example, if detection of a small lesion is important). How can the imaging protocol be modified to ensure that all portions of the aorta are completely imaged?

2. For gadolinium-enhanced MR angiography, a 3D gradient echo sequence is needed. Consider the effects of different gradient strengths on receiver bandwidth, sampling frequency, and imaging times.

   a. With a 10 mT/m maximum gradient strength, the TR of the sequence is 8 msec and TE is 2.4 msec. For a field of view of 50 cm (0.5 m), what is the receiver bandwidth when the maximum frequency-encoding gradient is used?

   b. What will be the receiver bandwidth following a gradient upgrade to 20 mT/m?

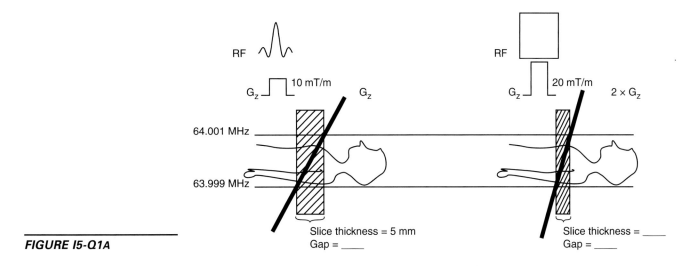

FIGURE I5-Q1A

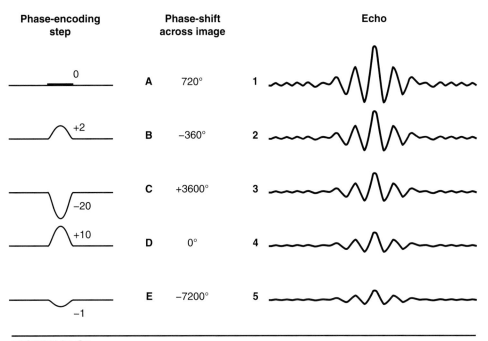

FIGURE I5-Q3

c. The minimum TR and TE for the same sequence and stronger 20 mT/m gradient are now 5 msec and 1.6 msec. Explain why.

3. In Figure I5-Q3, match the phase-encoding step to the resulting phase shift of magnetic moments in the y direction and to the corresponding echo measured for an image with 128 voxels in the phase-encoding direction.

k-Space

k-space is the name of the place where MR echoes are stored. As introduced in Chapter I-1, one of the miracles of MRI is that k-space turns out to be the Fourier transformation of the original tissue slice. Because of the duality property (as discussed in Chapter I-1), taking the Fourier transformation of k-space then gives back a representation of the tissue slice, called the MR image (Figure I6-1).

So far, the pulse sequence diagram has been explained with the sole purpose of addressing spatial localization. To grasp many of the more advanced concepts in MR physics, a more profound understanding of k-space and its relationship with the pulse sequence diagram is necessary. This chapter focuses on how the application of the gradients described in the pulse sequence diagram produces echoes that represent the Fourier transform of the tissue slice. With this knowledge, more innovative and complex ways of filling k-space can be explored. Combined with a greater understanding of the relationship between k-space and the image discussed in Chapter I-7. The reader will then be equipped to understand the fast imaging techniques that are commonly used in cardiovascular MRI, the "k-space shortcuts," to be presented in Chapter I-8.

KEY CONCEPTS

▶ k-space is the Fourier transformation of the tissue slice and of the MR image.

▶ A simplified version of the Fourier transformation $H(k_x, k_y)$ of an image $h(x, y)$ can be expressed in terms of its mathematical formula, $H(k_x, k_y) = \int_{-\infty}^{\infty} h(x, y)\cos(k_x x + k_y y)dxdy$.

▶ Gradient-induced phase shifts can be represented as a sinusoidal modulation of the phases of magnetization vectors. The modulation can be expressed as $\cos k_x x$ or $\cos k_y y$, where k_x and k_y are proportional to the areas under the gradient waveforms, G_x and G_y, respectively. During application of a gradient, such as G_x, the value of k_x changes continuously, since k_x is proportional to $G_x \times t$.

▶ Application of gradients and summation of signal using receiver coils effectively generate the Fourier transform of an image.

▶ Pulse sequence diagrams describe the recipe for generating an MR image in terms of the k-space trajectory.

▶ To improve the efficiency of a k-space trajectory, portions that do not involve data sampling should be traversed as rapidly as possible.

▶ k-space trajectories can be designed to suit different demands for efficiency and image quality.

WHAT IS k-SPACE?

In this chapter, k-space is defined as the Fourier transform of the tissue slice or the MR image. The reader is encouraged to review the part in Chapter I-1 on Fourier transformations and, in particular, Figures I1-28 and I1-29, for a qualitative understanding of Fourier transforms as spatial frequency maps. This section presents a more quantitative definition of the Fourier transformation.

In two dimensions, the Fourier transform $H(k_x, k_y)$ of an image $h(x,y)$ can be expressed as

$$H(k_x, k_y) = \int_{-\infty}^{\infty} h(x,y)\cos(k_x x + k_y y)dx\,dy$$

This equation describes how to obtain the Fourier transform of an image. (Strictly speaking, the full form of the Fourier transform is

$$H(k_x, k_y) = \int_{-\infty}^{\infty} h(x,y)e^{-i(k_x x + k_y y)}dxdy$$
$$= \int_{-\infty}^{\infty} h(x,y)\,[\cos(k_x x + k_y y)$$
$$- i\sin(k_x x + k_y y)]dx\,dy$$

where i is the imaginary number $\sqrt{-1}$. The sine term has imaginary values and is ignored in this book to simplify the equation.) Before the meaning and implications of this equation are explored, the terms $h(x,y)$ and $H(k_x, k_y)$ must be explained in greater detail.

The expression $h(x, y)$ refers to the spatial distribution of signal intensities in an image, for example, a tissue slice

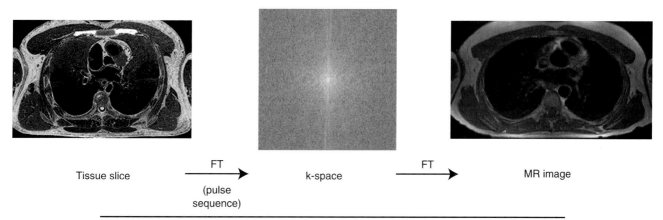

Tissue slice $\xrightarrow[\text{(pulse sequence)}]{\text{FT}}$ k-space $\xrightarrow{\text{FT}}$ MR image

FIGURE I6-1. k-space. MR image generation involves filling k-space with the intensities of measured echoes, followed by a Fourier transformation that recreates an image representation of the original tissue slice. (Note that, as discussed in Chapter I-1, for simplicity, the Fourier transformation and inverse Fourier transformation are considered identical.)

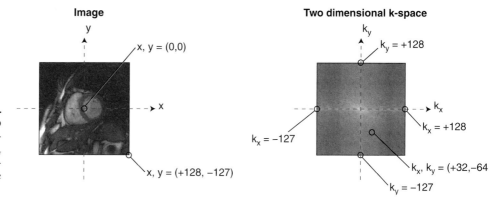

FIGURE I6-2. k-space in two and three dimensions. In k-space, the axes are k_x and k_y (and k_z) representing spatial frequencies with units of inverse distance.

or an MR image. Either can be thought of as a grid or array of numbers, where at each pair of coordinates in the array, (x,y), the value of the intensity at that location has a value equal to h(x,y). In the case of an MR image, the intensity values at each location h(x,y) depends on the interplay between intrinsic tissue properties such as T1 and T2 relaxation times and MR pulse sequence parameters such as TR, TE, and flip angle. The coordinates of the image space, h(x,y), are usually centered at location (x,y) = (0,0), so that for a 256 × 256 matrix image, x values would range from −127 to +128, and y values would also range from −127 to +128 (Figure I6-2). Based on the size of each voxel, x and y can also be expressed in units of distance (cm, for example).

The expression for k-space, $H(k_x,k_y)$, similarly refers to a grid or array of numbers (Figure I6-2). The coordinates in k-space are defined in terms of (k_x, k_y), where k_x corresponds to the spatial frequency $\cos k_x x$ and k_y the spatial frequency $\cos k_y y$. The units of the spatial frequencies, k_x and k_y, are usually given in inverse distance (1/cm or cycles per cm). At each coordinate in the grid, the value of the intensity at that point equals $H(k_x,k_y)$ and reflects how much of the spatial frequency component, $\cos(k_x x + k_y y)$,

is contained in the image. The coordinates of k-space are usually centered at location (k_x,k_y) = (0,0), so that for a 256 × 256 k-space matrix, k_x would range from −127 to +128 and k_y also from −127 to +128 (Figure I6-2).

To illustrate the relationship between h(x, y) and $H(k_x,k_y)$, consider the image of a wavy potato chip or piece of corrugated cardboard tilted off axis depicted in Figure I6-3. Mathematically, this image can be defined by the following function:

$$h(x, y) = 9 \cos (3x + 5y)$$

which means that the value of the intensity of the image at every location (x,y) can be calculated by plugging in values of x and y into the expression 9 cos (3x + 5y).

To derive the Fourier transformation or spatial frequency map of this image, observe that the overall spatial variation in the image is defined simply as cos (3x + 5y). This means that the only spatial frequency that is needed to describe this function has k_x = 3 and k_y = 5. That is, the Fourier transformation has only a spike at one location, (k_x,k_y) = (3,5). The value of $H(k_x,k_y)$ at that location, H(3,5), would be equal to the amplitude of the sinusoidal

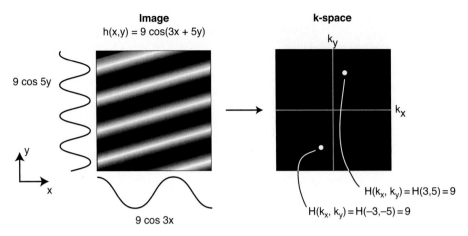

Image
h(x,y) = 9 cos(3x + 5y)

9 cos 5y

9 cos 3x

k-space

k_y

k_x

H(k_x, k_y) = H(3,5) = 9

H(k_x, k_y) = H(−3,−5) = 9

FIGURE I6-3. Image of the function h(x, y) = 9 cos(3x + 5y) (left) and its corresponding Fourier transform (or k-space) map (right). The amplitudes of the values throughout k-space, (k_x,k_y), equal zero except where (k_x,k_y) = (3,5) and (−3,−5), where the values are 9.

function in the image, which reflects how high the peaks and deep the grooves are in the surface. In the example, the amplitude is 9, and therefore H(k_x, k_y) = H(3, 5) = 9. Note that because of the symmetry of cosine functions (cos(−x) = cosx), there is another nonzero value in k-space at (−3,−5), as shown in Figure I6-3.

In the Fourier transform equation, the integral sign, $\int_{-\infty}^{\infty}$, indicates that the expression between the $\int_{-\infty}^{\infty}$ and the dx dy should be summed for all values of x and y. Therefore, the equation says that the value of the Fourier transform, H(k_x,k_y), of an image, h(x,y) can be calculated by multiplying each intensity value in the image by a sinusoidal function, cos (k_xx + k_yy), and then taking the integral for all values of x and y.

Translated into words, this equation says that *to determine the value of k-space at a particular frequency, k_x, k_y, the image must be multiplied by cos(k_xx + k_yy) and then summed up for all values x and y across the entire image.*

The next section will show how the gradients and receiver coil are used to perform the calculation.

> **IMPORTANT CONCEPT**: By definition, the value of k-space at a particular k_x, k_y can be determined by performing two steps: (1) multiplying the image by cos(k_xx + k_yy) and then (2) summing the value of all the signal across the entire image.

HOW AN MR PULSE SEQUENCE CONVERTS A TISSUE SLICE INTO ITS FOURIER TRANSFORM (k-SPACE)

There are two steps to getting the Fourier transform of a tissue slice, that is, k-space. The first step is to apply frequency- and phase-encoding gradients. The second step is to use the receiver coil to collect all of the signal across the tissue slice, that is, to sum up all the signal from all the protons in the slice. This section will show how applying gradients effectively multiplies the image by

cosine functions and how the receiver coil essentially integrates or sums the resulting product.

Application of a Gradient = Multiplying the Image by a Cosine Function

With the application of a linear gradient across the field of view, the varying magnetic field strength causes protons to precess at different frequencies, and consequently a phase shift across protons accumulates. As illustrated in Figure I6-4, phase shifts can be expressed as a sinusoidal modulation of the phases, so that the effect of a gradient can be seen as multiplying the original magnetization vectors by a cosine function along the direction of the gradient. In Figure I6-4, the gradient induces a phase shift of 720° along the column of tissue. The resulting pattern of magnetization vectors is simply equal to the original magnetization vectors multiplied by the function, cos 2y. Note that the amplitudes of the magnetization vectors reflect the relationship between tissue properties and MR pulse sequence parameters and are unaffected by the gradient. Only their orientations or directions are modulated.

For the purposes of translating this concept into an understanding of k-space, the frequency of the sinusoidal change in phase is called "k." For example, in Figure I6-4, k_y = 2.

The longer the gradient stays on, the greater phase dispersion. Initially, the phase shifts will be slight, corresponding to a low-frequency cosine modulation of phases. If the gradient is strong, then the phase shifts will increase more quickly over time (Figure I6-5). Translated in terms of k, which is defined as the frequency of the sinusoidal function that is induced by the gradients, the longer the gradient is left on, the larger the k. The stronger the gradient, the faster k will increase.

CHALLENGE QUESTION: What is the effect of applying no phase-encoding gradient?

Answer: Multiplying cos 0y or cos 0 is the equivalent to multiplying by 1. (Recall from Chapter I-1 that cos 0 equals 1.) This reflects the

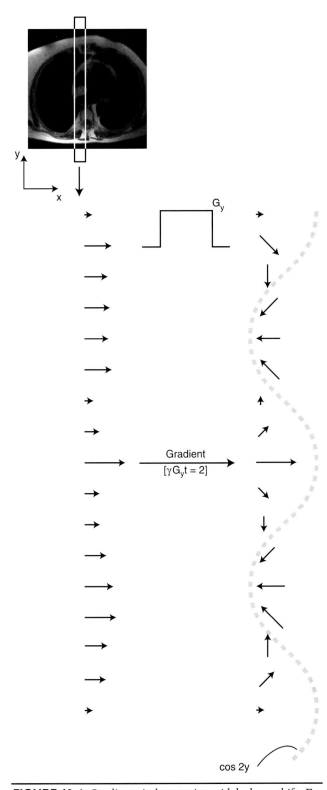

FIGURE I6-4. Gradients induce a sinusoidal phase shift. For example, a gradient in the y direction that causes phase shift of 720° (two full cycles of 360°) has the effect of multiplying the original magnetization vectors by cos 2y. The magnitudes of the vectors along the column of tissue vary, according to the signal intensities of the tissues.

fact that magnetic moments retain their original magnitude and phase with zero phase-encoding gradient.

> **IMPORTANT CONCEPT:** Gradients cause dephasing. The gradient-induced phase shifts can be represented as a sinusoidal modulation in phase. The stronger the gradient and the longer its duration, the greater the sinusoidal variation.

The observations about gradients in the y direction also hold true for gradients in the x direction. With G_x, the dephasing across the x direction can be expressed as the original magnetic moments being multiplied by cos $k_x x$, where the coefficient k_x describes the sinusoidal variation of the cosine function in the x direction. k_x will progressively increase the longer the gradient G_x is left on.

$k_{x,y}$ Proportional to the Area under the $G_{x,y}$ Gradient Curve

As discussed in Chapter I-4 (Figure I4-3), the amount of dephasing caused by a gradient is proportional to the area under the gradient curve. The gradient pulse is of constant strength, described by its strength, G, and has duration, t. The net effect of any gradient is $G \times t$.

In this chapter, dephasing is expressed more specifically in mathematical terms as a multiplication of the original signal by a sinusoidal function, cos $k_x x$ or cos $k_y y$, where the coefficients, k_x and k_y, represent the frequency of the sinusoidal modulation. It follows that, as measures of dephasing, k_x and k_y are proportional to the areas under their respective gradient curves (Figure I6-6):

$$k_x = G_x \times t \times \gamma$$
$$k_y = G_y \times t \times \gamma$$

Each gradient acts independently by modulating the dephasing in different directions. The gradients can be applied simultaneously or sequentially. Gradients can have reversed polarity and cause phase shifts that are reversed in direction, corresponding to negative values of k. With negative gradients, the stronger the negative gradient, the more negative the k values.

The Elusive, Ever-Changing k

While a gradient is on, the dephasing is cumulative, and k values (k_x or k_y) will continuously change. When the gradient is positive, k progressively increases over time. When the gradient is negative, k progressively decreases. When the gradient is turned off, the phase differences are maintained because the protons return to precessing at

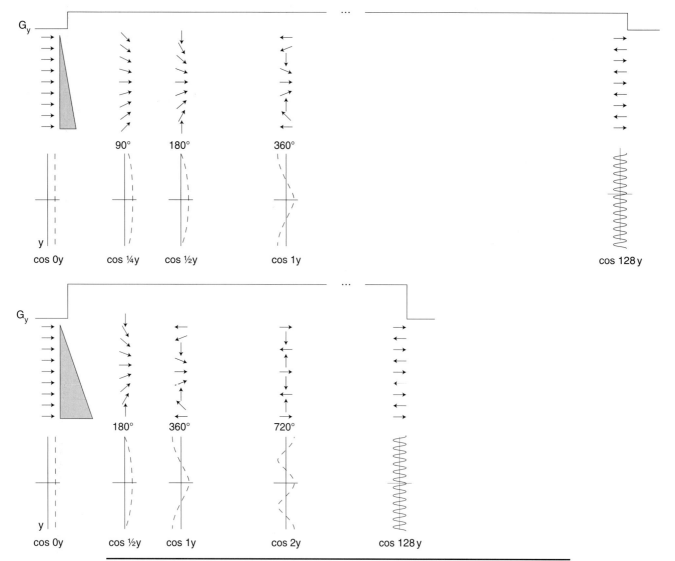

FIGURE I6-5. Gradients and sindusoidal modulation of phase shifts. Phase shifts can be represented as the original magnetic moments multiplied by a sinusoidal function whose frequency increases as the gradient strength and duration increase. Using a gradient that is twice as strong, the maximum phase shift is achieved in half the time (below). As depicted in Figure I6-4, the magnetic moments will vary in amplitude, depending on properties such as proton density, T1 relaxation, and T2 relaxation. For simplicity these variations are ignored.

the same 64 MHz frequency. Given that their phase dispersion stays the same, k maintains the same value it had at the instant the gradient was turned off.

> **IMPORTANT CONCEPT:** The dephasing effect of a gradient is equivalent to modulating the phase by a sinusoidal function, $\cos k_x x$ or $\cos k_y y$, where k_x and k_y are proportional to the area under the gradient waveforms, G_x and G_y, respectively. While a gradient such as G_x is on, the value of k_x changes continuously, because k_x is proportional to $G_x \times t$.

Integration by the Receiver Coil

During the readout period, as the echo is being formed, data are collected by the receiver coil. The measured signal depends on the cumulative contributions of all protons in the field. The coil effectively *sums* all signals from all protons.

The signals being emitted by the protons represent the magnetization vectors modulated by the sinusoidal function induced by the gradients. Therefore, when the receiver coil records signal, it is equivalent to measuring the sum of signals from the original tissue multiplied by a cosine function. These words ring some bells. They are the definition of the Fourier transform!

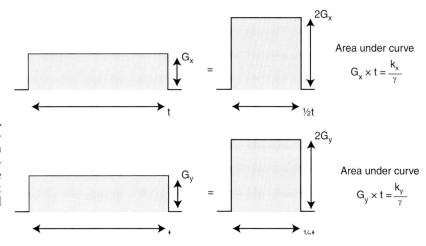

FIGURE I6-6. Relationship between gradients and the resulting sinusoidal modulation of the signal by cos $k_x x$ or cos $k_y y$. The frequency of the sinusoidal modulation of phase is proportional to the area under the gradient curve, which depends on its amplitude and duration.

Summary: Gradients + Receiver Coil = Fourier Transform

By applying gradients in the x and y directions and by using a receiver coil to collect or sum up all of the signal, the MR system creates a Fourier transform of the tissue slice.

> **IMPORTANT CONCEPT:** Applying gradients is the same as multiplying the image by cosine functions, while the receiver coil effectively sums the resulting product. The combination of gradients and receiver coils generates the Fourier transform of the tissue slice, or k-space.

READING PULSE SEQUENCE DIAGRAMS: THE k-SPACE TRAJECTORY

To fill k-space, values for all combinations of k_x and k_y are needed. For example, for a 256 × 256 image matrix, a full k-space matrix with dimensions of at least 256 × 256 must be filled. How can this be achieved?

k_x and k_y are proportional to the areas under the G_x and G_y gradient waveforms. To fill k-space, signal must be collected by the receiver coil at times when areas under G_x cause sinusoidal modulations of frequency k_x varying from −127 to +128 and areas under G_y cause k_y to vary from −127 to +128, and all combinations thereof. The different ways in which this can be achieved define the *k-space trajectory*.

The term *k-space trajectory* refers to the manner in which k-space is filled (Figure I6-7). For example, horizontal lines of k-space may be filled one at a time, as introduced in the previous chapter, known as a *linear k-space trajectory*. Each line of k-space represents a separate echo collected during a given phase-encoding step with application of a frequency-encoding gradient. With conventional linear k-space trajectories, the sampling of data is evenly distributed across k-space. Other k-space

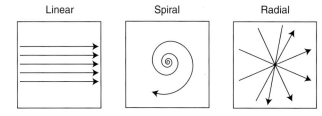

FIGURE I6-7. k-space trajectories. Alternative approaches to filling k-space, such as spiral or radial trajectories, provide advantages over linear filling.

trajectories may offer more efficient or desirable ways of collecting k-space data. For example, a *spiral k-space trajectory* describes the filling of k-space along a spiral pattern. This trajectory can be used to *oversample* the center of k-space relative to the periphery. Another approach is to fill k-space with a series of diagonal lines traversing near or through the center, a method referred to as a *radial k-space trajectory*. These alternative strategies favor sampling of the center of k-space and can be used to improve the efficiency of k-space filling compared to linear trajectories.

Since the rectilinear trajectories are the simplest, this section will start with these conventional approaches before presenting newer methods. The analysis will proceed by way of examples.

Linear k-Space Trajectories

Following are three examples of linear k-space trajectories.

■ Example 1

Consider the pulse sequence diagram in Figure I6-8, which depicts a gradient echo sequence. In this example, no phase-encoding gradient is applied ($G_y = 0$). The frequency-encoding gradient, G_x, has a positive lobe. Let k-space have dimensions of 256 × 256. The

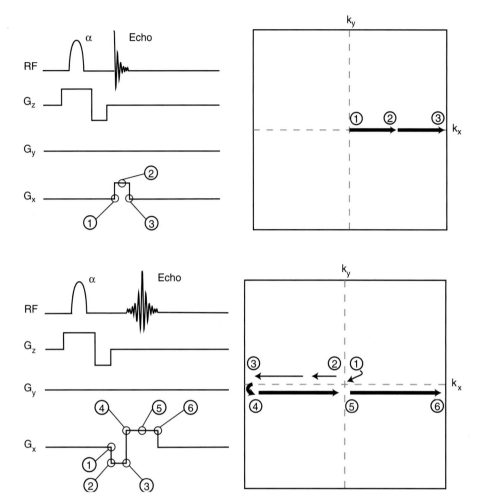

FIGURE 16-8. Pulse sequence diagram and corresponding k-space trajectory for no G_y and simple positive G_x.

FIGURE 16-9. Pulse sequence diagram and corresponding k-space trajectory for a gradient G_x with a dephasing lobe, one step of a typical gradient echo sequence.

k-space trajectory for this portion of a pulse sequence is shown in the k-space diagram at the right of the figure.

Time Point 1: At time point 1, since no gradients have been applied in either the x or y direction, $G_x = 0$ and $G_y = 0$; therefore k_x and k_y (corresponding to areas under their respective gradient curves) are both equal to zero. Hence, the k-space trajectory starts in the center of k-space. Because there is no G_y gradient, k_y is equal to zero for this trajectory.

Time Point 2: Once the G_x gradient is applied, the value of k_x will start to increase. Its value will be proportional to $G_x \times t$, the area under the G_x curve. Midway through the pulse, at time point 2, k_x will be +64.

Time Point 3: At the end of the pulse, time point 3, $k_x = +128$.

In summary, the k-space trajectory for this portion of the pulse sequence diagram will start in the center of k-space and then traverse along the x axis to the right (positive) edge of k-space. If the echo is sampled during the application of the G_x gradient, then the values can be used to fill k-space from $k_x = 0$ to $+128$. The value of k_y remains 0. ■

■ Example 2

For a typical gradient echo pulse sequence, the readout gradient has a dephasing lobe before the positive gradient. Figure 16-9 describes the k-space trajectory of this part of a typical gradient echo sequence.

Time Point 1: At time point 1, no gradients have been applied in either the x or y direction, so k_x and k_y are both equal to zero. The k-space trajectory again starts in the center of k-space. Because no G_y gradient is applied, k_y is always equal to zero for this trajectory.

Time Point 2: In this example, G_x starts with a dephasing lobe, and therefore the value of k_x will start to decrease to a negative value starting from time point 2. k_x will be proportional to $G_x \times t$, where G_x has a negative value.

Time Point 3: If the G_x gradient pulse is designed properly, then at the end of the dephasing lobe, at time point 3, the value of k_x will be -127.

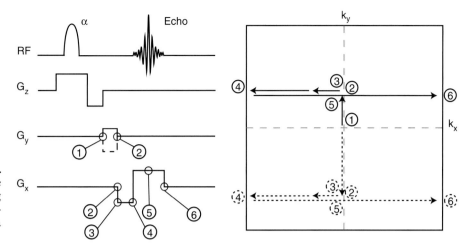

FIGURE I6-10. Pulse sequence diagram and corresponding k-space trajectories for two different phase-encoding steps of a typical gradient echo sequence.

Time Point 4: The G_x is now reversed. Because it is positive, the cumulative area under the G_x gradient pulse will now start to increase, starting at time point 4.

Time Point 5: When the area under the positive lobe of G_x equals the area under the negative lobe of G_x, the k-space trajectory will again pass through the center of k-space because the net area under the G_x curve will be zero (time point 5).

Time Point 6: The k-space trajectory will continue in the positive x direction until the gradient is turned off. This would typically be at the point where the cumulative area under the G_x curve is proportional to $k_x = +128$.

In summary, in this example, the k-space trajectory will start in the center of k-space and then traverse along the negative direction along the x axis out to the left edge of k-space. With gradient reversal, the trajectory reverses direction and moves in the positive direction along x until it reaches the right edge of k-space. It is during the positive lobe of G_x that the echo is sampled (time points 4, 5, and 6) and used to fill the single line of k-space (bolded line). The portion of the trajectory from time point 1 through time point 3 does not contribute to filling of k-space. This travel to the leftward most part of k-space is made in preparation for collection of the echo. ∎

■ Example 3

Now consider two parts of a conventional gradient echo pulse sequence, one with a positive phase-encoding gradient (solid line in Figure I6-10) and another with a negative phase-encoding gradient (dashed line). Figure I6-10 analyzes the corresponding two k-space trajectories.

Time Point 1: At time point 1, since no gradients have been applied, k_x and k_y are both equal to zero. The phase-encoding gradient, G_y (solid line), is first applied with positive amplitude for a short duration, causing k_y to increase in value proportional to $G_y \times t$, say, $k_y = 50$.

Time Point 2: At the end of the phase-encoding pulse, k_x is still 0. While G_y is off, k_y will remain at a value of $+50$ and will not change.

Time Points 3–6: As in Example 2, the trajectory of k_x will take a negative course with the dephasing lobe (time points 3–4). Then, during the readout period, while the positive G_x is applied, the trajectory will span the extent of k_x from -127 to $+128$ (time points 4–6).

Time Points 1–6, G_y Negative: In the second case, the negative phase-encoding gradient results in $k_y = -100$. The trajectory is shown as a dashed line in Figure I6-10. ∎

What Is Filling k-Space?

The path of the k-space trajectory depends on the gradients. During some or most of the trajectory, data are collected and used to fill k-space. However, other parts of the trajectory may be considered simply as travel time, when no signal is sampled. During data sampling, k-space is filled with the values of the spin echo or gradient echo as measured by the receiver coil and subsequently digitized by the ADC (Figure I6-11), as discussed in Chapter I-5.

k-space is a 2D array of numbers, and values occupying each point in k-space are often depicted as dots of varying brightness (as in Chapter I-1, Figures I1-30 and I1-31). The brighter the dot, the higher that value of k-space. Because the center of the echo usually corresponds to the center of k-space, it usually has the brightest dots or highest values.

For complete filling of k-space with a linear trajectory, the total number of k_y lines, N_{PE}, determines the number of times the pulse sequence must be repeated. For each repetition, the phase-encoding gradient is varied to achieve the desired range of k_y values. Negative G_y lobes accomplish the filling of the lower half of k-space, while positive lobes fill the upper half (as in Example 3).

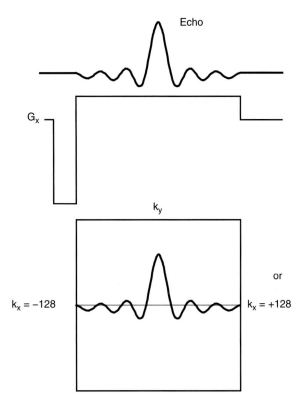

Echo

G_x

k_y

$k_x = -128$ $k_x = +128$

or

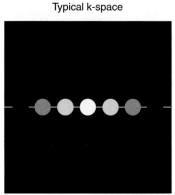

Typical k-space

FIGURE I6-11. The sampled echo is used to fill a line of k-space. The values that fill k-space are sampled from the spin echo or gradient echo, measured using the receiver coil. The magnitude of the sampled signal can be represented as dots with varying intensity (right).

Making the k-Space Trajectory More Efficient

During portions of the k-space trajectory when no data are being collected, such as the dephasing lobe of a linear trajectory, the time spent does not contribute to the resulting image quality. The sole purpose of the dephasing lobe is to get to the left hand edge of k-space; no signal measurements are taken. In terms of efficiency, to get to a k_x value of -127 in the shortest possible time, G_x should be maximized. In Example 2, the dephasing lobe should use the maximum gradient strength to minimize the time needed for dephasing.

CHALLENGE QUESTION: How can the pulse sequence illustrated in Figure I6-10 be modified to further reduce the imaging time?

Answer: The duration and timing of the phase- and frequency-encoding gradients add to the imaging time with fast gradient echo sequences. Both the dephasing lobe of the frequency-encoding gradient (G_x) and the phase-encoding lobe (G_y) are "downtime" during which no echoes are sampled. Therefore, it makes sense to shorten these as much as possible. Both gradients, G_x and G_y, can also be applied at the same time (Figure I6-12). To arrive at $k_x = -127$ and $k_y = +50$ as fast as possible, both gradients can be applied simultaneously and at maximum strength so that the trajectory follows a diagonal course from $k_x, k_y = (0,0)$ to $(-127,50)$. With a gradient echo sequence, a more efficient trajectory can reduce the echo times, and consequently the repetition times, enough to make a difference in the overall acquisition times.

IMPORTANT CONCEPT: Portions of the k-space trajectory that do not involve data sampling should be traversed as rapidly and efficiently as possible.

Centric versus Sequential Linear k-Space Trajectories

A linear trajectory can be designed in different ways. As shown in Figure I6-13, the central portions of k-space can be filled first and the edges last, or k-space can be filled linearly from one edge through the center to the other edge. The former is described as *centric* k-space filling, while the latter is termed *sequential*.

CHALLENGE QUESTION: How would the pulse sequence diagrams for centrically ordered versus sequentially ordered linear filling of k-space differ?

Answer: The order of filling is determined by the order in which the different phase-encoding gradients are applied. For centric ordering, the first echo collected would be generated with zero phase-encoding gradient. The second would have a small phase-encoding gradient ($k_y = +1$), the third, a small negative phase-encoding gradient ($k_y = -1$), then a more positive, slightly stronger gradient ($k_y = +2$), a slightly more negative gradient ($k_y = -2$), and so on until $k_y = -127$ and $k_y = +128$. For sequential linear filling of k-space, the first phase-encoding gradient would be at its maximum, $k_y = +128$, and then subsequently would

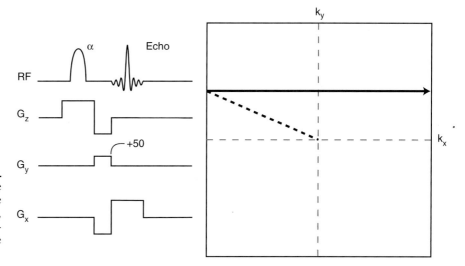

FIGURE I6-12. By synchronizing the rephasing lobe of G_z, the dephasing lobe of G_x, and the phase-encoding blip in G_y, the pulse sequence time can be shortened further, and consequently, the image acquisition time can be reduced.

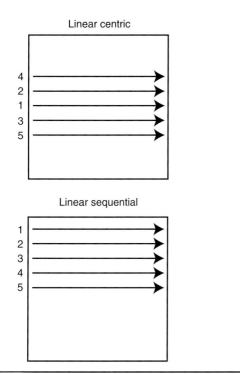

FIGURE I6-13. Linear centric versus linear sequential filling of k-space.

decrease, $k_y = +127$, $k_y = +126,\dots$, $k_y = 0$, $k_y = -1$, $k_y = -2,\dots$, $k_y = -127$.

Other k-Space Trajectories

Once the relationship between gradients and k-space trajectories is understood, many creative ways of designing pulse sequences can be considered. Some of these are discussed here, and others in the Review Questions at the end of this chapter.

Single-Shot Echo Planar Imaging

With single-shot *echo planar imaging (EPI)*, multiple echoes are sampled following a single RF pulse. Rather than filling only one line per RF pulse, all 64 or 128 lines needed for an image are collected following a single RF excitation. The filling of k-space must be highly efficient, otherwise T2* decay will lead to loss of any measurable signal. Hence, the pulse sequence is designed to minimize travel time of the k-space trajectory. One solution is shown in Figure I6-14, which describes a single-shot echo planar trajectory for 128 × 128 image.

Time Point 1: At time point 1, the negative gradients in G_x and G_y bring the trajectory to the lower left corner of k-space ($k_x = -63$, $k_y = -63$).

Time Interval 2: During time interval 2, G_y is off, so k_y remains −63. The positive lobe of G_x (with area +128) causes the trajectory to pass from $k_x = -63$ to $k_x = +64$.

Time Point 3: A small positive "blip" in G_y (area = +1) shifts the value of k_y from −63 to −62. Since G_x is zero, k_x stays at 64.

Time Interval 4: The G_x gradient now reverses. Because it is negative, the cumulative area under the G_x gradient pulse will now start to decrease, passing to through zero and reaching −63.

Time Interval 5: Following another blip in G_y, the trajectory fills the $k_y = -61$ line, and so on.

The trajectory starts in one corner of k-space and uses small phase-encoding gradients to "blip" from one line to the next. The readout gradient along x alternates between the positive and negative directions. The echo planar trajectory is extremely efficient. Except for the initial negative lobes of G_x and G_y and the short G_y blips, echoes are sampled almost continuously throughout this k-space trajectory.

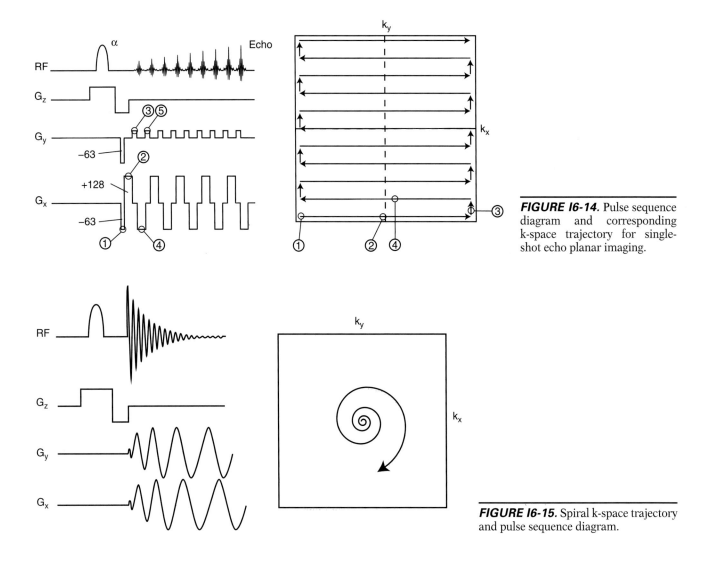

FIGURE I6-14. Pulse sequence diagram and corresponding k-space trajectory for single-shot echo planar imaging.

FIGURE I6-15. Spiral k-space trajectory and pulse sequence diagram.

Spiral Trajectory

The central portions of k-space contain most of the information about image contrast, while the periphery of k-space encodes high-resolution details. As will be shown in the next chapter, most of the information content of an image is contained in the low-spatial-frequency portion of k-space. Therefore, many sequences have been designed to sample the central portions of k-space preferentially over the periphery for better image quality in shorter acquisition times. One highly efficient and elegant way of doing this is with a spiral k-space trajectory. A typical pulse sequence diagram and k-space trajectory are shown in Figure I6-15. In addition to oversampling the center of k-space, this method has the advantages that data are collected during the entire k-space trajectory and there is no travel time. Another important attribute is that the sampling of k-space starts at the center of k-space. The interested reader is referred to Question 6 in the Review Questions.

Extrapolating to 3D Imaging

Once the concept of 2D k-space is understood, the extension to 3D comes quite naturally. Before discussing 3D k-space, consider the reasons why 3D imaging might be preferred over 2D imaging.

3D versus 2D Imaging

3D imaging has several advantages over 2D imaging. Because the entire volumetric slab is excited and imaged (Figure I6-16), the slices or partitions that are reconstructed can be thin and without problems of cross-talk and without need for interslice gaps. The thinner partitions also lend themselves well to reconstructions in oblique planes (multiplanar reconstructions).

The primary disadvantage of 3D imaging is time. Because the acquisition times are increased by a factor equal to the number of phase-encoding steps in the second phase-encoding dimension, N_{PE2}, TR times must be

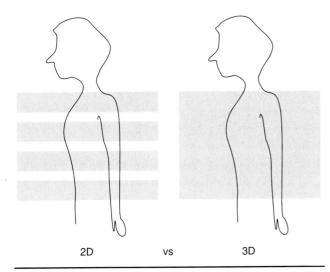

FIGURE I6-16. 2D versus 3D imaging.

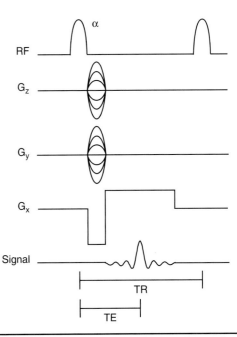

FIGURE I6-17. 3D pulse sequence diagram for gradient echo imaging.

extremely short for sequences to be performed in a reasonable time.

3D Pulse Sequences

For 3D MR imaging, a 3D k-space must be filled, that is, all values for (k_x, k_y, k_z) must be determined. The gradients, G_x and G_y, are typically used in the same way as in a conventional 2D pulse sequence diagram. The third gradient, G_z, is considered a second phase-encoding gradient in the so-called partition direction and is similar to G_y.

A typical pulse sequence diagram for a 3D gradient echo acquisition is shown in Figure I6-17.

Filling k-Space in 3D

The matrix of the 3D k-space typically has the same dimensions as the desired image. For example, to make an image with $256 \times 256 \times 64$ voxels, a k-space with dimensions of at least $256 \times 256 \times 64$ must be filled. The properties of k-space in 3D are the same as those in 2D. The central areas of k-space determine image contrast, and the edges of k-space (defined as the concentric spheres within increasing distances from the center) contain the high-resolution details of the image.

The same relationship between the areas under the gradient curves and locations in k-space apply with 3D as with 2D imaging. In 3D, the area under the third gradient curve, G_z, defines the position along k_z in k-space.

> **IMPORTANT CONCEPT:** In 3D, the area under G_z (partition-encoding gradient) defines positioning along the k_z direction in k-space.

Compare and contrast the following two examples of ways in which 3D k-space can be filled using the same pulse sequence shown in Figure I6-17.

■ 3D Gradient Echo Example 1

If the desired k-space filling order is shown in Figure I6-18, how would the pulse sequence drawn in Figure I6-17 have to be performed? Partition 1, $k_z = +128$, is filled first, then partition 2 ($k_z = +127$) and so on through the 256th partition ($k_z = -127$). The total k-space matrix is $256 \times 256 \times 256$.

Answer: The pulse sequence diagram summarized in Figure I6-17 would need to be played out as shown in Figure I6-19. To fill the first partition, the first G_z would have a maximum positive value so that $k_z = +128$. G_z would have this value for all of the 256 phase-encoding (G_y) steps for the first partition. These 256 steps, known as a *partition loop*, would be configured just like a 2D pulse sequence diagram, with incrementally changing G_y pulses for each step (starting, in this case, with a maximum G_y so that $k_y = +128$, then $+127$, $+126$,..., 0,..., -127) and a standard G_x readout gradient. The next 256 steps of the pulse sequence diagram would be used to fill the second partition, which would have a value of $k_z = +127$. For a $256 \times 256 \times 256$ matrix, this process is repeated 256 times. The acquisition time for a 3D image would be 256 times as long as the corresponding 2D image, provided the TR was kept the same. ■

■ 3D Gradient Echo Example 2

In contrast to 3D Gradient Echo Example 1, what if the desired k-space filling is as shown in Figure I6-20?

Answer: The 3D gradient echo pulse sequence would need to be played out as shown in Figure I6-21.

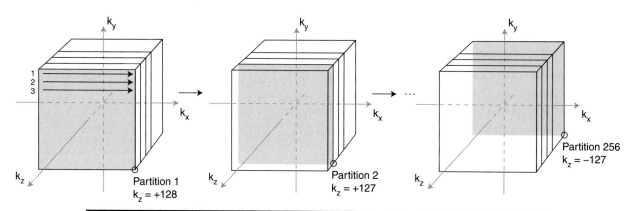

FIGURE I6-18. Linear sequential 3D k-space filling where the desired order of partition filling is shown with shading. Within each partition, the order of phase-encoding steps is sequential, labeled 1, 2, 3,...

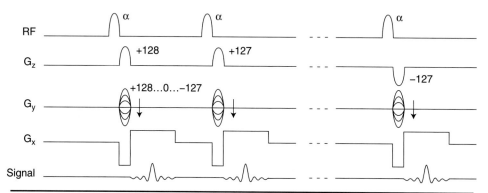

FIGURE I6-19. Pulse sequence diagram for 3D gradient echo sequence with k-space trajectory shown in Figure I6-18. Each set of 256 echoes corresponds to the pulse sequence for a partition, which is referred to as a partition loop. Within each partition loop, the phase-encoding steps are ordered from highest G_y (+128) to lowest G_y (−127), as indicated by the downward arrow.

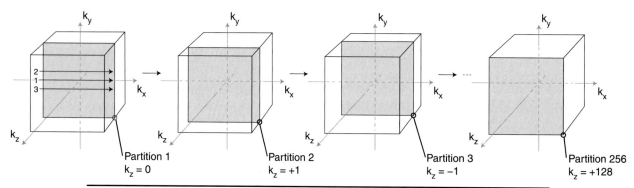

FIGURE I6-20. Linear centric 3D k-space filling where the desired order of partition filling is shown with shading. Within each partition, the order of phase-encoding steps is centric, labeled 1, 2, 3,....

In this case, the ordering of the filling of partitions is centric rather than sequential. The first partition loop would have no G_z ($k_z = 0$). G_y would incrementally change in a centrically ordered fashion (starting, in this case, with a G_y of zero or k_y of zero, $k_y = +1$, $k_y = -1$, and so on), and a G_x would be a conventional readout gradient. The second partition would correspond to a $k_z = 1$, and the next 256 steps of the pulse sequence diagram would be used to fill it, again in a centrically ordered fashion. Then the next partition loop filled would have a $k_z = -1$, followed by $k_z = +2$, −2, +3, and so on until $k_z = +128$. ■

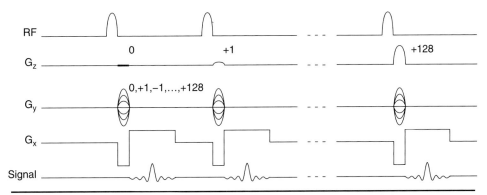

FIGURE I6-21. Pulse sequence diagram for 3D gradient echo sequence with k-space trajectory shown in Figure I6-20. Each set of 256 echoes corresponds to one partition loop (G_z). Within each partition loop, the phase-encoding steps (G_y) are centrically ordered.

Acquisition Times for 2D versus 3D

For a 2D image, the total time required to fill k-space is the number of phase-encoding steps multiplied by the TR ($N_{PE} \times TR$).

With a 3D image, the time required to fill 3D k-space is the time required to fill each partition loop ($N_{PE} \times TR$) multiplied by the number of partitions (N_{PE2}), or $N_{PE} \times TR \times N_{PE2}$. With phase-encoding dimensions in the range of hundreds, the acquisition times for 3D imaging can become daunting. Yet, because there are a number of important applications for which 3D imaging is essential (vascular imaging, for example), a great deal of work has gone into reducing acquisition times to an acceptable range for clinical implementation.

The next two chapters focus on strategies for reducing acquisition times. In Chapter I-7, a more detailed discussion of the relationship between k-space and images is presented in order to explain the principles on which some of the acquisition time-reducing strategies are based. Then some of the techniques commonly used to reduce acquisition times in cardiovascular MR imaging are reviewed in Chapter I-8.

REVIEW QUESTIONS

For the following questions, design the pulse sequence diagram on the right to produce the k-space trajectory shown, similar to the example shown in Figure I6-Q0. Note that for simplicity, the echoes resulting from the pulse sequence are plotted on the same line as the RF pulse.

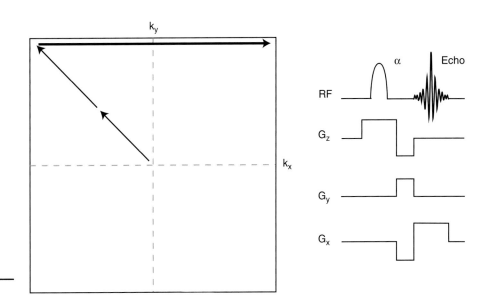

FIGURE I6-Q0.

Example:

1.

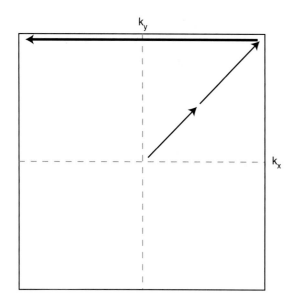

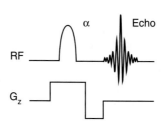

FIGURE I6-Q1

2.

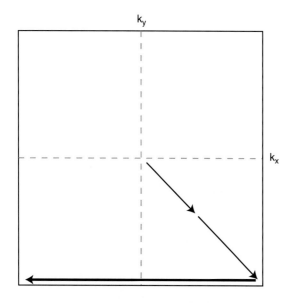

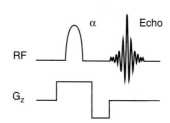

FIGURE I6-Q2

3.

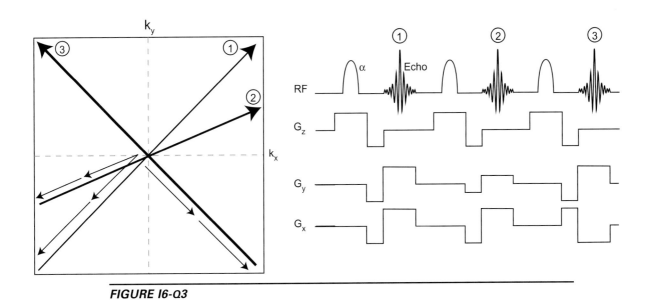

FIGURE I6-Q3

For Questions 4–6, for the pulse sequence diagram provided, draw the k-space trajectory.

4.

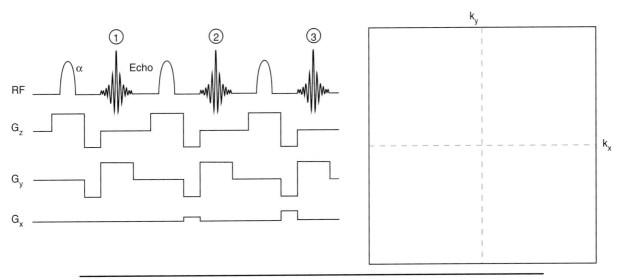

FIGURE I6-Q4

5. 128×128 matrix

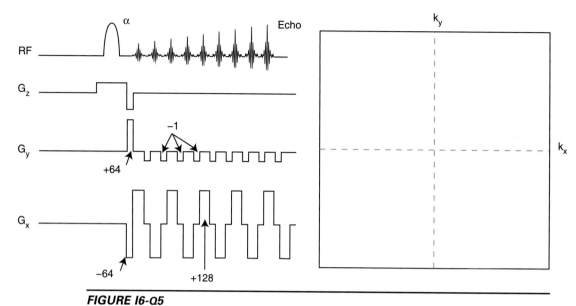

FIGURE I6-Q5

6.

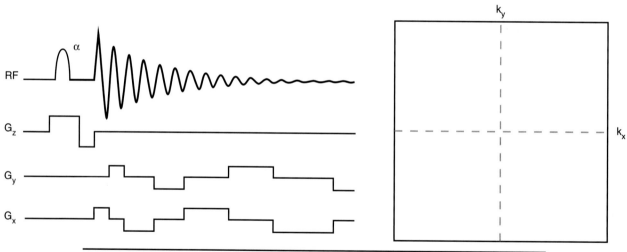

FIGURE I6-Q6

7. Consider the following 3D k-space filling order desired and complete the pulse sequence diagram for a 256 × 256 × 256 image.

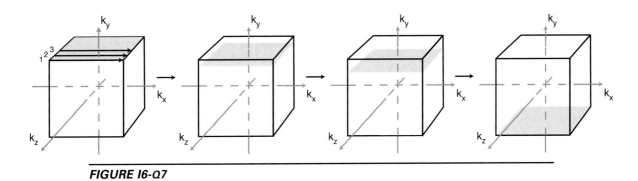

FIGURE I6-Q7

Chapter 7

More k-Space: The Relationship between k-Space and the Image

The previous chapter concentrated on how the pulse sequence diagram defines the k-space trajectory. This chapter focuses in more detail on specific properties and characteristics of k-space and their relationship to the quality of the image. With the ability to understand their consequences, some ways to "shortcut" k-space are introduced in this chapter. The next chapter then focuses on how these and other strategies are routinely used to reduce acquisition times in clinical cardiovascular MR imaging.

KEY CONCEPTS

▶ k-space is the Fourier transform of the image: the center of k-space holds low-spatial-frequency information (image contrast), whereas the periphery of k-space holds high-spatial-frequency information (image details).

▶ The real and imaginary components of k-space reflect symmetric and asymmetric components of the image, respectively, and MR images are generated using both.

▶ The symmetric properties of k-space facilitate shortcuts in data collection.

▶ Asymmetry or truncated sampling of echoes creates Gibbs ringing artifacts in the image.

▶ Zero filling of k-space increases the apparent spatial resolution of the image but not the true resolution.

▶ The dimensions of k-space and field of view (FOV) of the image are inversely related; the spacing of k-space data is inversely related to image size or FOV.

▶ Rectangular FOV manipulates the spacing of k-space data to generate images in reduced acquisition times without sacrificing spatial resolution.

▶ Oversampling of k-space can prevent wraparound artifacts associated with fields of view that are smaller than the imaged object.

k-SPACE AS THE FOURIER TRANSFORM OF THE IMAGE: A REVIEW

As discussed extensively in Chapters I-1 and I-6, k-space is the Fourier transform, or spatial frequency histogram, of the tissue slice or volume. The center of k-space consists of information about the lowest spatial frequencies in the image, while the periphery contains the high-spatial-frequency data. It may be obvious, but is probably still worth stating:

> IMPORTANT POINT: The center of k-space does not reflect the content of the center of the image.

The low-spatial-frequency data in the center of k-space reflect the overall shades of white, gray, or black in the image. If the image overall is bright or has a lot of high signal, then the center of k-space will have high amplitude. The high-spatial-frequency data at the edges of k-space contain information about fine details in the image including high-resolution definition of edges of large and small structures. Figure I7-1 illustrates this point with an MR image of the heart shown together with its k-space map. To highlight their contributions to the image, various amounts of the central and peripheral portions of k-space are extracted and their corresponding images shown. From the figure, it is apparent that most of the image information is in the central-most portion of k-space.

SYMMETRIC AND ASYMMETRIC COMPONENTS OF k-SPACE

In the preceding chapters, k-space and the definitions of the Fourier transform are expressed in terms of cosine functions. However, that story is incomplete. Because cosine

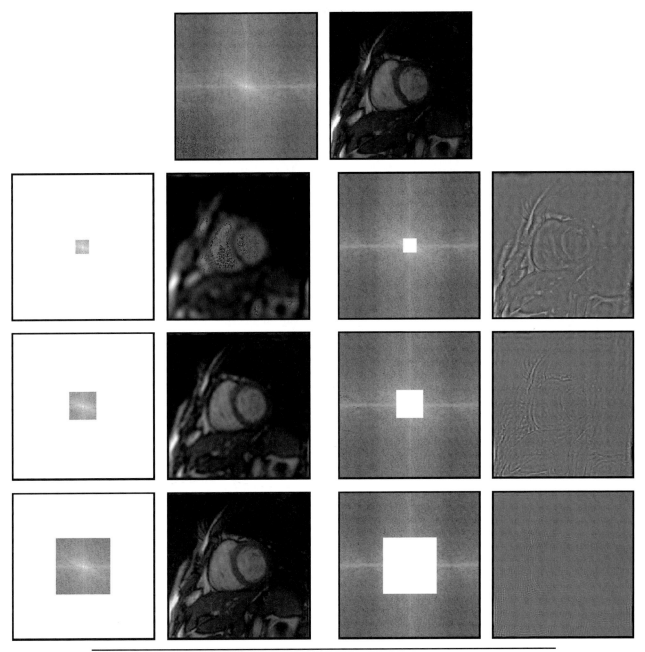

FIGURE I7-1. k-space contribution to an MR image of the heart. At top, the full k-space map and original image are shown. Below, k-space is divided into the central 1% (left)/peripheral 99% (right) at top, central 4% (left)/peripheral 96% (right) in the middle, and central 15% (left)/ peripheral 85% (right) portions at bottom, along with the corresponding images for each subset of k-space. The peripheral portions of k-space (right two columns) primarily provide information about fine details and edges, while the overall image contrast information is contained in the central portions of k-space (left two columns).

functions are symmetric functions (see Figure I1-14)— that is, they are the mirror images of themselves—they can describe only the symmetric components of images. Real medical images are asymmetric, so cosine functions alone are not sufficient to describe them. To complement the cosine functions, sine functions are needed. As asymmetric functions, sine functions can be used to describe asymmetric parts of the image (see Figure I1-14). Using the full complement of sine and cosine functions, images can be completely represented in terms of spatial frequencies.

How can both the sine and cosine frequency maps be expressed in k-space? To make it possible to record both sine and cosine frequency information, k-space must consist of *two* sets of numbers—one representing the cosine spatial frequency component, and another the sine spatial frequency component. These two numbers can be expressed together as a *complex number*. Complex numbers are numbers that have two components, typically written as

$$a + ib$$

where a and b are real numbers, and b represents the coefficient of the imaginary component, i, defined as the square root of -1 ($\sqrt{-1}$). Recall the full Fourier transform definition given in Chapter I-6:

$$H(k_x, k_y) = \int_{-\infty}^{\infty} h(x,y)e^{-i(k_x x + k_y y)} dx \, dy$$
$$= \int_{-\infty}^{\infty} h(x,y)[\cos(k_x x + k_y y)$$
$$- i\sin(k_x x + k_y y)] dx \, dy$$

That is, the Fourier transform is a complex number in which the real term contains the cosine frequencies and the imaginary term contains the sine frequencies. The real and imaginary terms for each pair of k-space coordinates (k_x, k_y) is stored in seperate maps. The cosine frequency map is referred to as the *real component of k-space*, while the sine frequency map is the *imaginary component of k-space* (Figure I7-2). The imaginary component is necessary to specify asymmetries in the image and is critical for localizing objects in the image, differentiating left, right, superior, or inferior.

Real, Imaginary, Magnitude (Modulus), and Phase Images

Taking the Fourier transform of the real component of k-space generates a *real image*, which is symmetric. Taking

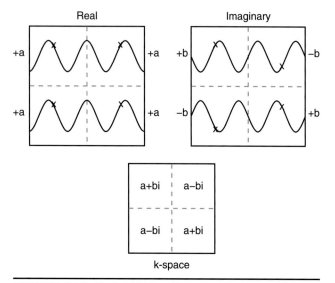

FIGURE I7-2. Real and imaginary components of k-space leading to symmetric and asymmetric properties of k-space, respectively.

the Fourier transform of the imaginary component generates an *imaginary image*, which is asymmetric.

Most commonly, the MR images that are used clinically are combinations of the real and imaginary data and are referred to as *magnitude (modulus) images*:

$$\text{Magnitude image} = \sqrt{\begin{array}{c}(\text{Real image})^2 \\ + (\text{Imaginary image})^2\end{array}}$$

The complement to the magnitude or modulus image is the *phase image*. The phase image reflects the relationship between the real and imaginary images and is defined mathematically as

$$\text{Phase image} = \arctan\left(\frac{\text{Imaginary image}}{\text{Real image}}\right)$$

where phase values range from $-180°$ to $+180°$, and arctan (arctangent, $\tan^{-1}$) is the inverse of the trigonometric tangent function ($\tan x = \sin x / \cos x$; $\arctan(\tan x) = x$). The phase image is critical in phase contrast imaging (Chapters II-3 and III-6).

Symmetry in k-Space

As illustrated in Figure I7-2, k-space has a particular symmetry that reflects the relationship between the real and imaginary components. This pattern of symmetry is referred to as *Hermitian conjugate symmetry*, in which the upper right and lower left quadrants of k-space are theoretically identical, while the upper left and lower right are also theoretically identical. An important consequence of this symmetry is that it is not always necessary to sample k-space fully to make an image. If only part of k-space is collected, the other portion can be inferred based on the symmetry of k-space. Note that the symmetry of k-space assumes a perfectly homogeneous magnetic field. Inhomogeneities lead to phase errors so that symmetry is no longer perfect.

> **IMPORTANT CONCEPT:** Only about half of k-space is needed to generate an image, because the uncollected lines can be calculated based on the Hermitian symmetry of k-space.

ASYMMETRIC k-SPACE

Many fast imaging strategies in MRI take advantage of the Hermitian conjugate symmetry of k-space to reduce acquisition times. Half-Fourier acquisition single-shot turbo spin echo imaging (HASTE, described in Chapter I-4)

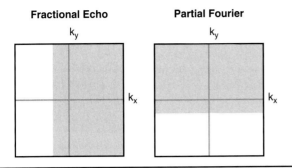

FIGURE I7-3. Two types of asymmetric k-space filling approaches, where the shaded areas depict collected data. Partial Fourier methods are also referred to as partial Nex.

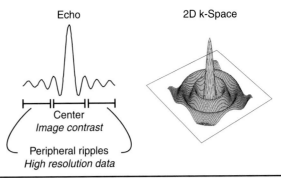

FIGURE I7-4. A single echo and a complete collection of echoes forming k-space (depicted in 3D). The center of the echo or k-space contains image contrast information, while the peripheral ripples hold the high-spatial-resolution information.

is one example. With HASTE sequences, just over half of the phase-encoding lines of k-space are collected. The missing half is approximated mathematically, and the computer-generated data are used to complete k-space. Half-Fourier imaging is an example of a *partial Fourier* or *partial Nex* (*number of excitations*) technique, meaning that the phase-encoding lines are partially collected. To correct for the phase errors caused by magnetic field inhomogeneities, a few more than half of the lines of k-space are collected with HASTE methods.

Collection of asymmetric portions of k-space can also be implemented in the frequency-encoding direction, where it is referred to as *fractional echo* or *partial echo* imaging (Figure I7-3). In both cases, the missing data can be calculated, as with HASTE sequences. Alternatively, in many implementations, zeroes are substituted for the missing data. To understand the effects of asymmetries of k-space filling on images, the sinc function and its Fourier transform need to be reviewed again.

Sinc Function and k-Space Revisited

Gradient echoes and spin echoes are sinc functions because they contain a composite of signal across a range of frequencies (receiver bandwidth). k-space represents a full set of echoes and has the appearance of a two-dimensional sinc function, as illustrated in Figure I7-4.

As discussed in Chapter I-5, the central peaks of both k-space and any given echo contribute predominantly to defining image contrast, while the periphery of k-space (or, in the case of an echo, the peripheral ripples) contain high-resolution information about fine details. Practical constraints limit the duration of the echo and its sampling. This results in an imperfect rendering of the Fourier transformation of the tissue slice in k-space. The effects of truncation of the echo on the spatial representation of the tissue in the MR image are explored in the next section.

> **IMPORTANT CONCEPT:** The central peaks of an echo or of k-space contain image contrast information while the peripheral ripples of an echo or of k-space contain higher-spatial-resolution information.

Effect of Truncating k-Space on Image Quality

The degree to which each echo or the entire k-space represents all spatial frequencies in the image determines how well they represent its true Fourier transformation. It is useful to focus in particular on the high-frequency, peripheral ripple, components because they are, by necessity, always at least partially truncated with MR imaging. With the loss of high-spatial-frequency information, the effects of truncation are primarily seen in terms of reduced edge definition and fine details in the MR image. Figure I7-5 illustrates two scenarios: (a) a perfectly and completely sampled echo and the resulting perfect image representation of the tissue and (b) the typical situation of an imperfectly sampled echo and the resulting image representation. In the perfect scenario, with a completely sampled sinc function, the edges of all of the structures are defined perfectly so that even small lesions, such as the tiny right renal cyst shown in the figure, are accurately depicted. If the echo is undersampled, image quality deteriorates, because the echo no longer represents the perfect Fourier transformation of the tissue slice. Truncation of the echo results in decreased spatial resolution and increased ringing artifacts.

The concept of an undersampled echo and its effect on image quality is analogous to the truncation of the RF pulse and its effect on slice profile, as discussed in Chapter I-5. For example, consider Figure I7-6, which focuses on the delineation of the abdominal aorta in Figure I7-5. With complete sampling of a sinc function that makes up

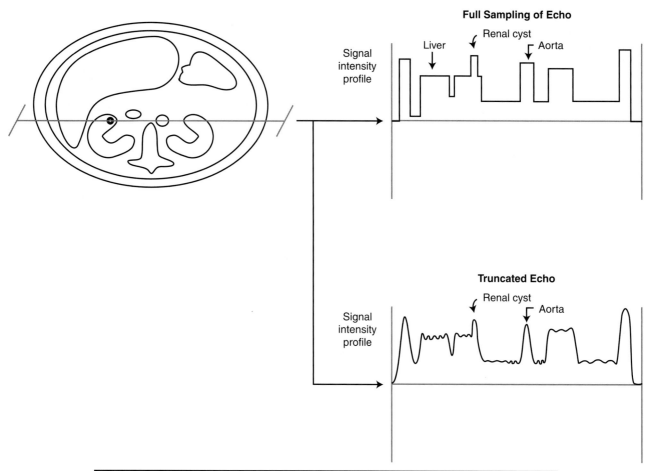

FIGURE I7-5. Signal intensity profiles through the kidneys and aorta with perfect (above) and reduced sampling (below) of the echo resulting in perfect and reduced spatial resolution. Reduced spatial resolution impairs accurate measurements of aortic diameter and detection of small lesions such as the renal cyst.

an echo, all the spatial frequency components of the image would be completely represented in k-space. Hence, the Fourier transformation of k-space would result in an image that perfectly depicts anatomic structures. For example, the signal intensity in the aorta would be uniformly high and its edges sharply defined. Truncating the echo leads to loss of high-spatial-frequency information, producing images with blurred edges and ringing artifacts around the edges of objects, called *Gibbs truncation artifact* or *Gibbs ringing artifact*. The greater the truncation, the greater blurring and ringing artifacts (Figures I7-6 and I7-7).

On clinical MR systems, a post-processing filter may be applied to minimize the ringing artifact. However, if the truncation of the echo is severe, the filter will not be able to eliminate the ringing entirely. In any case, the filters do not recover high-spatial-frequency information and can, at times, contribute to worsening of the image quality.

Zero Filling k-Space

Truncated sinc functions are a recurring theme in fast MR imaging because they are associated with shortened acquisition times. Rather than collect the full number of phase-encoding steps, commercial systems frequently employ a strategy called *zero filling* or *zero padding* to reduce the number of phase-encoding steps by up to one-half. The uncollected, peripheral lines of k-space are filled with zeroes to maintain the *apparent* resolution of images, but the acquisition times are reduced substantial. This approach is frequently used in 3D imaging applications such as 3D MR angiography.

With zero filling, a 512-point imaging matrix can be generated with only 256 phase-encoding steps. The periphery of k-space is simply "padded" with a rim of zeroes (Figure I7-8). Taking the Fourier transform of this modified k-space will create an image with 512 × 512 voxels. With finer voxels, the image may have the appearance of being higher in spatial resolution than a 256 × 256 matrix

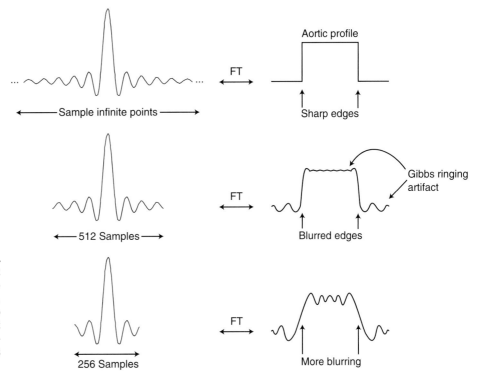

FIGURE I7-6. Effect of different samplings of the echo on the signal intensity profile of the aorta. With decreased sampling, the echo no longer represents the perfect Fourier transformation of the tissue slice, and blurring and Gibbs ringing artifacts result.

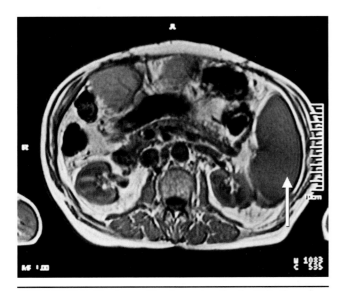

FIGURE I7-7. Ringing artifact best visualized within the spleen (arrow) as fine, subtle striations paralleling the outer margin of the organ.

image, but in fact, the extra voxels are merely *interpolated*. Interpolation is roughly the equivalent of taking the average value of two adjacent voxels to make a new voxel in between the two. The addition of zeroes in k-space does not actually improve the spatial resolution at all (see discussion later in this chapter), but it does reduce the effect of volume averaging in 3D images and hence is frequently used in 3D applications. On commercial systems this is often referred to as *zero interpolation, zip interpolation, zero padding,* or *sinc interpolation*.

IMPORTANT CONCEPT: Zero filling can be used to increase the number of voxels in the image and may make the images appear to have more details. However, spatial resolution is not improved.

Asymmetric k-Space Filling

An alternative and commonly used way of increasing the apparent resolution of an image without a proportional increase in acquisition time is to use a combination of *asymmetric sampling of the echo* (fractional echo) and zero filling (Figure I7-9). This approach takes advantage of the inherent symmetry of the sinc function that makes up the echo. Rather than using 256 data points to sample 128 points on either side of the central peak of the echo, an asymmetrically sampled echo might include 64 points to the left and 192 to the right. By sampling further out (192 rather than 128) from the center, more peripheral ripples are included in the echo, and the spatial resolution is higher than with symmetric sampling. In fact, the spatial resolution of the image approaches that of an image with a 384×384 matrix (192 samples on either side of the echo). Consequently, the spatial resolution will be better, and the Gibbs ringing artifact less, for the asymmetric case than for a symmetrically sampled echo (with 256 samples), even though the acquisition time is the same.

In k-space, the central peak of the measured echo is usually in the center of k-space. If there is an asymmetric echo, the symmetry of k-space is maintained by filling in

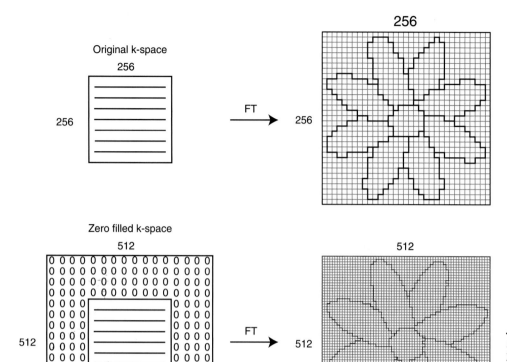

FIGURE I7-8. Zero filling of a 256 × 256 matrix to 512 × 512 and the effect of interpolation on the image. Although voxel size decreases with zero filling, true spatial resolution is not improved.

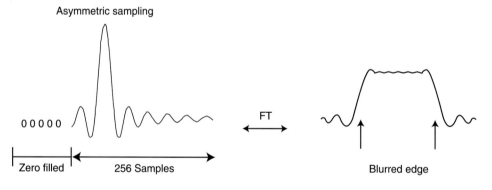

FIGURE I7-9. Asymmetric sampling of the echo using 256 samples and zero filling. Corresponding Fourier transform demonstrates that the blurred edges and Gibbs ringing artifact will be intermediate between those for symmetrically sampled echoes using 256 and 384 points.

the uncollected portion of k-space with "fake" data. The easiest "fake" data to generate are zeroes, and most fractional echo applications (Figure I7-3) use zero filling. For the example in Figure I7-9, each row of k-space would contain at least 384 data points—192 on either side of the central peak—where 128 of 192 points to the left of the sampled echo would be filled with zeroes.

If the asymmetry of k-space is in the phase-encoding rather than frequency-encoding direction, then the method is referred to as partial Fourier. Partial Fourier applications (Figure I7-3) can also use zero filling. Alternatively, in some applications such as HASTE, the Hermitian properties of k-space are used to extrapolate the uncollected portions of k-space.

Truncated and Asymmetric k-Space Filling: Effects on Spatial Resolution

What is the spatial resolution for truncated and asymmetric k-space filling with zero padding?

Without interpolation or zero padding, the spatial resolution of an image is the image voxel size. With zero filling, and particularly with asymmetric k-space filling, spatial resolution becomes more complicated.

Consider the examples in Figure I7-10. For simplicity, assume that the image FOV is 500 mm. For a fully sampled 512 × 512 k-space matrix, assume that the corresponding image will be 512 × 512 voxels. Then the spatial resolution will be equal to the size of the voxels, about 1 mm (500 mm/512 voxels). The examples discussed below

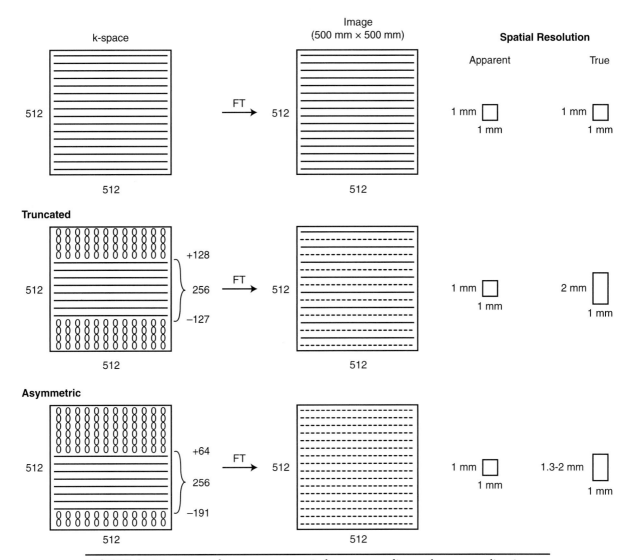

FIGURE I7-10. Truncated versus asymmetric k-space sampling and corresponding images. The true and apparent (interpolated) spatial resolutions are also shown.

assume that asymmetric sampling and undersampling are performed in the phase-encoding direction, as is typically the case in clinical applications to reduce acquisition times.

First, consider the case of symmetric k-space sampling with zero filling. If only the central 256 lines of data are collected and the outer 256 lines are padded with zeroes, then the voxel size in the 512 × 512 image will still be 1 mm × 1 mm. However, the spatial resolution depends on the actual data collected and so will be 500 mm/256 or 2 mm. In this case, the "interpolated" resolution is 1 mm, but the true spatial resolution in the phase-encoding direction is still 2 mm.

CHALLENGE QUESTION: What will be the difference in acquisition times between the fully sampled and zero-filled examples?

Answer: The zero-filled acquisition, by sampling only half the number of phase-encoding steps, will be half as long.

When k-space is sampled in an asymmetric fashion and zero filled, spatial resolution becomes much more difficult to ascertain. If 256 lines of k-space are collected asymmetrically, and the rest of the 512 × 512 matrix is filled with zeroes, then the interpolated resolution will again be 1 mm. The true spatial resolution in the phase-encoding direction depends on how asymmetrically k-space is sampled. It cannot be determined precisely, but it must be somewhere between 1 and 2 mm. For example, if at least one side of k-space spans 192 data points (Figure I7-10, bottom), then the spatial resolution can be expected to approach 1.3 mm (500 mm/384) at best.

IMPORTANT CONCEPT: With zero filling, the image spatial resolution can no longer be assumed to equal the image voxel size.

The specific techniques used to obtain asymmetric k-spaces filling and examples of applications are covered in detail in the next chapter.

THE DIMENSIONS AND SPACING OF k-SPACE

Other strategies to reduce acquisition times that will be discussed in this and the next chapter take advantage of properties of k-space related to its dimensions and the spacing of data points within k-space. This section introduces the concepts of voxel size and field of view.

Like the MR image, k-space itself has measurable dimensions and an overall size that are meaningful. The array of values that make up k-space can be thought of as an image with voxels that have specific dimensions Δk (Δk_x, Δk_y, Δk_z, Figure I7-11). For each dimension, Δk is a measure of the spacing between adjacent data points in k-space. The overall size of k-space, k_{total} ($k_{x,total}$, $k_{y,total}$, $k_{z,total}$), is the product of each voxel size, Δk, times the number of k space points. For a 256 $\times$ 256 k-space matrix,

$$k_{x,total} = \Delta k_x \times 256$$
$$k_{y,total} = \Delta k_y \times 256$$

The data in k-space furthest from the center contain the highest-spatial-resolution information. Consequently, larger k-spaces contain higher-spatial-resolution information than smaller k-spaces. This is explored further in the next section.

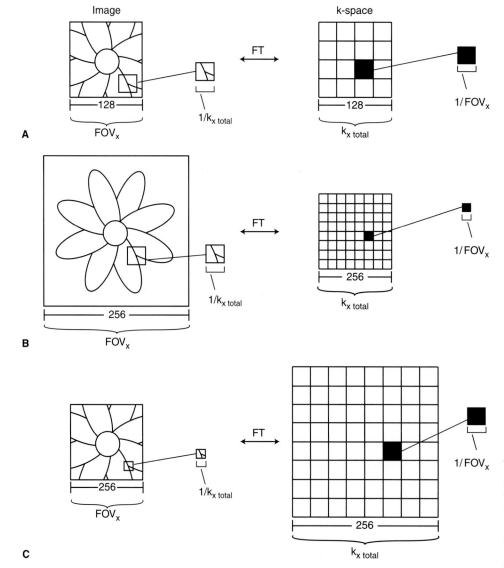

FIGURE I7-11. Examples of three different k-spaces. The dimensions of k-space are inversely related to the voxel size of the image, and the dimensions of the image are inversely related to the voxel size of k-space (Δk).

Inverse Relation of k-Space Voxel Size and Image Voxel Size

The matrix of k-space is usually equal in size to the matrix of the image. For example, if the image has 256×256 voxels, then k-space will typically also be a 256×256 matrix.

Figure I7-11, parts a and b, show that the spacing of the voxels in k-space is inversely related to the overall size of image (FOV).

$$\text{voxel size}(k_x) = \Delta k_x = \frac{1}{\text{FOV}_x}$$

Similarly, Figure I7-11, parts a and c illustrate that there is an inverse relationship between the voxel size in the image (spatial resolution) and the overall size of k-space:

$$\text{voxel size}(x) = \frac{1}{k_{x\,\text{total}}}$$

In Figure I7-11, parts a and b, the images have the same spatial resolution but different FOV. Because spatial resolution is the same, the overall size of k-space is the same. However, doubling the FOV makes each k-space voxel half the size.

Next, compare Figure I7-11, parts a and c, where the images have the same FOV but different spatial resolutions. Where the resolution is doubled (that is, the image voxel size is halved), the overall dimensions of k-space are doubled. Each k-space voxel is the same size in the two cases, since the FOV is unchanged.

The inverse relationship between the image and k-space intuitively makes sense. k-space is a spatial frequency map (where spatial frequency is a function of 1/distance, cycles/cm), while the image is a spatial map (a function of distance, cm). When the image is small, much higher spatial frequencies and a larger k-space are needed to describe the details within the image.

> **IMPORTANT CONCEPTS:** The spacing of voxels in k-space is inversely related to the size of the image. The spacing of voxels in the image is inversely related to the overall size of k-space.

The Relationship between k-Space Dimensions, Gradients, and Sampling Frequencies

How do k-space dimensions relate to pulse sequence diagrams and sampling frequencies?

From the previous chapter, the k-space trajectory can be described in terms of areas under the gradient lobes on a pulse sequence diagram, where $k_x = \gamma G_x t$. Traversal of the width of k-space, $k_{x\,\text{total}}$, is accomplished by a gradient pulse with area $G_x \times t_{\text{echo}}$, where t_{echo} equals the duration of

the echo. The size of each k-space voxel, Δk, is proportional to the area under the corresponding gradient curve divided by the total number of k-space samples. In other words, Δk is proportional to the area under the gradient curve during the sampling time needed for a given k-space data point:

$$\Delta k_x = \frac{k_{x,\text{total}}}{\text{matrix size}_x} = \frac{\gamma \times G_x \times t_{\text{echo}}}{\text{matrix size}_x}$$

Gradient diagrams that might result in different k-space sizes are shown in Figure I7-12.

The dimensions of k-space depend on the area under the G_x curve. For example, for a 256 matrix, Δk_x is proportional to the area under 1/256 of the G_x curve. If G_x is doubled, then the height of the gradient curve is doubled, and the width is halved. For Δk_x to remain constant, the duration of sampling for each k-space value must be halved. Independently of gradient strength, the dimensions of k-space for this image will remain constant. This is consistent with the receiver bandwidth and sampling frequency principles discussed in Chapter I-5.

As illustrated in Figure I7-12, different gradient strengths can be used to generate the same k-space configuration. In fact, it turns out that for an image with a given FOV, changing the gradient strength does not affect the overall size of k-space nor the spacing of voxels in k-space. Gradients affect only the duration of the echo sampling process.

> **IMPORTANT CONCEPT:** The dimensions and spacing of k-space are unaltered by gradient strength.

Asymmetry in Δk Spacing: Rectangular Field of View (RecFOV)

An appreciation of the relationship between the spacing of k-space data points and image spatial resolution is necessary to understand a very commonly used tool in MR imaging—*rectangular field of view (recFOV)*. With rectangular FOV, lines of k-space in the phase-encoding direction are undersampled by increasing the spacing between k-space lines (Δk_y) while still maintaining the overall size of k-space.

CHALLENGE QUESTION: What effect does increasing Δk_y have on the resulting image?

Answer: Since

$$\Delta k_y = \frac{1}{\text{FOV}_y}$$

increasing Δk_y will decrease the FOV in the y direction (Figure I7-13).

Undersampling k-space in the phase-encoding direction results in a reduced FOV in the phase-encoding

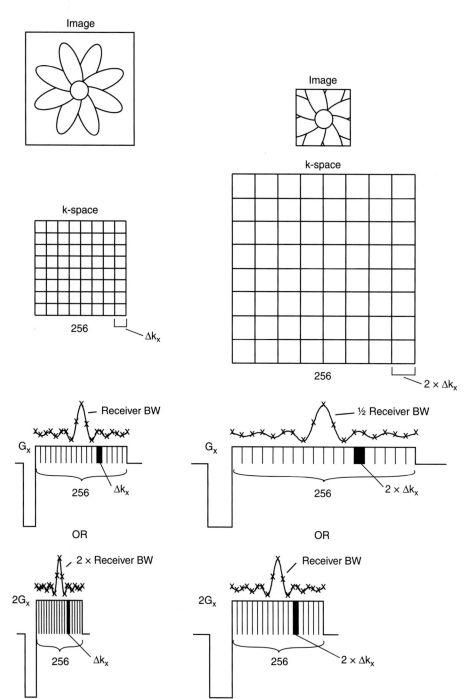

FIGURE I7-12. The spacing of voxels in k-space is proportional to the area under the gradient curve. The same k-space can be generated with gradients of different strengths.

direction (Figure I7-13). For example, with 50% rectangular FOV, only every other phase-encoding line is collected so that Δk_y is doubled. The imaging FOV is then half as large in the phase-encoding direction as in the frequency-encoding direction. Fewer phase-encoding lines means shorter acquisition times.

Rectangular FOV is applicable in the setting of a body part that is narrower in the phase-encoding direction than in the frequency-encoding direction. For example, in the

chest, the anterior-posterior dimension is usually much smaller than the left-to-right dimension, and therefore rectangular FOV can be implemented using phase-encoding in the anterior-posterior direction.

How does rectangular FOV affect spatial resolution of the image? The undersampling of k-space results in fewer voxels in the phase-encoding direction of the image. However, because the FOV_y is also decreased by half, the spatial resolution in the y direction is not diminished at

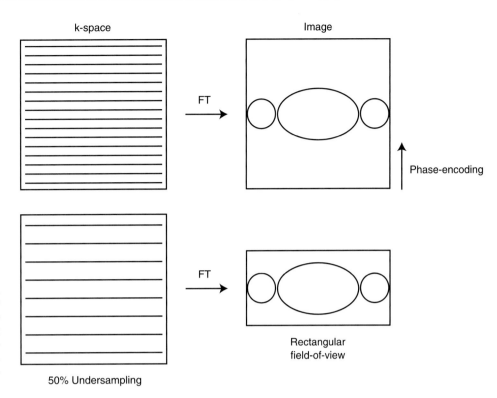

FIGURE 17-13. Rectangular FOV. An undersampling of k-space in the phase-encoding direction creates a rectangular-shaped image, which is well suited for imaging the chest and abdomen.

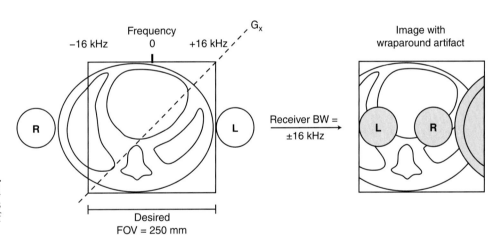

FIGURE 17-14. Wraparound artifact. Tissue that extends beyond the desired FOV of 25 cm wraps into the image.

all. This is consistent with the fact that the overall k-space dimension stays the same. With rectangular FOV, there is a corresponding loss in signal-to-noise ratio compared to full FOV imaging. This loss is related to the decreased time necessary to produce the image.

> **IMPORTANT CONCEPT:** To utilize rectangular FOV, the phase-encoding direction should be defined along the narrower dimension of the body. Rectangular FOV results in no loss in spatial resolution but can substantially reduce the image acquisition time.

WRAPAROUND ARTIFACT AND OVERSAMPLING

What happens if the FOV is smaller than the dimension of the body? The tissue that extends beyond the FOV can appear within the FOV, itself, creating an artifact called *wraparound artifact* or aliasing artifact.

Wraparound artifact is a consequence of the undersampling of high-frequency signals. Recall that the Nyquist theorem says that to sample accurately a signal of a particular frequency f, the sampling frequency must be at least two times as great as f (2f).

Consider the example shown in Figure I7-14, where the desired FOV is limited to the heart. In this case, the receiver bandwidth that spans the horizontal width of the heart with the frequency-encoding gradient G_x is ±16 kHz. The Nyquist theorem says that for this bandwidth, the sampling frequency must be at least twice as great as 16 kHz, or 32 kHz. What about the tissue that lies beyond the FOV? Protons from outside the FOV, although not desired, are nevertheless still exposed to higher ends of the gradient and will therefore contribute signal at higher frequencies than the expected bandwidth. In Figure I7-14, tissue from the right arm will precess at approximately −24 kHz, and tissue from the left arm will be at about +20 kHz.

As illustrated in Chapter I-5 (Figure I5-19), frequencies that are higher than half the sampling frequency are imperfectly represented. For example, signal at −24 kHz from the right arm is undersampled when the sampling frequency is 32 kHz (accurate sampling would require a sampling frequency of at least 48 kHz). Sampling the −24 kHz signal at a frequency of 32 kHz results in a signal that has the appearance of an 8 kHz signal. The protons precessing at 8 kHz will be mismapped or "wrapped" into the FOV. Signal from the right side of the body will therefore appear in the image at the left (Figure I7-14). Conversely, signal at +20 kHz from the left arm, when undersampled, will appear to have a frequency of −12 kHz and therefore will be localized in the right half of the image.

Wraparound artifact can occur in both the frequency-encoding and phase-encoding directions. One simple solution to avoid wraparound artifact is to increase the FOV to match the body size (Figure I7-15). For example, in the case shown in Figure I7-15, an FOV that is twice as large will result in an image with no wraparound artifact. However, spatial resolution will deteriorate by a factor of two, and consequently, detectability of small or subtle lesions will be reduced.

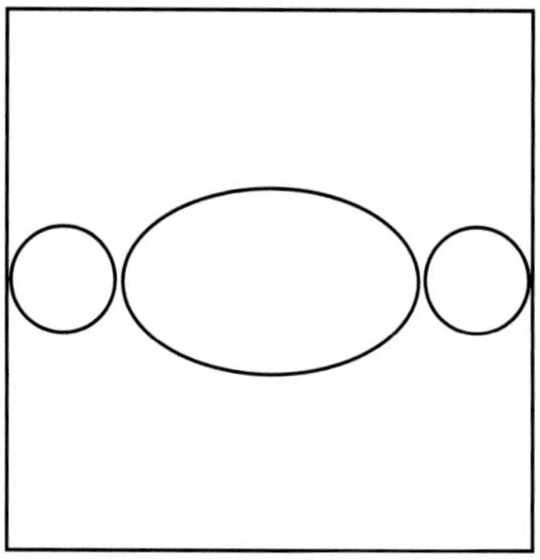

FOV = 500 mm

FIGURE I7-15. Increasing the FOV to avoid wraparound artifact can be performed at the expense of reduced spatial resolution.

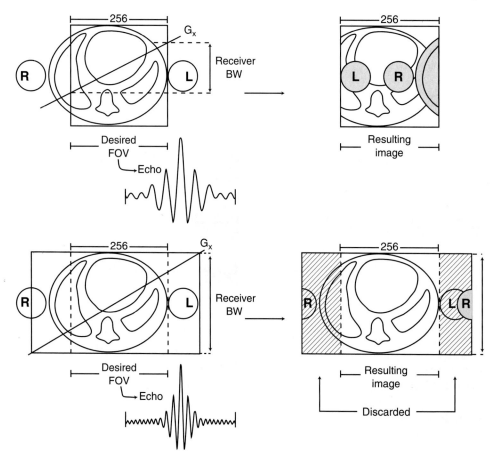

FIGURE I7-16. Frequency oversampling eliminates wraparound artifact without an increase in echo duration or acquisition time.

CHALLENGE QUESTION: In the case of Figure 17-15, how could spatial resolution be preserved despite the increase in field of view and without increasing acquisition time?

Answer: In the original configuration, the spatial resolution is approximately 1 mm (250 mm/256). With the larger FOV of 500 mm, the spatial resolution would be decreased to 2 mm (500 mm/256). By increasing the matrix from 256 to 512 and then using a rectangular FOV (assuming phase-encoding is in the anterior-posterior direction) to reduce the number of phase-encoding steps by 50% back to 256, the spatial resolution would be preserved without increasing the acquisition time. The overall FOV would have dimensions 250 mm × 500 mm, and the matrix would be 256 × 512, for a spatial resolution of 1 mm × 1 mm.

An alternative solution to wraparound artifact is to perform *oversampling*. When the wraparound artifact is in the frequency-encoding direction, oversampling in the k_x direction is a better solution than increasing the FOV because there is no increase in imaging time and no loss of resolution. To avoid wraparound artifact in the phase-encoding direction, oversampling in the k_y direction can be performed, but unlike frequency oversampling, phase oversampling requires increased imaging times. Specifics about oversampling in the two directions are given next.

Frequency Oversampling (No Frequency Wrap)

In the clinical setting, *frequency oversampling* or *no frequency wrap* is routinely implemented. With frequency oversampling, the number of data points sampled in the echo is doubled. This is achieved by doubling the receiver bandwidth or sampling frequency so that twice the number of samples can be measured in the same time. Doubling the receiver bandwidth, but keeping the gradient constant, results in double the FOV (Figure I7-16).

For example, consider an image of the chest with 256 voxels in the frequency-encoding direction (Figure I7-16). With 100% frequency oversampling, the sampling frequency is doubled, and consequently, 512 data points are sampled instead of 256 in the same sampling time. Consequently, the FOV in the left-to-right direction is doubled (Figure I7-16). The image is reconstructed with doubled FOV and doubled number of voxels. Spatial resolution is therefore unaffected. When the MR image is displayed, the outer half of the image is discarded.

Frequency oversampling ensures that there is no wraparound artifact in the frequency-encoding direction when the FOV is smaller than the body dimension. Unlike phase oversampling, frequency oversampling does not increase the acquisition time because there is no increase in echo sampling time. For this reason, many clinical sequences have 100% frequency oversampling built into most acquisitions as a default setting.

> **IMPORTANT CONCEPT:** Frequency oversampling reduces wraparound artifact in the frequency-encoding direction without an increase in acquisition time. With frequency oversampling, the FOV in the frequency-encoding direction can be smaller than the dimension of the body in that direction.

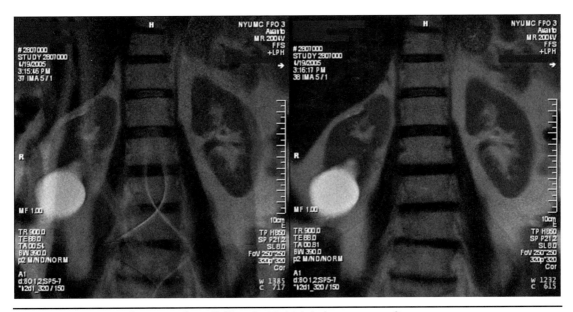

FIGURE I7-17. Coronal image without (left) and with (right) phase oversampling.

Phase Oversampling (No Phase Wrap)

Phase oversampling or *no phase wrap* is performed for similar reasons that frequency oversampling is performed—to prevent wraparound artifact in the phase-encoding direction from tissues outside the FOV interfering with the image. The cost of phase oversampling is significantly greater because acquisition times are increased in proportion to the oversampling. Doubling the number of phase-encoding steps will result in a doubling of acquisition time.

From a k-space perspective, the concept of phase oversampling is the same as frequency oversampling. To perform phase oversampling, the number of phase-encoded data points in k-space is increased. For example, for 100% phase oversampling, the number of phase-encoding steps is doubled, say from 256 to 512. The image is reconstructed with twice the FOV in the phase-encoding direction and 512 voxels, maintaining the same spatial resolution. Then the outer half of the image is discarded.

Despite increased acquisition times, judicious use of phase oversampling can be helpful in some applications. For example, for coronal imaging of the torso, where the frequency-encoding direction is typically superior to inferior (craniocaudal) while the phase-encoding direction is left to right, phase oversampling can be used to prevent wraparound artifact from the arms (Figure I7-17).

REVIEW QUESTIONS

1. Recognizing that the image is a post-processed image from an MR angiogram, match the Fourier transforms (left) with the images (Figure I7-Q1).

2. In the above example,
   a. Where in Fourier space ("k-space") are the data points that best describe the overall shade of gray or white in the image?
   b. Where in Fourier space ("k-space") are the data points that best describe the abdominal aorta?
   c. Where in Fourier space ("k-space") are the data points that best describe the lumbar arteries?

3. Consider an MR image of the chest in which the total span of the body including both arms is 425 mm, the left-to-right span of the chest is 300 mm, and the anterior-posterior dimension of the chest is 225 mm (Figure I7-Q3A).
   a. Initially the imaging FOV is set up to be 500 mm × 500 mm using a 256 × 256 matrix, and the acquisition time is 20 sec. What is the spatial resolution of this image?
   b. Your first intervention is to reduce the FOV to 300 mm, since you are only interested in pathology in the chest and not the arms. What technique must be used to avoid wraparound artifact? Which directions should phase encoding and frequency encoding be? What will be the acquisition time with these modifications? What will be the spatial resolution?

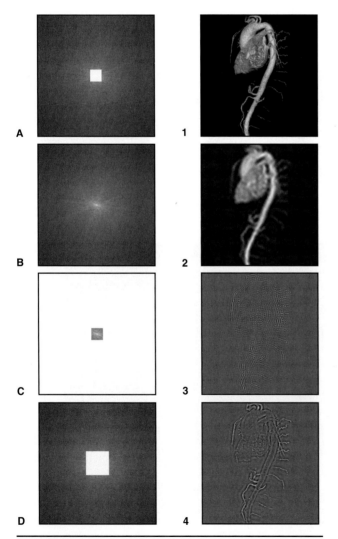

FIGURE I7-Q1

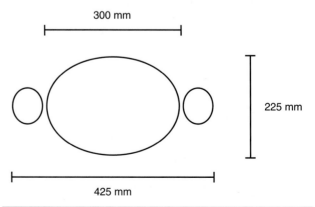

FIGURE I7-Q3A

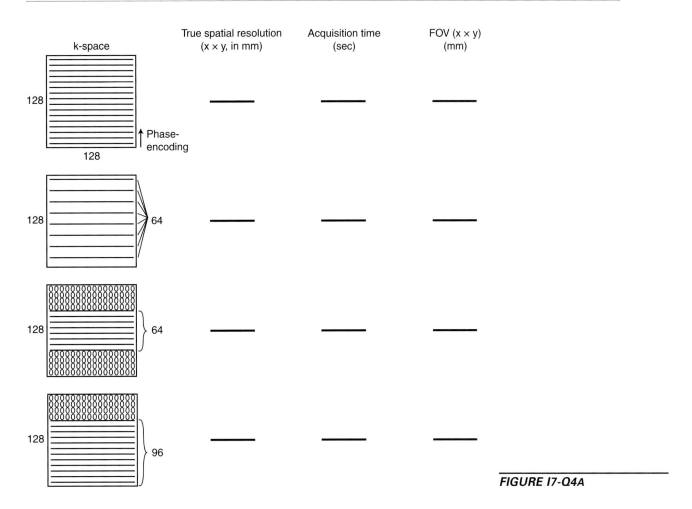

FIGURE I7-Q4A

c. The subject is unable to suspend respiration for the full 20 sec acquisition time. What modification can be implemented to reduce the acquisition time? What effect will this change have on the image size, image resolution, and acquisition time?

4. For the patterns of k-space filling shown in Figure I7-Q4, complete the table for image spatial resolution and acquisition times, assuming a 25 cm FOV and 10 msec TR.

Fast Scanning and k-Space Shortcuts

Cardiovascular MRI demands fast imaging and, at the same time, requires collection of sufficient data for high-quality images. The development of fast imaging techniques has long been the focus of intensive research; many methods have been described, and many implemented in routine clinical practice. This chapter considers the main ways in which acquisition times can be reduced: by decreasing TR, by increasing the number of echoes collected per TR, and by reducing the number of phase-encoding steps, N_{PE}. The image qualities of different methods are evaluated. Particular emphasis is placed on a new field of fast imaging, called parallel imaging. Lessons learned are applied in a detailed case study of how to reduce the acquisition time of a 3D gradient echo MR angiography sequence. The chapter closes with a brief discussion of "dynamic" MR imaging, where acquisitions are repeated over time to follow the temporal course of events, such as patterns of contrast enhancement or cardiac motion.

KEY CONCEPTS

▶ Reductions in acquisition times can be achieved by decreasing TR, by increasing the number of echoes per TR, and by decreasing N_{PE}.

▶ TR can be reduced by decreasing the RF duration and the readout duration.

▶ Increasing the number of echoes per TR requires fast refocusing to maintain sufficient signal amplitude before T2 or T2* decay.

▶ N_{PE} can be decreased in several ways: directly, via partial Fourier methods, using nonrectilinear k-space trajectories, and by parallel acquisition techniques.

▶ Parallel acquisition techniques use coil sensitivity variations to reconstruct images from incomplete or partially filled k-space. They can substantially reduce acquisition times, at the cost of lower signal-to-noise ratios.

▶ To fill multiple k-spaces for dynamic MR imaging, keyholing or view-sharing approaches can be used to reduce acquisition times and improve temporal resolution.

ACQUISITION TIMES AND IMAGE QUALITY

Before discussing how to make images faster, consider the factors that determine acquisition time for 2D imaging:

$$\text{Acquisition Time (2D)} = \frac{TR \times N_{PE} \times N_{acq}}{ETL}$$

where TR = repetition time, N_{PE} = number of phase-encoding steps, N_{acq} = number of acquisitions (or number of signals averaged), and ETL = echo train length or number of echoes sampled per RF excitation.

In 3D imaging, phase-encoding steps in two directions contribute to the acquisition time:

$$\text{Acquisition Time (3D)} = \frac{TR \times N_{PE1} \times N_{PE2} \times N_{acq}}{ETL}$$

where N_{PE1} and N_{PE2} represent the number of phase-encoding steps in the two phase-encoding directions. Because of time constraints, N_{acq} is usually equal to one for most cardiovascular 3D imaging.

From these equations, it follows that to reduce acquisition times, the three main areas of focus should be to reduce TR, to reduce the number of phase-encoding steps, and to increase the echo train length (defined as the number of echoes sampled per TR). Before considering each in turn, it should be emphasized that the price of faster imaging is usually reduced signal-to-noise ratio (SNR), since, as discussed in Chapter I-1, SNR is proportional to the square root of the time necessary to collect the data (sample all echoes) for an image.

REDUCING TR (FOR GRADIENT ECHO IMAGING ONLY)

For spin echo imaging, because the TR directly affects image contrast, it is often not practical to consider shortening TR to make imaging more efficient. Recall, for example, that TR must be relatively long for T2-weighted image contrast.

For gradient echo imaging, however, it is practical to decrease TR. The components that make up TR (Chapter I-4, Figure I4-10) are RF duration, TE, and echo duration (or sampling time). Each of these three components can be shortened. The effects of reducing each component on image quality are discussed next.

Decreased RF Time

The RF duration can be shortened by "compressing" the energy of the RF pulse into a shorter time by using higher transmitter bandwidths with stronger slice-select gradients or by using an asymmetric RF pulse. Both approaches can be implemented simultaneously—a compressed asymmetric RF pulse gives the shortest RF duration.

Shortened Symmetric RF Pulses

If the RF duration is shortened by truncating the sinc-shaped RF pulse, for example, by reducing it from four periods to two periods (Figure I5-9), the slice profile will worsen considerably without much time savings.

However, with higher transmitter bandwidth and increased slice-select gradient strength, a given slice thickness can be excited with a much shorter RF pulse without any degradation in slice profile (Figure I8-1). The maximum transmitter bandwidth is constrained by the maximum gradient strength and the thickness of the slice desired. MR pulse sequences are typically configured to operate by default to minimize RF durations.

Asymmetric RF pulses

Similar to an asymmetric or partial echo (see Chapter I-7), an asymmetric RF pulse can also be used for RF excitation. Asymmetric RF pulses provide a compromise between full and truncated RF pulses. For a given excitation time, they produce better slice profiles than symmetric pulses (Figure I8-1).

CHALLENGE QUESTION: What is the effect of shortening RF pulse duration on image SNR?

Answer: RF pulse duration does not affect signal sampling time and therefore does not affect SNR much. However, shorter RF pulses do reduce the sharpness of the slice profile and therefore can reduce the overall amount of signal if the desired imaging slice is imperfectly excited.

> **IMPORTANT CONCEPT:** Increased transmitter bandwidth shortens RF excitation time. Asymmetric RF pulses can further reduce RF excitation time with less impact on slice profile than symmetric truncation of the RF pulse.

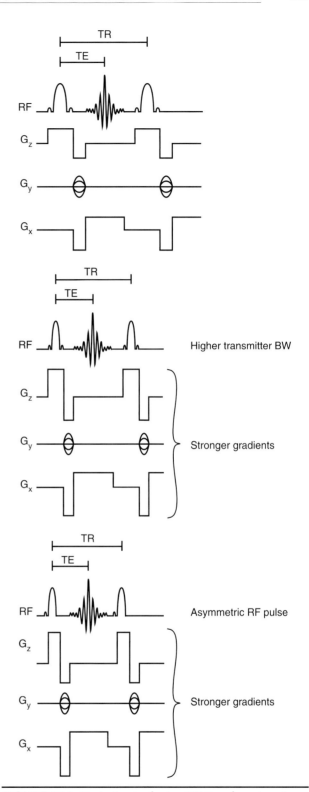

FIGURE I8-1. Strategies to shorten RF time by using strong slice-select gradients and high transmitter bandwidth together with asymmetric RF pulses.

Decreased TE

The echo time is defined as the time between the center of the RF pulse and the peak of the echo. In some cases, the TE is constrained by the desired image contrast. However, in most cardiovascular applications, such as 3D MRA, a shorter TE is advantageous. It reduces not only acquisition times but also T2* effects.

The most direct way to shorten TE in a gradient echo sequence is through stronger frequency-encoding gradients or faster slew rates (Figure I8-2). A stronger gradient will shorten the duration of dephasing and readout lobes of the frequency-encoding gradient. Shortening the dephasing lobe does not reduce SNR. However, shortening the readout lobe does decrease SNR because SNR is proportional to the square root of the sampling time.

An additional way to reduce TE is to use asymmetric or partial echoes with zero filling (Figure I8-2), as discussed in Chapter I-7. With asymmetric echoes, the center of k-space is filled earlier during the acquisition, and hence the effective TE is shorter. Also, because the dephasing lobe is shorter, TR is also decreased slightly (Figure I8-2).

Decreased Echo Sampling Time

The strategies that reduce the readout duration parallel those that decrease TE (Figure I8-2). Stronger gradients and higher receiver bandwidths shorten the readout duration by increasing the sampling frequency. Additionally, an asymmetric echo can be used to reduce the number of samples. The loss in spatial resolution is lower with asymmetric truncation than symmetric truncation (Chapter I-7). The shorter the sampling time, however, the lower the SNR for the image, and therefore these strategies are not practical when the SNR is already at its critical limits.

> **IMPORTANT CONCEPT:** Increased receiver bandwidth shortens TE and TR. The use of asymmetric echoes can further shorten TE and TR without as much sacrifice in image quality as is caused by symmetrically truncated echoes. Shortening the duration of echo sampling reduces image SNR.

INCREASING EFFICIENCY WITH MULTIPLE ECHOES PER RF EXCITATION

Increasing the number of echoes sampled per TR improves the imaging efficiency. This can be achieved with both spin echo imaging and gradient echo imaging. Each approach is discussed in the following subsections.

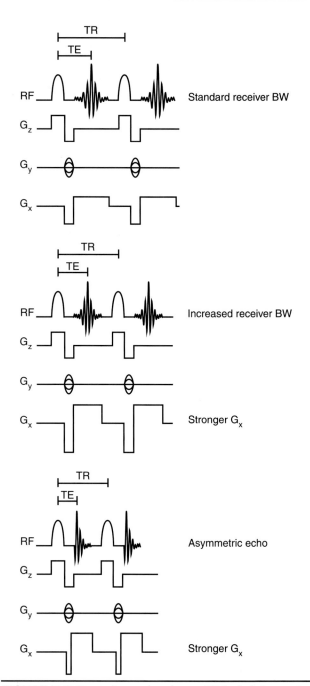

FIGURE I8-2. Strategies used to shorten TE include increasing receiver bandwidth, use of asymmetric echoes, and a combination of both techniques.

Spin Echo ETL

With fast spin echo imaging, multiple 180° refocusing pulses are applied to generate multiple echoes for each 90° RF excitation (Chapter I-4). The improvement in efficiency of fast spin echo over conventional spin echo sequences is directly proportional to the number of echoes generated per RF excitation, or the echo train length (ETL) (Figure I8-3). The placement and ordering of

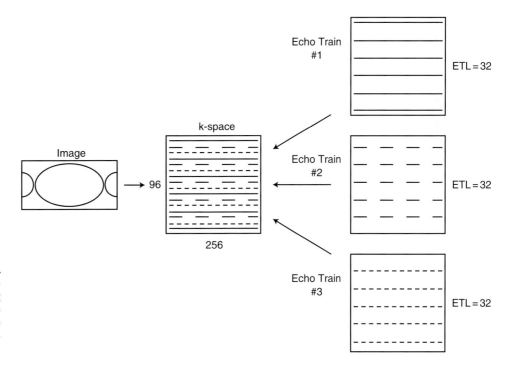

FIGURE I8-3. Filling of k-space for fast spin echo imaging with ETL = 32 and a total of 96 phase-encoding steps. Note that this acquisition uses rectangular FOV.

the multiple echoes in k-space influences image contrast. The echoes with the desired TE should be used to fill the central lines of k-space. As discussed in Chapter I-4, the TE of the echo used to fill the central line of k-space is called the effective TE or TE_{eff}.

Fast spin echo imaging is commonly used to assess the anatomy of blood vessels and the heart. Typical ETL values are between 16 and 32. If higher ETLs can be achieved, by use of fast 180° pulses and very short readout durations, then all of the data needed to generate a single image can be achieved in a single RF pulse. This is referred to as single-shot imaging and is typically implemented in the clinical setting in conjunction with partial Fourier methods. As discussed in Chapter I-4, a half-Fourier acquisition single-shot turbo spin echo (HASTE) sequence with an ETL of 68 can produce a 128×256 image matrix following a single RF excitation pulse. The remainder of k-space is extrapolated by assuming the Hermitian symmetry of k-space. With a short interecho spacing of 4–5 msec, a 256×128 image can be generated with TEs ranging from 10 msec to 300 msec. The effective TE of the HASTE sequence is typically 60 to 120 msec.

CHALLENGE QUESTION: What is the acquisition time for a single-slice HASTE image with a matrix of 512×256, an ETL of 132, and an interecho spacing of 3.2 msec?

Answer: As a half-Fourier technique, HASTE requires only 132 of 256 lines of k-space to generate an image with 512×256 matrix. The remaining 124 lines of k-space are calculated from the measured data. The total time to acquire 132 echoes is 132×3.2 msec or 421 msec.

The effects of echo train imaging on image quality depend on the time spent sampling echoes. For full-Fourier methods, fast spin echo techniques may reduce image SNR because higher receiver bandwidths are needed to shorten the echo sampling time so that echoes can be sampled before T2 decay. Partial Fourier methods, such as HASTE, are even more signal-poor because the total time spent collecting signal is only about half that of full-Fourier methods.

Gradient Echo Methods of Accelerating Imaging

Multiple echoes can also be sampled following a single RF pulse with gradient echo imaging (Chapter I-4). Rather than using 180° pulses, the readout gradient is reversed repeatedly to refocus the protons and generate additional echoes. One critical difference between spin echo and gradient echo methods is that with spin echo the multiple echoes follow T2 decay of the signal, while with gradient echo the multiple echoes follow T2* decay. T2* decay is quicker than T2 decay, and therefore the time constraints are much greater for multiecho gradient echo sequences.

One of the fastest approaches with gradient echo imaging is echo planar imaging (EPI), discussed in Chapter I-6. In EPI, the readout gradients are rapidly reversed, and the phase-encoding gradient is typically blipped to step through k-space with each echo. When all lines of k-space are collected in a single excitation (say, 64 to 128 echoes), the sequence is called single-shot EPI. Alternatively, the lines of k-space can be collected in multiple sets with fewer echoes each (for example, four sets of 32). This is

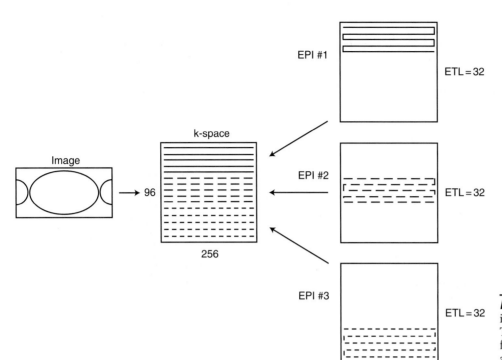

FIGURE I8-4. Filling of k-space in segmented or multi-shot EPI. The multiple echoes obtained following each excitation are acquired in sequential groups.

termed multi-shot EPI or *segmented* EPI (Figure I8-4). The key parameter, equivalent to spin echo ETL, is often referred to as the *number of lines per segment*.

The very high receiver bandwidths that are necessary to collect enough echoes before T2* decay mean that fast gradient echo techniques such as EPI have low SNR compared with conventional gradient echo methods. This is why EPI is not usually implemented with half-Fourier methods—reducing the already low SNR further would result in uninterpretable images.

REDUCING N_{PE}: CONVENTIONAL RECTILINEAR k-SPACE TRAJECTORIES

The third way to shorten acquisition time is to reduce the number of phase-encoding steps. A decrease in N_{PE} reduces the acquisition time proportionately. In general, lowering N_{PE} reduces SNR (SNR is proportional to the square root of N_{PE}). Three approaches to reduce N_{PE} will be discussed: conventional strategies with rectilinear k-space trajectories, nontraditional k-space trajectories, and parallel imaging.

Decreasing N_{PE} and Lowering Spatial Resolution

An obvious method to reduce the acquisition time is to decrease the number of phase-encoding steps without changing any other parameters. As a result, spatial resolution in the phase-encoding direction will be reduced. For example, if the phase-encoding steps are reduced from

200 to 150 for an image with FOV 300 mm, then the 25% decrease in acquisition time will be associated with an increase in the voxel size from 1.5 mm to 2 mm in the phase-encoding direction. In other words, spatial resolution will be reduced by 25%, and the ability to resolve a small (1 mm) lesion will diminish as a result.

RecFOV: Decreasing N_{PE} with a Concomitant Change in Field of View

As discussed in Chapter I-7, a more clever approach, when feasible, is to decrease the number of phase-encoding steps in parallel with a decrease in the FOV in that direction, resulting in a rectangular field of view (recFOV). The phase-encoding direction should be along the narrower dimension of the body. In the example discussed in the previous section, if the anterior-posterior dimension of the body is 225 mm or less, then 75% (225/300) recFOV can be performed. The acquisition time will be reduced by 25%.

CHALLENGE QUESTION: What is the effect of recFOV on spatial resolution?

Answer: Spatial resolution is unchanged because the FOV and the N_{PE} are both reduced by 25%.

Partial Fourier

Partial Fourier methods refer to the acquisition of a limited number of k-space lines and then use of one of the two methods to fill the remainder of the data space: zero filling or calculating the missing data (based on the Hermitian conjugate symmetry of k-space; see Chapter I-7). In 3D spoiled gradient echo applications for contrast-enhanced MRA, k-space is usually zero-filled in at least one, and typically both, phase-encoding directions. The reduction in the number of phase-encoding steps directly decreases acquisition time. As discussed in Chapter I-7, the number of data points sampled in k-space and the degree of asymmetry determine the spatial resolution and Gibbs ringing artifact in the image.

REDUCING N_PE: NONTRADITIONAL k-SPACE TRAJECTORIES

An alternative strategy to reduce the number of phase-encoding steps is to consider different k-space trajectories. Most conventional MR pulse sequences use a rectilinear approach with either sequential or centric k-space filling. Linear trajectories have several intrinsic disadvantages. First, the time spent collecting data is evenly distributed across k-space without regard for the greater importance of the central regions (see Figure I7-1, for example). Second, the trajectory is not very efficient; the dephasing lobes of the frequency-encoding gradients are necessary for each echo but are used only to travel within k-space and not for data collection. Also, with a rectilinear

approach, the time at which the central area of k-space is collected is not always well controlled relative to events such as arrival of a gadolinium contrast bolus in the aorta.

Two alternative k-space trajectories reduce acquisition times with fewer of these limitations.

Spiral Trajectory

Chapter I-6 introduced the spiral trajectory and the corresponding pulse sequence diagram. The spiral trajectory has several advantages over fast rectilinear k-space filling: First, the center of k-space is sampled better than its periphery. Second, the center of k-space is acquired immediately after the RF excitation, when very little dephasing has occurred. Third, the k-space trajectories are smooth, in contrast to EPI, and do not require ultrafast gradient switching. And fourth, because the center is collected first, timing of specific events (such as contrast bolus arrival) is more precise.

Spiral trajectories are well suited for fast imaging applications because a substantial portion of k-space can be sampled in one extended readout. Single-shot spiral imaging can be sufficient for low-spatial-resolution imaging. Alternatively, several spiral trajectories can be interleaved (Figure I8-5) to produce high-spatial-resolution images. Because the data are not collected on a square

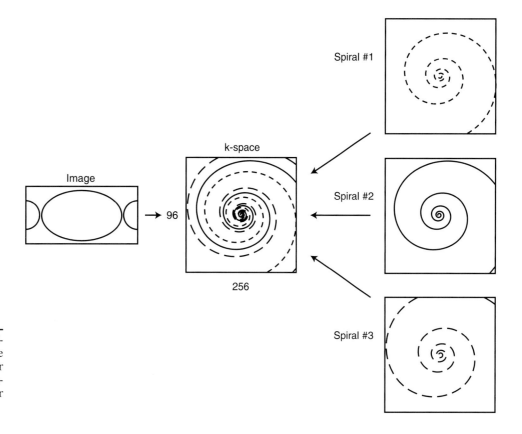

FIGURE I8-5. Interleaved spiral k-space trajectory. k-space is typically filled with fewer RF excitations with spiral trajectories than with rectilinear trajectories.

grid, they must first be interpolated to fit the k-space matrix before the Fourier transform. The acquisition time depends on the number of interleaves, $N_{interleaves}$, and the time needed to make each spiral pass through k-space. Since the latter is given by TR, the equation is

$$\text{Acquisition Time (2D)} = \text{TR} \times N_{interleaves}$$

Although the acquisition times are reduced, long readout times for spiral trajectories can lead to greater sensitivity to magnetic field inhomogeneity.

Spiral-like trajectories can also be used for 3D imaging. Spiral or elliptical-centric trajectories through 3D k-space are especially useful in 3D MRA sequences, when it is beneficial to collect the center of k-space at the beginning of the acquisition. Interpolation of data to fit the k-space grid can be cumbersome. One method to simplify this approach is to collect data on a Cartesian grid in a spiral-like fashion.

Radial Trajectory

With radial trajectories, the readout gradient is oriented obliquely and rotated after each readout to create a linear trajectory that traverses the center of k-space with every acquisition. This method oversamples the center of k-space at the cost of undersampling its periphery. Allowing for data undersampling, the number of RF excitations (TRs) is typically reduced compared with rectilinear trajectories, resulting in shorter acquisition times (Figure I8-6). Radial k-space filling can be performed for both 2D and 3D imaging. Areas of application include fast perfusion imaging and MR angiography.

REDUCING N_{PE}: PARALLEL ACQUISITION TECHNIQUES

One of the most exciting and important recent advances in MR has been the development of parallel acquisition techniques, which enable N_{PE}, and consequently acquisition times, to be reduced by factors of 2, 4, 8, and more with no loss of spatial resolution. Parallel acquisition methods exploit the differences in signal detected by receiver coils positioned over different parts of the body. Instead of relying solely on the phase-encoding steps, spatial localization can in part be derived from differences in sensitivity of multiple coils to pick up signal from the same source. Reducing the need for phase-encoding steps allows acquisition times to be reduced accordingly.

Parallel imaging can be understood from the starting point of the concept of rectangular FOV, where undersampling of k-space in the phase-encoding direction results in a decrease in the FOV in the same direction (Chapter I-7). If the body is narrower in the phase-encoding direction, rectangular FOV is a handy technique for reducing image acquisition times without sacrificing spatial resolution. But what happens if the body is not asymmetric? As discussed in Chapter I-7, if the field of view is smaller than the object being imaged, then aliasing, or image wraparound artifact, will occur (Figure I8-7).

Parallel acquisition techniques make clever use of the coil sensitivity profiles to solve the aliasing problem and "unwrap" the image. For parallel acquisition techniques to work, more than one receiver coil must be used, each with its own receiver channel (Chapter I-1). The coils ideally are oriented side by side in the phase-encoding direction. The factor by which phase-encoding steps are

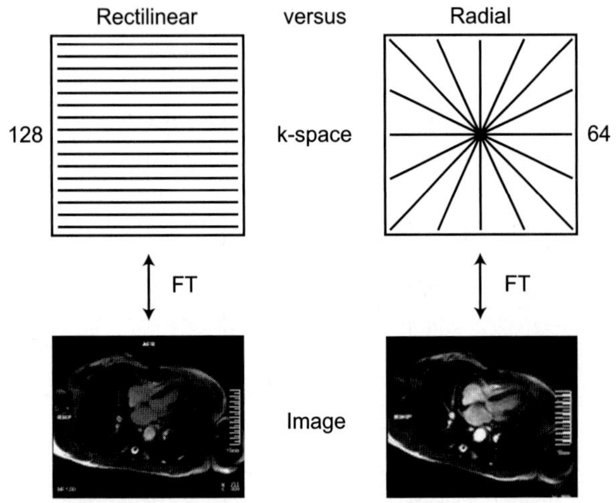

FIGURE I8-6. Radial k-space trajectory. The oversampling of the center of k-space means that fewer RF excitations are required for comparable image quality, although data undersampling results in streak artifacts.

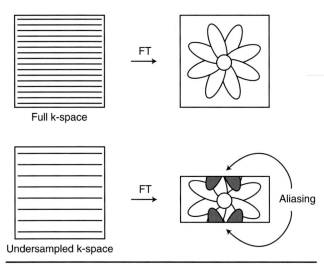

FIGURE I8-7. Undersampling of k-space leads to a rectangular field of view. If the image is not rectangular and the FOV is smaller than the imaged object, then aliasing (wraparound artifact) occurs.

undersampled is sometimes referred to as the *R factor* (for example, a factor of two in Figure I8-7). For successful unwrapping the R factor generally can be no more than the number of independent coil elements in the phase-encoding direction with separate receiver channels.

> **IMPORTANT CONCEPTS:** Parallel imaging uses the spatial information derived from differences in detected signal from different coils. If multiple coil elements are aligned in the phase-encoding direction, their spatial information can be used to overcome aliasing, or wraparound artifact, which is caused by undersampling the phase-encoding steps.

Parallel acquisition methods can be thought of in two general categories—pre-Fourier transform and post-Fourier transform. The pre-Fourier method is commonly called *SMASH* (for *SiMultaneous Acquisition of Spatial Harmonics*), and the post-Fourier method is called *SENSE* (for *SENSitivity Encoding*).

With SENSE, knowledge of the sensitivity profiles is used to unwrap images. With SMASH, the profiles are used to fill in the missing or undersampled lines of k-space. Common to both parallel imaging methods is the use of coil sensitivity profiles, which are introduced next before each method is discussed.

Phased-Array Coils and Coil Sensitivity Profiles

Phased-Array Coils

Cardiovascular MR applications use phased-array coils to receive the signal produced by the protons in the body. As introduced in Chapter I-1, phased-array coils are composed of several (typically 4 to 8) coils that can each receive signal simultaneously and independently. The image produced with phased-array coils reflects the sum of the signals from all of the individual coil elements.

If there are enough receiver channels to match the number of coil elements, then signals from each of the coils can be processed separately. Parallel imaging can be fully implemented. If there are not enough receiver channels, then signals from multiple coils are combined or multiplexed, to each receiver channel. The degree to which parallel imaging can be used to reduce N_{PE} depends on the number of coils in the phase-encoding direction with its own receiver channels.

Coil Sensitivity Profiles

All coils have varying sensitivity to signal. Other characteristics being equal, protons that are closest to a coil are detected the best, while those that are farther away produce weaker signal. The depth and breadth of the sensitivity are related to the diameter of the coil (Figure I8-8).

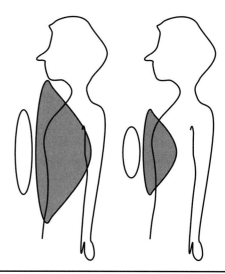

FIGURE I8-8. Coil sensitivity profiles. Larger coils provide broader and deeper coverage.

Measured MR signal from a particular region can be expressed as the product of the signal in that region and the sensitivity of a receiver coil to that region:

Measured signal = Proton signal × Coil sensitivity

When multiple coil elements are combined in a phased-array coil, the overall coil sensitivity has uniformity better than each individual element and can be relatively uniform across the imaging field.

CHALLENGE QUESTION: How are surface coils such as torso phased-array coils used to image a volume of tissue such as the thorax?

Answer: Typically two sets of phased-array coils are used, one placed anteriorly and the other posteriorly. Provided that depth penetration is adequate relative to the thickness of the subject, a relatively uniform sensitivity can be achieved across the thorax.

Note that despite, the use of coil sensitivity correction filters, coil nonuniformity is still apparent in most MR images: Signal intensity is higher in the superficial tissues close to the coils than deeper in the body.

Parallel imaging exploits the differences in coil sensitivities. Rather than being combined straightaway, the measurements from the different coils are kept separate at first. Then, together with separate coil sensitivity maps for each of the coils, their individual signal contributions are used to aid spatial localization.

> **IMPORTANT CONCEPT:** With parallel imaging, signal intensity from the field of view must be separately measurable from each of the coil elements. Additionally, coil sensitivity profiles must be measured for each of these coils.

The ways in which coil sensitivity profiles are used to achieve parallel imaging for SENSE and SMASH are described next, with simplified examples to illustrate the principles.

SENSE

With SENSE, the wraparound artifact that results from undersampling k-space is corrected at the level of the image, rather than in k-space. Since the correction is applied after the Fourier transformation, SENSE is referred to as a post-Fourier, or image domain, approach (Figure I8-9).

To unwrap the image, the signal intensity of the aliased portions must be separated into two components: the signal from the image proper and the signal contribution from the aliased portion from the opposite end of the image. Consider the example in Figure I8-10, where the signal is separated into the image proper (□) and the signal that is wrapping from the top and bottom of the image (⊡). The unwrapping of the image relies on differences in sensitivity of each coil to the proper and wrapped portions, which in turn depends on the proximity of each coil to each region.

Unwrapping of the image is achieved by considering measured signal from each coil individually. In fact, for SENSE to work, the signal intensity must be measured separately for each coil, expressed as SI(Coil 1) and SI(Coil 2).

Consider first the signal intensity measured using Coil 1 only. With Coil 1, the signal intensity of the voxel labeled in Figure I8-10 will have contributions from the image proper and from the aliased component. The contributions of each to the image depend both on the amounts of signal from those parts of the image and on the coil sensitivity to each location. For example, for Coil 1, the contribution from the protons in the image proper (top petal of the flower) should be greater than that from the aliased portion.

Coil 2, because of its lower position, will have greater signal contribution from the aliased portion than from the image proper.

Expressed in terms of the coil sensitivity profile, the contributions to signal measured by Coil 1 can be expressed as follows:

$$SI(Coil\ 1) = (\square \times [coil\ 1\ sensitivity\ to\ \square]) \\ + \boxdot \times [coil\ 1\ sensitivity\ to\ \boxdot])$$

Similarly, the SI from Coil 2 can be expressed as

$$SI(Coil\ 2) = (\square \times [coil\ 2\ sensitivity\ to\ \square]) \\ + \boxdot \times [coil\ 2\ sensitivity\ to\ \boxdot])$$

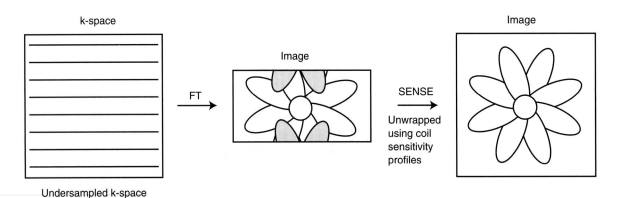

FIGURE I8-9. SENSE technique. The aliasing caused by undersampling of k-space is corrected by manipulating the image using coil sensitivity profiles.

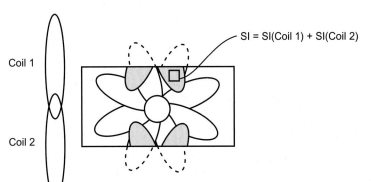

FIGURE I8-10. SENSE parallel acquisition technique. SI from each coil in the measured square includes a component from the image proper and a component from the aliased portion originating from the lower petal of the flower.

If separate receiver channels are available to keep the signal from each coil separate, then SI(Coil 1) and SI(Coil 2) can be measured. With knowledge of the coil sensitivity profiles for Coils 1 and 2, then the problem of SENSE imaging becomes that of solving two equations for two unknowns, □ and □.

Consider some sample values. Assume the coil sensitivity measurements give the following values:

$$\text{Coil 1 sensitivity to } \square = 0.9;$$
$$\text{Coil 2 sensitivity to } \square = 0.1$$

$$\text{Coil 1 sensitivity to } \square = 0.2;$$
$$\text{Coil 2 sensitivity to } \square = 0.8;$$

consistent with the expected higher sensitivity for Coil 1 at □ than □, and vice versa for Coil 2.

Suppose the signal in the voxel in question is measured as 37 from Coil 1 and 43 from Coil 2, then the equations to describe the true □ and aliased □ components would be

$$\text{SI(Coil 1)} = 37 = (\square \times 0.9) + (\square \times 0.2)$$
$$\text{SI(Coil 2)} = 43 = (\square \times 0.1) + (\square \times 0.8)$$

In this example, the two equations can be solved using algebra to find that □ = 30 and □ = 50.

CHALLENGE QUESTION: What is the overall measured signal intensity in the voxel?

Answer: The measured signal intensity is the sum of the signals measured from Coils 1 and 2. If SI(Coil 1) = 37 and SI(Coil 2) = 43, then the sum of these two values is 80. Note that by knowing the coil sensitivity profiles, the contribution to the voxel from the image proper can be calculated as 30, while the wrapped portion adds another 50 to the image signal intensity.

The voxel in the aliased portion of the image would then be reassigned a value of 30 instead of 80. A voxel that corresponds to the tissue outside the original field of view would be created with a signal intensity of 50. By repeating this process for all voxels, an image with a full field of view and no aliasing is reconstructed.

For a SENSE R factor greater than 2, then the process is conceptually the same, only slightly more complicated. For example, if SENSE is applied with an R factor of 3, using three coils, each with its own sensitivity profile, then k-space can be undersampled by a factor of 1/3. To unwrap the resulting image, each voxel signal intensity must be expressed in terms of three equations, based on signal measured from each of the three coils, with three unknowns, reflecting the more complex patterns of aliasing associated with undersampling of k-space by 1/3. Again, different sensitivity profiles for the three coils would be essential to unwrap the image.

> **IMPORTANT CONCEPT:** With SENSE imaging, images are constructed from data collected from each coil individually with only a fraction of the phase-encoding steps. Then, using coil sensitivity profiles, the image can be unwrapped to produce a full FOV image.

SMASH

The goal of SMASH is the same as of SENSE: to undersample the phase-encoding lines and then to solve the aliasing problem by using measurements from each individual coil and their different coil sensitivity profiles. Whereas SENSE solves the problem in the spatial domain of the image, SMASH calculates the missing lines of k-space before applying the Fourier transformation (Figure I8-11).

To understand how SMASH works, it is necessary to revisit how phase-encoding gradients cause phase shifts across the field of view (Chapter I-5).

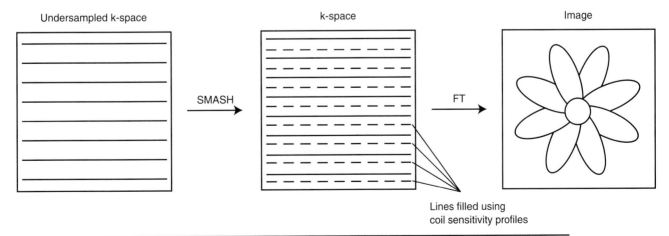

FIGURE I8-11. SMASH technique. The aliasing caused by undersampling of k-space is avoided by filling in the missing k-space data using information from coil sensitivity profiles.

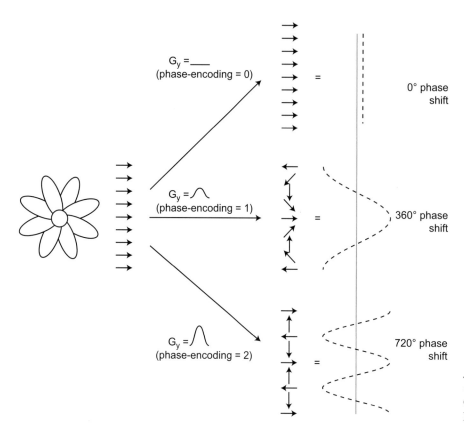

FIGURE I8-12. Consecutive G_y gradients introduce specific phase shifts for protons in the y direction.

Consider the difference between the echo measured with a zero phase-encoding gradient, and then with the first and second phase-encoding steps (review Figure I5-26, Figure I8-12). With no phase-encoding gradient, there is no phase shift across the field of view in the phase-encoding direction; that is, the relative phase shift is zero. With the first step of the phase-encoding gradient, the protons across the field of view in the phase-encoding direction will experience a slight phase dispersion so that the net phase shift from one end of the image to the other will be 360°. With the next increment in phase-encoding gradient, the phase shift across the image will increase to 720°.

The important observation is that the only difference between the zero phase-encoding step and the first phase-encoding step is a 360° phase shift or phase modulation across the image. Given the data from the zero phase-encoding step, one could synthesize the first phase-encoding step signal by applying a phase modulation to the zero phase-encoding signal. With SMASH, the coil sensitivity profiles are used to generate the desired phase modulation.

Consider the example of two coils in the phase-encoding direction used to produce SMASH images with R = 2. First, an echo is collected without a phase-encoding gradient. The measured signal represents summed signal from both coils. The echo that would correspond to the first phase-encoding step is skipped. Then the echo with the second phase-encoding gradient is collected. The third

is skipped, and so on, so that the total number of phase-encoding steps is reduced by one-half.

With SMASH, the data originally collected from the zero phase-encoding step is used to synthesize an echo for the first phase-encoding step. How is this achieved? If the signal from Coil 2 is inverted (made negative) while the signal from Coil 1 is kept positive, then the resulting signal will resemble the zero phase-encoding step data modulated by a 360° phase shift in the phase-encoding direction (Figure I8-13). This signal is used to fill the missing first phase-encoding line of k-space:

Phase-encoding step 0 = Measured data
= Coil 1 + Coil 2 from phase-encoding step 0

Phase-encoding step 1 = Synthesized data
= Coil 1 − Coil 2 from phase-encoding step 0

Therefore, with SMASH, the collected lines are formed by the sum of signals from both coils, and the missing lines (every other line of k-space) are then filled with the difference in measured signal between Coils 1 and 2.

An example of how three coils could be used to reduce k-space sampling by a factor of 3 is shown in Figure I8-14, where combinations of signals from the coils can be used to fill in the missing data:

Phase-encoding step 0 = Measured data
= Coil 1 + Coil 2 + Coil 3 from phase-encoding step 0

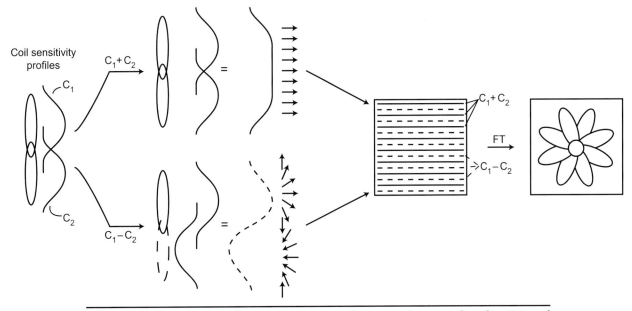

FIGURE 18-13. SMASH implemented with two coils in the phase-encoding direction and undersampling of k-space by a factor of 2. C_1 and C_2 refer to signals sampled separately from Coils 1 and 2, respectively. The missing lines of k-space can be computed by subtracting signal of Coil 2 from Coil 1.

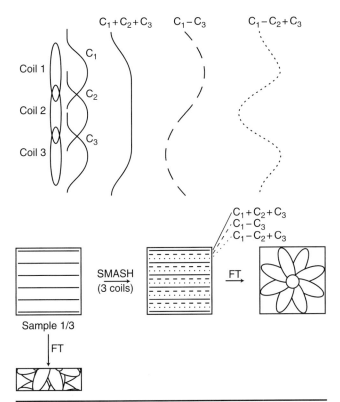

FIGURE 18-14. SMASH implemented with three coils in the phase-encoding direction and threefold undersampling of k-space.

Phase-encoding step 1 = Synthesized data
= Coil 1 – Coil 3 from phase-encoding step 0

Phase-encoding step 2 = Synthesized data
= Coil 1 – Coil 2 + Coil 3 from phase-encoding step 0

In other words, phase modulations of 360° and 720° are obtained by manipulating the coil data and taking advantage of different coil sensitivities.

With SMASH, the coil sensitivity profiles must be measured to ensure that assumptions about the phase modulations are valid. That is, for SMASH to work, Coil 1 – Coil 2 in Figure 18-13 must closely approximate the effect of a phase-encoding gradient that induces a 360° phase shift across the phase-encoding direction. Measurement of the coil sensitivity profiles enables corrections or modified weighting of the signal from each coil as needed to approximate the desired phase modulation.

> **IMPORTANT CONCEPT:** With SMASH imaging, a fraction of the k-space data is collected. The unsampled lines of k-space are calculated by synthesizing phase modulations using coil sensitivity profiles. The Fourier transformation produces a full FOV image.

Tradeoffs and Challenges of Parallel Imaging

Parallel imaging faces many technical challenges.

The key requirement of parallel imaging is coil sensitivity profiles. Accurate coil sensitivity measurements can be challenging, particularly in applications in the torso, where subject breathing can alter the relationship between the phased-array coil and the body—and consequently the sensitivity profile—from one breath hold to another. Whereas original implementations required separate acquisitions for sensitivity maps and imaging, new commercially available sequences incorporate the sensitivity profile mapping into the same acquisition as the imaging sequence. This can be achieved with SENSE or SMASH by fully sampling the central lines of k-space (for example, the central 24–36 lines) and using the resulting low-spatial-resolution image as a sensitivity map. The remainder of k-space is then undersampled and SENSE or SMASH algorithms applied. The tradeoff to this approach is that the full R-fold reduction in acquisition time is not achieved.

CHALLENGE QUESTION: With a 256 × 256 image, an R factor of 2 with parallel imaging should reduce the acquisition time by a factor of 2, from 40 sec to 20 sec. What is the actual reduction in acquisition time if the central 36 lines are fully sampled?

Answer: If the central 36 lines are fully sampled, then the total number of phase-encoding steps increases from the expected 128 to 146 (128 + 18). Therefore, the effective reduction in acquisition time is a factor of 256/146 = 1.75 rather than 2.

Another challenge to parallel imaging is the need for extensive computations. Constant refinements in computational algorithms are being proposed to reduce these demands.

Parallel imaging methods require that signals from multiple coils aligned in the phase-encoding direction be independently measurable. The R factor, the degree to which k-space is undersampled, cannot exceed the number of coils in the phase-encoding direction. This presents technical challenges. Most phased-array coils have a limited number of coils in each direction. With conventional designs more coil means smaller coils. The smaller the coils, the lower their depth sensitivity (Figure I8-8). Second, most systems have a limited number of receiver channels. The trend is now toward larger numbers of receiver channels and specially designed receiver coils with multiple independent elements. Performance of these new systems will determine the clinical use of parallel imaging.

Parallel imaging permits fast image acquisition without a reduction in spatial resolution. Nonetheless, there is a loss in SNR, because k-space is undersampled. SNR is also reduced by a factor called g, for *geometric factor*, which reflects the lack of total spatial independence of coil profiles. The geometric relationships between individual coils result in g values greater than 1. SNR in parallel imaging is reduced by a factor that is proportional to the square root of the R factor and proportional to the g factor:

$$SNR_{parallel} = \frac{SNR}{g\sqrt{R}}$$

Since g varies spatially within the image, routine SNR measurements with parallel imaging techniques are challenging.

> **TRADEOFFS AND CHALLENGES IN PARALLEL IMAGING:**
> - Need for coil sensitivity maps
> - Need for intensive computation
> - Requirement for special coil design with large numbers of independent coil elements and separate receiver channels for each
> - Reduced SNR

The dramatic savings in acquisition times, however, make parallel imaging techniques attractive. When implemented in conjunction with sequences that can tolerate the reduction in SNR (Figure I8-15) particularly at higher magnetic field strengths, parallel imaging methods currently represent the best approach for reducing acquisition times. Active development of improved MR hardware and image reconstruction algorithms that take advantage of parallel imaging promise further advances in coming years.

SUMMARY OF FAST IMAGING STRATEGIES

A summary of the techniques described so far in this chapter is given in Table I8-1.

FAST IMAGING EXAMPLE: OPTIMIZING A 3D MRA ACQUISITION

In this section, many of the principles discussed in the chapter are put to practice in the problem of designing a 3D MR angiography sequence. Starting with an arbitrary coronal 3D spoiled gradient echo pulse sequence, the goal is to apply strategies presented in this chapter to produce

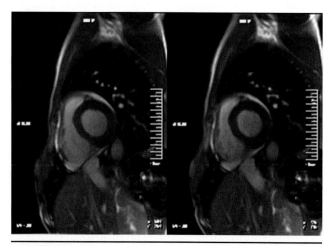

FIGURE I8-15. Single image from steady-state free precession cine acquisition without (left, 6 heartbeat acquisition time) and with (right, 4 heartbeat acquisition time) parallel imaging. Image quality is comparable despite the 33% decrease in acquisition time.

TABLE I8-1

Strategy	Approach
Reduce TR	Shorten RF with higher transmitter BW or asymmetric RF pulses increase receiver BW and use of asymmetric echoes
Increase ETL	Multiple echoes per RF pulse with spin echoes or gradient echoes
Reduce N_{PE}	Lower N_{PE} with lower spatial resolution
	Lower N_{PE} with rectangular field of view
	Partial Fourier imaging
	Nontraditional k-space trajectories (spiral, radial)
	Parallel imaging (SENSE, SMASH)

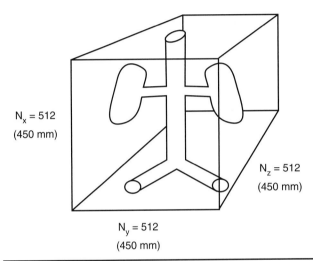

FIGURE I8-16. Initial parameters for a coronal 3D gradient echo acquisition.

a 3D MRA sequence with high spatial resolution (≤2 mm voxels) and an acquisition time of less than a breath hold (<20 sec).

The following parameters define the starting point in this example (Figure I8-16):

TR = 6.0 msec, TE = 2.5 msec, flip angle = 25°

FOV = 450 mm × 450 mm × 450 mm (x, y, z)

Matrix = 512 × 512 × 512

Voxel size = 0.9 mm × 0.9 mm × 0.9 mm

where the number of signal averages is 1, the RF pulse is symmetric, and the two phase-encoding directions are left to right (y direction) and anterior to posterior (z direction).

CHALLENGE QUESTION: What is the acquisition time for this 3D gradient echo sequence?

ANSWER: $T_{acq} = N_{PE1} \times N_{PE2} \times TR$. The other potential contributors to the equation—the number of signals averaged and the echo train length—are both equal to 1 for this class of sequences. Therefore, $T_{acq} = 512 \times 512 \times 6$ msec = 1,572,864 msec = 1573 sec = **26 min**!

Step 1: Reduce TR

CHALLENGE QUESTION: What approaches can be used to reduce TR?

Answer: For gradient echo imaging, the TR is constrained by the duration of the RF pulse, the TE, and the duration of the readout. The RF pulse duration can be reduced by use of higher transmitter bandwidth and an asymmetric RF pulse (Figure I8-17). The TE and readout duration can be reduced by increasing the receiver bandwidth and use of an asymmetric echo (Table I8-1).

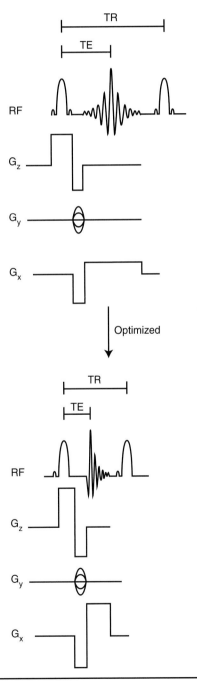

FIGURE I8-17. Minimizing TR and TE by increasing transmitter and receiver bandwidths.

Three steps can be taken to reduce the TR.

First, the RF pulse duration can be potentially reduced by increasing the high transmitter bandwidth. An asymmetric RF pulse is also an option.

Second, if the receiver bandwidth is increased, then the sampling frequency will increase, and the echo will be compressed. By decreasing TE and the readout duration, the TR will decrease. As a result, the TR will be shortened from 6 msec to about 4.2 msec, while the TE drops from 2.5 msec to 1.6 msec. Note that these examples assume high maximum gradient strengths and rapid gradient rise times. Practically speaking, there is a limit to how high the receiver bandwidth should go. As bandwidths increase, the loss in SNR increases more than the gain in speed. In most clinical applications, the maximum receiver bandwidth used is between 500 and 800 Hz/voxel.

Third, an asymmetric echo can be used for the readout. This results in the center of k-space being filled earlier, and hence a shorter TE and readout duration. Now the minimum TR is, say, 3.6 msec, and the TE about 1.2 msec.

Result of Step 1: Assume that the above steps result in TR = 3.6 msec (TE = 1.2 msec). What is the corresponding T_{acq}?

$$T_{acq} = 512 \times 512 \times 3.6 \text{ msec} = 944 \text{ sec}$$
$$= \mathbf{15.7 \text{ min}}$$

CHALLENGE QUESTION: What is the effect of Step 1 on SNR?

Answer: The reduction in acquisition time is almost all due to reduced echo sampling times (RF shortening is modest by comparison). Echo sampling times are reduced by about 40%. SNR is proportional to the square root of sampling time, and hence the shorter acquisition has 0.77 as much SNR. That is, the SNR after Step 1 is 23% lower than the starting value.

> **IMPORTANT CONCEPT:** TR can be reduced by using an asymmetric RF pulse, higher receiver bandwidth, and asymmetric echo sampling.

Although a 40% reduction is substantial, the acquisition time is still much too long for clinical implementation. Further steps must be taken.

Step 2: Reduce the Number of Phase-Encoding Steps

Since the area of imaging interest is not cube-shaped, the FOV can be refined to fit the area of interest, taking advantage of rectangular FOV options to reduce the number of phase-encoding steps in each phase-encoding direction.

The longest direction is in the cephalocaudal direction, and therefore the frequency-encoding direction is defined as such.

In this example, assume that because of the subject's size, the left-to-right dimension can be reduced to

350 mm and the anterior-to-posterior dimension to 112 mm.

For the numbers given, the left-to-right dimension is reduced from 450 mm to 350 mm, which represents use of 77.8% (350 mm/450 mm) rectangular FOV. Therefore, $N_y = 77.8\% \times 512 = 398$. In the anterior-to-posterior dimension, 25% (112 mm/450 mm) rectangular field of view can be used so that N_z is 128 (25% × 512). These changes are shown in the upper part of Figure I8-18.

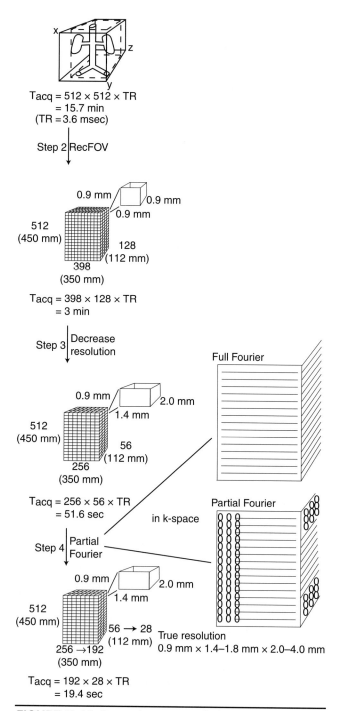

FIGURE I8-18. Successive steps applied to 3D gradient echo sequence optimization.

Result of Step 2:

$$N_y = 398, N_z = 128 \, (TR = 3.6 \, msec)$$
$$T_{acq} = 398 \times 128 \times 3.6 \, msec = 183 \, sec = \textbf{3 min}$$

CHALLENGE QUESTION: Using rectangular FOV, how is spatial resolution or voxel size affected?

Answer: The spatial resolution is unchanged. Voxel dimension remains 0.9 mm $\times$ 0.9 mm $\times$ 0.9 mm.

Step 3: Decrease the Number of Phase-Encoding Steps at the Expense of Resolution

Although for static body imaging the higher the spatial resolution, the better the imaging, in cardiac and vascular applications spatial resolution can be sacrificed for corresponding reductions in acquisition time to help minimize notion artifact. The resolution can be maintained in the frequency-encoding direction without an effect on acquisition time. Decreased resolution in both phase-encoding directions will directly reduce the acquisition time.

For example, in this case, if the number of voxels in the left-to-right direction is decreased from 398 to 256 (reduced by 36%) without a change in FOV, then the resolution or voxel size in that dimension increases from 0.9 to 1.4 mm (350 cm/256). Similarly, in the anterior-posterior direction, if the number of voxels is reduced from 112 to 56 (50%) while the FOV remains 112 mm, then the voxel size in that direction increases from 0.9 mm to 2 mm (112 mm/56). These changes are shown in the middle part of Figure I8-18.

Result of Step 3:

$$N_y = 256, N_z = 56 \, (TR = 3.6 \, msec),$$
$$\text{voxel dimension } 0.9 \, mm \times 1.4 \, mm \times 2 \, mm$$
$$T_{acq} = 256 \times 56 \times 3.6 \, msec = \textbf{51.6 sec}$$

Step 4: Use Partial Fourier to Reduce the Number of Phase-Encoding Steps

In both phase-encoding directions, partial Fourier methods can be used to collect asymmetric data and to fill the uncollected parts of k-space with zeroes. Because the edges of k-space are still collected (albeit only at one end and not the other), fine details are still relatively well visualized. However, the true spatial resolution no longer is represented by the voxel size (as discussed in Chapter I-7). If 75% asymmetric filling is used in the left-to-right direction, then N_y is reduced from 256 to 192. In the anterior-posterior direction, zero padding is typically used to reduce N_z by one-half, from 56 to 28. The acquisition times are reduced proportionately. In the left-to-right

direction, the spatial resolution is degraded beyond 1.4 toward 1.8 mm, while in the anterior-posterior direction it is between 2 and 4 mm. These changes are illustrated at the bottom of Figure I8-18.

Result of Step 4:

$$N_y = 192, N_z = 28 \, (TR = 3.6 \, msec)$$
$$\text{Voxel dimension } 0.9 \, mm \times 1.4 \, mm \times 2 \, mm$$
$$\text{Spatial resolution } 0.9 \, mm \times 1.4 - 1.8 \, mm \times 2 - 4 \, mm$$
$$T_{acq} = 192 \times 28 \times 3.6 \, msec = \textbf{19.4 sec}$$

Alternative Step 4: Parallel Imaging

An alternative or additional approach to reducing the number of phase-encoding steps is to use a parallel acquisition technique such as SMASH or SENSE. For example, if there are three independent coils aligned from left to right across the y direction, then the N_y can in theory be undersampled by one-third. Depending on the SNR limitations, it is also possible to reduce not just N_y but also N_z whereby parallel acquisition techniques are applied in both phase-encoding directions.

Instead of using zero filling, parallel imaging in the N_y direction with three coils in the y direction will result in a reduction of N_y from 256 to 97. This corresponds to undersampling by a factor R = 3, plus full sampling in the central 24 lines of k-space (for the coil sensitivity profiles). The remainder of the parameters are the same, $N_z = 56$ and TR = 3.6 msec. As a consequence, the acquisition time is reduced to 20.6 sec. One great benefit of this approach over the zero-filling techniques is the maintenance of voxel size and spatial resolution with parallel techniques. However, the SNR is reduced because of the decrease in acquisition time with fewer phase-encoding steps and imperfect coil geometry.

Result of Alternative Step 4:

$$N_y = 97, N_z = 56 \, (TR = 3.6 \, msec)$$
$$\text{Voxel dimension = spatial resolution:}$$
$$0.9 \, mm \times 1.4 \, mm \times 2 \, mm$$
$$T_{acq} = 97 \times 56 \times 3.6 \, msec = \textbf{20.6 sec}$$

CHALLENGE QUESTION: What if parallel imaging were combined with partial Fourier methods? Compute the acquisition time if, in addition to Step 4, parallel imaging were implemented using R = 3 and full sampling of the central 24 lines of k-space.

Answer: The number of phase-encoding steps, N_y, would be reduced from 192 to 80 (192/3 + 16 extra lines).

Result of Alternative Step 4 plus Step 4:

$$N_y = 80, N_z = 28 \, (TR = 3.6 \, msec)$$
$$\text{Voxel dimension } 0.9 \, mm \times 1.4 \, mm \times 2 \, mm$$

Spatial resolution 0.9 mm × 1.4–1.8 mm × 2–4 mm

$$T_{acq} = 80 \times 28 \times 3.6 \text{ msec} = \textbf{8.1 sec}$$

Although the reduction in acquisition time is highly desirable, the concomitant reduction in signal-to-noise ratio could make this strategy impractical.

Summary of Optimization and Further Considerations:

In this example, the acquisition time was reduced from 26 min to 19.4 sec (or 8.1–20.6 sec with parallel imaging) by use of several strategies: reducing TR by shortening the RF and echo durations and decreasing the number of phase-encoding steps using a combination of recFOV, zero filling, and parallel imaging. In the example used, the selection of specific parameters was arbitrary but representative.

Different optimization strategies can be selected or emphasized according to the imaging needs, subject size, time constraints, and so forth. For example, for a smaller patient, the entire FOV could be reduced and spatial resolution maintained with a reduction in the number of phase-encoding steps. Alternatively, if the subject is unable to hold their breath adequately for these imaging parameters, then N_{PE} can be reduced further and spatial resolution decreased. Alternatively, a higher receiver bandwidth can be used to reduce TR, at the cost of lower SNR. Parallel acquisition techniques, in one or both phase-encoding directions, can be used to reduce imaging times considerably. In real clinical practice, the imaging protocols (see Chapter II-4) are set up with default values. The user can then make desired changes. The information in this chapter and case study will help the reader to understand the tradeoffs associated with each kind of modification.

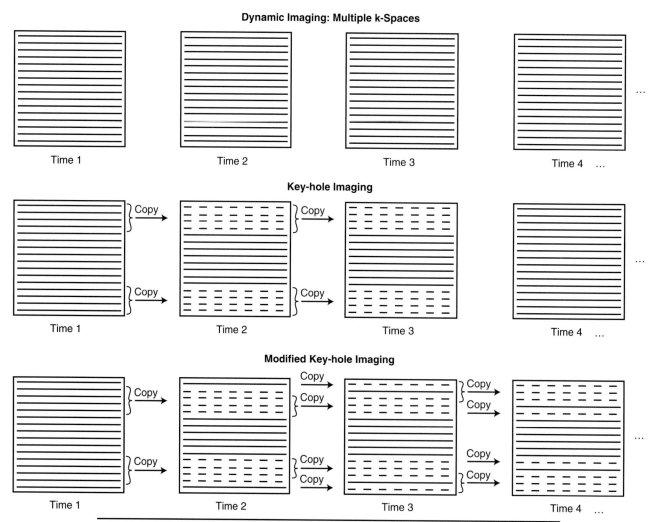

FIGURE I8-19. Two keyholing techniques. Solid lines are newly collected lines of k-space, while dashed lines are copied from other time points. Acquisition times for the second and third acquisitions are but a fraction of the full acquisition time. Copying can be performed forward (as shown) or backward across time points.

FILLING MULTIPLE k-SPACES

There are several cardiovascular applications in which images at the same location are acquired repeatedly over time. For example, in cine gradient echo imaging (Chapter III-4), a slice of the heart is viewed at multiple time points across the cardiac cycle in order to assess its motion and contractility. Velocity-encoded phase contrast imaging (Chapter II-3) is performed to measure blood velocities in vessels across the cardiac cycle. In gadolinium-enhanced MRA (Chapter II-4), fast repeated MRA acquisitions enable assessment of the hemodynamic properties of vessels. For cardiac perfusion (Chapter III-7), tissue slices are viewed during the course of enhancement by an exogenous contrast agent.

In most of these applications, the speed of each individual acquisition is important because it determines the temporal resolution of the dynamic imaging. The faster the acquisitions, the better the temporal information that

can be obtained from the images. In the preceding sections, methods to reduce acquisition times for each image were discussed. This section considers ways in which multiple k-spaces can be collected more efficiently by sharing data across time points. In all examples, rectilinear k-space trajectories are used, but the principles apply also to other trajectories.

Keyhole Imaging Approaches

Common to *keyhole imaging* is the notion that most of the information content of an image is represented in the central portions of k-space (see Figure I7-1). Therefore, only the central lines of k-space need to be updated with high temporal resolution. The periphery of k-space is still sampled, but much less frequently than the central part (Figure I8-19). For example, following a full collection of k-space, the next two to four acquisitions may perform only central k-space data collection. The remainder of

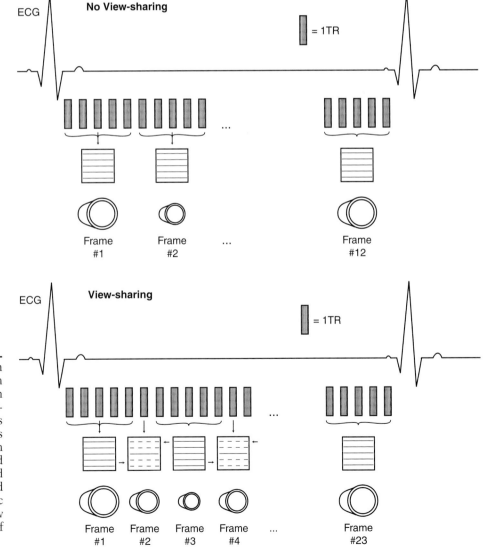

FIGURE I8-20. View sharing. In this example, five echoes from five TRs are added to each k-space frame during one heartbeat. Sharing k-space data across time frames (below) increases the apparent temporal resolution of electrocardiographically gated images of cardiac motion. Solid lines are collected, while dashed lines are copied. (Schematic drawings reflect a short-axis view of the heart at different stages of contraction and relaxation.)

k-space for the partial acquisitions can be filled by copying data from the first acquisition.

Another approach to keyhole imaging is to supplement with the sampling of a few lines in the periphery of k-space across the various time points. The periphery of k-space is still undersampled relative to the center of k-space but the additional updating of perephereal k-space lines improves the temporal representation of high resolution data.

The true temporal resolution of keyholed data is difficult to ascertain. The effective temporal resolution may be given as the average time per acquisition. For example, in the keyhole example in Figure I8-19, if a full k-space acquisition requires 21 sec and the second and third acquisitions require only 7 sec, then the effective temporal resolution is approximately (21 + 7 + 7)/3 = 11.7 sec.

View Sharing

A different approach to dynamic imaging, called *view sharing*, is typically reserved for cardiac cine gradient echo imaging and cardiovascular velocity-encoded cine phase contrast imaging, techniques that will be discussed in later parts of this book. The goal is to improve the temporal resolution of the images, where temporal resolution refers to the number of frames of the cardiac cycle that are imaged. Although the method can be implemented in a number of ways, one classic example is shown in Figure I8-20.

To increase the number of frames of the cardiac cycle that are imaged, data are shared between adjacent k-spaces. Typically, with view sharing, alternate frames contain only a limited sampling of k-space data. For these frames the remanders of k-space is copied from preceding and subsequent frames. As a result, the number of frames can be nearly doubled with no change in acquisition time. The true temporal resolution of these view-shared acquisitions is difficult to estimate but lies somewhere between the original temporal resolution and the view-shared version.

REVIEW QUESTIONS

1. Consider the effects of increasing receiver bandwidth across the following range of values for an imaging matrix of 256 × 128 × 32 voxels (Figure I8-Q1).

a. First, complete Table I8-2A:
b. Discuss the relative benefits of increasing receiver bandwidth from 250 Hz/voxel (64 kHz) to 500 Hz/voxel (128 kHz).
c. How do the benefits in b) compare to the transition from 500 Hz/voxel (128 kHz) to 1000 Hz/voxel?

2. With multislice spin echo imaging, the time following each echo before the next RF pulse is used to image other

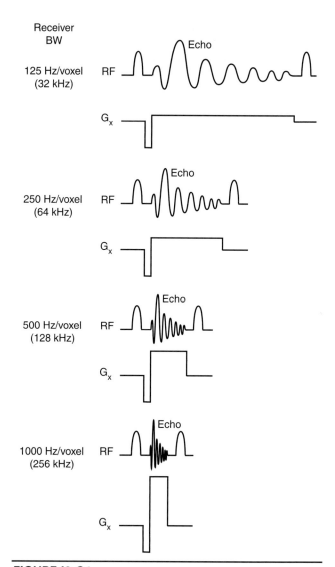

FIGURE I8-Q1

▶ **TABLE I8-2A**

Receiver Bandwidth		Echo sampling duration (msec)	TR (msec)	TE (msec)	Acquisition Time	Relative SNR
125 Hz/voxel	32 kHz	8	10	4		1
250 Hz/voxel	64 kHz	4	6	2		
500 Hz/voxel	128 kHz	2	4	1.5		
1000 Hz/voxel	256 kHz	1	3	1		

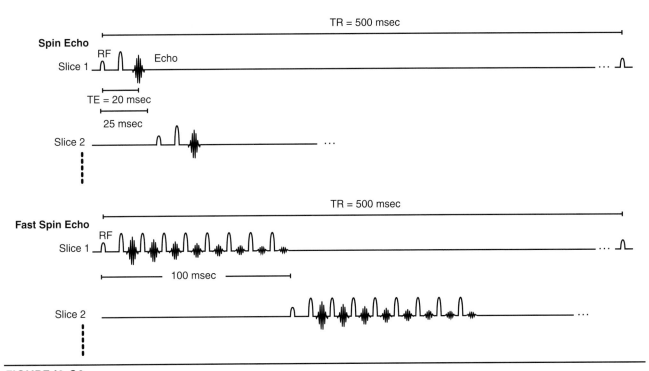

FIGURE I8-Q2

slices. In fast spin echo imaging, on the other hand, multiple echoes are generated with every RF pulse, so the number of slices that can be imaged is reduced.

For a spin echo sequence, if the TR = 500 msec and TE = 20 msec, then there is time for about 20 slices to be imaged during the TR (Figure I8-Q2), because the time from the start of an RF pulse to the end of the echo is about 25 msec. For an imaging matrix of 256×256, the time for a single acquisition is 256×500 msec = 128 sec.

If the sequence is modified so that eight echoes are sampled following each TR, with an interecho spacing of 10 msec, the total time from start of the RF to end of the echo is now 100 msec.

a. How many slices can be imaged in a single acquisition?
b. What will the acquisition time be?
c. Discuss the relative benefits and drawbacks of the two approaches in the clinical setting if 20 slices are desired.

3. You wish to perform a gadolinium-enhanced MR angiogram of the carotid arteries and thoracic aorta. Consider the following two protocols and determine which set of parameters is preferable for imaging. For both acquisitions, the 3D MRA sequence has the following parameters: TR = 4 msec, TE = 1.2 msec, flip angle = 40°.

Coronal acquisition (Figure I8-Q3). Coronal positioning of the imaging volume (dashed lines) with depiction of two representative axial cross sections

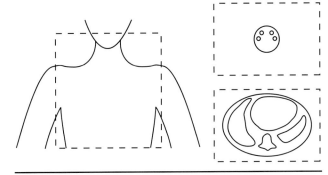

FIGURE I8-Q3

(right) through the neck and chest. The imaging matrix is

$$N_x = 512$$
$$N_y = 160$$

$N_z = 32$ (zero-filled or interpolated to 64)

The FOV is

$$FOV_x \text{ (craniocaudal)} = 400 \text{ mm}$$
$$FOV_y \text{ (left-right)} = 400 \text{ mm}$$
$$FOV_z \text{ (anterior-posterior)} = 128 \text{ mm}$$

Sagittal acquisition (Figure I8-Q4). Sagittal positioning of the imaging volume (dashed lines) with depiction of two representative axial cross sections (right) through the neck and chest. The imaging matrix is

$$N_x = 512$$

▶ **TABLE I8-3A**

	FOV$_x$	FOV$_y$	FOV$_z$	N$_x$	N$_y$	N$_z$	x (mm)	y (mm)	z (mm)	Time
Coronal	400	40	128	512	160	32(64)				
Sagittal	400	400(250)	96	512	160(100)	48(96)				

$$N_y = 160 \rightarrow recFOV \text{ to } 100$$
$$N_z = 48 \text{ (interpolated to 96)}$$

The FOV is

$$FOV_x \text{ (cranio-caudal)} = 400 \text{ mm}$$

$$FOV_y \text{ (anterior-posterior)} = 400 \text{ mm} \rightarrow 250 \text{ mm recFOV}$$

$$FOV_z \text{ (left-right)} = 96 \text{ mm}$$

Complete Table I8-3A, where x, y, z refer to true spatial resolution. Also calculate the voxel size and total time for each acquisition. Which acquisition approach is preferable and why?

4. For the phased-array coil shown in Figure I8-Q5, what is the maximum R factor (undersampling of phase-encoding steps) that can be achieved for 2D imaging using parallel acquisition techniques, assuming that each coil element is independent and with its own receiver channel? What direction must phase-encoding be for this to occur? What about a 3D sequence?

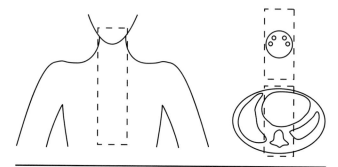

FIGURE I8-Q4

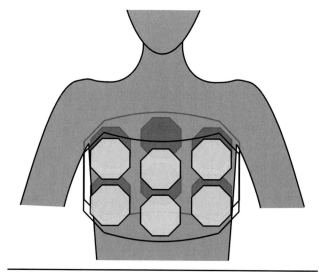

FIGURE I8-Q5

Chapter 9

Selectively Saturating, Nulling, and Exciting Protons

Up to this point, RF pulses and tissue image contrast considerations have assumed that all of the protons in the field of view, including both water and fat, contribute to the image. However, in some cases, only signal from some tissues and not others is desired. For example, to enhance conspicuity of pathology in a fatty surrounding or to characterize fat-containing lesions, a sequence that selectively eliminates signal from fat protons is useful. Alternatively, suppressing certain types of signal that cause artifacts (such as ghosting or wraparound) can improve image quality. In MRI, tissue suppression or selective excitation can be performed in several ways. These techniques are grouped here under common themes: saturation (spatial and frequency), nulling by inversion recovery, and selective excitation.

REVIEW OF RELEVANT MR PHYSICS CONCEPTS

Before discussing each of the selective imaging methods, a brief review of some relevant MR concepts that were covered in earlier chapters may be helpful. The chapters in which these topics were discussed are noted for each concept.

Invisibility of Longitudinal Magnetization (Chapter I-2)

Recall that all magnetization vectors, regardless of their orientation, can be expressed in terms of their longitudinal and transverse components. Magnetization aligned longitudinally with the main magnetic field (1.5 T) is invisible to the receiver coils. Longitudinal magnetization is considered to be potential rather than measured signal. On the other hand, transverse magnetization is measurable.

Dephasing by Gradients (Chapter I-4)

Immediately following RF excitation, magnetization in the transverse plane is coherent. When gradients are applied, as needed for frequency and phase encoding, precessional frequencies begin to vary spatially across the field of view (remember the Larmor equation!). The protons rapidly lose their coherence and dephase. For most of the discussion so far, this dephasing has been considered undesirable. However, it can be useful for eliminating unwanted signal.

Differences between Fat and Water Protons (Chapter I-1)

Fat and water protons placed in the same field experience slightly different local magnetic fields because of their different molecular environments. As a result, fat protons precess slightly slower than water protons. At 1.5 T, the difference is about 220 Hz, tiny when compared to the Larmor frequency of about 64 MHz (64,000,000 Hz). If water protons are precessing at 63,775,820 Hz, fat protons in the same 1.5 T magnetic field will precess at 63,775,600 Hz. Two important consequences arise from these differences in precessional frequencies:

1. *Differences in resonance frequency:* For resonance, the RF pulse must have the same frequency as the precessional

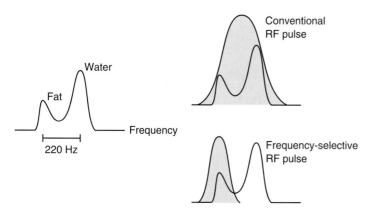

FIGURE I9-1. Resonance peaks for fat and water. Conventional excitation is performed using a broad-bandwidth RF pulse that excites all hydrogen protons, including both fat and water. A slight difference in precessional frequencies between fat and water allows for frequency-selective RF excitation using a narrow bandwidth RF pulse that can be used to image fat or water protons selectively.

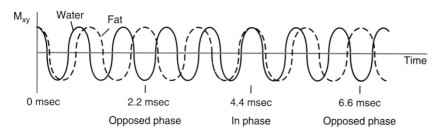

FIGURE I9-2. Slight differences in their precessional frequencies cause fat and water proton magnetization vectors to point in opposite directions in the transverse plane 2.2 msec after RF excitation (assuming 1.5 T). At 4.4 msec, the vectors are realigned, and hence signal from fat and water is additive.

frequency of the protons to cause excitation. Because fat and water precess at different frequencies, it is possible to excite one and not the other selectively, provided the RF pulse has a narrow enough bandwidth. With a bandwidth of less than ±100 Hz, the RF pulse can selectively excite only water or only fat (Figure I9-1). As will be discussed below, these pulses can be used for excitation or suppression.

2. *In-phase and opposed-phase imaging (chemical shift artifact of the second kind):* Immediately after the RF excitation, the transverse magnetization of the protons are coherent. However, because of differences in precessional frequencies, the fat and water protons gradually become dephased (Figure I9-2). At predictable time points, fat and water protons precessing in the transverse plane will be completely out of phase or opposed phase; that is, they will have a phase difference of 180° and point in opposite directions. Consequently, their signals will cancel. Voxels that contain purely fat or water are not affected by the relative phase difference, but voxels that have fat and water in roughly equal proportions will appear black because of the cancellation of signal. This is referred to as *chemical shift artifact of the second kind* or the *India ink artifact* (Figure I9-3).

CHALLENGE QUESTION: If the frequency difference between fat and water protons at 1.5 T is 220 Hz, at what time intervals would you expect their respective signals to become in and out of phase?

Answer: If the frequency difference is about 220 Hz or 220 cycles/sec, then the fat and water protons would become in phase about every 4.4–4.5 msec (since 1000/220 = 4.5).

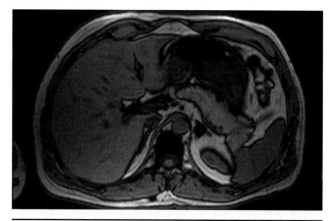

FIGURE I9-3. Chemical shift artifact of the second kind, or India ink artifact, associated with the opposed phases of fat and water protons. At 1.5 T, this artifact is best seen at TE 2.2 msec or TE 6.6 msec. Voxels that contain equal amounts of fat and water, such as at the interfaces of solid organs and fat, demonstrate signal loss that resembles India ink lines around the organs.

For a frequency difference of 220 Hz at 1.5 T, fat and water protons are out of phase first at about 2.2 msec after RF excitation. Then at 4.4 msec, the fat and water protons are in phase again. By 6.6 msec, they are out of phase again. This phase-varying behavior is exploited in some gradient echo imaging applications in order to help characterize fat-containing lesions, such as adrenal adenomas or fatty tumors. It is also used in water excitation sequences, as will be discussed later in this chapter.

Spatially Selective versus Nonselective RF Excitation (Chapter I-5)

With nonselective RF excitation, the RF pulse is applied without use of any gradients. Because the entire volume of tissue in the magnet is precessing at approximately the same frequency, the RF pulse will excite the entire volume. Application of a slice-selective gradient during a narrow bandwidth RF pulse causes protons in only one slice of tissue to be excited. Aside from slice-selective imaging, spatially selective RF excitation can also be used to saturate tissues in specific locations, as will be discussed in the next section.

SATURATION

To suppress specific tissue, a common approach, known as saturation, is used. First a 90° RF pulse excites the tissues to be suppressed by tipping their magnetizations into the transverse plane. Then, a gradient called a dephasing gradient or crusher gradient dephases the signal so that it can no longer contribute to subsequent imaging. The RF pulse is typically referred to as a prepulse because it precedes the routine RF excitation of spin echo and gradient echo sequences. The suppressing effect of the prepulse lasts until the tissue recovers its longitudinal magnetization, which depends on its T1 relaxation time. Once the tissues recover coherent longitudinal magnetization, they again contribute signal to the images. The saturation process needs to be reapplied before this happens.

Saturation can be either spatially defined for specific slices or blocks within the field of view, or tissue selective, such as in the preferential saturation of fat and not water protons.

Spatial Presaturation

Saturation pulses to achieve suppression of signal from different regions of the body are extremely useful tools for clinical MR imaging. In time-of-flight imaging (as will be discussed in Chapter II-2), the inflow of protons into the slice causes increased signal. Saturation prepulses can be used to suppress signal from protons flowing in one direction, such as venous blood, in order to image selectively arterial protons flowing in the opposite direction (Figure I9-4).

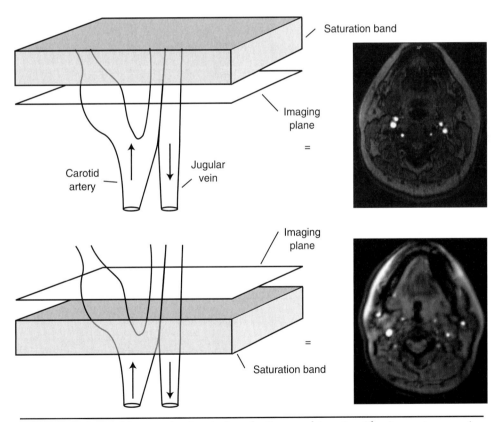

FIGURE I9-4. Spatial saturation bands for selective vessel imaging. Flowing protons moving through the imaging slice in time-of-flight imaging cause high signal intensity. Application of a saturation band, shown in gray, above the imaging slice will eliminate the signal from the venous protons entering the slice downward, where the protons flowing upward into the slice from the carotid artery still contribute to high signal in the image. Below, the converse is true, and the carotid artery signal is suppressed.

In clinical practice, spatial presaturation pulses are also commonly used to reduce signal from protons that are the source of imaging artifacts such as wraparound artifacts (Figure I9-5) and motion artifacts from tissues such as the chest or abdominal wall (Figure I1-36).

How does spatial presaturation work? Before the spin echo or gradient echo sequence is initiated, 90° RF prepulses are applied with the appropriate spatially localizing gradients so that they affect only the selected regions. For example, in the case shown in Figure I9-5, prepulses are designed to affect only two sagittal slabs of tissue to the left and right of the field of view to include both arms. The dephasing gradient causes complete dephasing of the transverse magnetization. Protons from these regions do not contribute to the subsequent signal until they recover following T1 relaxation.

CHALLENGE QUESTION: How could a spatial presaturation band reduce the motion artifacts apparent in Figue I1-36?

Answer: The artifacts arise primarily from the high signal of the fat in the skin of the anterior chest wall. A coronal saturation band placed over the skin would reduce the artifact.

When a prepulse is used for suppressing artifacts, the location of the saturation bands is typically constant over the course of the image acquisition. For time-of-flight sequences, on the other hand, the saturation bands may move or travel with the acquisition slices. For each transverse imaging slice, the saturation band may be positioned immediately above the slice to suppress venous signal, keeping the same position relative to the slice and therefore also moves (Figure I9-6).

CHALLENGE QUESTION: What is the benefit of having traveling saturation bands for time-of-flight imaging?

Answer: Following application of the saturation pulse, the signal from the blood protons in the slab is suppressed until T1 recovery occurs. If the saturation band is far from the imaging slice, and if the flow is sufficiently slow, then there will be time for the protons that were saturated to recover before entering the imaging slice. Keeping the saturation band immediately adjacent to the imaging slice ensures that the venous protons will be completely saturated as they enter and traverse the imaging slice.

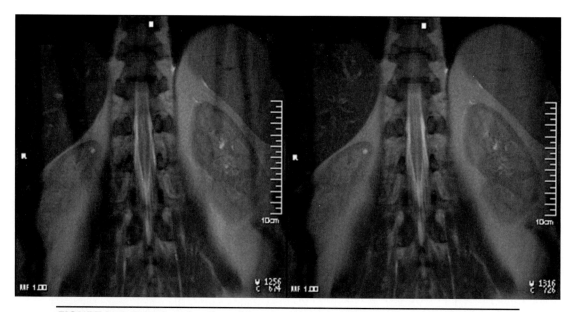

FIGURE I9-5. Wraparound artifact of the arms in an image (left) can be reduced by application of spatial presaturation pulses over the region of the arms to minimize their signal (right).

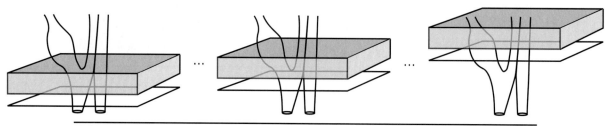

FIGURE I9-6. Traveling saturation band with time-of-flight imaging of the carotid arteries.

IMPORTANT CONCEPT: Spatial presaturation is commonly used to minimize several different types of artifacts including wraparound, ghosting, and motion artifact. It is also useful in time-of-flight imaging to image arterial or venous blood flow selectively.

Fat Saturation

The difference between fat and water precessional frequencies, illustrated in Figure I9-1, is exploited with frequency-selective *fat saturation* or *fat suppression*. With most sequences, a fat suppression option can be implemented by adding a frequency-selective fat suppression pulse to the beginning of the pulse sequence. This consists of a 90° RF prepulse centered on the fat frequency. Typically no gradients are applied during this RF pulse, so that the fat across the entire field of view is excited. The RF pulse is immediately followed by application of a crusher or dephasing gradient, which results in total dephasing of the fat protons (Figure I9-7). During the rest of the routine pulse sequence (gradient echo or spin echo), only the water protons contribute to the measured signal.

CHALLENGE QUESTION: With the aim of reducing acquisition times, you consider shortening the duration of the fat saturation pulse. Why is this a bad idea?

Answer: To achieve frequency-selective excitation, the fat saturation pulse must, by definition, have a narrow bandwidth, typically around 100 Hz, which means the pulse must be relatively long, say 10–20 msec (Figure I5-7). A shorter fat saturation pulse would mean a wider bandwidth and more inadvertent suppression of signal from water protons. Note that in addition to the duration of the pulse, an additional 5–20 msec of dephasing is typically required. This component can be shortened with use of stronger crusher gradients.

In the standard implementation, the fat suppression pulse and crusher gradient are applied before each RF pulse; that is, once every TR in the pulse sequence. As such, the addition of fat saturation adds considerably to the acquisition time. However, this degree of repetition of fat saturation pulses is not always necessary. With some pulse sequences such as fast 3D gradient echo imaging, the TR times are very short, as short as 3–4 msec. From one RF pulse to the next, fat does not have time to recover its longitudinal magnetization and remains suppressed.

CHALLENGE QUESTION: How long would fat signal be expected to remain suppressed after a fat suppression pulse?

Answer: As the longitudinal magnetization of fat recovers, the effect of the fat suppression is lost. If the T1 of fat is 250 msec, then 250 msec after the RF pulse, the fat signal will have recovered about 63% of its longitudinal magnetization.

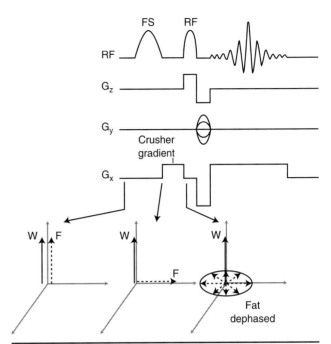

FIGURE I9-7. Frequency-selective fat suppression. A frequency-selective fat saturation (FS) prepulse selectively excites fat protons. When the crusher gradient is applied (G_x), the fat protons are dephased in the transverse plane and will not contribute subsequently to signal resulting from the RF excitation.

The fat signal begins to be measurable only when its longitudinal magnetization has recovered sufficiently. Because the T1 relaxation time of fat is about 250 msec, this would not be expected to occur to a significant degree until at least 100 msec. This means that a fat suppression pulse can be applied only intermittently. If the TR is 3 msec, then a fat suppression pulse need only be added every 30–40 TRs (Figure I9-8). In fact, if the central lines of k-space are collected immediately after the fat suppression pulse, while the peripheral lines of k-space are collected later, one can apply a fat suppression pulse even less frequently. With some commercially available centrically ordered 3D gradient echo sequences, the fat suppression pulse is applied only once every partition (slice) to produce fat suppressed images with minimal addition to the acquisition time.

CHALLENGE QUESTION: How is frequency-selective fat saturation affected by magnetic field in homogeneises?

Answer: Frequency-selective fat saturation is very susceptible to field inhomogeneity because it relies on precise excitation of fat protons and not water protons, and the frequency difference, 220 Hz, is very small relative to the Larmor frequency. If the magnetic field is not uniform, deviations in Larmor

3D GRE Intermittent Fat Saturation

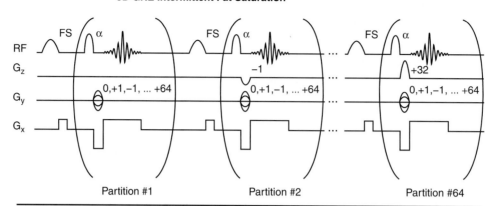

FIGURE I9-8. Intermittent fat suppression applied once every partition. Where each partition includes 128 excitations and TR = 3 msec, the fat suppression pulse is applied every 384 msec. While this is longer than the T1 of fat, centric k-space filling ensures that fat appears adequately suppressed, since recovery of fat magnetization during the filling of the peripheral lines of k-space has little effect on image contrast.

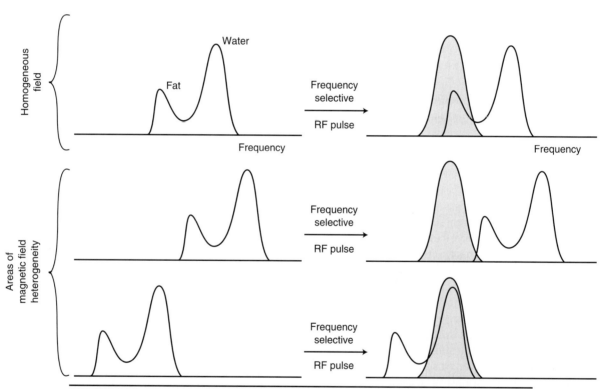

FIGURE I9-9. Magnetic field inhomogeneity limits the success of frequency-selective fat saturation (gray area). In areas of magnetic field inhomogeneity, the RF pulse may fail to suppress fat (middle) or it may inadvertently suppress water signal (bottom).

frequency of 100–200 Hz or more can dramatically impact fat suppression (Figure I9-9). If the field happens to be a bit weaker than the expected 1.5 T, so that water protons precess 220 Hz more slowly than expected, then it is possible that water may be inadvertently suppressed instead of fat.

IMPORTANT CONCEPT: Fat saturation pulses can be applied intermittently by taking advantage of the relatively slow recovery of longitudinal magnetization of fat protons compared with TR. Fat saturation pulses need to be applied even less frequently when centric k-space filling is used. Frequency-selective fat saturation requires good field homogeneity.

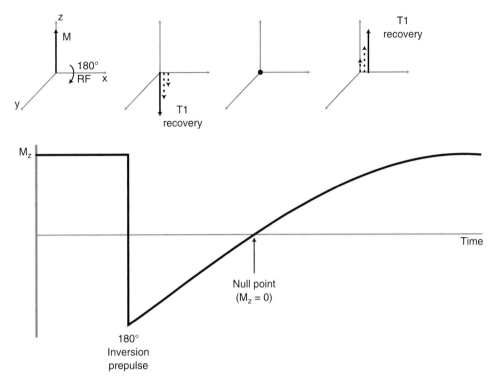

FIGURE I9-10. Inversion recovery pulse for signal nulling. The inversion time (TI) is defined as the time between the 180° inversion prepulse and the null point of the tissue that is to be suppressed. The RF excitation pulse for the sequence is applied at the null point.

NULLING (INVERSION RECOVERY)

Inversion recovery sequences can suppress signal from certain tissues based on their T1 recovery times. As with suppression pulses, the aim is to eliminate longitudinal magnetization from undesirable tissues prior to RF excitation. Unlike saturation techniques, which rely on a special 90° prepulse, inversion recovery sequences apply a 180° prepulse to invert the magnetization and then wait for the longitudinal magnetization to recover (Figure I9-10). At specific points partway through recovery, each tissue will have no longitudinal magnetization. These moments are considered the *null points*.

CHALLENGE QUESTION: What determines the time it takes to reach the null point?

Answer: Recovery of longitudinal magnetization depends on the T1 of a tissue. Recall from Chapter I-2 that the expression of longitudinal magnetization in terms of T1 is exponential. After a 180° pulse, it will take 0.693T1 to reach the transverse plane. For example, if the T1 of a tissue is 1000 msec, then, 693 msec following a 180° pulse, the longitudinal magnetization of this tissue will be negligible.

Nulled tissue will not contribute to the echo generated by the subsequent RF excitation pulse. The time between the 180° inversion prepulse and the RF excitation of the pulse sequence is referred to as the *inversion time* (TI). For both spin echo and gradient echo imaging, the RF excitation pulse is usually applied at this inversion time to achieve

tissue nulling. Where frequency-selective methods can be used specifically for fat or water suppression, inversion recovery methods are less specific and will suppress any tissue with a T1 relaxation time equal to the selected value.

Unlike frequency-selective methods, the inversion recovery technique affects all the protons in the image. At the inversion time, the magnetization vectors of some tissues have experience varied longitudinal recovery and may still be inverted. For most routine imaging, MR systems consider only the absolute value or amplitude of the magnetization vectors, thereby confusing negative and positive signal (Figure I9-11). The variable state of longitudinal magnetization has interesting implications for image contrast, as will be discussed below. Several different inversion recover applications frequently used in cardiovascular MR imaging are introduced in the following section.

> **IMPORTANT CONCEPT:** Inversion recovery sequences can produce tissue suppression by imaging at the appropriate inversion time following a 180° inversion prepulse. The inversion time should occur when the magnetization of the tissue to be suppressed has zero longitudinal magnetization (its null point).

Short Tau Inversion Recovery (STIR)

Short tau inversion recovery, or *STIR*, sequences are commonly used in a number of clinical indications including cardiovascular MR imaging. STIR sequences are long-TR

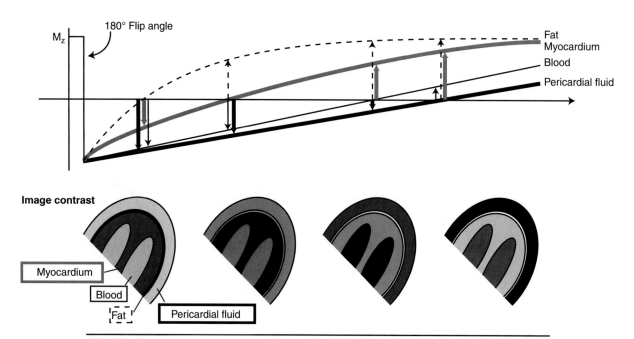

FIGURE I9-11. Image contrast at different inversion times when different tissues (from left to right: fat, myocardium, blood, and pericardial fluid) are nulled because of their different T1 values. Image signal intensity represents the absolute value (magnitude) of the longitudinal magnetization.

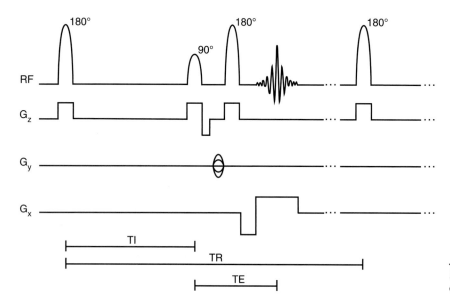

FIGURE I9-12. Inversion recovery spin echo sequence.

and long-TE spin echo or fast spin echo sequences that produce T2-weighted image contrast (Figure I9-12). With STIR, the inversion prepulse is timed for fat suppression. It also provides additive T1 and T2 image contrast, as will be illustrated below.

STIR imaging is typically performed with an inversion time of about 160 msec to null fat at 1.5 T.

CHALLENGE QUESTION: What should the null point for fat be, and why is this not used for STIR imaging?

Answer: With a T1 of about 250 msec, the TI should be 0.693 × 250 or about 175 msec. However, it is important to realize that with repeated excitations, there is incomplete longitudinal recovery between RF pulses. The inverted magnetization after each RF pulse is therefore less than the full magnetization. Hence, the null point will be reached earlier than if there were full magnetization after the inversion.

With an inversion time selected to null fat, the STIR sequence is often referred to as a fat-suppressed sequence.

CHALLENGE QUESTION: Is fat the only tissue suppressed on a STIR sequence?

Answer: No. Fat is not the only tissue that can be nulled on a STIR sequence. Other tissues that have a similarly short T1 relaxation time, such as proteinaceous fluid or hemorrhage, will be nulled together with fat. Consequently, STIR is a less than optimal method to differentiate between fat and other tissues that are have short T1; a frequency-selective fat suppression pulse is more specific for fat.

STIR versus Frequency-Selective Fat Saturation (for T2-Weighted Fast Spin Echo Imaging)

As discussed in Chapter I-4, with fast spin echo or turbo spin echo imaging, fat appears bright, both for T1- and T2-weighted imaging, because of J-decoupling. In some applications, the conspicuity of pathology can be improved by reducing signal from fat. Two methods are commonly used to achieve fat suppression: STIR and frequency-selective fat saturation. The two methods are compared side by side in Table I9-1.

Frequency-selective fat suppression assumes that the magnetic field is homogeneous (Figure I9-9), and it fails in areas of inhomogeneity. Field inhomogeneities have negligible effect on T1 relaxation times, and hence STIR achieves fat suppression regardless of field inhomogeneities. This robustness comes at the cost of decreased specificity and increased time. Fat is not definitively characterized by its nulling on STIR. Other tissues with similarly short T1 relaxation times will also be nulled at an inversion time of about 160 msec. Another disadvantage of STIR is the requirement of the inversion pulse and inversion time which add substantially more to the

▶ TABLE I9-1

STIR	Frequency-Selective Fat Saturation
Relies on T1 relaxation for nulling	Relies on specific precessional frequency of fat
Robust even with field inhomogeneities	Fails if field is inhomogeneous
Longer acquisition times due to inversion times	Faster, especially with intermittent fat suppression pulses
Not specific for fat (other tissues with short T1 also are suppressed)	Specific for fat (if field is homogeneous)
Typically T2-weighted sequence with additive T1- and T2-weighted image contrast	Works with any T1-weighted images or any fast spin echo images
Can be achieved on any MR system	Requires narrow transmitter bandwidth for the fat saturation pulse

acquisition time than the fat suppression RF pulse and crusher gradient (<20–50 msec).

CHALLENGE QUESTION: As discussed in Chapter I-3, at higher field strengths fat appears even brighter relative to other tissues on T1-weighted images. How would the magnetic field strength, for example, 3 T versus 1.5 T, affect the consideration of STIR versus frequency-selective fat saturation for fat suppression?

Answer: Because the T1 relaxation time of fat is not significantly different at 3 T, the STIR sequence is implemented similarly at the higher field. Based on the Larmor equation, the difference between fat and water frequencies at 3 T will be 440 Hz. With a larger frequency difference, the fat saturation RF pulse can have a broader bandwidth and therefore a shorter duration. Therefore, assuming comparable magnetic field homogeneity, frequency-selective suppression may be preferable at higher field strengths.

> **IMPORTANT CONCEPT:** STIR sequences rely on differences in T1 relaxation for fat suppression. They are robust in the setting of field inhomogeneity, but acquisition times for STIR are lengthened by the inversion time. Frequency-selective fat suppression pulses are more specific for fat but require a homogeneous magnetic field.

Image Contrast with STIR: Additive T1 and T2 Weighting

As explored in Chapter I-4, with conventional spin echo imaging, T1 and T2 relaxation times tend to have opposite effects on the image. A longer T1 tends to cause tissues to be lower in signal intensity (since less T1 recovery occurs from RF pulse to RF pulse), whereas a longer T2 tends to cause tissues to be higher in signal intensity (less signal decay over time). This inverse relation is unfortunate, because long T1 and long T2 times tend to go hand in hand with most pathological and fluid-filled structures. With STIR, the 180° prepulse changes this relationship. At short inversion times, the magnetization vectors of most tissues are still inverted. (Recall from the earlier discussion and Figure I9-11 that the MR reconstruction software does not usually distinguish between magnetization vectors that are inverted or upright.) Consequently, the effect of T1 relaxation times on image signal intensity is now the opposite of what is seen with conventional spin echo imaging (Figure I9-13). Tissues with longer T1 times (such as most pathology) now have more magnetization, or greater signal, while tissues with shorter T1 times are lower in signal. Coupled with a fairly long echo time to bring out T2 differences, the STIR sequence can provide additive T1- and T2-weighted image contrast. Pathological tissues that have long T1 and long T2 relaxation times will now

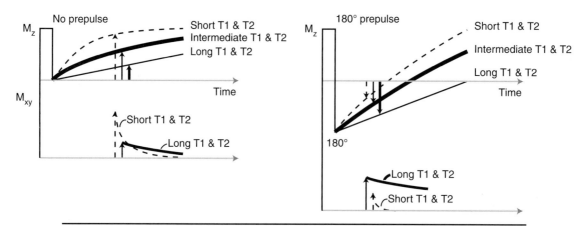

FIGURE I9-13. Difference in image contrast without (left) and with (right) a 180° prepulse. Note that most pathologic and fluid-filled structures have long T1 and T2 times relative to normal tissues. The effects of these long times are additive with a T2-weighted short-TI inversion recovery sequence. Tissues with long T1 and T2 times are much higher in signal intensity than tissues with short T1 and T2 times.

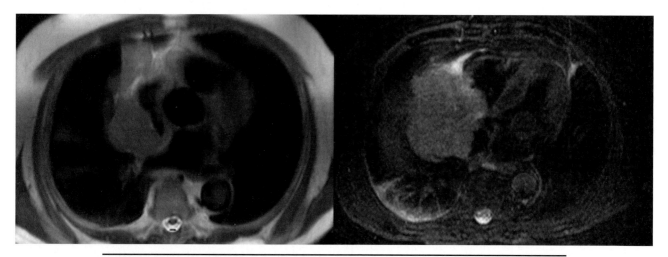

FIGURE I9-14. Additive T1 and T2 weighting with STIR imaging. Lymphomatous mass invading the right heart is slightly hyperintense on T2-weighted imaging (left). STIR imaging at a lower level (right), by virtue of its fat suppression and additive T1 and T2 weighting, causes significantly greater contrast between the mass and the heart.

have even more signal compared with background tissues (Figure I9-14).

Viability or Myocardial Infarct Imaging

Inversion recovery imaging is useful in the evaluation of myocardial infarcts using delayed contrast-enhanced imaging (see Chapter III-5). Following gadolinium contrast administration, infarcted myocardium demonstrates a delayed pattern of enhancement and washout. At 10–15 min after injection, the infarcted myocardium has more gadolinium contrast than uninfarcted myocardium. The difference in T1 is slight and typically subtle or even imperceptible on conventional T1-weighted imaging.

To improve image contrast and hence the detectability of infarcted regions, an inversion recovery sequence is used to null the uninfarcted myocardium so that infarcted myocardium appears bright by comparison (Figure I9-15).

The inversion time to achieve nulling of the uninfarcted myocardium depends on the amount of gadolinium contrast material in the tissue, which, in turn, depends on factors such as the amount of contrast material used, the time after injection, and the subject's cardiac function. The specific value of the inversion time also depends on whether the sequence is centrically or sequentially encoded. Typical values for the inversion times to null uninfarcted myocardium at 1.5 T following a single dose of gadolinium contrast are 200–350 msec.

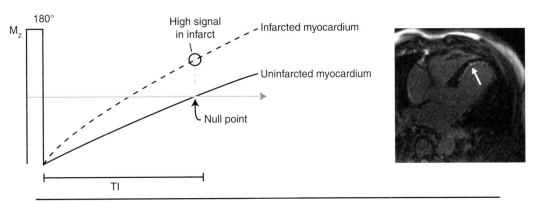

FIGURE I9-15. Inversion recovery sequence used to suppress signal from uninfarcted myocardium by imaging at its null point. The infarcted myocardium, which has more gadolinium contrast at 10–15 min after injection, and therefore a shorter T1 time, appears bright (arrow) relative to the suppressed myocardium.

CHALLENGE QUESTION: How and why does the optimal inversion time for suppressing uninfarcted myocardium change with time after injection?

Answer: As the gadolinium contrast material continues to wash out of the uninfarcted myocardium, its T1 relaxation time increases, and hence the optimal inversion time also increases.

Double Inversion Recovery for Black-Blood Imaging

There is often a need for suppressing signal from the blood, as flowing blood can be difficult to distinguish from vessel wall pathology such as an intramural hematoma or dissection and myocardial abnormalities in the heart. The flow of blood into and out of an imaging slice adds another level of complexity to the saturation problem. Most routine anatomic imaging of the heart and vessels uses a double inversion recovery sequence to ensure that the blood signal is nulled (Figures I9-16 and I9-17).

The prepulse portion consists of *two* 180° RF pulses: a *non*selective 180° pulse, which inverts all of the protons in the field, immediately followed by a slice-selective 180° pulse, which reverts the protons in the imaging slice back to their original alignment, leaving all protons outside of the imaging slice inverted (Figure I9-16).

For stationary tissues in the imaging slice, the net effect of the two prepulses is negligible because the net 360° RF excitation returns magnetization to its original longitudinal state. By the time the imaging sequence begins, the blood in the imaging slice will have been completely replaced by blood containing protons that originated outside the slice, which have only experienced the nonselective 180° prepulse. At a certain point following the inversion prepulse, the magnetization vectors for the blood will cross their null point. If the imaging portion of

the pulse sequence begins at this point, blood signal will be nulled.

Blood has a T1 relaxation time of about 1200 msec, so the null point will be at about 830 msec (0.693 × 1200 msec) after the inversion. In fact, as with STIR imaging, because of the incomplete recovery of longitudinal magnetization from slice to slice, the actual inversion time is usually shorter. Also, to ensure that blood is nulled, the early echoes collected at around the null point are usually used to fill the center of k-space. Sequences with such a pair of inversion recovery prepulses are often referred to as *black-blood* sequences. More details about black-blood fast spin echo imaging are provided in Chapter III-3.

> **IMPORTANT CONCEPT:** Double inversion recovery prepulses can suppress signal from moving blood. This is useful for imaging of vascular wall pathology and myocardial disease.

SELECTIVE EXCITATION

Another way to suppress fat is to tip water magnetization into the transverse plane but return fat magnetization to the longitudinal axis. These approaches, usually referred to as selective excitation, take advantage of differences in phase between fat and water that result from their different precessional frequencies. If RF pulses are timed to occur when the transverse components of fat and water are opposed phase, then their effect on magnetization of each tissue type will be different. Selective excitation is achieved with a series of RF pulses of varying amplitude, separated by the time delay needed for fat and water magnetization to reach opposing phase (2.2 msec at 1.5 T). These RF pulses are called *binomial pulses* because the pattern is that of the coefficients of an expression that represents a binomial raised to a power, such as "1–2–1," which corresponds to the coefficients in $(a + b)^2 = a^2 + 2ab + b^2$. Patterns for

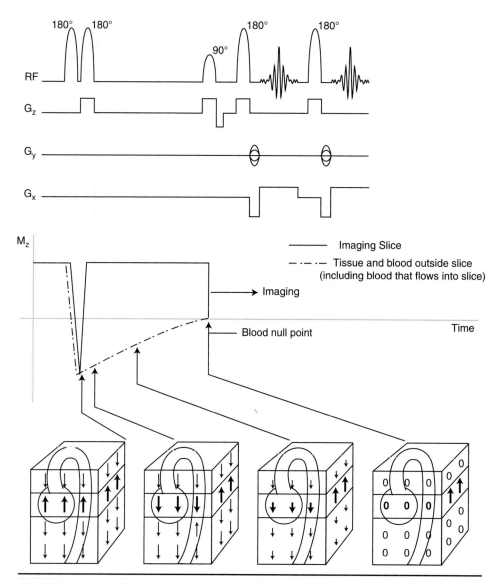

FIGURE I9-16. Double inversion recovery spin echo pulse sequence. The effect of two consecutive 180° RF pulses on the protons within the slice (→) is negligible. All protons outside the slice are inverted only by the first 180° pulse and therefore will recover over time. At an appropriate inversion time, all of the blood protons will cross their null point ("0"), including those passing through the imaging slice (heart and aorta).

some of the simplest binomial RF trains are shown in Table I9-2. The simplest example, "1–1," is illustrated in Figure I9-18.

At the end of an RF pulse that tips the magnetization vectors 45°, all protons will precess coherently. However, immediately thereafter, fat and water will precess at slightly different frequencies (a difference of 220 Hz at 1.5 T). At 1.5 T, after 2.2 msec the fat and water protons are opposed phase (Figure I9-18). A second RF pulse of 45° will then have different effects on the two species, tipping water protons fully into the transverse plane and returning

▶ **TABLE I9-2**

Binomial Pattern	RF Pulse Train	Typical Flip Angles
"1–1"	RF → 2.2 msec → RF	45°–45°
"1–2–1"	RF → 2.2 msec → 2RF → 2.2 msec → RF	22.5°–45°–22.5°
"1–3–3–1"	RF → 2.2 msec → 3RF → 2.2 msec → 3RF → 2.2 msec → RF	12.5°–37.5°– 37.5°–12.5°

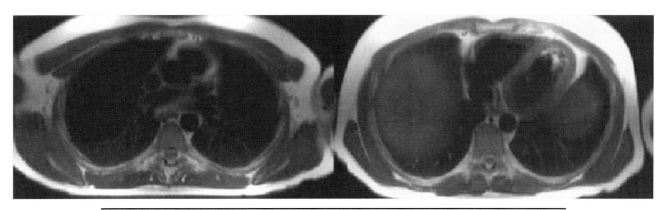

FIGURE I9-17. Double inversion recovery single-shot fast spin echo images demonstrate successful nulling of signal in flowing blood in the great vessels and heart.

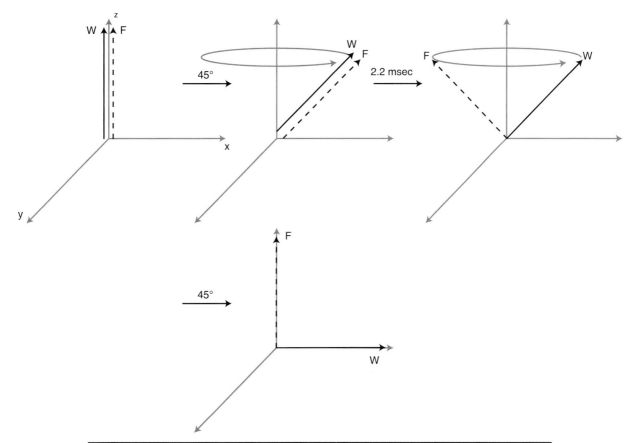

FIGURE I9-18. Water excitation. By using two α/2 (45°) (a "1–1" binomial pattern in Table I9-2), water is excited to α (90°) and fat undergoes no net excitation (0°).

fat into the longitudinal axis. As shown in Figure I9-18, the net effect of the two RF pulses is 90° excitation for the water protons and 0° for the fat. Consequently, water has been selectively excited. This example illustrates the concept, but more complex versions are usually implemented.

Frequency-Selective Fat Suppression Compared with Water Excitation

For frequency-selective fat suppression, the narrow transmitter bandwidth of the RF pulse intended to suppress fat requires a relatively long pulse duration to avoid suppression of water protons. The longer the fat suppression RF pulse, the more precisely fat is selectively suppressed. Selective water excitation pulses can be much shorter because they are not frequency selective and do not need to be slice selective. However, the requirement for more than one RF pulse separated by delay times to accumulate 180° phase differences between fat and water lengthens the pulse sequence. Both methods are sensitive to B_0 field inhomogeneities.

CHALLENGE QUESTION: How does imaging at higher field strengths such as 3 T affect frequency-selective fat suppression and water excitation?

Answer: Because the frequency shift between fat and water is twice as great at 3 T compared with 1.5 T, the transmitter bandwidth of the fat suppression pulse can be broader at 3 T. Consequently, the frequency-selective fat suppression RF pulse can be shorter in duration. With water excitation, the time between consecutive RF pulses is reduced by one-half to 1.1 msec because of the doubling of frequency difference between fat and water at 3 T. Assuming comparable field homogeneity, fat suppression at 3 T is superior to 1.5 T.

> **IMPORTANT CONCEPT:** Water excitation uses a series of binomial RF pulses separated by intervals of 2.2 msec (at 1.5 T) to allow fat and water protons to become opposed phase so that fat protons are returned to the longitudinal axis whereas water protons are excited to the desired flip angle.

REVIEW QUESTIONS

1. What sequence or modification should be used to answer the following clinical questions or to improve the image quality? Specifically, which of the following selective techniques would be most appropriate: frequency-selective saturation, spatially-selective saturation, inversion recovery, or selective excitation?

   a. A subject is referred for evaluation of suspected vasculitis involving the carotid arteries. You wish to perform a fat-suppressed T2-weighted image through the neck in order to improve conspicuity of the vessel wall, since high signal intensity in the wall would reflect inflammatory changes, even in the absence of luminal abnormalities. During past cervical spine surgery, the subject had metallic hardware placed.

   b. A subject has a hyperintense mass in the heart on T1-weighted images. You wish to determine whether this mass is a solid fatty mass or a complex hemorrhagic mass.

   c. When trying to suspend respiration, a subject inadvertently moves his chest during each acquisition. As a result, subcutaneous fat signal from the chest wall propagates through the image, degrading its quality.

2. A small-field-of-view image is desired over the heart as shown in Figure I9-Q2. As discussed in Chapter I-8, the

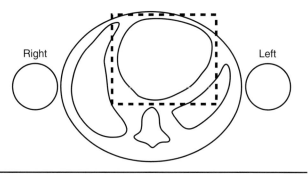

FIGURE I9-Q2

tissue that lies outside the FOV will cause wraparound artifact unless measures are taken. Weigh the relative merits of using spatially selective saturation bands versus frequency or phase oversampling to eliminate this artifact.

3. An example of a water excitation pulse sequence was demonstrated in this chapter using the following RF pulses: 45° → 2.2 msec → 45°. What happens with a series of RF pulses:

   22.5° → 2.2 msec → 45° → 2.2 msec → 22.5°?

   Draw the fat and water magnetization vectors through the course of the sequence (Figure I9-Q3A).

4. A binomial train of RF pulses can be used for water excitation as discussed in this chapter. Consider the variant of binomial pulses shown in Figure I9-Q4A. What is the effect of this sequence of fat and water protons?

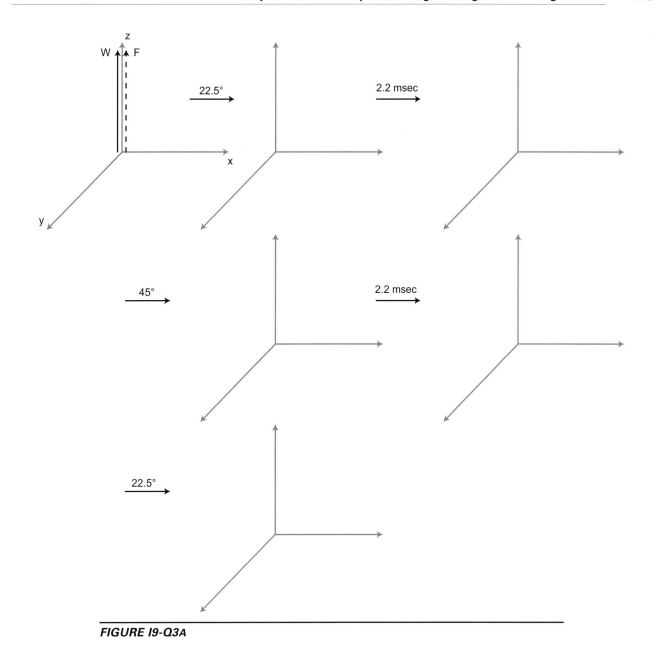

FIGURE I9-Q3A

5. What are the problems with the following images and how can you improve image quality?
   a. Gadolinium-enhanced myocardial infarct imaged with the aim of nulling uninfarcted myocardium, leaving infarcted myocardium hyperintense (Figure I9-Q5A).
   b. Half-Fourier acquisition turbo spin echo (HASTE) imaging of the aorta for assessment of descending aortic wall pathology (Figure I9-Q5B).

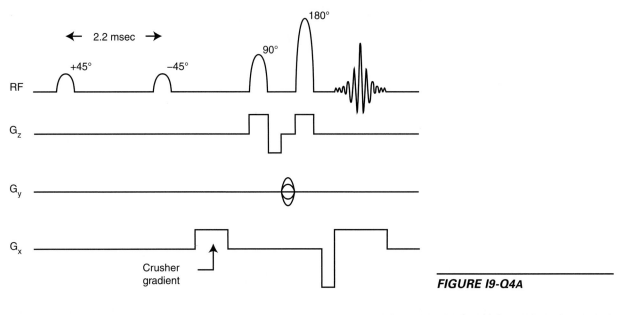

FIGURE I9-Q4A

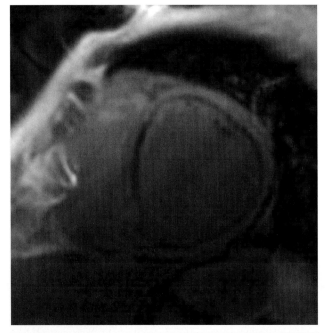

FIGURE I9-Q5A

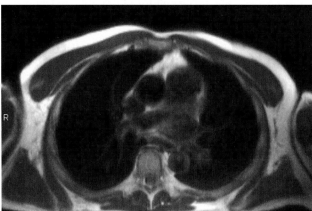

FIGURE I9-Q5B

Safety and Cardiovascular MRI

Concerns about MR safety are not confined to cardiovascular studies; however, there are specific issues that should be considered in the population of patients undergoing cardiovascular MRI. This chapter reviews general MR safety issues, emphasizing compatibility of cardiovascular devices and the safety of performing stress studies. A sample safety form is provided at the end of the chapter.

This chapter is intended to serve as an overview of safety topics, but it is by no means comprehensive. The information could become outdated quickly, given the rapid changes in the field. For updates and for more detailed information about MR safety, the reader is referred to several recent references and two Web sites (1–5).

KEY CONCEPTS

▶ Short-term exposure to the static magnetic fields, B_0, used for medical imaging has not been shown to cause adverse biological effects.

▶ Risks of exposure to B_0 magnetic fields are primarily related to implanted or foreign metallic objects and external ferromagnetic objects that become projectile near the magnet.

▶ Built-in controls of absorption of RF energy, quantified as specific absorption rate, ensure that maximum changes in tissue temperature are kept below FDA limits.

▶ For medical devices and equipment, safety within the magnetic environment cannot be assumed; frequently updated safety information should be consulted before devices are allowed beyond the 5 G line.

BIOLOGICAL EFFECTS AND HAZARDS OF MRI

Biological effects of MRI can be considered in terms of the static B_0 magnetic field, RF pulses, time-varying gradients, and the acoustic noise resulting from the gradient coil vibrations.

Static Magnetic Field (B_0)

For cardiovascular MR imaging, most systems use magnetic field strengths of 1 to 3 T. Research systems are being installed for human use that are 8 T and higher. Short-term exposures to static magnetic fields have not been shown to result in harmful biological effects in humans. The FDA has categorized clinical MR systems with a static magnetic field of up to 8 T as posing "nonsignificant risk" for patients >1 month old. (Current FDA guidelines can be found at their Web site: www.fda.gov.)

The fringe field around the MR scanner decreases with distance from the magnet. The static magnetic field strength that is thought to be totally risk-free for all individuals is 5 gauss (recall that 1 tesla = 10,000 gauss, so 5 G is 0.0005 T), or about 10 times the strength of the earth's magnetic field. For safety purposes, the *5 G line* is demarcated with signage and physical barriers that exclude access by members of the public who have not been screened appropriately.

The hazards to a subject resulting from the static magnetic field within the 5 G line primarily result from metallic projectiles and implanted or foreign metallic objects, including defibrillators and pacemakers. Ferromagnetic material behaves like a magnet when placed in a magnetic field, B. If the field is uniform, the material will tend to align itself with the direction of B and remain stationary. In the presence of a gradient, such as the fringe field outside of the magnet, ferromagnetic items will travel toward increasing B.

The attraction of objects such as non-MR-compatible oxygen tanks, intravenous fluid poles, floor polishers, and medical instruments to the MR scanner can result in their transformation to deadly projectiles. Several incidents of ferromagnetic projectiles causing injury or death have been reported. Careful testing, verification, and labeling of external devices form a significant component of any safety management program in a clinical MR facility.

Note also that damage to magnetic data storage devices (computer disks), credit cards, cameras, watches, and other electronic devices can occur in the magnetic field area within the 5 G line. As mentioned in Chapter I-1, it is important to realize that once the MR system is installed and brought to field, the superconducting magnet is always on. These risks exist 24 hours a day, regardless of whether the MR computer console or system lights are on or off.

Specific considerations about implanted medical devices are reviewed in subsequent sections of this chapter.

Exposure of flowing blood, which is essentially a fluid filled with charged particles, to the static magnetic field causes a *magnetohydrodynamic effect*. The resulting voltage changes that occur across the diameter of a vessel are not considered physiologically significant, although they can manifest as an elevated T wave on the electrocardiogram. This effect does have the potential to interfere in the monitoring for ischemia in subjects inside the MR system, as will be discussed in Chapter III-1.

> **IMPORTANT CONCEPTS:** The static magnetic field is not known to cause adverse biological effects when subjects are exposed for short durations. The risks of exposure to magnetic fields higher than 5 G are primarily related to implanted or foreign metallic objects and to ferromagnetic objects becoming projectiles when inadvertently brought in the vicinity of the MR system.

RF Pulses

RF pulses result in power deposition in human subjects that is transformed into heat. MRI-related heating depends on a variety of factors including the nature of the exposure, the subject's thermoregulatory system, certain underlying health conditions and medication use, and ambient conditions such as temperature, humidity, and airflow. The measurement used to describe the absorption of RF energy is the specific absorption rate (SAR), which is expressed in watts per kilogram. The SAR for an MR sequence is usually expressed in terms of whole-body averaged SAR or peak SAR. Current U.S. FDA guidelines limit whole-body SAR exposure to 4 W/kg for subjects with normal thermoregulatory function and 1.5 W/kg for all subjects regardless of their condition. Roughly speaking, the guidelines are based on levels that produce a maximum change in tissue temperature of less than 1°C. It is important to realize that the RF power deposition increases with the square of the B_0 field strength, so that a doubling of B_0 from 1.5 T to 3 T results in a fourfold increase in SAR. Commercial MR systems have built-in controls to limit SAR exposures safely below FDA limits (Table I10-1).

Hazards associated with RF fields are typically related to exposed wires or electrical cables or loops of conductors in which current is generated, causing burns. Therefore it is essential to avoid looping electrical wires or cables within the magnetic field or allowing them to cross each other. Sheets or other insulating material should be

placed between the wires and the subject's skin to avoid direct contact. Generally, loose wires should be secured and and positioned to run down the bore of the magnet, exiting from the center of the magnet, and not along the sides. Additionally, burns can occur when subjects are in direct contact with the body RF coils or other RF transmit coils, so it is recommended that insulating material be placed between the subject's skin and the transmit RF coil if the coil itself is not padded.

Even without extrinsic devices, closed loops can occur when body parts are in contact, such as when a subject touches his/her hands together or when a subject's calves are touching. Skin-to-skin contact points while the patient is in the magnet should be eliminated by using sheets or other insulating materials.

> **IMPORTANT CONCEPT:** Specific absorption rate (SAR) limits are incorporated in the design of commercial MR pulse sequences. Exposed, crossed, or looped wires should be avoided. Direct contact between subject's skin and RF transmit coils should be minimized to reduce the risk of burns. Skin-to-skin contact points that create closed loops should also be avoided.

Time-Varying Magnetic Field Gradients

The rapid switching of magnetic field gradients used in certain types of pulse sequences can stimulate muscle and nerve tissue. Mean thresholds for stimulations of different tissues are given in Table I10-2, where subject-to-subject variability is well known.

▶ **TABLE I10-1 FDA SAR Guidelines (2003)**

Site	Dose Calculation	Time (min) equal to or greater than	SAR (W/kg)
Whole body	Averaged over	15	4
Head	Averaged over	10	3
Head or torso	Per gram of tissue	5	8
Extremities	Per gram of tissue	5	12

▶ **TABLE I10-2 Mean Stimulation Thresholds for Gradient Switching**

Organ	Mean Threshold for Stimulation (T/sec)
Heart	3600
Respiratory system	900
Pain	90
Peripheral nerves	60

Interestingly, the stimulation thresholds vary depending on the gradient direction. The gradient G_z, along the long axis of the body, has the lowest stimulation threshold. The stimulation sites of peripheral nerve stimulation also vary depending on the gradient direction, but in general they occur at bony prominences such as the iliac crest, upper and lower back, and scapula.

CHALLENGE QUESTION: Which pulse sequences are the most likely to push the limits of gradient switching rates?

Answer: Echo planar imaging and other fast gradient echo sequences.

Very strong and/or rapidly switched gradients have the potential to cause dangerous cardiac stimulation. However, given that the threshold for cardiac stimulation is a couple of orders of magnitude greater than current FDA guidelines, this risk remains hypothetical in the clinical setting.

Acoustic Noise

One unfortunate consequence of gradient switching is the generation of substantial forces on the gradient coils. These oscillating forces result in tappng or knocking noises that can exceed occupational safety guidelines. The FDA has indicated that MR-related noise levels must be kept below a peak of 140 dB. Hearing protection should be offered to sensitive subjects and when the systems are operating above 90 dB. Disposable earplugs or MR-compatible headphones are most commonly used. People who remain in the scanner room with the subject should also be required to use hearing protection. Recently, several vendors have developed strategies for reducing acoustic noise by use of insulation material and special construction of the gradient coils.

IMPORTANT CONCEPTS: Time-varying gradients can result in peripheral nerve stimulation and, at their extremes, even cardiac stimulation. However, when operating within commercially implemented limits, these risks are minimized. Additionally, acoustic noise generated from the gradient switching warrants routine use of hearing protection for those in the scanner room.

DEVICES, IMPLANTS, AND OTHER PATIENT-SPECIFIC RISKS

One of the most important hazards associated with MR imaging is the attraction of implanted ferromagnetic objects to the magnet. Before specific devices and situations are considered, it may be helpful to review the general effects of MR systems on ferromagnetic objects.

Within the bore of the magnet, the B_0 magnetic field is relatively homogeneous. The effect of the uniform magnetic field on ferromagnetic objects in the bore is to make them into small magnets that will, like protons, align with the direction of the field. Depending on its size and shape, the object may cause damage to surrounding tissues because of the rotational movement.

Outside the bore of the magnet, the magnetic field is spatially varying. The strength of the magnetic field decreases further from the magnet. Ferromagnetic objects outside of the magnet are attracted to the bore and thus can experience both rotational and translational forces, causing them to accelerate toward the magnet's isocenter. These forces are strongest around the ends of the magnet. Therefore, as a subject enters into and exits out of the magnet bore, the effects of the magnetic field on ferromagnetic material in the body are likely to be greatest.

RF and gradient effects on implants and devices can also lead to adverse results. The risks include induction of electric currents in electronically activated devices, their excessive heating, and movement of objects made from ferromagnetic materials.

With the burgeoning field of medical implants and devices, evaluation for MR safety is a vast topic that requires constant updating. Several publications and Web sites are devoted to providing updated information on new devices and testing at higher magnetic field strengths. The reader is directed to those sources for more detailed information. Below, an overview of considerations specific to the cardiovascular patient population is provided. Most comments apply to 1.5 T; data on safety at 3 T is rapidly emerging.

Implants and Devices

Pacemakers and Other Electronically Activated Devices

Pacemakers have been considered strictly contraindicated in the MR suite. However, recently, several reports have described the safe performance of MR in subjects with cardiac pacemakers who are considered non-pacemaker-dependent. It is conceivable that in the future, restrictions on subjects with pacemakers may be modified, provided they are non-pacemaker-dependent and certain precautions are carefully attended to. Recently some electronically activated devices have been labeled as "MR-safe" by the FDA, including certain neurostimulation systems, cochlear implants, and programmable drug infusion pumps. To date, there are no implantable cardioverter defibrillators that have been designed to be MR compatible.

Heart Valve Prostheses and Annuloplasty Rings

The forces exerted by the beating heart far exceed the magnetic field-related forces on prosthetic valves and annuloplasty rings. Therefore, MR imaging up to 1.5 T is considered safe for a patient with any of these devices, including the Starr-Edwards model Pre-6000 heart valve prosthesis.

Coils, Stents, and Filters

The variability in construction of these devices mandates that specific documentation about the device, material, and manufacturer be obtained to determine MR safety. In general, for those tested and found to have no magnetic field interactions, the MR procedure can be performed immediately after insertion. For implants made from weakly ferromagnetic materials, a waiting period of at least 6 to 8 weeks is typically advised to allow sufficient tissue ingrowth to prevent motion or loosening of devices during the MR study.

Cardiac Pacing Wires

Cardiac pacing wires that are retained after surgery have never been reported to cause an incident or injury associated with an MR procedure. However, theoretically, there is a risk of inducing electrical current or heating, and therefore in many centers these are considered a relative contraindication for MR procedures. Similarly, the safety of imaging subjects with temporary pacing wires, disconnected from the external pulse generator, must be considered carefully. In both cases, safety of subjects, if imaged, is best ensured at systems of 1.5 T or below and using MR pulse sequences that do not involve rapid gradient switching or high RF energy deposition.

Brain Aneurysm Clips

Implanted intracranial aneurysm clips that are ferromagnetic are contraindicated because motion may displace the clips and cause injury or even death. However, many aneurysm clips are now nonferromagnetic and have been tested and shown to be safe for MR imaging, particularly those that are purely titanium or titanium alloy types. Clips manufactured after 1995 may have manufacturer's product labeling to assure MR compatibility. Careful determination and identification of brain aneurysm clips should be a routine part of all screening procedures for MR imaging.

Thermal Injury from Medical Devices and Monitoring Equipment

One hazard of MR imaging results from the inductive heating of conductors and subject monitoring leads by RF energy. Injuries have been reported related to burns from conductive leads placed against bare skin, blisters from a non-MR compatible pulse oximeter, and a burn from an electrocardiographic cable. Care must be taken to avoid loops of conductors within the magnet bore, because the rapidly changing magnetic field will induce a current, causing heating and burns. The maximum induction results when the conducting loop is positioned in a plane perpendicular to the direction of the changing magnetic field. No wires, whether looped or not, should be in direct contact with skin. Some insulation can be achieved using a sheet or other insulating materials. To avoid these risks, fiber optic cables are preferred.

RF energies can also cause heating in the tips of long wires or leads, such as Swan-Ganz catheters, and therefore these are considered at risk if the body coil is used for RF transmission over the region of the lead.

> **IMPORTANT CONCEPT:** For medical devices and equipment, safety within the magnetic environment cannot be assumed. Frequently updated device safety information should be maintained in the clinical MR environment. All implants, devices, and equipment must be verified as MR safe before being allowed beyond the 5 G line.

Other Patient-Related Safety Considerations

- *Metal in the eye:* Retained metallic foreign bodies in the eye have the potential to cause injury. Subjects who have a history of orbital trauma by a potentially ferromagnetic object for which they sought medical attention are suggested to have the orbits evaluated by radiographic images (x-rays).
- *Skin staples and metallic sutures of the skin* are considered safe provided they are nonferromagnetic and also not in the volume of tissue to which the RF pulse is applied. However, if the staples or sutures do not meet these conditions, then the MR study may be performed, provided the patient is instructed to report warmth or burning during the study. Also, placing cold compresses or ice packs along the staples during the study may reduce the risks of RF exposure.
- *Tattoos and permanent cosmetics:* Another potential source of thermal heating resulting from RF deposition relates to the use of iron oxide and other metal-based pigments in traditional and cosmetic tattoos. As a precaution, an ice pack or cold compress may be applied to the tattoo during the procedure, if the tattoo is in the imaging volume.
- *Drug-delivery patches:* Some patches contain metallic foil, which can result in thermal injury in the MR scanner. Management options include removal of the patch or placement of an ice pack on the patch.
- *Pregnancy:* To date, there has been no evidence that non-contrast-enhanced MR imaging has produced deleterious effects in pregnancy. Therefore, if the procedure is considered to be warranted in the medical care of the mother or fetus, MR imaging may be performed,

regardless of the trimester. However, the use of gadolinium contrast agents must be considered carefully, because the agents do cross the placenta and enter the fetal circulation.

CARDIAC STRESS MRI

Aside from the safety issues that apply to all patients, evaluation of patients with ischemic heart disease by means of pharmacologic stress raises additional safety concerns. Experience with dobutamine-enhanced stress studies using cine gradient echo imaging and vasodilator-enhanced perfusion studies is growing, and serious adverse events are uncommon. The transition of stress MR imaging to widespread clinical implementation depends not only on its accuracy for detection of significant coronary artery disease but also on acceptance of its safety.

A more thorough discussion on the safety of stress MR is provided in Chapter III-7.

SAFETY MANAGEMENT

A program for safety management is essential for any clinical MR facility. Among the requirements for a safe clinical MR setting, one of the most important on a day-to-day basis is the screening of individuals who are planning to enter the MR environment. A sample MR screening questionnaire is provided in Figures I10-1 and I10-2. Adequate training of personnel and proper control of access to the MR areas are also critical. The specific guidelines for the operation of a safety program for a clinical MR imaging facility are beyond the scope of this book, but thoroughly reviewed in a number of references (1–5).

REFERENCES

1. Kanal E. www.radiology.upmc.edu/MRsafety.
2. Kanal E, Borgstede JP, Barkovich AJ, et al. American College of Radiology White Paper on MR Safety: 2004 update and revisions. AJR Am J Roentgenol 2004; 182:1111–1114.
3. Price RR. The AAPM/RSNA physics tutorial for residents. MR imaging safety considerations. Radiological Society of North America. Radiographics 1999; 19:1641–1651.
4. Shellock FG. www.mrisafety.com.
5. Shellock FG, Crues JV. MR procedures: Biologic effects, Safety, and Patient Care. Radiology 2004; 232: 635–652.

MRI SAFETY SCREENING FORM   Date _____

Name _____ ACC Number _____

Height _____ Weight _____ Birth Date _____/_____/_____

```
┌──────────────────────────────────────┐
│          ✳ IMPORTANT ✳                │
│                                        │
│   For your safety, this form must be   │
│   completed and signed before your     │
│            MRI study.                  │
└──────────────────────────────────────┘
```

Before your MRI exam, please remove all metallic objects. You will be given a locker for your belongings. If you have any questions, please consult the Technologist, Doctor, Nurse or Front Desk Staff *before* entering the MRI area.

YES	NO	
☐	☐	Have you ever worked with metal (grinding, fabricating, etc.) or ever had an injury to the eye involving a metallic object (e.g., metallic slivers, shavings, foreign body)? If yes, please describe: _____
☐	☐	Are you pregnant or experiencing a late menstrual period? Date of last menstrual period: _____/_____/_____
☐	☐	Are you breast feeding?
☐	☐	Do you have drug allergies? if yes, please list: _____
☐	☐	Have you ever had a surgical procedure or operation of any kind? If yes, which type? _____
☐	☐	Have you ever had asthma, allergic reaction, respiratory disease, or prior reaction to contrast used for an MRI examination? If yes, please describe: _____

FIGURE I10-1. MRI safety questionnaire, front.

✳DO NOT ENTER THE MRI ROOM WITHOUT CLEARANCE FROM THE TECHNOLOGIST✳

Some of the following items may be hazardous to your safety and some can interfere with the MRI examination.
Do you have?

YES	NO		
☐	☐	Cardiac pacemaker	
☐	☐	Previous cardiac pacemaker removed	
☐	☐	Implanted cardiac defibrillator	
☐	☐	Carotid artery vascular clamp	
☐	☐	Aneurysm clip(s) in Brain	
☐	☐	Implanted drug infusion device	
☐	☐	Bone growth/fusion stimulator	
☐	☐	Neurostimulator (TENS-Unit)	
☐	☐	Any type of Biostimulator	
☐	☐	Cochlear, otologic, or ear implant	
☐	☐	Hearing aid *(Remove before MRI)*	
☐	☐	Nitroglycerin Patch	
☐	☐	Any other implanted item _____	
☐	☐	Any type of prosthesis (Heart Valve, Eye, Penile, etc.)	
☐	☐	Artificial limb or joint	
☐	☐	Electrodes (on body, head, or brain)	
☐	☐	Intravascular stents, filters, or coils (i.e. Gianturkle, Greenfield)	
☐	☐	Shunt (spinal or intraventricular)	
☐	☐	Vascular access port and/or catheter	
☐	☐	Swan-Ganz catheter	
☐	☐	Any implant held in place by a magnet	
☐	☐	Transdermal delivery system (Nitro)	
☐	☐	IUD or diaphragm	
☐	☐	Any metal fragments – Shrapnel or Bullet	
☐	☐	Internal pacing wires	
☐	☐	Aortic clip	
☐	☐	Metal or wire mesh implants	
☐	☐	Wire sutures or surgical staples	
☐	☐	Harrington rods (spine) or metal rods on bones	
☐	☐	Joint replacement _____	
☐	☐	Bone/joint pin, screw, nail, wire, plate	
☐	☐	Tattooed makeup (eyeliner, lips, etc.)	
☐	☐	Body piercing(s)	
☐	☐	Dentures or Dental Braces	
☐	☐	Removable dental item *(Remove before MRI)*	
☐	☐	Claustrophobia, Anxiety, Motion Disorder	

Please mark on the drawing any metal inside your body.

Right   **Left**

I attest that the above information is correct to the best of my knowledge.

_____   _____
Patient Signature   Date

_____   _____
Guardian   Date

Safety form reviewed by:

Front Desk _____   Technologist _____

Expediter _____

FIGURE I10-2. MRI safety questionnaire, back.

Vascular MR Imaging

Flow

Blood flow can create different kinds of effects on MR images. Some are highly desirable and can be used to image vessels, while others are undesirable and lead to artifacts. This chapter introduces a few basic principles of blood flow in the body. Then the different kinds of effects that flow has on MR images are reviewed. Chapter II-1 concludes by discussing artifacts and ways to minimize them. The specifics of vascular MR sequences, such as time-of-flight imaging (Chapter II-2), phase-contrast angiography, flow quantification (Chapter II-3), and gadolinium-enhanced MR angiography (Chapter II-4), are considered in subsequent chapters.

KEY CONCEPTS

▶ Flow patterns vary depending on vessel geometry and contour.

▶ Flow can cause signal loss or signal gain on both spin echo and gradient echo sequences.

▶ Spin echo sequences are typically used for black-blood imaging; parameters that favor signal loss due to flow include a longer TE and thin slices oriented perpendicular to flow.

▶ Gradient echo sequences are often used for bright-blood imaging; flow-related enhancement is maximized with a longer TR and thin slices oriented perpendicular to flow.

▶ Flow-related dephasing can be reduced by minimizing TE or by using flow compensation (gradient moment nulling), which requires longer TE.

▶ Artifacts related to flow include pulsation artifacts and overestimation of stenoses.

BLOOD FLOW IN VESSELS

Types of Flow

The study of blood flow in the vessels of the body is a vast and complex topic. The behavior of blood depends upon several factors, including its velocity and geometry of the vessels. In long, large, widely patent vessels, the flow usually can be described as *laminar flow*. The velocity profile across the vessel is parabolic—negligible velocity at the wall (Figure II1-1) and maximum velocity in the center. With laminar flow, the maximum velocity is equal to twice the average velocity across the vessel.

At the entrance of an aortic branch vessel such as the renal artery, the flow across the orifice starts as *plug flow*, that is, the velocity across the entire vessel is constant. With plug flow, the maximum velocity and mean velocity are identical.

A stenosis within a vessel causes blood to flow at high velocities through the narrowing. Beyond it, flow is nonlaminar, with vortices or eddies, reflecting *turbulent flow*. Turbulent flow causes signal dephasing in MR and contributes to an overestimation of vessel stenosis. Some distance beyond turbulent flow, the flow regains laminar behavior (Figure II1-1).

One special consideration in blood flow is what happens at vessel bifurcations, such as the bifurcation of the common carotid artery into the internal and external carotid arteries (Figure II1-1). As a consequence of *flow separation*, the laminar flow is disturbed in the branches, and small vortices may form. On MR imaging, these areas can cause signal loss and be misinterpreted as areas of vessel stenosis even in the absence of disease. These areas are challenging because regions of flow separation are prone to the formation of atherosclerotic plaque. Flow is further disturbed in the setting of stenoses, thereby worsening the signal loss.

Measures of Flow

By definition, the *velocity* of blood is the distance traveled per unit time (typically in units of centimeters/sec or meters/sec). In general, the velocity of blood in a vessel is not uniform across its lumen. The maximum velocity is typically near the center of the vessel, while slower velocities are measured toward the vessel wall (Figure II1-1). In addition to the spatial variation, arterial flow in the body is pulsatile, with a period defined by the cardiac cycle.

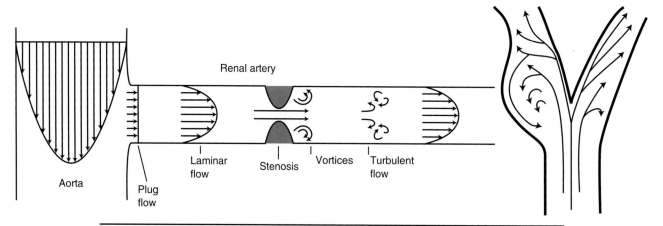

FIGURE II1-1. Flow patterns illustrated in the aorta and renal artery, including a renal artery stenosis (left), and in the carotid bifurcation (right).

Velocities change over time, typically higher during systole and lower during diastole. One of the most commonly used measurements of velocity in the clinical setting is the absolute maximum velocity, also known as the *peak systolic velocity*, which represents the highest velocity across the vessel cross section during peak systolic flow.

Velocity is commonly called "first-order flow." What are referred to as "higher-order" flow patterns include acceleration and jerk. Acceleration ("second-order flow") is defined as a constant change in velocity over time. Jerk ("third-order flow") is a constant change in acceleration over time. Because of the complex geometry of vessels, combined with the pulsatility of blood, flow in most vessels can be characterized as including higher-order flows. However, for many applications of MR, constant velocities are assumed.

Blood flow, or flow rate, on the other hand, refers to the volume of blood moving through a vessel in a given time (typical units of mL/sec or mL/min). Typically, with MRI, instantaneous flow is measured by assuming a constant velocity of blood over a short measurement period. To determine the instantaneous flow rate in a vessel, the average luminal velocity of blood at that time (cm/sec) is multiplied by the cross-sectional area of the vessel (cm²):

Flow (cm³/sec or mL/sec) = Average velocity (cm/sec)

× Cross-sectional area (cm²)

Often the total average flow over a specified period, such as one heartbeat, is reported. Examples of useful flow measurements include the measurement of total flow through the ascending aorta per heart beat (as a measurement of stroke volume) and the determination of intracardiac shunt fractions by comparing flow rates through the ascending aorta and main pulmonary artery. These are usually calculated by determining the average luminal velocity over one heartbeat and multiplying it by the cross-sectional area.

▶ TABLE II1-1 Typical peak velocities of blood in normal vessels

Vessel	Range of Peak Velocity (cm/sec)
Internal carotid artery	70–125
Aorta	70–100
Pulmonary artery	30–60
Common femoral artery	90–140
Popliteal vein	5–12

> **IMPORTANT CONCEPTS:** Flow patterns in blood vessels vary depending on vessel geometry and the presence of pathology such as atherosclerotic plaque

Typical velocities

Normal peak velocities of blood in different vessels of the body are listed in Table II1-1.

Arterial blood flow is pulsatile, and therefore velocities vary considerably across the cardiac cycle (Figure II1-2). The thoracic aorta normally has a large diastolic flow reversal that is equivalent to approximately 15% of the forward flow; the reversal is responsible for diastolic filling of the coronary arteries. In the peripheral arteries, a triphasic velocity waveform is normally seen, caused by the relationship between the pulsatility of blood, the distensibility of vessel walls, and the high resistance to circulation of the distal vessels in the musculature. In the setting of arterial stenosis, measured velocities can greatly exceed values given in Table II1-1. When stenoses become nearly occlusive, velocities decrease.

In the venous system, the flow is nearly constant except for mild variations related to breathing where intrathoracic pressure changes affect venous return.

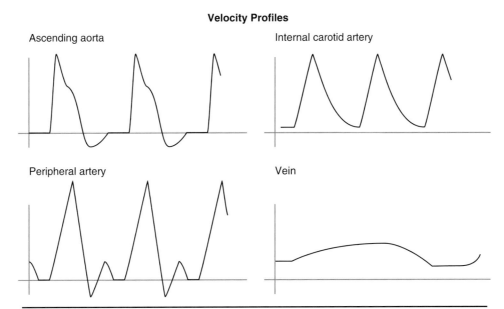

Velocity Profiles

Ascending aorta

Internal carotid artery

Peripheral artery

Vein

FIGURE II1-2. Representative velocity versus time curves in different vessels. While arterial vessels are pulsatile at a rate dependent on the cardiac cycle, venous flow typically has minimal variation, due to changes in intrathoracic pressure with respiration.

Types of Flow Effects

Flow can cause signal gain or signal loss depending on the nature of the pulse sequence and the nature of the flow (Table II1-2). Both effects are exploited in MR imaging. Techniques that rely on signal loss or signal void are referred to as *black-blood imaging* methods. Those that maximize flow-related enhancement are called *bright-blood imaging* techniques. It is important to understand the different causes of signal gain and loss so that each approach can be designed to minimize the factors that cause the opposite effect. Additionally, an understanding of these relationships can help avoid errors in interpretation that may arise from unintended flow-related effects. In the following sections, each flow effect is described first, then the concepts are synthesized in a discussion on how to perform bright-blood or black-blood *MR angiography (MRA)*.

> **IMPORTANT CONCEPT:** Flow can cause signal loss or signal gain on MR images. Opposing factors should be minimized in designing pulse sequences that emphasize one flow pattern over the other.

FLOW-RELATED SIGNAL LOSS

Flow Voids on Spin Echo

The loss of signal in moving blood on spin echo imaging has given rise to the alternative term used to describe spin echo imaging in the heart and vessels: "black-blood" imaging. The signal loss occurs because to generate a spin

▶ **TABLE II1-2 Flow Effects in MRI**

Signal Loss	Flow voids (spin echo imaging)
	Turbulence/disturbed flow
	Dephasing
	Intravoxel dephasing
Signal Gain	Flow-related enhancement (gradient echo imaging)

echo, protons must experience both the 90° and 180° pulses, both of which are typically slice selective. Blood that moves quickly through the slice of interest will not experience both RF pulses and therefore will not generate any signal (Figure II1-3).

Whether a complete signal void is produced by moving blood depends on the slice thickness and the time between the 90° and 180° pulses, or TE/2. Blood that traverses the slice thickness in the time TE/2 will not see both pulses. The minimum velocity needed to generate a signal void, V_{void}, is therefore

$$V_{void} \geq \frac{\text{Slice thickness}}{\text{TE/2}}$$

Conditions favorable for generating a signal void are thinner slices and longer TE.

For example, if the slice thickness is 5 mm and the TE is 50 msec in a spin echo sequence, then the minimum velocity for complete signal void is

$$V_{void} = \frac{5 \text{ mm}}{25 \text{ msec}} = 0.2 \text{ m/sec} = 20 \text{ cm/sec}$$

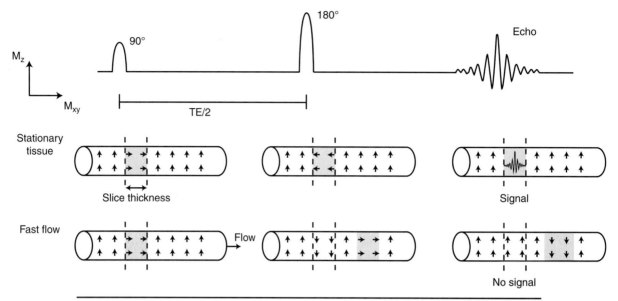

FIGURE II1-3. Effect of flowing blood on spin echo generation. Small arrows within the vessels indicate the net magnetization of protons in the blood. Only protons that are tipped into the transverse plane by the 90° pulse and then refocused within the transverse plane by the 180° pulse can generate an echo.

However, if the slice thickness is 10 mm, then the minimum velocity for a signal void is

$$V_{void} = \frac{10\ mm}{25\ msec} = 0.4\ m/sec = 40\ cm/sec$$

From Table II1-1, for a 5 mm slice, V_{void} is sufficiently low to ensure that almost all vessels, including all arteries and most veins, will demonstrate complete signal void on this sequence provided the images are gated to systole. Note that with a thicker slice, veins may have some visible signal intensity.

A sequence with a longer TE is more likely to generate a signal void than a sequence with short TE because there is more time for the blood to flow out of the slice during the pulse sequence.

Because blood flow is pulsatile, the timing of the acquisition relative to the cardiac cycle impacts the MR signal. Flow voids are greater in systole and less in diastole. Additionally, if images are acquired in the plane of flow rather than perpendicular to it, some protons, despite rapid flow, may still experience both 90° and 180° pulses. Complex patterns of signal intensity may result.

> **IMPORTANT CONCEPT:** To ensure that flowing blood produces negligible signal on a spin echo sequence, thiner slices, longer TEs, and slice orientation perpendicular to the direction of flow should be used.

CHALLENGE QUESTION: Other than adjusting slice thickness and TE, what other strategy can be used with spin echo or fast spin echo imaging to null signal from moving blood?

Answer: As discussed in Chapter I-9, double inversion recovery prepulses can be used to null signal from blood.

Flow-Related Dephasing (Spin Echo and Gradient Echo)

One recurring theme in MR physics is that gradients cause dephasing. To compensate for dephasing, most gradients are applied in two parts: a dephasing lobe and a rephasing lobe. When the area under the dephasing lobe equals the area under the rephasing lobe, protons are assumed to be in phase.

One assumption that has been implicit in these discussions is that the protons are stationary in the magnetic field. That is, for the rephasing lobe to cancel out the effects of the dephasing lobe, the protons must stay in the same location for each gradient. Protons that experience a stronger magnetic field than 1.5 T during dephasing gradient will experience a weaker magnetic field than 1.5 T during the rephasing gradient, and vice versa.

But what if protons are moving?

If protons are moving along the direction of the frequency-encoding gradient, then they will not necessarily experience dephasing and rephasing in the manner intended. That is, the dephasing will not equal the rephasing. In fact, moving protons will accumulate a net phase

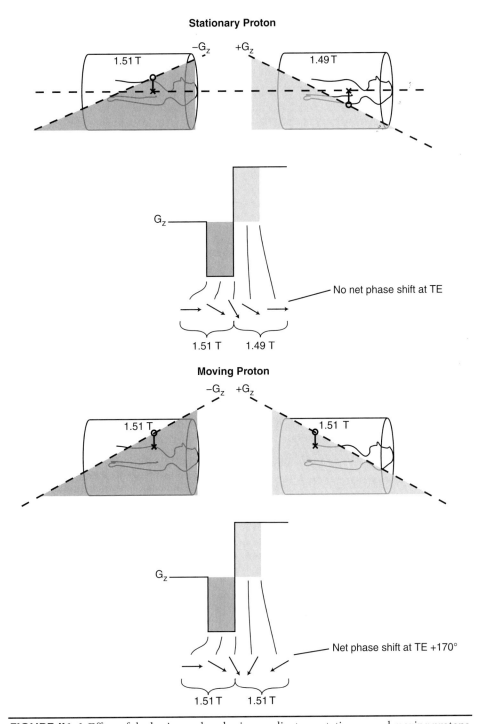

FIGURE II1-4. Effect of dephasing and rephasing gradients on stationary and moving protons. When the area under a positive gradient lobe equals the area under the negative lobe, a stationary proton will experience no net phase shift, but a moving (arterial) proton will. It starts in a region of the gradient that causes a positive phase shift. With gradient reversal, the proton has now moved nearer the feet and therefore again experiences a positive phase shift. Consequently, with the bipolar gradient, the moving proton experiences a net positive phase shift.

shift relative to stationary protons that is dependent on their velocity and direction. Figure II1-4 illustrates two scenarios—stationary versus moving protons—in a gradient echo pulse sequence. In this example, if a proton moves from the head to the feet (arterial flow), the net phase shift will be positive, while a proton moving in the opposite direction (venous flow) will accumulate a negative net phase shift. The gradients shown are G_z but the same principles apply to gradients in any direction, and most often refer to those in the readout derection (GA).

> **IMPORTANT CONCEPT:** Protons moving in the direction of the frequency-encoding gradient will acquire a net phase shift that is either positive or negative, depending on the direction of flow, and its magnitude will relate to velocity.

CHALLENGE QUESTION: What effect would switching the polarity of the gradient (first positive, then negative) in Figure II1-4 have on the phase shift of moving protons?

Answer: The magnitude of the phase shift will be the same, but the sign of the phase shift will be opposite. In other words, protons moving from the head to the feet (arterial flow) would have a negative phase shift, while protons moving from the feet to the head (venous flow) would have a positive phase shift.

The amount of phase shift that a proton experiences as a result of moving through the field is proportional to the gradient applied, for example G_x, the velocity of the protons, v, and to the square of the time, t, during which the gradients are applied. If the direction of flow is reversed, the phase shift will be opposite in sign as well. Because the phase shift is proportional to the square of the gradient duration, the longer the TE, the more flow-related dephasing.

> **IMPORTANT CONCEPT:** The phase shift experienced by moving protons is proportional to the square of the duration of the gradients; the longer the TE, the more flow-related dephasing.

There are two major implications of flow-related dephasing:

1. *The bad news:* Flow in the readout or frequency-encoding direction causes dephasing. Protons that are dephased cancel each other, and therefore there will be signal loss in the image due to flow. Unless measures are taken, flow in the frequency-encoding direction always leads to signal loss, whether the sequence is spin echo or gradient echo.
2. *The good news:* MR signal changes can be used to obtain information about flow direction or flow velocity. Not only is flow direction determinable by the sign of the phase shift, but the amount of phase shift is proportional to the velocity moving in the frequency-encoding direction. *Phase-contrast imaging* uses the phase information to measure blood velocities and flow (see Chapters II-3 and III-6).

Intravoxel Dephasing

Dephasing may also occur within a voxel because of flow effects. Within a given voxel, individual protons may have varying velocities, which give rise to phase dispersion of the protons within the voxel and consequently cause signal loss. This is referred to as *intravoxel dephasing*. Factors other than flow also contribute to intravoxel dephasing, including magnetic field inhomogeneity and susceptibility effects. The smaller the voxel, the less the intravoxel dephasing. Also, the less time there is for accumulation of phase differences (that is, the shorter the TE), the less dephasing.

Turbulence

Turbulent flow causes the flow patterns of protons to become randomly dispersed in multiple directions. The phase differences of protons result in signal nulling. Shorter TEs and smaller voxel sizes reduce the effects of turbulence.

> **IMPORTANT CONCEPTS:** Flow-related dephasing can occur within individual voxels, called intravoxel dephasing, or across voxels. Its effects depend on the flow patterns within vessels. Turbulent flow causes random, unpredictable patterns of signal loss.

Flow Compensation (Gradient Moment Nulling)

For MR imaging approaches that rely on flow-related enhancement, it is imperative that flow-related dephasing be minimized. The simplest solution is to minimize the TE. A more sophisticated and popular strategy uses more complex gradient pulses, called *flow compensation* or *gradient moment nulling*, to reduce the phase shift from moving protons. Flow compensation gradients can be thought of as two pairs of bipolar gradients of opposite polarity applied sequentially. The net effect of flow compensation gradients is to spare both stationary protons and those with relatively constant velocity from flow-related dephasing.

The way flow compensation gradients work is as follows. With a bipolar gradient (say, negative lobe first, then positive lobe), a proton moving with constant velocity along the direction of the gradient will develop a phase shift that is proportional to its velocity. The reversed bipolar gradient (positive lobe and then negative lobe) will cause a similar proton to experience a net phase shift with the same magnitude but opposite sign. By applying the two sets of bipolar gradients back to back, the phase shifts of each will cancel out. There will be no net phase shift for protons moving at a near-constant velocity. Ways in which a combination of bipolar gradients are implemented are illustrated in Figure II1-5.

CHALLENGE QUESTION: What is the effect of a pair of bipolar gradients of opposite polarity on stationary protons?

Answer: After each set of bipolar gradients, stationary protons will have no net phase shift because the dephasing and rephasing lobes have equal areas. After the two pairs, there will still be no net phase shift.

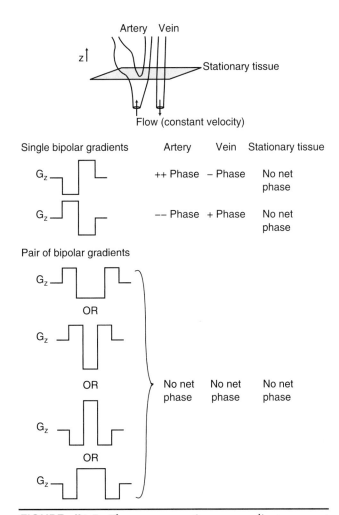

FIGURE II1-5. Flow compensation or gradient moment nulling. For stationary tissues, the net phase shift following application of gradients with equal positive and negative lobes will be zero. The sign of the phase shift for a moving proton with constant velocity depends on the gradient polarity. By combining two bipolar gradients of opposite polarity, the net phase shift for a moving proton will be canceled out.

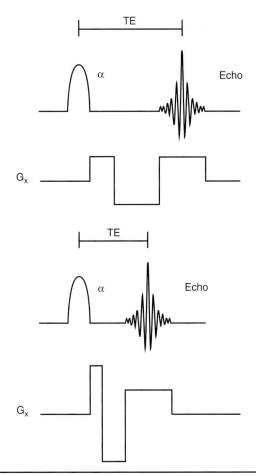

FIGURE II1-6. Flow compensation gradients in the frequency-encoding direction. With flow compensation, the net area under the gradient lobes should be equal at the center of the echo. To minimize TE, stronger gradients should be used for the non-readout lobes, as shown in the lower half of the figure.

> **IMPORTANT CONCEPT:** Very short TE or flow compensation gradients help minimize flow-related dephasing. Flow compensation results in longer TE and, consequently, longer acquisition times.

Flow compensation gradients can be applied in one direction or in multiple directions, depending on the nature of the flow relative to the slice orientation. Figure II1-6 illustrates two implementations of flow compensation for a frequency-encoding readout gradient. Because this more complicated three-lobed gradient pattern requires more time, efforts are made to maximize gradient strengths to minimize TE.

By reducing flow-related dephasing, flow compensation increases the signal intensity of flowing blood. It is therefore commonly used in time-of-flight imaging (Chapter II-2) and in bright-blood cine gradient echo imaging for evaluation of myocardial function (Chapter III-4). One disadvantage of flow compensation is the increase in TE caused by the extra gradient lobes.

The flow compensation gradients illustrated in Figure II1-6 result in first-order gradient moment nulling. Such gradients minimize dephasing caused by first-order flow. This strategy is inadequate to eliminate dephasing of blood that is undergoing acceleration or changing velocities.

Higher-Order Flow

In most arterial systems, blood flow is pulsatile, with periodic acceleration and deceleration. For limited acceleration, slow enough that velocity is almost constant within the time frame of the flow compensation gradients, first-order flow compensation can be sufficient for imaging. For most normal vessels, flow compensation with first-order gradient moment nulling is adequate to minimize flow-related dephasing.

When there is marked acceleration, higher-order flow, or turbulence, dephasing will occur despite first-order flow compensation gradients. Short TEs are the best solution for minimizing flow-related dephasing in these settings. Higher-order flow-related dephasing is very sensitive to TE, more than first-order flow is. When TE shortening is not an option, more complex gradient schemes can also eliminate dephasing that results from acceleration (second-order flow compensation) or jerk (third-order flow compensation). However, the additional gradient lobes with these methods come at the cost of even longer TE (and consequently longer TR and acquisition times) and therefore are not commonly used.

CHALLENGE QUESTION: Can high-order flow compensation reduce the flow-related dephasing effects of turbulent flow?

Answer: No flow compensation schemes, no matter how high the order, can reduce the dephasing effects of turbulence.

> **IMPORTANT CONCEPT:** Dephasing due to higher-order flow patterns, such as acceleration and jerk, can be minimized by using shorter TEs or higher-order flow compensation techniques. Dephasing due to turbulent flow is not reduced with flow compensation.

FLOW-RELATED ENHANCEMENT

While the previous section reviewed the problem of signal loss due to flow, this section focuses on signal *gain* due to flow. Usually observed with gradient echo imaging, *flow-related enhancement* occurs because the flow of fresh protons into the imaging slice provides a source of unsaturated protons. These protons have full longitudinal magnetization, in contrast to the relatively saturated protons in the imaging slice due to the short TRs associated with gradient echo sequences. Following an RF pulse, their echoes have greater amplitude than those of the saturated background tissues (Figure I4-6). Factors that affect the degree of saturation of tissues with gradient echo imaging include flip angle, T1 relaxation times, and TR (Table II1-3).

Flow-related enhancement is the basis for time-of-flight (TOF) MR angiography (Chapter II-2) and for ECG-gated cine spoiled gradient echo imaging of the heart (Chapter III-4). For these bright-blood techniques, sequences should be optimized for flow sensitivity and dephasing should be minimized.

Time-of-Flight

In a given imaging slice, partial replacement of the saturated spins with unsaturated spins results in increased signal intensity (Figure II1-7). Arrival of "fresh" protons is the basis for *time-of-flight* MR imaging. If the velocity is fast enough to replace all blood contained within the slice during a TR interval, then the maximum signal intensity—that is, maximum flow-related enhancement—will be achieved.

The velocity of blood associated with *maximum flow-related enhancement*, $V_{max\ FRE}$, depends on the distance to

> **TABLE II1-3 Tissue Saturation with Spoiled Gradient Echo Imaging**

More Saturation	Less Saturation
High flip angle	Low flip angle
Short TR	Long TR
Long T1	Short T1

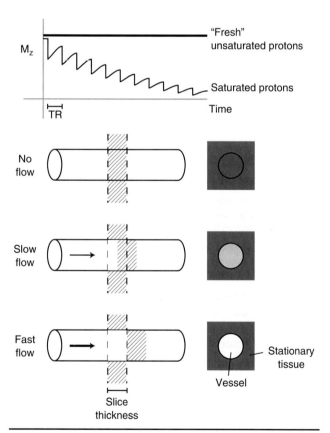

FIGURE II1-7. Flow-related enhancement is the basis for time-of-flight imaging. Stationary protons become saturated, that is, their longitudinal magnetization is reduced following multiple excitations. Arrival of fresh protons causes flow-related enhancement, increasing the signal intensity to a maximum value when there is complete replacement of protons in the slice during each TR.

be traversed by blood within a slice relative to the time interval between RF pulses (TR). If the vessel is perpendicular to the slice, then

$$V_{maxFRE} = \frac{Slice\ thickness}{TR}$$

That is, conditions favorable for generating flow-related enhancement include thinner slices, slices being oriented perpendicular to the direction of flow, and a longer TR.

This relationship reflects the fact that the thicker the slice, the faster the blood protons have to flow to replace those in the slice within the same time period. For example, if the slice thickness is 5 mm, and the TR is 25 msec, then

$$V_{maxFRE} \geq \frac{5\ mm}{25\ msec} = 0.2\ m/sec = 20\ cm/sec$$

That is, any flow above 20 cm/sec will cause maximum flow-related enhancement. This is achieved in most arteries and veins. If the slice thickness were 10 mm, then

$$V_{maxFRE} \geq \frac{10\ mm}{25\ msec} = 0.4\ m/sec = 40\ cm/sec$$

Consequently, sluggish veins will not show as much flow-related enhancement in a 10 mm as in a 5 mm slice.

Alternatively, the longer the TR, the more time there is for the protons in the vessel to be replaced with fresh spins. For detection of very slow flow, a longer TR should be used.

> **IMPORTANT CONCEPT:** Thinner slices oriented perpendicular flow and longer TRs make a gradient echo sequence highly sensitive to slow flow.

CHALLENGE QUESTION: What is the effect of higher flip angle on these gradient echo images?

Answer: Recall from Chapter I-4 (Figure I4-6) that the higher the flip angle, the greater the suppression of signal from stationary tissues. Also, as will be discussed further in Chapter II-2, fresh protons will generate high signal with high flip angles. Therefore, provided the velocity of blood exceeds $V_{max\ FRE}$, higher flip angles will result in greater image contrast between the flowing blood and background tissues.

Entry Slice Phenomenon

When imaging is performed one slice at a time, each slice will show flow-related enhancement as discussed in the previous section of this chapter. However, multiple slices or an entire volume are often imaged in a single acquisition. In these cases, the flow-related enhancement is most

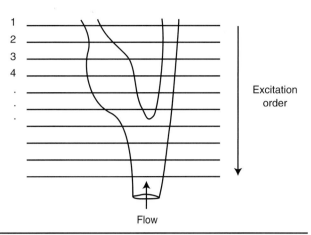

FIGURE II1-8. Imaging the carotid artery with slice order countercurrent to flow direction. Slice excitation will not saturate the inflowing protons, so flow-related enhancement is maximized.

prominent at the first slice, or *entry slice*. The effect is reduced deeper into the imaging volume, where even the moving protons will have experienced RF excitations before reaching the imaging slice. The order of excitation of slices can be adjusted to increase or decrease entry slice phenomenon. For example, if the imaging order is countercurrent to the flow, then more slices will show flow-related enhancement than if the imaging is performed concurrent to the flow (Figure II1-8).

Selective Flow-Related Enhancement

With TOF imaging, any inflow of unsaturated protons into the imaging slice will cause increased signal. This means that both arteries and veins will appear bright. In most clinical applications, as will be discussed in Chapter II-2, only certain vessels (for example, the arteries) are of interest. To suppress signal from the undesired vessels, a saturation band can be applied just to one side of the imaging slice. The choice of side depends on whether arterial or venous flowing protons are to be suppressed. As illustrated in Figure I9-4, for imaging the carotid arteries, a saturation band above each imaging slice will eliminate flow-related enhancement from the veins, leaving only the arteries to show flow-related enhancement.

GENERAL STRATEGIES FOR CLINICAL FLOW-RELATED IMAGING

In the clinical setting, most cardiovascular imaging protocols include both a black-blood imaging spin echo sequence and a bright-blood gradient echo sequence. Black-blood imaging relies on flow-related signal loss and aims to minimize flow-related enhancement. Bright-blood imaging has the opposite goals. Summary strategies for each are reviewed in the following paragraphs.

Black Blood Imaging

Black-blood imaging is used in cardiovascular MRI to visualize vessel wall pathology such as atherosclerotic plaque, intramural hematoma and dissection, and extraluminal disease, including thrombosed portions of aneurysms and vasculitides. Common applications include aortic and carotid artery imaging as well as coronary artery imaging. When flowing blood has low signal intensity, the wall and extraluminal structures are well defined and pathology more easily discernible.

To ensure good black-blood imaging, slices should be thin and oriented perpendicular to flow. Pulse sequences are typically spin echo sequences.

CHALLENGE QUESTION: Would flow-compensation gradients be useful for black-blood spin echo sequences?

Answer: No. Flow-compensation gradients are intended to reduce flow-related dephasing. This dephasing is desirable in black-blood imaging.

Where blood velocity is slow relative to V_{void} and blood generates signal despite use of spin echo-based approaches, additional double inversion prepulses can be applied to ensure blood nulling (Chapter I-9).

Bright-Blood Imaging

Bright-blood imaging applications include time-of-flight MR angiography and cine spoiled gradient echo sequences for cardiac function. Generally, bright-blood sequences are gradient echo sequences. To maximize flow-related enhancement in spoiled gradient echo imaging, thinner slices, oriented perpendicular to flow, should be used. Longer TRs allow time for more unsaturated protons to enter the slice. All efforts should be made to minimize flow-related dephasing, using either short TEs or flow compensation. Smaller voxels and shorter TE times also help to minimize intravoxel dephasing.

> **IMPORTANT CONCEPTS:** For black-blood imaging, techniques to reduce signal from moving blood are used and flow-related enhancement is avoided. Conversely, for bright-blood imaging, techniques to increase flow-related enhancement, while minimizing flow-related dephasing, are used.

ARTIFACTS

Pulsation Artifact

Any periodic motion, such as those caused by breathing, vascular pulsation, or CSF pulsation, can cause artifacts

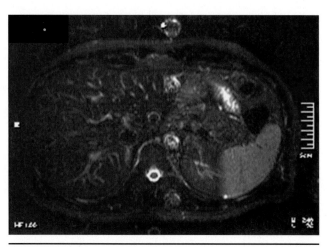

FIGURE II1-9. Pulsation artifact producing columns of ghost images of the aorta and spinal canal.

in the phase-encoding direction. The artifacts seen are frequently referred to as *ghosting artifacts*. In cardiovascular applications, the most common cause is aortic or arterial pulsation, hence the specific term *pulsation artifact* (Figure I1-36 and Figure II1-9). Pulsation artifacts are caused by phase mismapping. With each phase-encoding step, the total signal changes are assumed to be due to different degrees of dephasing caused by the phase-encoding gradient. If signal decreases are due to other effects, such as flow, then the resulting measured signal will be attributed to phase-encoding gradient effects. The signal will be attributed to another voxel that lies some distance away from the flow-affected voxel. There are no pulsation artifacts in the frequency-encoding direction.

For pulsation artifacts to occur, the time frame for phase encoding must exceed the duration of one pulsation. The distance between adjacent ghosts depends on the relationship between the acquisition time and the duration of the motion:

$$\text{Distance between ghosts (voxels)} = T_{acq}/T_{motion}$$

For the inversion recovery fast spin echo image shown in Figure II1-9, the acquisition time is 22 sec. If the pulse rate is 80 beats per minute or $T_{motion} = 0.75$ sec, then the ghosts will occur separated by

$$\text{Distance between ghosts} = 22/0.75 \cong 29 \text{ voxels}$$

Across the 128 voxels in the phase-encoding direction, approximately 3–4 ghosts will be evident, as shown in Figure II1-9. If the subject's heart rate goes up, T_{motion} decreases, and the distance between ghosts will become greater. The distance between ghosts will also increase if the acquisition time increases.

Strategies to Minimize Pulsation Artifacts

Several approaches can be used to minimize the consequences of pulsation artifacts:

1. Vary the phase-encoding direction. Ghosting occurs only in the phase-encoding direction. If the artifact interferes with visualization of vital structures that happen to be aligned with the aorta in the phase-encoding direction, it is possible to reorient the ghosts by swapping the phase- and frequency-encoding directions. Since phase encoding defaults to the narrowest dimension of the body, the price of swapping phase- and frequency-encoding directions is usually longer acquisition times because more phase-encoding steps are needed after the swap.
2. Saturation bands. A saturation band placed upstream through the pulsating vessel (or other sources of motion artifact) will suppress inflowing signal, and pulsation artifacts will seem less conspicuous. For example, in the imaging of patients with arrhythmogenic right ventricular dysplasia (see Chapter III-5), a saturation band can be placed over the left ventricle to minimize ghosting related to left ventricular motion. As another example, for patients with respiratory motion arising from the chest wall, saturation bands can be placed over the subcutaneous tissues to reduce the signal from those structures and eliminate the ghosting artifacts. As discussed in Chapter I-9, saturation bands usually require only a minor increase in acquisition times.
3. Electrocardiographic gating. Synchronization of acquisitions with the cardiac cycle may help reduce pulsation artifacts. The drawback of electrocardiographically gated or peripherally gated sequences is much longer acquisition times.
4. Image post-processing. In some applications, post-processing software can eliminate motion or pulsation artifact from the displayed image. For example, in time-of-flight imaging, by confining the reconstructed volume to the region immediately around the vessel of interest, ghosting artifacts can be excluded from the processed images.

> **IMPORTANT CONCEPTS:** Solutions to pulsation artifacts include (1) swapping phase- and frequency-encoding directions, (2) saturation bands, (3) cardiac gating, and (4) image-processing tools to exclude artifacts from reconstructed images.

Overestimation of Stenoses

The luminal diameter even of normal vessels is difficult to assess with accuracy on MRI. The differences in velocities along the wall of the vessel lead to dephasing, and consequently vessel size is typically underestimated on MRI.

In the setting of stenosis, the effects of flow on MR imaging cause the degree of narrowing almost always to be overestimated. Accelerated velocities through areas of stenosis cause dephasing, both across voxels and within voxels. Nonlaminar flow profiles, including vortices or eddies and areas of turbulence, further exacerbate dephasing and signal loss. Where vessels are tortuous or where there is stream separation, such as at the carotid bifurcation (Figure II1-1), signal loss may mimic or exaggerate stenosis. Finally, as will be discussed in Chapter II-4, image post-processing algorithms, such as maximum intensity projection, can further worsen the overestimation of stenoses with MR angiography.

Stenosis overestimation can be improved by reducing TE, decreasing the voxel size, and using flow compensation. First-order flow compensation is a standard technique in MR angiography.

> **IMPORTANT CONCEPTS:** The overestimation of stenoses that inevitably occurs with MR angiography can be minimized by shortening TE and by using higher-spatial-resolution imaging. First-order flow compensation gradients, despite lengthening TE, are usually desirable.

REVIEW QUESTIONS

1. To image a patient with suspected intramural hematoma, the following spin echo sequence has been implemented for black-blood imaging: TR = 1000 msec, TE = 10 msec, slice thickness 12 mm. The resulting images show undesirable signal in the lumen of the aorta (Figure II1-Q1).

   Which of the changes listed in Table II1-4A might help improve the image by reducing the signal from blood flow in the aorta?

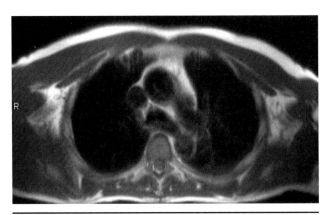

FIGURE II1-Q1

▶ **TABLE II1-4A**

Proposed Changes	Check Which Apply
a. Electrocardiographic gating to systole	
b. Electrocardiographic gating to diastole	
c. Change TE to 5 msec	
d. Change TE to 20 msec	
e. Change slice thickness to 8 mm	
f. Change slice thickness to 15 mm	
g. Add flow compensation gradients to frequency-encoding gradients	
h. Add double inversion recovery prepulses	

▶ **TABLE II1-5A**

Proposed Changes	Check Which Apply
a. Change the slice orientation to axial	
b. Change the slice orientation to coronal	
c. Electrocardiographic gating to systole	
d. Electrocardiographic gating to diastole	
e. Change TR to 20 msec	
f. Change TR to 30 msec	
g. Change TE to 5 msec	
h. Change TE to 12 msec	
i. Change flip angle to 5°	
j. Change flip angle to 25°	
k. Add flow compensation gradients to frequency-encoding gradients	
l. Add double inversion recovery prepulses	

2. The spoiled gradient echo image in Figure II1-Q2 is generated in a subject with an aortic dissection. TR = 25 msec, TE = 10 msec, flip angle = 15°.

You see the suggestion of an intimal flap in the aorta but lament the poor contrast between the flap and surrounding blood. Which of the changes in Table II1-5A should be implemented to improve the contrast?

3. What causes the signal loss, seen only during systole, in this patient with aortic stenosis (Figure II1-Q3)? Will use of first-order flow compensation gradients eliminate this signal loss?

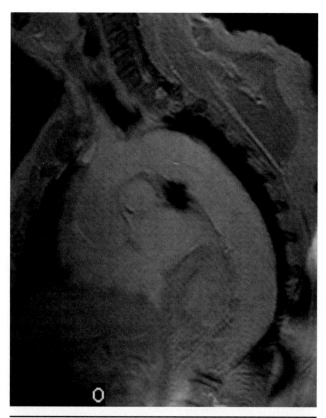

FIGURE II1-Q2

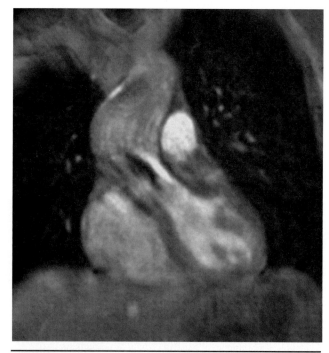

FIGURE II1-Q3

4. What would be the fastest way to prevent the ghosting artifact shown in Figure II1-9?

Time-of-Flight MR Angiography

The three main techniques for clinical MR angiography are time-of-flight (TOF), phase-contrast, and gadolinium-enhanced imaging. TOF techniques rely on flow-related enhancement and do not use exogenous contrast material. Methods that are used include 2D and 3D gradient echo techniques and a combined approach called *multiple overlapping thin-slab acquisition (MOTSA)*. 2D TOF is the most commonly used technique for most cardiovascular imaging. Applications include MR imaging of the carotid arteries; some peripheral vascular MR angiography, particularly in the calves and feet; and MR venography. At the conclusion of this chapter, sample TOF MR protocols are provided for carotid artery imaging and MR venography. Gadolinium-enhanced carotid and peripheral MR angiography protocols are contained in Chapter II-4.

KEY CONCEPTS

▶ 2D TOF imaging is sensitive to slow flow moving through the slice plane.

▶ With TOF imaging, strategies to reduce background signal must be balanced against saturation of flowing protons.

▶ Saturation bands can be combined with TOF to create selective MR arteriography or venography.

▶ Flow compensation, together with reduced TE and small voxel size (high spatial resolution), reduce overestimation of stenoses.

▶ 3D TOF has higher spatial resolution and is less susceptible to turbulent flow than 2D TOF, but it is also less sensitive to slow flow.

▶ Clinical Protocols:
   ▶ Carotid MRA without gadolinium contrast
   ▶ Pelvic MR venography without gadolinium contrast

2D TIME-OF-FLIGHT MR ANGIOGRAPHY

The goals of time-of-flight imaging are to produce high-spatial-resolution images where flow-related enhancement is maximized, flow-related dephasing is minimized, and background tissue is suppressed. Background tissue suppression is achieved because TOF imaging is a gradient echo technique; so exposure to repeated excitation pulses in rapid succession saturates most tissue in an imaging slice (Chapter I-4). Flowing blood enters the slice fully magnetized (not having experience any excitation pulses), so it can generate high signal following the RF pulse. This creates bright signal in vessels with flowing blood relative to a dark background of stationary tissues. To maximize flow-related enhancement, the imaging slices are positioned perpendicular to the direction of blood flow. Flow compensation gradients (see Chapter II-1), applied in one or more directions, reduce flow-related dephasing. A typical pulse sequence diagram for 2D TOF imaging is shown in Figure II2-1.

With TOF, any inflow of unsaturated protons will produce signal. Therefore, both arteries and veins are bright. A spatially selective saturation band is usually applied to saturate venous signal when MR arteriography is desired.

Sequence parameters that can be manipulated to optimize TOF imaging are described in the following paragraphs.

Parameter Selection

TR

One challenge in TOF angiography is the need to balance flow-related enhancement and background tissue suppression. Selection of TR is the key to the nature of this balance.

Recall from Chapter II-1 that a long TR and thin slices favor flow-related enhancement. With thinner slices, shorter TRs can be used. The gain in time with shorter TR compensates for the need to image more slices for the same anatomic coverage. However, thinner slices result in higher spatial resolution, and shorter TR achieves greater background suppression, and so this strategy can be advantageous.

In the typical setting, TRs vary in the range of 25 to 50 msec. Longer TRs make the sequence more sensitive to slow flow, at the cost of longer acquisition time.

IMPORTANT CONCEPT: Long TR favors flow-related enhancement, decreases background suppression, and increases acquisition times.

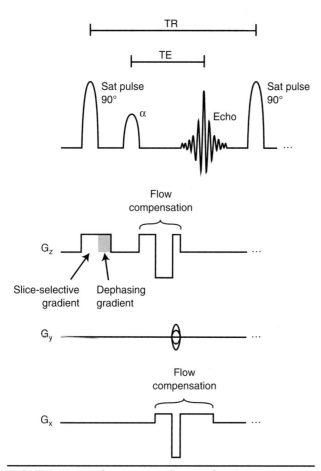

FIGURE II2-1. Pulse sequence diagram for 2D TOF imaging. Flow compensation gradients are shown in both the slice-select and frequency-encoding directions.

Flip Angle

Selection of the flip angle is important for TOF angiography. Recall from Chapter I-4 (Figure I4-6) that when the TR is less than the T1 relaxation time, the flip angle significantly affects the magnetization available to generate signal. Specifically, the higher the flip angle, the greater the suppression of background tissue (Figure II2-2).

Higher flip angles produce more signal and consequently greater contrast between flowing and stationary tissues, provided that the flow into the slice is sufficiently fast for all spins in the vessels to be completely replaced with each excitation. However, with slow-flowing protons, higher flip angles will cause partial saturation. Typical flip angles vary from 45° to 60°, but flip angles can be as low as 30° or as high as 90°.

IMPORTANT CONCEPT: Higher flip angles are advantageous with fast-flowing vessels because they lead to more signal from flowing blood and less signal from the background stationary tissue.

Voxel Size

Decreases in voxel size reduce intravoxel dephasing and improve spatial resolution. Smaller voxels are achieved by increasing the number of phase-encoding steps (N_{PE}) or reducing the field of view. Higher N_{PE}, together with thinner slices, usually come at the expense of increased acquisition times and lower SNR.

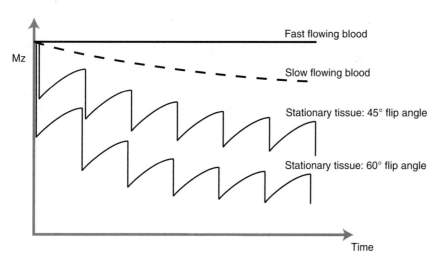

FIGURE II2-2. Effect of flip angle on TOF imaging. Higher flip angles cause greater saturation of background tissues. Note that slowly moving blood has signal intermediate between those of fast-moving blood and stationary tissues.

TE and Flow Compensation

To minimize flow-related dephasing, TE can be shortened or flow compensation used. Flow compensation gradients in read and slice-select directions (as shown in Figure II2-1) minimize effects of velocity on phase dispersion. Higher-order flow effects are minimized by keeping TE as short as possible (allowing for the flow compensation gradients). TE values are typically on the order of 8 to 9 msec.

Acquisition Times

For a typical TR of 25 msec and a 256 × 128 imaging matrix, the acquisition time per slice is 3.2 sec. To image a slab of 64 2D slices would require approximately 3 minutes of imaging time. With 2D TOF, contiguous slices are typically imaged with a small degree of overlap. This facilitates image reconstruction (as described subsequently) by avoiding imaging artifacts associated with discontinuities at the slice edges. For example, if the slice thickness is 3 mm and a 1 mm overlap is used, then the total slab thickness for 64 slices is 64 × (3 mm − 1 mm) = 128 mm.

Other Considerations

In vessels with pulsatile blood flow, imaging during systole can improve quality of TOF images. As will be discussed in Chapter III-1, synchronization can be achieved using central electrocardiographic gating or peripheral gating. The acquisition times increase considerably with gating, because imaging is performed only during a short portion of each cardiac cycle.

TOF images have a component of T1 weighting, so tissues other than vessels, such as subcutaneous fat and bone marrow, will increase the signal. One solution is to suppress signal from fat, using either a frequency-selective fat saturation pulse, selective water excitation, or a 180° inversion pulse to null fat (Chapter I-9). Because each of these options lengthens acquisition times, it is common to rely on post-processing methods to reduce the effects of unwanted fat signal (as described subsequently). Another option for suppressing background tissue, particularly for intracranial angiography, uses magnetization transfer pulses (Chapter I-3).

Arteriography vs Venography

If a sequence is sensitive to slow flow, then both venous and arterial structures will appear bright on 2D TOF images. As discussed in Chapter I-9, typically only one type of vessel is of interest. In such a case, the other vessel type can be suppressed by application of a saturation band distal (for arteriography) or proximal (for venography) to the imaging slice (Figure I9-4). For most reliable suppression, the saturation band should travel with the imaging slice, remaining adjacent to the slice (Figure I9-6).

CHALLENGE QUESTION: What parameters should be changed to convert a typical MR angiographic 2D TOF sequence to a useful MR venographic sequence?

Answer: First, the position of the saturation bands relative to the imaging slice should be switched to ensure that the arterial signal is suppressed for MR venography. Second, to increase sensitivity to slower blood flow, the TR can be lengthened, slice thickness reduced, and the flip angle decreased.

Chapter II-4 contains a more detailed discussion of MR venography, using both gadolinium-enhanced and non-enhanced MR techniques.

Image Post-Processing

With 2D TOF imaging, slices are oriented perpendicular to the direction of flow for maximum flow sensitivity. These images are commonly post-processed to allow a more realistic view of the vessel, similar to conventional angiography. Image post-processing techniques, such as maximum intensity projections, are reviewed in detail in Chapter II-4. Frequently a range of coronal, sagittal, and oblique reconstructions of the axial images is produced to enable better visualization of atherosclerotic plaques and stenoses (Figure II2-3). To eliminate signal from unwanted tissues in the field of view, the imaging volume can be selectively cropped so that only the vessels of interest are visible in the post-processed image (see also Chapter II-4).

Pitfalls

In-Plane Flow and Reversal of Flow Direction

Because TOF imaging relies on the inflow of unsaturated spins, the slice position must be perpendicular to the

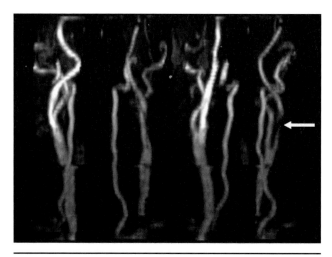

FIGURE II2-3. Selected 2D TOF source images and coronal (left) and oblique coronal (right) maximum-intensity projection reconstructions of the left carotid artery, depicting stenosis of left internal carotid artery (arrow), better seen on the oblique view.

direction of flow. Where vessels are particularly tortuous or, worse yet, if flow direction reverses, 2D TOF imaging may not be successful and, in fact, may even be misleading. In-plane flow results in saturation and signal loss, which can mimic stenosis. Reversal of flow direction will result in inadvertent suppression by the traveling saturation band. The latter is particularly problematic in the setting of stenoses or occlusions, where retrograde filling or the development of collaterals may be overlooked by TOF imaging (Figure II2-4).

> **IMPORTANT CONCEPT:** TOF imaging, when performed with saturation bands to achieve selectivity in imaging arteries or veins, can result in inadvertent suppression of signal in the case of flow reversal.

Overestimation of Stenosis

As discussed in Chapter II-1, all MRA methods overestimate vascular stenoses because of flow-related dephasing and limited spatial resolution. With 2D TOF imaging, the best

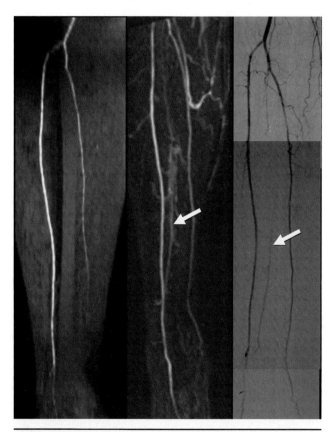

FIGURE II2-4. Comparison of 2D TOF MRA (left), gadolinium-enhanced MRA (middle), and digital subtraction angiography (DSA, right). Retrograde (caudal to cranial) filling of the peroneal artery, seen on gadolinium-enhanced MRA and DSA, is not seen on 2D TOF MRA. On the 2D TOF MRA, the caudal saturation band suppressed signal from blood flowing toward the head in the peroneal artery.

strategies to avoid this artifact are flow compensation, TE minimization, and reduction of voxel size. Because TOF acquisitions require acquisition times approaching 10 min, image quality is also sensitive to motion artifacts. Subject motion can result in uninterpretable TOF images with severe overestimation of disease (Figure II2-5).

> **IMPORTANT CONCEPT:** To reduce overestimation of stenosis, use flow compensation, shorter TEs, and smaller voxel sizes.

3D TIME-OF-FLIGHT MRA

While many of the concepts of 2D TOF apply to 3D TOF, there are some important differences. With 3D TOF imaging, an entire slab of tissue is imaged using thin partitions (typically less than 1 mm in thickness). Because the entire slab experiences each RF pulse, the inflow effect of fresh spins is seen best where the spins enter the slice and diminishes with distance into the slab. 3D TOF is best used in the setting of vessels with high velocities and with parameters that do not saturate the signal from flowing blood. Flip angles with 3D TOF are typically between 10° and 30°, lower than with 2D TOF. The most common clinical application is intracranial angiography. Use of 3D TOF for extracranial vascular imaging is less common. Some centers use 3D TOF to supplement 2D TOF in carotid MRA.

Table II2-1 summarizes the differences between 2D and 3D TOF imaging.

Multiple Overlapping Thin-Slab Acquisition (MOTSA)

To take advantage of the strengths of both 2D and 3D TOF, the technique of multiple overlapping thin-slab acquisition (MOTSA) has been implemented. Multiple overlapping 3D

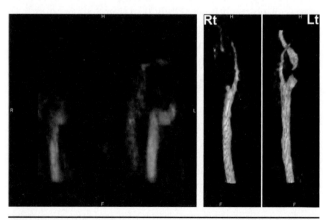

FIGURE II2-5. Overestimation of stenosis on TOF (left) secondary to subject motion during the acquisition. Gadolinium-enhanced MRA shows long-segment severe stenosis of the right internal carotid artery (Rt) and focal high-grade stenosis of the left ICA (Lt).

> **TABLE II2-1** 2D vs 3D TOF MR Angiography

Attribute	2D TOF	3D TOF
Acquisition time	Shorter	Longer
Sensitivity to slow flow	More	Less
Sensitivity to intravoxel dephasing	More	Less
Susceptibility to turbulence	More	Less
Spatial resolution	Thicker slices	Thinner partitions
Tortuous vessels or reversed flow	Poor	Better
Signal-to-noise ratio	Less	More
Example of advantage in carotid MRA	Visualize slow flow beyond stenosis	Grade percent stenosis

slabs are used to improve the sensitivity to slow flow over conventional 3D imaging while still enabling coverage of an extended area of interest. The overlapping slices are discarded to eliminate slices that typically have low signal at the two ends of 3D TOF slabs. MOTSA is most commonly implemented with intracranial MRA.

REVIEW QUESTIONS

1. A subject is referred for MR evaluation of the carotid and vertebral arteries because of vertigo that worsens with right arm exertion. A 2D TOF image through the neck with saturation band placed above the slice is shown in Figure II2-Q1A.
   a. What abnormality is seen on this image? What are the differential diagnoses?

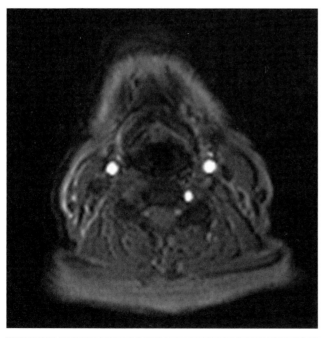

FIGURE II2-Q1A

b. How could you determine which of the differential diagnoses most likely applies in this case?

2. A patient complaining of right leg claudication has a peripheral MR angiography examination using 2D TOF imaging. The maximum-intensity projection reconstruction of the right calf is shown in Figure II2-Q2A. The referring physician reviews the images and questions a right anterior tibial artery origin stenosis.

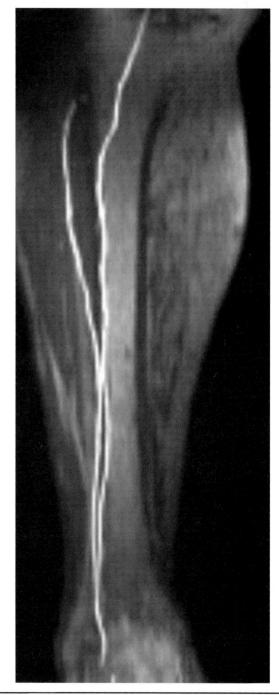

FIGURE II2-Q2A

a. Do you agree or disagree with her finding?
b. How could you modify the MR acquisition to prove your assessment?

3. Your MR system has a generic protocol for 2D TOF imaging. You wish to optimize the sequence for carotid artery imaging to evaluate for carotid artery stenosis. Which of the parameters or options in Table II2-2A should you implement, with the aim of minimizing overestimation of stenoses?

▶ **TABLE II2-2A**

Parameter Changes	Check Which Apply
a. Saturation bands superior to the imaging slice	
b. Decreased voxel size	
c. Increased TR	
d. Decreased TE	
e. Increased flip angle	
f. Flow compensation (gradient moment nulling)	

4. A patient is imaged using 2D TOF for evaluation of carotid artery disease. The maximum-intensity projection of the TOF images (cropped to show the left carotid artery) is shown in Figure II2-Q4A. Contrast-enhanced angiography is shown in Figure II2-Q4B. (Note that the contrast-enhanced images have been post-processed to depict only luminal gadolinium contrast material.) How do you explain the discrepant appearance of the left ICA between studies?

5. Discuss the artifact shown in the maximum-intensity projection schematic (Figure II2-Q5) of a series of axial 2D time-of-flight images of the carotid artery:

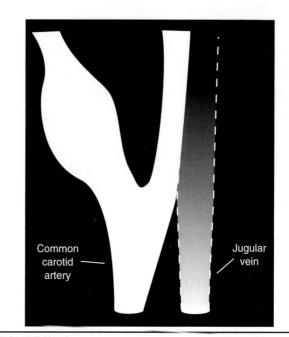

FIGURE II2-Q5

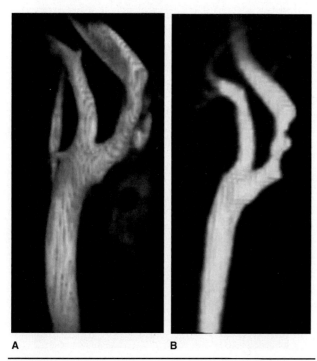

A   **B**

FIGURE II2-Q4A, B

▶ **PROTOCOL: Carotid MRA without Gadolinium Contrast**

Setup and Preparation	Notes
Coil	Neck phased-array (plus optional head coil)
Positioning tips	Supine, head first

Sequence	Imaging Plane	Parameters
1 Scout (true FISP or spoiled GRE)	Multiplanar	Default
2 2D TOF[1]	Axial	TR/TE/FA, 25/9/40°, 3–4 mm slices Flow compensation in slice select and frequency-encoding FOV < 250 mm Superior saturation band
3 2D TOF[2]	Axial	4 slices, inferior saturation band
4 3D TOF (Optional)	Axial	TR/TE/FA, 30/6/10°, 1–1.2 mm partitions 2 slabs with overlap Flow compensation in slice and frequency-encoding FOV < 250 mm Superior saturation band
5 T1 SE or TSE (Optional)[3]	Axial	Multislice imaging, typically with multiple signal averages and free breathing

[1]Images are post-processed, typically using maximum intensity projection reconstructions and selective cropping-out of unwanted tissues in the imaging volume.
[2]Second 2D TOF acquisition is performed using an inferior saturation band to determine flow direction in the vertebral arteries in case of possible subclavian steal. Only a limited number of slices is necessary.
[3]If dissection is suspected, high-resolution T1 TSE can be helpful to evaluate mural pathology in the carotid or vertebral arteries.

▶ **PROTOCOL: Pelvic MR Venography without Gadolinium Contrast**

Setup and Preparation	Notes
Coil	Torso phased-array
Positioning tips	Supine, head first

Sequence	Imaging Plane	Parameters
1 Scout (true FISP or spoiled GRE)	Multiplanar	Default
2 2D TOF[1]	Axial	TR/TE/FA, 25/9/40°, 4–5 mm slices with 0.5 mm overlap Flow compensation in slice and frequency-encoding Superior saturation band
3 2D TOF[2] (Optional)	Axial	Limited number of slices, inferior saturation band
4 T1-weighted gradient echo imaging (Optional)[3]	Axial	TE 4.4 msec (or dual echo TE 2.2 msec/4.4 msec) 6–8 mm slices, < 20 sec breath hold
5 STIR or T2-TSE with fat suppression (Optional)[3]	Axial/Coronal	TI 160 msec, TE > 80 msec 6–8 mm slices, < 20 sec breath hold

[1]Superior saturation bands should eliminate signal from arterial structures.
[2]Second 2D TOF acquisition may be performed using an inferior saturation band. If venous occlusion is suspected, this sequence is helpful to exclude the possibility of flow reversal mimicking thrombosis. Additionally, in suspected May-Thurner syndrome, this TOF acquisition can assess the relative positions of the iliac arteries and veins.
[3]T1-weighted gradient echo imaging and T2-weighted imaging with fat suppression can be useful to evaluate for extrinsic compression of veins by pelvic masses.

Phase Contrast MRI: Flow Quantification and MRA

Phase contrast imaging is primarily used to image blood flow, and therefore provides information that is more functional than anatomic. MR phase contrast data can be used for flow quantification by generating velocity maps, akin to Doppler ultrasound or echocardiography. They can also be used to make angiographic images as in phase contrast MR angiography. The first part of this chapter introduces the basic physics of phase contrast MR imaging. Applications to angiographic imaging and flow quantification are then discussed. Cardiac applications of phase contrast flow quantification are discussed separately in Chapter III-6.

KEY CONCEPTS

▶ With a bipolar gradient, protons moving in the direction of the gradient accumulate phase shift relative to stationary protons.

▶ Encoding velocity, or Venc, defines the range of velocities that can be measured with phase contrast flow quantification.

▶ Aliasing occurs if the tissue velocities exceed the Venc.

▶ Phase contrast angiography is sensitive to slow flow and features excellent background suppression.

▶ Phase contrast flow quantification sequences produce velocity-encoded images where signal intensity is proportional to the velocity of blood moving through or within the slice plane.

▶ The modified Bernouilli equation is used for estimating pressure gradients across stenoses based on the peak systolic velocity measured.

▶ Clinical Protocol:
   ▶ Aortic coarctation study.

PHASE CONTRAST MRI: THE PRINCIPLES

Recall from Chapter I-4 that for stationary protons, the dephasing caused by application of a gradient can be reversed by a gradient with opposite polarity. Such a pair of gradients with opposite polarity is referred to as a *bipolar gradient*.

Bipolar gradients have a different effect on depending on their motion along the direction of the gradient. This difference serves as the basis for phase contrast MR imaging and is used to generate image contrast between moving protons (such as blood in the vessels or heart) and stationary protons (most of the soft tissues).

The easiest way to understand phase contrast MRI is to consider the original implementation of the method using bipolar gradients, although, as will be discussed, other types of gradients are more commonly used now to make phase contrast images. The effects of bipolar gradients on stationary and moving protons are considered in turn.

Bipolar Gradients: Stationary Protons

A bipolar gradient is defined as a pair of gradient lobes with opposite polarity. For the discussion here, the amplitude of each lobe is equal but opposite in sign so that the areas under each lobe are assumed to be equal. As reviewed in Figure II3-1, a bipolar gradient causes no net phase shift for stationary protons (neglecting T2* decay).

Bipolar Gradients: Moving Protons

Now consider the effects of the bipolar gradient on protons moving in the direction of the gradient (Figure II3-2).

If a proton moves while the bipolar gradient is applied, then the amount of dephasing experienced will not equal the amount of rephasing. For example, consider a proton that moves from the neck to the pelvis during the course

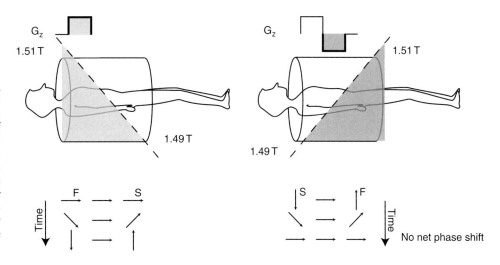

FIGURE II3-1. Bipolar gradient causes no net phase shift for stationary protons. Application of positive and negative gradients causes protons to precess relatively fast (F) and slow (S) depending on their position along the gradient. When the areas under the positive and negative gradient lobes are equal, stationary protons exhibit no net phase shift.

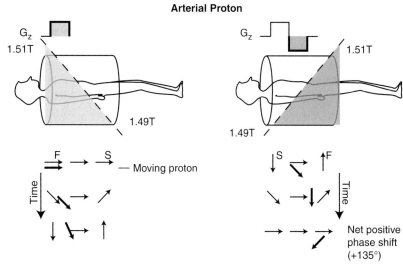

FIGURE II3-2. Bipolar gradient causes a net phase shift for moving protons. The arterial proton accumulates a positive phase shift during both lobes of the gradient and ends up with a net positive phase shift of 135°. The venous proton accumulates less phase shift than a faster-moving proton, and the phase shift is opposite in sign.

of the bipolar gradient application (Figure II3-2, top). During the positive lobe of the bipolar gradient, the proton in the neck will experience a stronger magnetic field, which causes a relatively large positive phase shift relative to the center of the magnet. It moves during this gradient, and by the time the gradient is reversed, it is in the lower abdomen and pelvis, where again it experiences a magnetic field that is greater than 1.5 T. Hence, during the reversed gradient, the proton continues to accumulate positive phase. At the end of the bipolar pulse, the moving proton will have a very large positive phase shift relative to the stationary protons in the field. The phase gain is directly proportional to the velocity along the direction of the gradient.

What happens if the proton moves half as fast and travels from the neck to the abdomen during the course of the bipolar gradient? Again, during the positive lobe of the gradient, the proton will accumulate a positive phase shift. But during the reversed gradient, the proton will experience little rephasing in the center of the magnet. This means that at the end of the bipolar pulse, this slower proton will still have a positive phase shift relative to the stationary protons, but it will not be as great as the faster-moving proton.

What if the proton moves in the opposite direction, for example a proton in the veins (Figure II3-2, bottom)? The relative phase of the proton will now be negative compared to the center of the magnet. During the reversed gradient, the rephasing will be minimal, and hence the venous proton will then have accumulated a negative phase shift.

These observations can be summarized as follows:

- Stationary protons accumulate no net phase shift following application of bipolar gradients, provided each lobe has equal and opposite area.
- The phase shift that is accumulated by moving protons is directly proportional to the speed of the protons moving in the direction of the bipolar gradient.
- The phase shift is also dependent on flow direction. As illustrated in Figure II3-2, arterial and venous protons accumulate phase shifts with opposite sign.

The exact relationship between phase shift and velocity of the protons can be predicted for a given bipolar gradient. In this way, phase contrast MR imaging can be used to convert maps of phase shifts into velocity maps.

Phase shifts accumulate for moving protons only if the protons are moving in the direction of the gradients. The direction of the bipolar gradients is referred to as the *flow sensitivity direction* or the velocity-encoding direction. Protons moving perpendicular to the gradients will not experience any phase accumulation.

> **IMPORTANT CONCEPTS:** Bipolar gradients cause protons moving in the direction of the gradients to accumulate a phase shift that is proportional to the velocity. Protons moving in opposite directions have phase shifts of opposite sign.

Two Bipolar Gradients Needed for Phase Corrections in Phase Contrast MRI

For a single bipolar gradient to provide accurate measurements of velocity based on phase differences, all phase shifts must be solely attributable to movement of protons during the gradients. The magnetic field must be perfectly homogeneous and the gradients perfectly linear.

CHALLENGE QUESTION: What factors other than motion can cause phase shifts?

Answer: Any factor that leads to differences in precessional frequencies across protons will produce phase shift. The most important contributor is magnetic field inhomogeneity.

Significant phase shifts are caused by magnetic field inhomogeneities, and these shifts are indistinguishable from those caused by motion. Consider the following example. If the main magnetic field is 1.5 T and the magnetic field gradient is intended to make the field at a particular location 1.51 T during the positive lobe and 1.49 T during the negative lobe, then a stationary proton would have no net phase shift after these two lobes of the bipolar gradient are applied. But what if the field is inhomogeneous, so that the magnetic field at a given location is 1.6 T instead of 1.5 T? Now the same bipolar gradient will cause the field at that location to be 1.61 T and 1.59 T during the two lobes. Relative to the protons that are at 1.5 T in the center of the magnet, the stationary protons in this region will experience a positive phase shift—a very positive phase shift—after the bipolar gradient. Thus, as a consequence of magnetic field inhomogeneity, these stationary protons would be misinterpreted as *very* fast-moving protons!

Therefore, without perfect field homogeneity it is impossible to do accurate phase contrast flow quantification using a single bipolar gradient. To correct for other causes of phase shifts, the collection of phase data with one bipolar gradient is repeated with following application of the mirror image of that bipolar gradient, and the two datasets subtracted (Figure II3-3).

The effect of field inhomogeneity on the net phase shift from each bipolar gradient will not be zero, but it will be the same for each bipolar gradient. In the example just described, the bipolar gradient that causes 1.61 T and 1.59 T would lead to a positive phase shift of, say, +160°. Then the second bipolar gradient, a mirror image of the first, would cause the field to be 1.59 T and 1.61 T, again resulting in a phase shift of +160°. Consequently, if the phase shifts from the two bipolar gradients are subtracted, then the net phase shift will be zero and the effects of an inhomogeneous magnetic field eliminated.

> **IMPORTANT CONCEPT:** To correct for magnetic field inhomogeneities, two separate sets of phase data using two different bipolar gradients are acquired and subtracted for phase contrast imaging.

For phase contrast flow quantification, two complete sets of echoes must be collected, one using each bipolar gradient. Having to repeat the acquisition and collect two sets of echoes makes phase contrast acquisitions twice as long as conventional gradient echo imaging.

CHALLENGE QUESTION: How many sets of acquisitions are necessary to generate a phase contrast image with flow sensitivity in three directions if bipolar gradients are used?

Answer: With standard bipolar gradients, a pair of bipolar gradients are necessary in each encoding direction. This means that six separate acquisitions are needed for flow sensitivity in three directions.

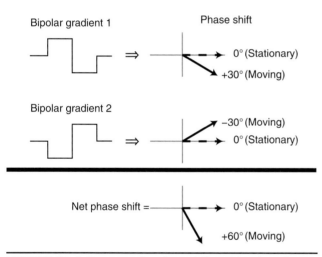

FIGURE II3-3. To correct for phase shifts arising from factors other than motion, two velocity-encoding gradients are applied and the two signals are subtracted. The phase shifts of moving protons will have opposite sign with the two sets of gradients, causing the net phase shift to double.

Use of Flow-Compensated and Flow-Encoded Gradients

Subtracting two datasets is necessary to cancel out the phase errors due to field inhomogeneities. But the pairs of gradients need not be mirror-image bipolar gradients. In fact, on most commercial systems, phase contrast MR images are generated with phase images acquired with (a) flow-encoding gradients and (b) flow-compensated gradients (Figure II3-4). As with bipolar gradients, using this pair of acquisitions and subtracting one set of phase data from the other helps to reduce artifacts due to other causes of phase errors, such as field inhomogeneity.

CHALLENGE QUESTION: How many sets of acquisitions are necessary to generate a phase contrast image with flow sensitivity in three directions if flow-compensated and flow-encoded gradients are used?

Answer: By using flow-compensated and flow-encoding gradients, only four acquisitions are necessary—one flow-compensated in all three directions and then three acquisitions with flow encoding, one in each of the three directions.

Use of flow-compensated gradients reduces the number of acquisitions necessary to generate flow sensitivity in three directions to four. With conventional bipolar gradients, six acquisitions (one pair per direction) would be needed.

Flow Sensitivity Direction versus Imaging Plane

With phase contrast imaging, there is an important distinction between the direction of flow sensitivity and the plane of imaging.

For phase contrast MR angiography, there is often a need for flow sensitivity to be three-dimensional. Consequently, flow-compensated gradients are acquired in all three directions, and the entire sequence requires collection of four sets of data. The imaging plane or slab can be two- or three-dimensional.

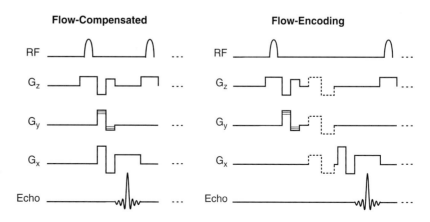

FIGURE II3-4. Phase contrast MR pulse sequences using flow-compensated and flow-encoded gradients.

Flow quantification acquisitions are typically 2D and set up to measure either *in-plane flow* or *through-plane flow*. Through-plane flow images are obtained by applying the velocity-encoding gradients in the slice-select direction (Figure II3-2), so that flow-sensitivity is in the through-plane direction, while the imaging plane is perpendicular to the direction of flow. Alternatively, the flow sensitivity desired may be in the plane of the image. In such cases, flow-encoding gradients are applied in both the frequency- and phase-encoding directions.

Three-dimensional phase-contrast flow quantification, with flow sensitivity in all three directions, is rarely used to image cardiovascular subjects because of the long acquisition times and complex image post-processing.

> **IMPORTANT CONCEPTS:** The direction of flow sensitivity and orientation of the imaging plane are independent parameters. With 2D flow quantification sequences, the direction of flow sensitivity can be either perpendicular to the imaging plane ("through-plane" with flow sensitivity in the slice-select direction) or in the plane of imaging ("in-plane" with flow sensitivity in the frequency- and phase-encoding directions).

If flow sensitivity is defined only in one direction, any flow perpendicular to that direction will not be detected by the sequence.

CHALLENGE QUESTION: What would be the effect on the estimates of velocities of flow that is oblique with respect to the flow-sensitivity direction?

Answer: If flow is oblique to the direction of flow sensitivity, its velocity will be underestimated (see Review Questions).

PHASE CONTRAST MRI: MAKING IMAGES

With phase contrast MRI, phase data are used to reconstruct either velocity-encoded flow quantification images or MR angiographic images. The reconstruction methods differ for the two applications.

For phase contrast MR angiography, the goal is to generate images that reflect the velocity of voxels, that is, depict flowing blood. For maximum signal, flow sensitivity should be three-dimensional. Net speed is calculated from velocities in each of the three directions, v_x, v_y, and v_z, and voxel signal intensity is calculated as

$$\text{voxel SI} = \sqrt{v_x^2 + v_y^2 + v_z^2}$$

The squares of the directional velocities ($v^2 = v \times v$) are always positive, and thus the signal intensity is always positive, independent of the direction of flow.

> **IMPORTANT CONCEPT:** For phase contrast angiography, the magnitude of velocity generates signal intensity, and flow direction information is usually ignored.

For flow quantification, velocity-encoded images or velocity maps are generated using the *net phase shift*, or *phase difference*. Phase difference is computed by subtracting the phase shifts generated by the two (flow-encoded and flow-compensated) acquisitions. On velocity-encoded images, the signal intensity in the image is directly proportional to the phase shift accumulated. Positive phase shifts appear with increasing brightness, while negative phase shifts have increasing darkness. Stationary protons are typically visualized as a mid-level gray. Most commercial implementations of phase contrast flow quantification sequences also reconstruct magnitude images to serve as anatomic reference images.

> **IMPORTANT CONCEPT:** On phase contrast images for flow quantification, net phase shifts are used to produce velocity maps. Flow direction is encoded by the gray scale: Faster flows in one direction are encoded as darker pixels, while faster flows in the other direction are brighter pixels. Stationary tissues are a medium gray.

ENCODING VELOCITY (Venc) AND ALIASING

With phase contrast imaging, the phase shift is proportional to the velocity of moving protons. However, the range of phase shifts that can be uniquely identified is limited to 360°. This means a limited range of velocities that can be measured with phase contrast imaging. For most MR sequences, the phase shifts are interpreted as ranging from +180° to −180°. The *encoding velocity* or *Venc* is the velocity of protons that will produce a phase shift of 180°. Protons moving at the Venc in one direction can accumulate phase shifts up to 180°, while protons moving in the opposite direction accumulate phase shifts down to −180°. If a proton moves faster than expected and accumulates a 181° phase shift, this will be interpreted as a −179° phase shift and correspond to a high velocity in the opposite direction from which it is really traveling. This is refered to as aliasing. A proton that accumulates +360° or −360° phase shift will be interpreted as stationary. This concept is illustrated in Figure II3-5.

What Does Aliasing Look Like?

It is important to be able to recognize aliasing quickly, preferably while the subject is still being imaged, so that,

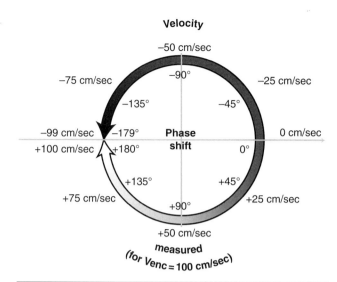

FIGURE II3-5. Encoding velocity (Venc). The range of velocities measured with phase contrast imaging is from +Venc (100 cm/sec in this example) to nearly −Venc (−99 cm/sec).

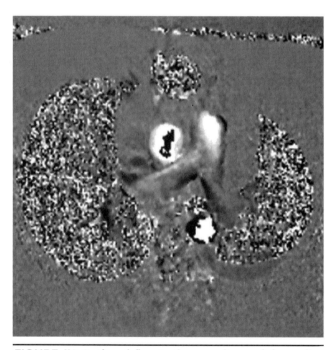

FIGURE II3-6. Aliased flow in the ascending and descending aorta in a phase contrast acquisition with Venc = 75 cm/sec. Immediately adjacent to the areas of brightest signal are areas of intensely dark signal in both the ascending and descending aorta.

if necessary, the acquisition can be repeated with higher Venc. In most cardiovascular applications, aliasing is easily recognizable on phase contrast images. On phase contrast images, the signal intensity should increase progressively with increasing velocities. When the velocity exceeds the Venc, the maximum phase shift will exceed 180°. Immediately adjacent to the areas of maximum brightness, the signal intensity will become intensely

dark. This is because velocities that just exceed +Venc will be interpreted as a velocity near the value of −Venc (Figure II3-6). For example, a phase shift of 181° will be displayed as a phase shift of −179°.

Aliasing: Problem Solving

Aliasing can be identified by a visual inspection of the phase contrast velocity-encoded images. If the subject is still in the MR scanner, the phase contrast acquisition can be repeated using a higher Venc. If the aliasing is not detected during the study, post-processing algorithms can often correct aliasing. As will be discussed below, aliasing is less of a problem with phase contrast MR angiography.

> **IMPORTANT CONCEPT:** Aliasing occurs when the measured velocity exceeds the user-assigned range of −Venc to +Venc. On phase contrast flow quantification images, aliasing appears as areas of extremely bright signal immediately adjacent to areas of intensely dark signal.

Choosing Venc

For phase contrast sequences, the Venc is a parameter defined by the user. What does the MR computer do with the number? It adjusts the amplitude and duration of the flow-encoding gradients, so that a proton moving at the encoding velocity will cause a phase shift of 180°. The lower the Venc, or the greater the desired sensitivity to slower-moving protons, the stronger the gradients that are needed.

What is the ideal Venc? The ideal Venc should be slightly greater than the maximum expected velocity. If the Venc is too low, then aliasing will occur. If the Venc is too high, then measurements of velocities will be less accurate because flows will be compressed to a narrow range of gray levels. The concepts are analogous to selecting velocity ranges in Doppler ultrasound or echocardiography. Typical Venc values for different vascular applications are shown in Table II3-1.

TABLE II3-1 Representative Vencs for phase contrast MR

Vessel	Typical Venc (cm/sec)	Stenotic Vessel Venc (cm/sec)
Aorta (normal)	250	500–1000
Internal carotid artery	150	300–500
Renal artery	150	200–300
Femoral artery	150	200–300
Veins	20	

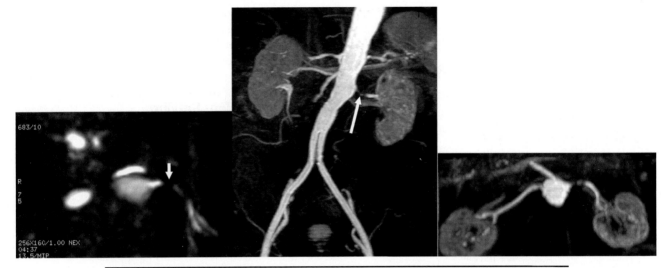

FIGURE II3-7. 3D phase contrast acquisition (left) viewed in the axial plane depicts bright signal in the initial part of a left renal artery stenosis, where flow is accelerating, and complete dropout of signal beginning at the most severe part of the stenosis and extending for 1 cm distally (small arrow). Corresponding 3D gadolinium-enhanced MRA images (middle and left) show a widely patent aorto-bi-iliac graft and and severe left renal artery stenosis (arrow). The signal dropout from spin dephasing on phase contrast images indicates that there is a pressure gradient across the stenosis. (Modified with permission from Zhang H and Prince MR, Magn Reson Imaging Clin N Am. 2004 Aug;12(3):487–503).

PHASE CONTRAST MR ANGIOGRAPHY

Phase contrast (PC) MR angiography is infrequently used in the clinical setting. Two potential applications are renal and cerebral angiography.

For both renal and cerebral applications, the direction of flow is complex, and therefore flow encoding in three directions is typically needed and 3D PC MR angiograms generated (Figure II3-7). Although synchronization of the acquisition to systole would provide greater flow-related signal, cardiac gating results in prohibitively long acquisition times. Therefore the signal in ungated PC angiograms reflects average flow during the cardiac cycle. The information from the different velocity-encoding directions is put together to provide a speed map. Thus the signal intensity is always positive, and flow-direction information is lost.

CHALLENGE QUESTION: What is the effect of aliasing on PC angiography?

Answer: Because signal intensity is based on the square of the measured velocity (v^2), only changes in the magnitude of the measured phases have an impact on the images. Consider an example where the Venc is 150 cm/sec. If the velocity in the x direction exceeds 150 cm/sec, say 155 cm/sec, then the aliasing will cause the recorded velocity to be -145 cm/sec. The signal intensity will reflect $\sqrt{145^2}$, rather than $\sqrt{155^2}$. Aliasing lowers the intensity of the voxel, but only slightly, and the effect is much less dramatic than for flow quantification velocity maps.

In most clinical settings, phase contrast angiography has been replaced by TOF or gadolinium-enhanced MRA,

mostly because of acquisition time constraints. However, there are some advantages to the PC method. First, because phase contrast relies on velocity to produce signal, there is excellent background suppression. With TOF or gadolinium-enhanced imaging, tissues with short T1 will also appear bright. On phase contrast images, all stationary tissues remain dark.

Although choosing the correct Venc can be challenging, this parameter does provide an additional degree of flexibility and sensitivity in MR angiography, not available with TOF imaging. For very slow flow imaging (as in CSF flow studies), using a very low Venc can enable exquisite sensitivity to slow-moving protons.

Last, phase contrast is extremely sensitive to higher-order flow patterns distal to stenoses. In renal MRA, it has been used to detect turbulent flow distal to a stenosis as a secondary sign of the severity of the narrowing (Figure II 3-7). This advantage can also be a disadvantage in that phase contrast angiography is extremely sensitive to flow disturbances, leading to overestimation of stenoses.

CHALLENGE QUESTION: Can phase contrast acquisitions be performed following administration of intravenous gadolinium contrast agents?

Answer: Yes. The gadolinium contrast does not affect the phase of protons.

IMPORTANT CONCEPT: Phase contrast angiography tends to be more time consuming, but it has the advantages of sensitivity to low-velocity flows and to turbulent flows. PC angiography also gives excellent background suppression.

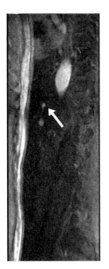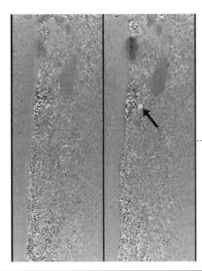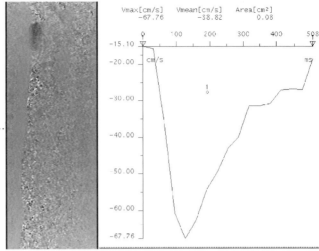

FIGURE II3-8. Phase-contrast acquisition to measure through-plane velocities of the left renal artery (arrow). A representative magnitude image is shown to the left. Three of the cine PC images are shown in the middle; note the greatest signal from the artery during peak systole (black arrow). A velocity versus time plot is shown based on a region of interest defined over the renal artery indicates a peak systolic velocity of 67.76 cm/sec.

PHASE CONTRAST MR FLOW QUANTIFICATION

Because flow in most arteries is pulsatile, blood velocities change continuously over the cardiac cycle. For meaningful flow and velocity measurements, phase-contrast acquisitions for flow quantification are typically gated to the electrocardiogram. Multiple images are acquired over each cardiac cycle. The images can be viewed in a cinematic loop and are referred to as *cine* phase contrast techniques. Velocity or flow rate versus time curves can then be plotted for a heartbeat (Figure II3-8).

The velocity-encoded images of phase contrast flow quantification techniques share a lot in common with Doppler ultrasonography, and their clinical applications are similar. For example, accelerated velocities distal to a stenosis in the carotid or renal arteries may be useful indirect measures of the severity of stenosis. Diminished velocities or flow beyond a stent may confirm stent occlusion.

ECG-Gated Cine Phase Contrast

With vascular stenoses, peak systolic velocity can be a useful parameter to grade severity of disease and to estimate the pressure gradient across a stenosis. To obtain a peak systolic velocity, the flow quantification acquisition must be electrocardiographically gated. The relationship between the MR pulse sequence and ECG signal is shown in Figure II3-9.

More details about segmented cine phase contrast acquisition will be discussed in Chapter III-6 after the principles of cine GRE imaging are discussed in Chapter III-4. The key

concept is that the temporal resolution of the images is defined as the time interval between each phase of the cardiac cycle. Ideally, temporal resolution is sufficient to allow accurate measurement of peak systolic velocities.

> **IMPORTANT CONCEPT:** Sufficient temporal resolution is necessary with ECG-gated cine phase contrast imaging for accurate measurements of peak systolic velocity.

Aliasing with Cine Phase Contrast Imaging

On ECG-gated cine phase contrast MR images, aliasing tends to occur during peak systole, when areas in the center of vessels or just distal to areas of stenosis get progressively brighter, and then suddenly appear intensely dark (Figure II3-10). On velocity versus time plots from phase contrast acquisitions, aliasing will have the same appearance as in Doppler ultrasound or echocardiography studies.

The acquisition can be repeated using higher Venc to remedy this problem. Alternatively, it may be possible to correct for the aliasing using post-processing software (Figure II3-11) that performs phase unwrapping.

PHASE CONTRAST FLOW QUANTIFICATION APPLICATIONS

For vascular applications, the most common indication for phase contrast flow quantification is the evaluation of stenoses.

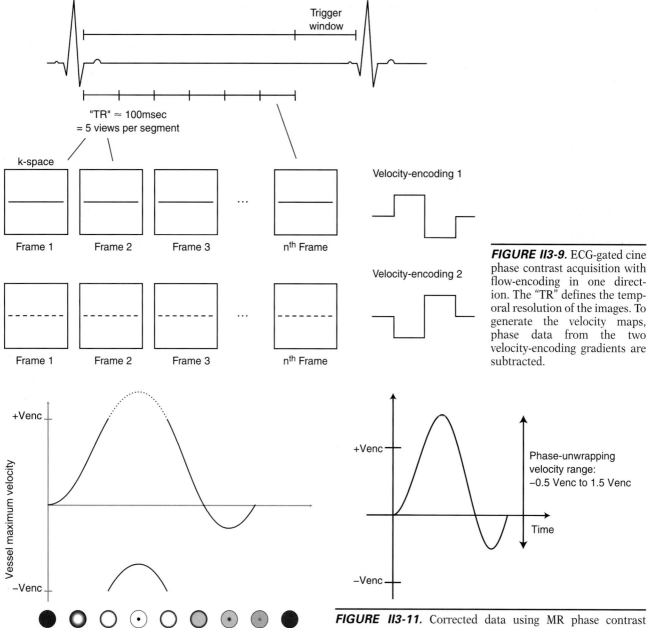

FIGURE II3-9. ECG-gated cine phase contrast acquisition with flow-encoding in one direction. The "TR" defines the temporal resolution of the images. To generate the velocity maps, phase data from the two velocity-encoding gradients are subtracted.

FIGURE II3-11. Corrected data using MR phase contrast imaging.

FIGURE II3-10. Systolic aliasing. Aliasing occurs at the fourth time point, when the velocity of blood moving in the direction of the velocity-encoding gradients exceeds the prescribed Venc, typically during systole.

One measure of the severity of stenosis is the peak pressure gradient that is generated across the area of narrowing. To estimate the pressure gradient, the *modified Bernoulli equation* can be used provided the peak systolic velocity through the stenosis is known:

$$\text{Pressure gradient (mm Hg)} = 4 \times v_{max}^2$$

where the peak systolic velocity, v_{max}, is measured in units of meter/sec (m/sec), while pressure gradient is in millimeters of mercury (mm Hg). Note that when commercial phase contrast software generates velocity maps in units of centimeters/sec (cm/sec), the measurements must be converted to m/sec before applying the equation. For example, 50 cm/sec must be converted to 0.5 m/sec.

CHALLENGE QUESTION: What is the pressure gradient in mm Hg across a stenosis if the maximum velocity across the lesion is measured to be 100 cm/sec? What velocity corresponds to a pressure gradient of 25 mm Hg?

Answer: Using the equation, velocity should be converted to units of m/sec. 100 cm/sec = 1 m/sec. The pressure gradient is then

$$\text{Pressure gradient (mm Hg)} = 4 \times v_{max}^2$$
$$= 4 \times 1 \times 1 = 4 \text{ mm Hg}$$

Working backward, for a pressure gradient of 25 mm Hg:

$$\text{Pressure gradient (mm Hg)} = 25 \text{ mm Hg} = 4 \times v_{max}^2$$
$$v_{max}^2 = 6.25$$
$$v_{max} = 2.5 \text{ m/sec}$$

or
$$V_{max} = 250 \text{ cm/sec}$$

Table II3-2 can be used to convert between maximum velocities and corresponding pressure gradients.

> **IMPORTANT CONCEPT:** The maximum pressure gradient across a vascular stenosis can be derived from the peak systolic velocity of blood across the stenosis using the modified Bernoulli equation.

Phase contrast acquisitions can be positioned through-plane or in-plane to estimate v_{max}. Positioning of the phase contrast imaging slice is critical for accurate estimates of the v_{max} and the pressure gradient. If the imaging slice does not pass through the area of maximum velocity, then the pressure gradient will be underestimated. To ensure that maximum velocities are correct, it may be necessary to perform several phase contrast acquisitions with variable positioning.

Phase contrast flow quantification has a variety of useful vascular applications, such as estimating the maximum carotid artery velocity in stenosis, and across a range of aortic diseases (Full protocol at end of chapter). Consider the following example.

■ **Example**

A young patient has a history of congenital postductal coarctation of the aorta that was repaired as a young child. She now has new signs of blood pressure discrepancies between the upper and lower extremities. Her gadolinium-enhanced MRA is shown in Figure II3-12.

A phase contrast acquisition with through-plane flow sensitivity is positioned perpendicular, and just distal to, the area of stenosis in the descending aorta. Because the stenosis involves the aorta, a Venc of 500 m/sec was used. The acquisition is ECG gated, and the temporal resolution is about 50 msec. Representative phase contrast magnitude and phase images are shown in Figure II3-13.

▶ **TABLE II3-2**

v_{max} at Stenosis (cm/sec)	Pressure Gradient (mm Hg)
0	0.0
25	0.3
50	1.0
75	2.3
100	4.0
125	6.3
150	9.0
175	12.3
200	16.0
225	20.3
250	25.0
275	30.3
300	36.0
325	42.3
350	49.0
375	56.3
400	64.0
425	72.3
450	81.0
475	90.3
500	100.0

Using the commercially available software to post-process the images, the maximum velocity throughout the cardiac cycle is plotted in Figure II3-13 and equals 300 cm/sec (or 3 m/sec) at its highest absolute value. Using the modified Bernoulli equation,

$$\text{Pressure gradient (mm Hg)} = 4 \times v^2$$
$$= 4 \times (3)^2 = 36$$

Thus the maximum pressure gradient across the stenosis is about 36 mm Hg. ■

Most of the discussion on flow quantification in this chapter has centered on measurement of velocities. Volume flow rates (measured in units such as mL/heartbeat or mL/min) can also be determined from the same phase contrast data by measuring the mean velocity of blood across its lumen (v_{mean}) and multiplying it by the cross-sectional area of the vessel lumen:

$$\text{Volume flow (mL/sec)} = v_{mean}(\text{cm/sec}) \times \text{area (cm}^2)$$

Again, phase contrast post-processing software can be used to determine volume flow rates. Because it is more commonly used in cardiac applications, this approach will be discussed further in Chapter III-6.

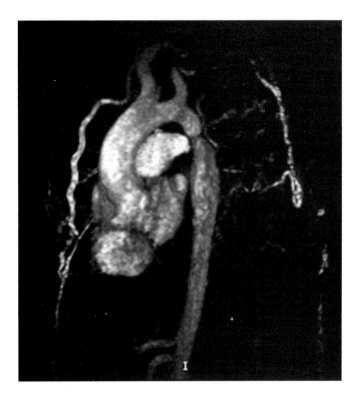

FIGURE II3-12. Gadolinium-enhanced MR angiography of the thoracic aorta in a subject who has had a coarctation repair.

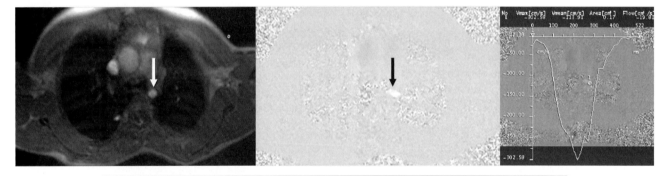

FIGURE II3-13. Phase contrast magnitude (left) and phase (middle) images through the proximal descending thoracic aorta (arrows), just distal to the level of narrowing seen in Figure II3-12. The plot of maximum velocity against time is shown to the right. Peak systolic velocity is −300 cm/sec or −3 m/sec. Velocities are negative because of the arbitrary nature in which caudal flow is defined as negative with this acquisition.

REVIEW QUESTIONS

1. Consider the gadolinium-enhanced MR angiogram shown in Figure II3-Q1A. There is mild to moderate stenosis of the left renal artery. Describe two ways in which phase contrast imaging could be implemented to assess whether this stenosis is significant enough to cause serious flow disturbances in the renal artery.

2. You wish to measure the maximum velocity of blood through the aorta, but inadvertently, the slice is positioned incorrectly, not exactly perpendicular to the vessel, but rather 30° off axis (Figure II3-Q2). What effect will this misangulation have on the accuracy of aortic blood velocity measurements? (Assume that flow

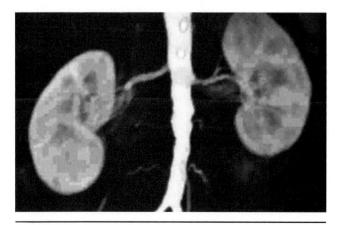

FIGURE II3-Q1A. Gadolinium-enhanced MR angiogram of the renal arteries.

sensitivity is perpendicular to the imaging plane.) *Extra challenging question*: What is the effect of this malpositioning on an estimate of the mean blood flow (mL/min) through the aorta?

3. Consider the example (Figure II3-12) of the recurrent stenosis in a patient with aortic coarctation. Phase contrast flow quantification was used to estimate the pressure gradient across the stenosis by measuring the maximum velocity just distal to the narrowing. An alternative approach to evaluating the severity of aortic coarctation is to determine the extent of collateral flow to the distal thoracic aorta via the intercostal arteries. How could phase contrast imaging be used to achieve this goal?

4. You have had a recent spate of cases in which phase contrast acquisitions have demonstrated aliasing. Fed up with this problem, you decide to fix the Venc on all acquisitions to be 500 cm/sec. Discuss the consequences of this decision.

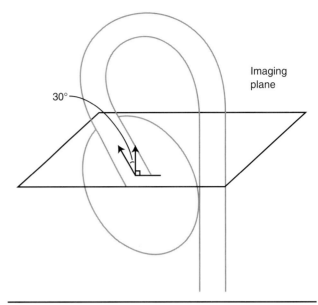

FIGURE II3-Q2. Error in positioning of the through-plane flow quantification slice. Instead of being perpendicular to the aorta, the slice is 30° off.

▶ **PROTOCOL: Aortic Coarctation Study**

Setup and Preparation	Notes
i.v.	22 G or larger
Gadolinium contrast	0.1–0.2 mmol/kg (20–30 mL)[1]
ECG leads	Necessary
Coil	Torso phased-array
Positioning tips	Supine, head first
Subject instructions	End - expiratory breath holding Supplemental oxygen by nasal canula optional

Sequence	Imaging Plane	Parameters
1 Scout (true FISP or spoiled GRE)	Multiplanar	Default
2 Double inversion recovery fast spin echo (single shot optional)	Axial ± Sagittal	ECG gated if possible 5–8 mm slices
3 Cine gradient echo[2]	Oblique sagittal through narrowing	ECG gated
4 Precontrast 3D MRA sequence	Oblique sagittal[3]	Min TR/TE, FA 25–40°, voxel size ≪ vessel diameter
5 Test bolus (optional)	Axial or sagittal	Images every 1–2 sec 1 mL contrast + 20 mL saline, 2–3 mL/sec

6 Postcontrast 3D MRA sequence
   (a) First acquisition timed using test
      bolus or bolus detection
   (b) Repeat acquisition a few sec after first acquisition
	Oblique sagittal	Same as precontrast
		20–30 mL contrast + saline,
		2–3 mL/sec

7 2D cine phase contrast flow quantification	Variable[4]	ECG-gated, segmented k-space, view-sharing, through-plane for flow quantification

[1]Gadolinium dose should be based on weight, particularly in pediatric subjects.
[2]Cine images depict areas of dephasing in the setting of physiologically significant stenoses (see Chapter III-4).
[3]The MRA portion of this study is detailed in Chapter II-4.
[4]Cine phase contrast flow quantification can be useful for assessing aortic coarctation (Figure II3-13,) either by estimating the pressure gradient at the level of stenosis based on the peak velocity through the stenosis or by determining the amount of collateral blood flowing to the descending thoracic aorta.

Gadolinium-Enhanced MRA

First-pass gadolinium-enhanced MRA has revolutionized the clinical use of MRA (1). It can be performed with just about any MR scanner and produces high-spatial-resolution images with broad anatomic coverage. The contrast agents are safe and provide a valuable alternative to conventional iodine-based contrast agents used in catheter-based and CT angiography, particularly in subjects allergic to iodinated contrast agents and in diabetic subjects or subjects with preexisting renal disease.

When compared with alternative approaches such as time-of-flight and phase contrast imaging, gadolinium-enhanced imaging has several advantages. The technique is fast, and it generates images of vessels independently of flow characteristics. Overestimation of severity of stenoses is generally less of a problem with gadolinium-enhanced MRA. Spatial coverage can be broad and, at the same time, spatial resolution of 2 mm or less can be achieved in the time frame of a single breath hold on high-end systems. The method is also versatile and can easily be applied to almost any body part. Disadvantages include the added cost of the contrast agent, requirement for intravenous access, lack of flow direction information (sometimes requiring supplemental time-of-flight imaging), and technical challenges of synchronizing bolus arrival with image acquisition. Despite these disadvantages, for most vascular imaging outside of the brain, gadolinium-enhanced MRA has become the technique of choice.

Although initial applications focused on imaging at a single station (typically a craniocaudal span of 35–45 cm), multistation bolus chase imaging following a single injection of contrast is now commonly used for indications that require greater spatial coverage, such as peripheral MR angiography. New commercial systems that integrate multichannel systems with moving-table technology can perform whole-body angiography from the head to the toes in under one minute. When temporal resolution is critical, ultrafast MR angiographic imaging methods can be used to generate fluoroscopic-type "time-resolved" views akin to conventional angiography. Contrast-enhanced methods can also be applied to image veins.

This chapter reviews the technical considerations for contrast-enhanced MR angiography and discusses pulse sequence optimization. A template for a standard single-station MR angiography protocol is presented. More advanced applications including multistation MR angiography, "time-resolved" imaging, and MR venography are then discussed. The chapter concludes with an overview of common artifacts and pitfalls of gadolinium-enhanced MR angiography.

A collection of gadolinium enhanced MR angiography protocols is listed at the end of the chapter. For some types of studies, multiple protocols are provided in this book; for example, a gadolinium-enhanced carotid MRA protocol is included at the end of this chapter, while an unenhanced TOF protocol is provided in Chapter II-2. Three peripheral MRA protocols for 1.5 T field strength are included; selection depends on the technology available.

KEY CONCEPTS

▶ First-pass contrast-enhanced MR arteriography requires synchronization of the MR acquisition with first-pass arterial enhancement.

▶ Interpolation and k-space ordering should match timing schemes for 3D acquisitions.

▶ Single-station protocols should include at least one black-blood pulse sequence for evaluation of mural and extraluminal pathology.

▶ Multistation MR angiography can be performed with repeated injections or using bolus chase methods.

▶ Fluoroscopic-type "time-resolved" MR angiography requires repeated fast acquisitions and is useful for understanding the temporal dynamics of contrast enhancement, including retrograde filling of proximally occluded vessels.

▶ Contrast-enhanced MR venography can be performed directly or with recirculation techniques.

▶ Pitfalls and artifacts of MR angiography can be avoided with careful attention to technique.

▶ Clinical Protocols:
  ▶ Carotid artery MRA with gadolinium contrast

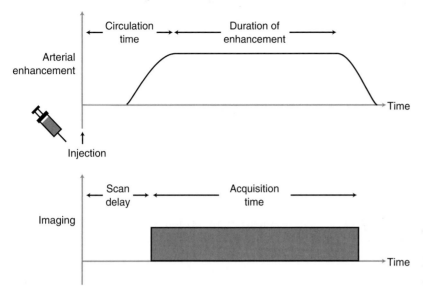

FIGURE II4-1. Kinetics of a contrast bolus injected into a peripheral vein. The data acquisition should be synchronized with the first pass of contrast material through the arteries.

> ▶ Thoracic aorta MRA with gadolinium contrast
> ▶ Abdominal aorta/renal artery MRA with gadolinium contrast
> ▶ Peripheral MRA with gadolinium contrast (three options)
> ▶ MR venography of chest with gadolinium contrast

FIRST-PASS CONTRAST-ENHANCEMENT: PRINCIPLES AND CHALLENGES OF TIMING

Principles

For routine contrast-enhanced MR angiography, a bolus of gadolinium contrast is injected intravenously followed by a saline flush, typically through an antecubital intravenous catheter. After passage through the venous circulation, right heart, pulmonary circulation, and left heart, the bolus fills the arteries of interest. The first time the bolus passes through the arterial circulation is referred to as *first-pass circulation*. Subsequently, after transit through the venous and cardiac circulation again, more dilute versions of the bolus will pass through the artery in concentrations almost equal to those in the veins.

To achieve high-quality gadolinium-enhanced MRA images, three conditions must be met: (a) the concentration of gadolinium contrast material in the arteries must cause sufficient T1 shortening to result in high signal on MR images, (b) the acquisition must be synchronized with the duration of arterial enhancement and precede significant venous enhancement, and (c) artifacts must be avoided. For the first two conditions, the rate of contrast injection, the amount of contrast material, the subject's cardiac output, and the MR acquisition time are important

parameters. Potential artifacts will be discussed at the end of this chapter.

A schematic of the relationship between contrast injection and MR acquisition is shown in Figure II4-1.

The transit time between intravenous injection and arterial enhancement is referred to as *circulation time*. Circulation times vary considerably, from as little as 8–10 sec in healthy subjects to as long as 50–60 sec in subjects with poor cardiac output. Not long ago, circulation time was used as a bedside index of a subject's cardiac output. For example, a fluorescent agent was injected intravenously, and the time for that agent to appear in the vasculature of the earlobe was used as an indicator of cardiac function. Variability in circulation times poses a challenge for contrast-enhanced MR angiography because the contrast is injected intravenously, while the vessels of interest are usually arterial and because the bolus volume is relatively small and so the duration enhancement is short.

Because contrast material is injected intravenously and mixes with unenhanced venous blood, a certain amount of dispersion of the contrast bolus occurs during its transit. The amount of dispersion determines the peak intensity of arterial enhancement. The higher the injection rate, the less dispersion, and the higher the peak gadolinium concentration in the arteries (Figure II4-2). Additionally, the higher the rate of injection, the faster the bolus appears in the artery or the shorter the circulation time. Although higher cardiac output leads to faster circulation, it also is associated with larger circulatory volumes that cause more dispersion of the bolus. Hence, with higher cardiac output, maximal arterial enhancement tends, paradoxically, to be lowered.

Several details related to contrast injection technique need to be considered when performing gadolinium-enhanced MRA, as discussed below.

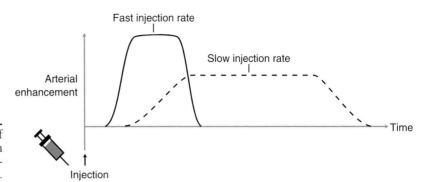

FIGURE II4-2. Faster rates of injection of contrast material result in shorter circulation times, higher intra-arterial gadolinium concentrations, and shorter durations of enhancement.

▶ **TABLE II4-1 Gadolinium Doses for MR Angiography Based on Subject Weight**

Body Weight	"Single Dose"	"Double" Dose	Maximum Dose
<100 lb	Weight-based	Weight-based	Weight-based
100–129 lb	20 mL	30 mL	30 mL
130–200 lb	20 mL	40 mL	40 mL
200–300 lb	20 mL	40 mL	60 mL

Contrast Dose

As introduced in Chapter I-3, doses of gadolinium contrast material are usually referenced to the subject's body weight in kilograms (kg). A single dose of gadolinium contrast material refers to 0.1 mmol of gadolinium contrast material per kg of subject body weight. Most commercially available contrast agents are supplied at a high concentration of 0.5 mol/L or 0.5 mmol/mL.

For vascular imaging, the gadolinium doses typically are rounded up based on weight guidelines, within the limit of 0.3 mmol/kg. For example, most adult subjects, regardless of weight, receive a dose of 20 mL for single-station MR angiography. This averages to be about 0.13–0.14 mmol/kg. Table II4-1 summarizes rough guidelines for single- and double-dose gadolinium contrast protocols for subjects of different weights, assuming a commercial preparation with gadolinium concentration 0.5 mol/L. A more detailed chart of precise weight-based gadolinium contrast doses is given in Table I3-1.

> **IMPORTANT REVIEW POINT:** For most adults, a "single dose" of gadolinium contrast material for MR angiography refers to 20 mL of the commonly available 0.5 mol/L preparation.

The optimal amount of contrast material for a given MRA examination depends on several factors. At the upper bounds, there are regulatory limitations for different contrast agents. The maximum recommended dose for a single gadolinium-enhanced examination is commonly 0.3 mmol/kg. Second, there are cost considerations.

Typically, vials of contrast are available in single-use 15 mL and 20 mL doses, and therefore a double dose of contrast material usually requires two bottles and is therefore twice as expensive. Aside from these issues, the tradeoffs between lower and higher doses largely pertain to the ability to fill the entire arterial structure of interest during the acquisition period before venous enhancement. Higher doses favor faster injection rates. For most single-station studies, such as renal artery MRA or carotid MRA, a single dose of contrast material is sufficient. When the vessel of interest is large, such as an abdominal aortic aneurysm, or when the desired field of view is broad, such as a full thoracic and abdominal aortic MRA, then a double dose is preferable. As will be discussed subsequently, multistation studies and recirculation MR venography studies typically require a double dose of contrast material. Time-resolved imaging can be performed with smaller doses, such as 0.05 mmol/kg (half-dose or less).

Special Considerations in the Pediatric Population

When the subject is a small child or infant, the volumes of contrast material can be quite small. For example, a single dose of contrast for a 4.5 kg (10 lb) infant is only 1 mL. Typically in studies of small children, doses of 0.2 mmol/kg are routinely used. The volumes of injection can be increased by diluting the gadolinium contrast drawn from the vial with sterile saline or D5W up to 100%. This allows larger volumes for injection that are easier to handle and ensure sufficient volumes for vascular imaging.

As a point of advice, when infants are mildly sedated, the injection of contrast material at room temperature can cause them to awaken and move during the acquisition. Warming the contrast material prior to injection helps to reduce the likelihood of the infant awakening.

> **IMPORTANT CONCEPTS:** For pediatric studies, gadolinium contrast doses can be diluted with sterile D5W or saline to increase the volume of injection. Warming the contrast material may reduce the chance of awakening a sedated subject.

Rate of Contrast Injection

The rate of contrast injection depends on the total amount of contrast to be administered and the duration of the imaging acquisition. In general, the faster the rate of contrast injection, the higher the gadolinium concentration in the arteries, and therefore the brighter the vessels (Figure II4-2). However, the duration of enhancement should match the acquisition times; very fast injections can mean durations of arterial enhancement that are too short for optimal imaging. Also, higher rates of injection require a larger-gauge intravenous catheter.

While injection rates vary among institutions, most centers use an injection rate of 2–3 mL/sec for routine single-station or double-station imaging studies. For multi-station studies, such as peripheral vascular MRA, a staged injection may be used, such as 2 mL/sec for the first 10 mL followed by 1 mL/sec for the remaining 20 mL. In theory, the prolonged injection period favors arterial enhancement of the distal vessels during imaging of the second and third stations. In fact, the truly optimized injection protocol probably varies for each individual.

For routine studies, a 22 gauge intravenous catheter placed in the antecubital fossa can be used to inject at a rate of 2–3 mL/sec of gadolinium contrast material.

Manual versus Automated Injections and Flush

Injections can be performed manually or automatically with commercially available MR-compatible power injectors. Because the gadolinium contrast is viscous, hand injections at rates above 2–3 mL/sec can be difficult depending on the strength of the person performing the injection. Warming the contrast material can reduce its viscosity and facilitate injection. With either manual or automated injections, it is important to follow the gadolinium contrast injection with a saline flush (20 mL) in order to ensure that all the contrast material is cleared from the tubing and veins. Typically the saline flush is administered at the same rate as the gadolinium contrast material. Commercially available MR-compatible injectors have two syringes—one for gadolinium contrast material and the other for saline—and rates of injection are programmable (Figure II4-3).

> **IMPORTANT CONCEPT:** For most MR angiography, contrast material and saline flush are injected at rates of 2–3 mL/sec.

The Timing Challenge

To accommodate the circulation time, most MRA acquisitions must be delayed from the start of the gadolinium injection by a time referred to as the *scan delay* (Figure II4-1). The appropriate scan delay must be determined so that peak arterial enhancement is synchronized with the filling

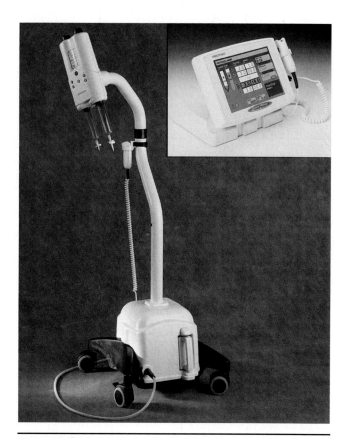

FIGURE II4-3. Commercially available MR-compatible injector. The dual syringe system enables automated injection of both the gadolinium contrast and saline flush. Photo courtesy of Medrad, Inc. © MEDRAD, Inc. All rights reserved.

of the central lines of k-space. In some applications, centric ordering is used, in which the central lines are acquired early in the acquisition, while in others, sequential ordering is used, and the central lines are collected in the middle of the acquisition (Figure II4-4). Strategies for synchronizing the acquisitions are discussed next.

Strategies for Optimal Timing

There are two main strategies to ensure optimal timing of the MR acquisition with arterial phase enhancement: a test bolus method and bolus detection method.

Test Bolus Method

The principle of the test bolus method is that circulation time can be measured for each individual subject using a small test bolus of the gadolinium chelate (2). By determining circulation time, an appropriate scan delay can be computed. Volumes of 0.5–2 mL are used for the test bolus followed by a 15–20 mL saline flush, both injected at the rate that will be employed for the full contrast bolus. With the start of the test bolus injection, images through the area of interest are acquired at known intervals, typically every second or every other second. The small bolus

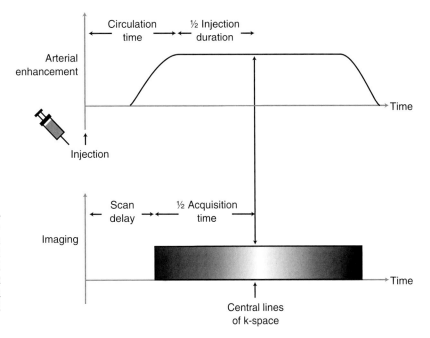

FIGURE II4-4. Synchronizing the MR acquisition with arterial enhancement. The duration of enhancement is assumed to be roughly equal to the duration of the injection. The central lines of k-space should be acquired during peak arterial enhancement. In this example the MR pulse sequence fills k-space in a sequential fashion.

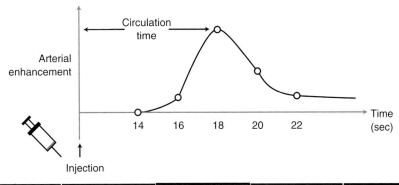

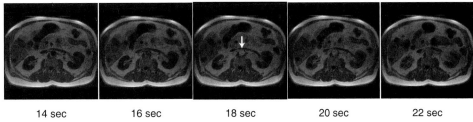

FIGURE II4-5. Measurement of circulation time for abdominal aorta using a test bolus timing examination. Imaging is initiated at the start of injection of the test bolus of contrast material. The time of peak aortic enhancement is 18 sec (arrow), so the subject's circulation time is 18 sec.

14 sec   16 sec   18 sec   20 sec   22 sec

of contrast can be visualized as a transient enhancement of the artery of interest. The subject's circulation time can be determined by identifying the image with maximum enhancement (Figure II4-5).

The circulation time is used to determine the scan delay. The specific relationship between the two parameters depends on whether the 3D MRA sequence is designed to fill k-space sequentially or centrically. Some of the formulas that have been offered in the literature are discussed in the following paragraphs.

Sequential k-Space Filling

If k-space is filled sequentially, the central lines of k-space are filled in the middle of the acquisition period (Figure II4-4).

Therefore, for a given scan delay, $T_{scan\,delay}$, the central lines of k-space will be filled at time $T_{scan\,delay} + \frac{1}{2} T_{acquisition}$. The midpoint of enhancement, or $T_{circulation} + \frac{1}{2} T_{Gd\,injection}$, should be synchronized with the filling of the central lines of k-space:

$$T_{circulation} + \frac{1}{2}T_{Gd\,injection} = T_{scan\,delay} + \frac{1}{2}T_{acquisition}$$

where $T_{Gd\,injection}$ refers to the duration of gadolinium chelate injection and is assumed to reflect the duration of arterial enhancement. Rearranging this formula

$$T_{scan\,delay} = T_{circulation} + \frac{1}{2}T_{Gd\,injection} - \frac{1}{2}T_{acquisition}$$

For example, consider the test bolus result shown in Figure II4-5, where the subject's circulation time is 18 sec. A routine 20 sec renal MRA acquisition uses 20 mL contrast volume and the rate of injection of both the gadolinium contrast and saline flush is 2 mL/sec. What should be the scan delay time?

If the contrast volume is 20 mL and it is injected at 2 mL/sec, then $T_{Gd\ injection}$ = 10 sec. If the acquisition time is typically about 20 sec, then the simple formula can be further simplified to

$$T_{scan\ delay} = T_{circulation} - 5\ sec$$

Using the simplified equation, the scan delay should be $T_{scan\ delay} = T_{circulation\ time} - 5\ sec = 13\ sec$.

CHALLENGE QUESTION: Consider the same subject shown in Figure II4-5. Consider if the subject weighs about 70 kg (154 lb) and is referred for imaging of a large abdominal aortic aneurysm. How would the gadolinium-enhanced MR angiogram be performed differently, assuming the same imaging sequence is used?

Answer: When the volume of the vessel of interest is large, a larger dose of gadolinium contrast should be used to fill that volume. With large aneurysms, a double dose of contrast may improve the image quality. Recall that doses are defined by subject weight. From Table II4-1, a double dose for this subject would be 40 mL. If the rate of injection is still 2 mL/sec, then $T_{Gd\ injection}$ = 20 sec. The circulation time and acquisition times are the same:

$$T_{scan\ delay} = T_{circulation\ time} + \frac{1}{2}T_{Gd\ injection}$$
$$- \frac{1}{2}T_{acquisition\ time}$$

$$T_{scan\ delay} = 18\ sec + 20\ sec - 10\ sec$$
$$T_{scan\ delay} = 28\ sec.$$

Centric k-Space Filling

For centrically-ordered k-space filling, the relationship between circulation time and scan delay is different. The central lines of k-space are filled during the first half of the acquisition period, at a time defined as $T_{center\ of\ k\text{-}space}$. Therefore, for a given scan delay, $T_{scan\ delay}$, the central lines of k-space will be filled at time $T_{scan\ delay} + T_{center\ of\ k\text{-}space}$. The midpoint of enhancement, or $T_{circulation} + \frac{1}{2}T_{Gd\ injection}$, should be synchronized with the filling of the central lines of k-space:

$$T_{circulation} + \frac{1}{2}T_{Gd\ injection} = T_{scan\ delay} + T_{center\ of\ k\text{-}space}$$

where $T_{Gd\ injection}$ refers to the duration of gadolinium chelate injection and is assumed to reflect the duration of arterial enhancement. Rearranging this formula,

$$T_{scan\ delay} = T_{circulation} + \frac{1}{2}T_{Gd\ injection}$$
$$- T_{center\ of\ k\text{-}space}$$

Again, assuming a contrast volume of 20 mL is injected at 2 mL/sec ($T_{Gd\ injection}$ = 10 sec), and the acquisition time is 20 sec, then the formula can be simplified by making the reasonable approximation that $T_{center\ of\ k\text{-}space}$ is 5 sec:

$$T_{scan\ delay} = T_{circulation}$$

The advantage of the test bolus method is that it can be implemented on any system without special software or hardware. It also allows for the opportunity to test the integrity of the intravenous catheter and vein. However, the test bolus approach does have the drawback of requiring an extra acquisition (typically 1 min) and a separate injection of contrast and saline flush. This is straightforward when an automated injector is available, but it can be cumbersome for manual injections. Residual gadolinium from the test dose also increases background signal for the subsequent MRA acquisition. For the test bolus to give an accurate guide to determining the best scan delay, the test bolus conditions must match those of the full contrast bolus—the rate of injection and amount of flush should be the same. It is also important to consider the effect of breath holding on circulation dynamics. When timing is critical and the MRA is to be acquired during suspended respiration, the test bolus should be given during the same phase of suspended respiration (end-expiration, for example, at least for the first 15–20 sec) as during the actual study.

IMPORTANT POINT: With use of a test bolus, a subject's circulation time for the organ of interest can be determined and used to optimize the scan delay time and ensure imaging during arterial enhancement.

For MRA sequences that fill k-space *sequentially*:

$$T_{scan\ delay} = T_{circulation} + \frac{1}{2}T_{Gd\ injection} - \frac{1}{2}T_{acquisition}$$

This simplifies to

$$T_{scan\ delay} = T_{circulation} - 5\ sec$$

in the typical case where the contrast volume is 20 mL, injection rate is 2 mL/sec, and the acquisition time is 20 sec. For MRA sequences that fill k-space *centrically*, the formula for a single-dose injection is simply

$$T_{scan\ delay} = T_{circulation}$$

provided the time to the center of k-space is approximately equal to $\frac{1}{2}T_{Gd\ injection}$.

Bolus Detection Methods

An alternative approach to the test bolus injection is to detect and monitor the appearance of the full contrast bolus in near real time. Fluoroscopic-type 2D images are acquired repeatedly in the vessel of interest. Once the leading edge of the bolus is seen in the aorta, the 3D MRA acquisition is initiated either by the operator or automatically (Figure II4-6). With automatic triggering, software repeatedly samples the signal intensity within a region of interest defined by the user (usually within the aorta). Once a predefined threshold is met, the acquisition is initiated by the system. For studies in the torso, the patient may be given a quick instruction to suspend respiration before starting the acquisition.

Because the bolus is already filling the vessels at the start of the acquisition, centric-ordered filling of k-space is usually performed. The bolus detection method is fast and efficient, but it requires software that may not be available on an MRI system. One slight disadvantage is the limited time for breath-holding instructions before the acquisition begins. However, the inability to hyperventilate is less of a problem if shorter acquisition times are used.

Guess Method

Some centers do not use any timing schemes, but rather rely on "guestimates" of a subject's circulation time based on age and cardiac history. For example, young, relatively healthy subjects would be expected to have circulation times of about 12 sec, while older subjects or those with poor circulation might be assumed to have circulation times of 24–30 sec. Guessing works in about 85–90% of cases. Mistiming may result in artifacts that are discussed at the end of this chapter. The guess method is more forgiving with larger and slower boluses, because the duration of enhancement (Figure II4-2) is longer. Therefore, centers that use the guess method often resort to a double dose of gadolinium contrast as the default dose.

3D SPOILED GRADIENT ECHO MRA SEQUENCES

Imaging Parameters

The 3D spoiled gradient echo MRA sequences are preset by most vendors. A receiver bandwidth is selected to allow reasonable signal-to-noise ratios, and the associated minimum TR and TE values are then defined based on the bandwidth. TE times are typically 1–2 msec, depending on the system characteristics. Typical TR values may be between 2–6 msec. As introduced in Chapter I-4, the flip angle depends on the desired degree of contrast between the vessels and the background tissue. The higher the flip angle, the greater the background

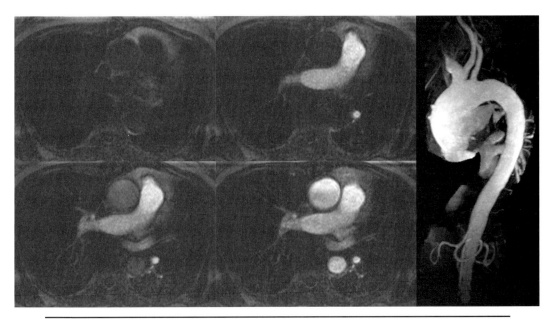

FIGURE II4-6. Bolus detection images showing the arrival of contrast in the pulmonary arteries and then the aorta (left). The 3D acquisition is triggered following the last image, either automatically or by the operator, to obtain a 3D MRA of the thoracic aorta (right). Although axial here, the "fluoroscopic" images can be positioned sagittally through the thoracic aorta.

suppression. However, higher flip angles also mean that the signal from gadolinium contrast material may become attenuated. In general, most MRA is performed with flip angles between 25°–40°.

Spatial Resolution and Isotropic Voxels

In setting up 3D MRA sequences, there are important tradeoffs among spatial coverage, resolution, and acquisition times. The ability of MRA images to depict accurately the degree of stenosis depends on the spatial resolution and contrast resolution. The smaller the vessels of interest, the higher the spatial resolution that is needed to diagnose and quantify the extent of vascular disease. In considering 3D MRA protocols, it is important to remember that the three dimensions are not interchangeable because one is a frequency-encoding direction and two are phase-encoding directions. Increasing the spatial resolution in the frequency-encoding direction does not increase acquisition time, but increasing the resolution in either phase-encoding direction does. Therefore, with 3D MRA, spatial resolution tends to be higher in one direction than in the other two. For MRA, the goal should be to attain *isotropic* spatial resolution. The 3D slab should be oriented with frequency encoding in the direction of largest field of view. The spatial resolution in the two phase-encoding directions should be adjusted to be approximately equal. As illustrated in the following example, with interpolated or partial Fourier 3D sequences, it is important to distinguish between the voxel size and the true spatial resolution.

■ EXAMPLE 1

Consider the case of a 3D renal MRA acquisition with partitions oriented in the coronal plane (Figure II4-7).

Scenario A: The field of view is 400 mm craniocaudally, 300 mm left to right, and the slab thickness is 96 mm. The matrix of collected data is 512 × 144 (with the 75% rectangular FOV from left-to-right) × 24. With asymmetric k-space filling and 75% partial Fourier in the left-to-right direction and zip interpolation in the partition direction, the interpolated imaging matrix is 512 × 192 × 48. What is the acquisition time for a TR = 4 msec? What are the true spatial resolution and voxel size for this acquisition?

Answer: The acquisition time is:

$$TR \times N_{PE1} \times N_{PE2} = 4 \times 144 \times 24 = 13.8 \text{ sec}$$

The voxel dimensions are calculated as follows:

Frequency encoding: 400 mm/512 = 0.8 mm
Phase encoding: 300 mm/192 = 1.6 mm
Partition (Phase encoding 2): 96 mm/48 = 2 mm

Although the voxel dimensions might give the misleading impression that the spatial resolution is isotropic in two dimensions, in fact, the true spatial resolution is:

Frequency encoding: 400 mm/512 = 0.8 mm
Phase encoding: 300 mm/144 = 2.1 mm
Partition (Phase encoding 2): 96 mm/24 = 4 mm,

which is definitely not isotropic.

Scenario B: To make the spatial resolution more isotropic, the number of phase encoding steps must be adjusted so that the matrix of collected data is 512 × 96 × 36 and the interpolated matrix is 512 × 128 × 72. With this modification, what are the new voxel dimensions, spatial resolution, and acquisition time?

Answer: The voxel dimensions are

Frequency encoding: 400 mm/512 = 0.8 mm
Phase encoding: 300 mm/128 = 2.3 mm
Partition (Phase encoding 2): 96 mm/72 = 1.3 mm

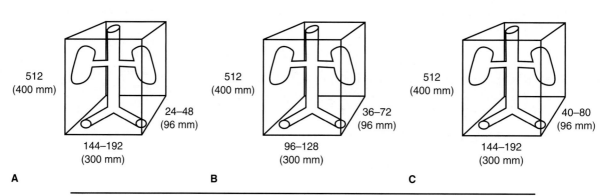

FIGURE II4-7. Scenarios A, B, C.

The true spatial resolution is:

Frequency encoding: 400 mm/512 = 0.8 mm

Phase encoding: 300 mm/96 = 3.1 mm

Partition (Phase encoding 2): 96 mm/36 = 2.7 mm

Acquisition time will be the same:

$$96 \times 36 \times 4 \text{ msec} = 13.8 \text{ sec}$$

Although the voxel size has become less isotropic in the two phase-encoding directions, the spatial resolution is closer to being isotropic than for Scenario A.

Scenario C: With an increase in acquisition time, Scenario A can be improved to generate an image with spatial resolution of less than 2.5 mm in all dimensions. For example, in Scenario C, consider a matrix of collected data of 512 × 144 × 40 which, using the same interpolation as in Scenarios A and B, would translate into an interpolated imaging matrix of 512 × 192 × 80. Compute the voxel size, true spatial resolution, and acquisition time.

Answer: The voxel dimensions are

Frequency encoding: 400 mm/512 = 0.8 mm

Phase encoding: 300 mm/192 = 1.6 mm

Partition (Phase encoding 2): 96 mm/80 = 1.2 mm

The true spatial resolution is

Frequency encoding: 400 mm/512 = 0.8 mm

Phase encoding: 300 mm/144 = 2.1 mm

Partition (Phase encoding 2): 96 mm/40 = 2.4 mm

One consequence of this change will be a higher acquisition time:

$$144 \times 40 \times 4 \text{ msec} = 23 \text{ sec}$$

Parallel imaging (Section I, Chapter 8) can help reduce acquisition times in this setting.

Discussion: These three scenarios emphasize the differences between voxel dimensions and true spatial resolution. Often, commercial systems provide information only about voxel dimensions, when in fact the true spatial resolution determines the ability to resolve fine details in the image—for example, small differences in vessel diameter. This example also demonstrates how spatial resolution (at least for the two phase-encoding directions) can be made more isotropic by adjusting the number of steps in each phase-encoding direction. ∎

IMPORTANT CONCEPT: Because atherosclerotic plaque, and other diseases of the vessels, can destributed circumferentially or eccentrically, it is important to strive for isotropic spatial resolution in cardiovascular MRI.

Slab Orientations and Targeted Isotropic Spatial Resolution

The orientation of a 3D acquisition depends on the geometry of the vessels of interest. Guiding principles are (a) to maximize use of rectangular field of view and (b) to have a minimum slab thickness—with the dual aim of reducing the number of phase-encoding steps while maintaining spatial resolution. The spatial resolution depends on the size of the vessels to be imaged and the importance of discriminating between different degress of stenosis. For example, because the internal carotid arteries are small and the distinction between 50% and 80% stenosis is clinically important, high spatial resolution is necessary. It can be achieved, in part, because the field of view in the neck is smaller and spatial coverage limited. For abdominal aortic aneurysm studies, the spatial resolution requirements are less stringent, but anatomic coverage must be considerably broader. Guidelines for slab positioning and targets for spatial resolution for different MRA applications are listed in Table II4-2.

THE BASIC MRA PROTOCOL (SINGLE-STATION)

A generic MRA protocol is given in Table II4-3. Protocols for specific MRA applications are provided at the end of this chapter.

For many MRA studies, following a series of scout images, some preliminary anatomic imaging is performed. For example, for renal MRA, T1-weighted images of the kidney and adrenal glands may be performed first. For peripheral MRA, scout images throughout the lower extremities using time-of-flight or true FISP techniques

▶ **TABLE II4-2 Guidelines for Slab Orientation and Targeted Isotropic Spatial Resolution for MRA**

MRA Application	Slab Orientation	Isotropic Spatial Resolution
Carotid arteries	Sagittal	1–1.5 mm
Subclavian arteries	Coronal	2 mm
Thoracic aorta	Oblique sagittal (parallel to aortic arch)	2–2.5 mm
Hand arteries	Coronal	1–1.5 mm
Abdominal aorta/mesenteric	Sagittal	2–2.5 mm
Abdominal aorta/renal arteries	Coronal	2 mm
Pelvic arteries	Coronal	2.5 mm
Peripheral arteries (including feet)	Coronal	1.5–2.5 mm
Feet alone	Sagittal	1–1.5 mm

▶ **TABLE II4-3 Generic MRA Protocol**

	Sequence	*Imaging Plane*	*Parameters*
1	Scout (true FISP or spoiled GRE)	Multiplanar	Default
2	Anatomic imaging/vascular scouts	Axial, other planes optional	2D TOF or true FISP (SSFP) as vascular scouts Other routine anatomic imaging
3	Pre-contrast 3D MRA sequence (30 spoiled GRE)	Variable	Minimum TR, TE, FA = 25–40°, voxel size << vessel diameter
4	Test bolus (optional)	Axial or sagittal	Images every 1–2 sec
5	Post-contrast 3D MRA sequence (a) First acquisition timed using test bolus or bolus detection (b) Repeat acquisition a few sec after arterial phase	Variable	Same as pre-contrast
6	Post-contrast T1-weighted imaging (optional)	Axial (or others)	2D or 3D spoiled GRE

are useful to guide positioning of the 3D slabs. For thoracic aortic studies, black-blood fast spin echo images should be performed to exclude intramural disease such as dissection or intramural hematoma (Chapter III-3).

Then the core of the MRA protocol is performed. First, the 3D MRA sequence is acquired without intravenous contrast. This acquisition is useful for several reasons: (1) to verify that slab positioning is reasonable (avoiding wraparound artifact, for example), (2) to confirm that the subject is able to suspend respiration for the acquisition (for studies in the torso), and (3) to serve as a mask for subtraction from the contrast-enhanced acquisition.

Then, for timing purposes, a test bolus (1–2 mL) can be injected to determine the subject's circulation time. This circulation time is used to calculate a scan delay for the contrast-enhanced acquisition using formulas described previously. Alternatively, if a bolus detection algorithm is used, the full contrast bolus is injected, and 3D imaging starts when the bolus has arrived in the arteries. It may be useful to acquire a second 3D acquisition immediately after the first one, or after a delay of about 6 seconds to allow the subject to breathe and suspend respiration again. The second image is often a useful backup in case of difficulties with the first acquisition. Also, occasionally the second acquisition will have useful diagnostic information regarding kinetics of enhancement, such as delayed enhancement of the false lumen of a dissection.

IMPORTANT POINT: For 3D MRA acquistions, it is often useful to acquire a second 3D image immediately after the first or after a delay of about 6 seconds to prepare for repeat breath holding.

Following the MRA, most protocols in the torso include a T1-weighted acquisition through the solid organs in the field of view. For example, for a renal MRA study, a contrast-enhanced acquisition through the abdomen facilitates characterization of incidentally detected renal masses. Mural enhancement in the setting of vasculitis can also be detected with this acquisition. Extraluminal pathology, such as extrinsic masses that compress blood vessels, can also be assessed. Considerations for specific gadolinium-enhanced MRA applications are discussed in more detail in specific protocols at the end of this chapter.

IMAGE PROCESSING

Image interpretation should always begin with a careful review of the source data. As will be illustrated later in this chapter, manipulated images such as subtracted images and angiographically-rendered images can lead to mistakes in interpretation. Nevertheless, when used to supplement source data, image processing tools can add valuable perspective for interpreting results. It is important to emphasize that *the key to accurate interpretation rests on optimized acquisitions rather than postprocessing.* Ideally, 3D MRA should be performed under optimized settings to achieve maximum spatial resolution, high signal-to-noise and contrast-to-noise ratios, full arterial enhancement without venous contamination, adequate fat and background suppression, and minimal artifacts.

Multiplanar Reconstructions

For analysis of 3D source images, *multiplanar reconstruction* (MPR) tools are critical. These enable the viewer to reconstruct 3D image datasets in any plane (Figure II4-8).

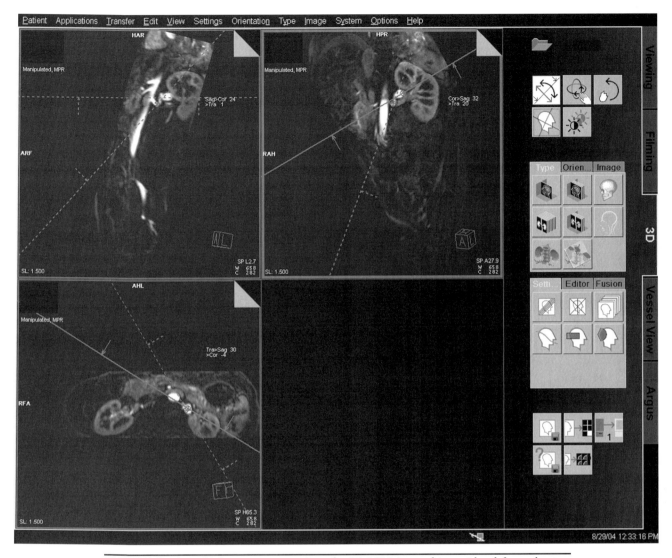

FIGURE II4-8. Multiplanar reconstruction of a 3D MRA in a subject with a left renal artery aneurysm. The dashed lines indicate the planes of reconstruction for the corresponding outlined boxes.

For example, if a 3D MRA of the renal arteries is performed with source images reconstructed coronally, the 3D MPR tool enables the images to be viewed in the axial plane for better appreciation of atherosclerotic plaque on the anterior and posterior walls, the so-called "en face" plaque, and other complex anatomy.

More advanced workstations can perform curved multiplanar reformatting, whereby the 3D image can be reconstructed along a surface that is not planar, but rather curved, for example, following a tortuous vessel (Figure II4-9).

Subtraction and the Importance of Reproducible Breath Holding

For angiographic reconstructions, the standard initial step is subtraction of the unenhanced or precontrast acquisition from the contrast-enhanced acquisition. Provided there is no significant motion between the two acquisitions, the resulting 3D data set will show only the enhanced vessels with virtually no background signal (Figure II4-10). Some manufacturers now provide automatic subtraction of the unenhanced from the enhanced 3D datasets as part of the image reconstruction process.

For imaging in the torso, acquisitions are performed during breath holding to minimize respiratory artifact. Because the unenhanced and enhanced acquisitions are performed during two separate breath holds, the quality of the subtracted data depends on the reproducibility of the breath holds. If, for example, the subject suspends respiration at end inspiration for one acquisition and at end expiration for the other, then the positions of the vessels will vary significantly between the two acquisitions, and, consequently, the subtracted images will have artifacts.

Given that the source images, and not the subtracted images, should be relied upon for interpretation, these artifacts should be inconsequential, but they do degrade the quality of the postprocessed images. The solution to this problem is to ask the subjects to breath hold in the same way for each acquisition. End-expiratory breath holding has been reported to be more reliable than end-inspiratory breath holding, but it is also more difficult to perform.

> **IMPORTANT CONCEPT:** All MRA acquisitions in the torso should be performed with breath holding, performed in a consistent way (e.g., all at end expiration or all at end inspiration). End-expiratory breath holding is more difficult but also more reproducible.

Angiographic Renderings

While radiologic interpretations rely on viewing the source data and multiplanar reconstructions, angiographic 3D renderings are routinely generated to enhance the perception of depth on an image displayed on a computer monitor and to summarize the imaging findings visually. The most commonly used computer graphics methods are described next (Figure II4-11), following a review of image segmentation .

Segmentation

Angiographic reconstructions are typically improved by limiting the data to the vessels of interest and excluding other tissues that hinder their visualization (Figure II4-12). Sources of high signal intensity on the MRA images that are frequently excluded include subcutaneous tissues, bone marrow, and bowel contents. Venous enhancement

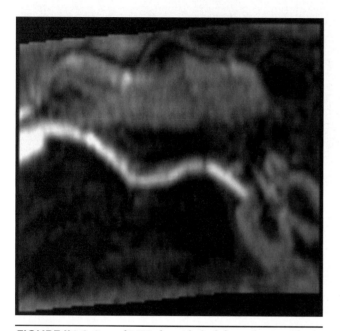

FIGURE II4-9. Curved MPR through the left renal artery of subject shown in Figure II4-8. Aneurysm is saccular and not shown in this view.

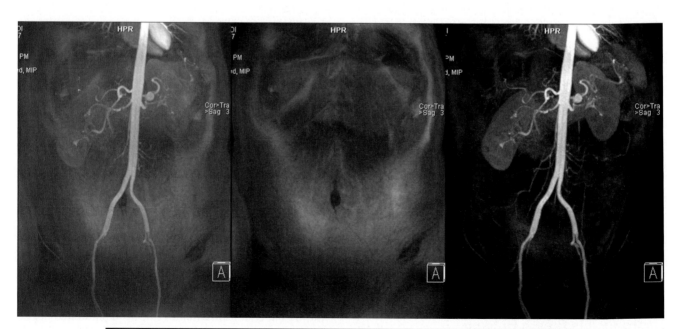

FIGURE II4-10. Image subtraction. The unenhanced acquisition (middle) is subtracted from the contrast enhanced acquisition (left) to generate an MRA with substantially decreased background signal.

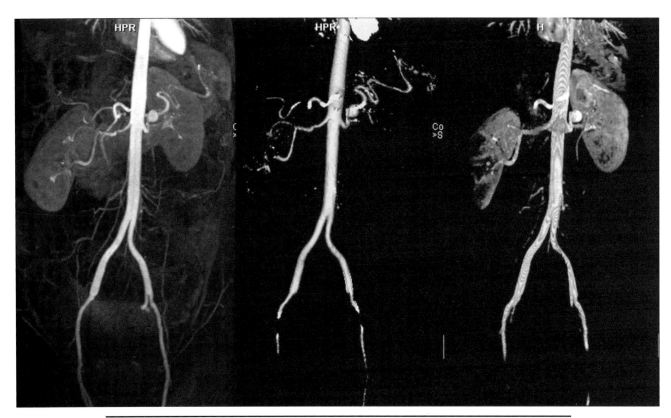

FIGURE II4-11. Examples of three types of 3D renderings: maximum intensity projection (MIP, left), surface shaded display (SSD, middle), volume rendering (right).

can also be excluded from the reconstructions using image segmentation. Since the source images should be relied upon to provide interpretations, the use of segmentation algorithms for MR angiography is primarily for cosmetic purposes.

Maximum Intensity Projection (MIP)

The most commonly used tool for angiographic rendering is the *maximum intensity projection (MIP)* algorithm (Figure II4-11). MIP capabilities are offered on most commercial MRI systems. MIPs are 2D projections of the angiographic data that can be generated from any viewer perspective. To make a MIP, the computer projects a grid of parallel rays through the data set along a user-specified direction. The brightest voxels along each ray are retained to generate the MIP. The MIP algorithm is most effective when the objects of interest are bright and there is little gradation in the image. High signal intensity from sources other than the vessels can interfere with visualization. Hence, with MIPs, subtraction of the unenhanced data from the enhanced data is critical to reduce signal from structures other than contrast-enhanced vessels. MIPs are simple and quick, but they retain only approximately 10% of the data from the original image. One consequence is that the relative positions of overlapping vessels (anterior versus posterior) are lost in a single MIP view. MIP images are frequently generated for multiple viewing angles, typically by rotating the 3D dataset in small increments to simulate a movie of a spinning body. Vessels near the center of the axis will remain stable, whereas those far off-axis will move around. The multiple viewing perspectives help the viewer to determine the relative positions of vessels and other structures.

Subvolume MIPs can also be performed by limiting the region to which the MIP is applied. This obviates some of the reliance on subtraction by allowing the viewer to exclude areas of extravascular high signal intensity from the MIP (Figure II4-12).

Surface Shaded Display (SSD)

An alternative rendering technique is to generate a *surface shaded display (SSD)*, which relies on a ray-casting algorithm that makes the surfaces of vessels opaque (Figure II4-11). With a simulated virtual light source, SSD provides the viewer with visual clues about the relative positions of vessels based on shading. Although SSD gives a more realistic three-dimensional appearance to vessels, it too uses only a small percentage of the original data to generate the reconstruction. With SSD, the original gray levels of the data are lost and only transitions (surfaces)

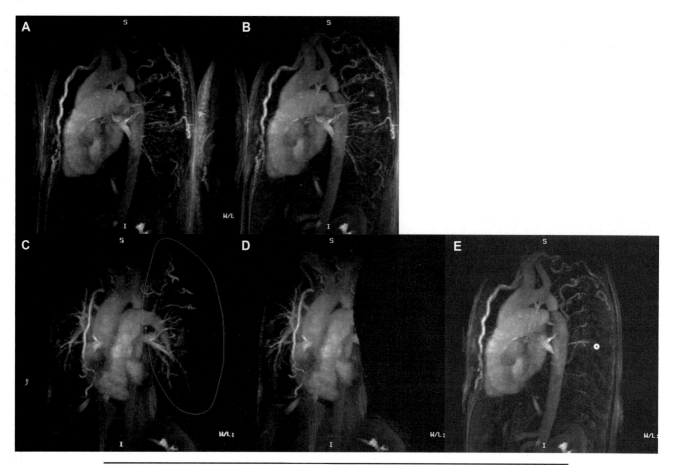

FIGURE II4-12. Segmentation of a 3D MRA dataset. The full dataset (**A**) viewed from a lateral perspective is first cropped anteriorly and posteriorly (**B**) to remove wraparound artifact from the chest wall. Then, using an oblique perspective, unwanted signal from the pulmonary vessels is segmented, or excluded by the user (**C, D**). The final reconstruction after segmentation (**E**) shows better visualization of the thoracic aorta and intercostal collateral arteries without overlying pulmonary vessels in this subject with aortic coarctation.

are viewed. Note that *endo*luminal SSDs have also been implemented for research applications in MR angioscopy.

Volume Rendering (VR)

Volume rendering (VR) methods have become widely available only recently, in part because they are computationally intensive. With VR, each voxel in the imaging volume is assigned a color (or gray level) and an opacity from 0 to 100%. The opacity controls the degree to which objects close to the user obscure objects further away. In other words, voxels with low opacities appear more transparent than those with high opacity. Unlike MIPs and SSDs, VR uses the entire imaging data set. It provides better visualization of small structures and a clearer depiction of the 3D relationship between structures, especially when confirmed with viewing at multiple angles.

More Advanced Post-Processing

New software tools are under development for ever more complex analysis of vascular disease including computer-aided diagnosis (Figure II4-13). For example, automatic and semiautomatic segmentation of the vessel wall can be used to provide quantitative measurements of vessel diameters and percent stenoses. Many of these tools still require validation, but they potentially will contribute to easier and maybe more accurate MR assessments of vascular disease.

> **IMPORTANT CONCEPT:** Although image post-processing tools can help to generate visually appealing MR angiograms, they should not replace a careful review of source data together with multiplanar reconstructions for accurate diagnosis of vascular disease.

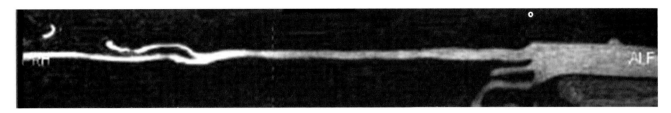

FIGURE II4-13. Image post-processing software automatically lays out the brachiocephalic and carotid arteries so that vessel calibers can be automatically calculated.

MULTISTATION MRA

Most clinical imaging systems are limited to a 40–50 cm field of view. To evaluate a more extended range of vasculature, multiple separate 3D acquisitions must be performed and the subject moved in or out of the scanner for each "station." For evaluation of the peripheral vasculature, imaging of the abdominal aorta (from the level of the renal arteries) to the knees or feet requires at least two to three stations. Other applications of multistation imaging include total aortic imaging for aneurysms, multistation imaging of vascular grafts (e.g., axillary-femoral grafts), and thoracic aorta-to-upper extremity imaging for embolic disease.

There are several options for acquiring multistation MRA. Which method is employed depends on the technology available. The options are discussed next, starting with the most basic and progressing to the more sophisticated methods currently available.

Separate Injections for Separate Stations

The simplest approach for multistation MRA is to treat each station as a separate examination, with separate contrast injections and subject (plus coil) repositioning for each station. This is possible on any system, without any special hardware or software. With judicious use of contrast doses, a two-station study can be accomplished in a single visit. The first station is imaged using the conventional 3D MRA protocol described previously. Following repositioning, the MRA protocol is repeated for the second station. For optimal image quality, a phased-array coil should be used for each station.

CHALLENGE QUESTION: Following the injection for the first station, residual gadolinium contrast will circulate in the arteries and veins. How is it possible to get high-quality arteriograms at the second station?

Answer: A pre-injection 3D acquisition should be performed at the second station to serve as a mask for the contrast-enhanced 3D image so that venous enhancement at the second station can be minimized by subtraction. Slightly higher doses of contrast material at the second station also help overcome the effects of residual circulating gadolinium contrast. Allocation of contrast

doses for the two stations might be 0.1 mmol/kg for the first station (about 15–20 mL) and 0.15 mmol/kg (25–30 mL) for the second station. The total dose must be less than 0.3 mmol/kg.

This protocol works well with separate chest/abdomen studies and abdomen/pelvis imaging. The simple multistation method is also suitable for imaging patients with claudication, where coverage of the abdominal aorta to trifurcation vessels may be all that is needed.

Because of limitations on total contrast doses that can be administered (typically up to 0.3 mmol/kg or triple dose) and large amounts of residual circulation, it can be challenging to acquire three or more station gadolinium-enhanced studies. Time-of-flight acquisitions at the third station can supplement the gadolinium-enhanced protocols, if necessary. Sample protocol options for peripheral MRA using separate station imaging are shown in Table II4-3. Detailed protocols at the end of this chapter give more information.

Protocol 1 (Table II4-4) starts with the third station (calves to feet) using 2D time-of-flight imaging and dedicated coils such as head and spine coils for the feet and calves, respectively. To get high-resolution images of the pedal vessels, separate positioning using the head coil is usually necessary. Then the subject is repositioned for the first and second stations for gadolinium-enhanced MRA using the torso phased-array coil. Total table time for the subject is typically on the order of 1½ hrs.

Alternatively (Protocol 2, Table II4-4), the third station can be performed with gadolinium-enhanced 3D interpolated MRA sequences. With repeated injections of gadolinium contrast, it is vital that pre-contrast acquisitions be performed at each station to serve as a mask for subtraction to eliminate residual venous enhancement. Because there is also residual gadolinium contrast circulating in the arteries, the subtraction process may diminish arterial enhancement. Therefore, progressively increasing doses of gadolinium contrast should be used for second and third injections (Table II4-4).

> **IMPORTANT POINTS:** With any MR system, multistation MRA can be performed by imaging each station sequentially with separate contrast injections. Typically, increased contrast doses are given at successive stations.

▶ **TABLE II4-4 Sample Full Peripheral MRA Protocols for Systems without Moving-Table Technology**

Protocol 1	Sequence	Gadolinium Dose	Coil
Station 3 (calves)	Time-of-flight		Spine array or torso phased-array coil
Station 4 (feet)	Time-of-flight		Head coil
Station 1 (pelvis)	3D interpolated spoiled GRE	0.1 mmol/kg (15–20 mL)	Torso phased–array coil
Station 2 (thighs)	3D interpolated spoiled GRE	0.15 mmol/kg (25–30 mL)	Torso phased-array coil
Protocol 2			
Station 3/4 (calves/feet)	3D interpolated spoiled GRE	0.08 mmol/kg (12–16 mL)	Torso phased-array coil
Station 2 (thighs)	3D interpolated spoiled GRE	0.1 mmol/kg (15–20 mL)	Torso phased-array coil
Station 1 (pelvis)	3D interpolated spoiled GRE	0.12 mmol/kg (18–24 mL)	Torso phased-array coil

Bolus Chase Imaging: Moving Patient Manually

As with conventional angiography, MRA can be performed using a bolus chase approach. By moving the subject quickly through the scanner bore between consecutive acquisitions, the bolus of gadolinium contrast material can be "chased" from the first station to the second, and from the second to the third. Hence, two or more stations can be imaged during the first pass of a single contrast bolus. For bolus chase imaging to work, the image acquisition times and time to move the patient between stations should match the transit time of the contrast material from station to station. Acquisition times less than 15–20 sec and table movement time of 5 sec or less are desirable.

To chase the bolus, the position of the patient within the magnet must change between the first and second and between the second and third acquisitions. With new commercially available systems, automatic moving tables can be controlled by the MR operator (see discussion in the next section). But even without moving-table technology, bolus chase imaging is still possible. There are generally two manual options:

1. On some systems, the MR table can be "unlocked" to be freely movable in and out of the magnet bore. The "floating" table can be constrained to move fixed distances with various homemade devices such as wooden blocks (e.g., 35 to 45 cm per station) (3).
2. With tables that cannot float, a separate device consisting of a plastic board can be used to move the subject (4). The board is placed onto the magnet table, and the subject positioned on it. Two people must be available to pull the board (and subject) 35 to 40 cm during the

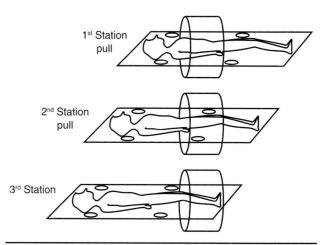

FIGURE II4-14. Peripheral MRA performed with the subject lying on a patient transfer board. Between each of the two or three acquisitions and the next, a 5 sec delay allows for the subject to be pulled a distance of 35 to 40 cm to the next station.

interval between acquisitions (Figure II4-14). Marking the table top and plastic board with distance labels helps to move the subject the correct distance between acquisitions, typically allowing at least 5 cm overlap between stations.

With both of these manual approaches, the scanner is not "aware" that anything has changed between acquisitions. The system does not shim at the second and third stations, and therefore field inhomogeneity may degrade image quality at these stations. The 3D acquisition orientation and parameters are not changed from one station to the next. Also, the body coil must be used for imaging, since the phased-array coils are not movable between acquisitions. This means that the image quality and spatial resolution are typically limited to imaging of larger vessels such as the popliteal artery and usually are not sufficient for the calves and pedal vessels.

There is one commercially available device to enable bolus chase imaging with a phased-array coil in the absence of moving-table technology. The AngioSURF product (MR-Innovation, Essen, Germany) consists of a rollerboard table insert, over which a phased-array coil is suspended. The subject is rolled to different positions beneath the fixed phased-array coil. Each acquisition is performed identically. Note that like the other methods described in this section, the moving-table technology is not integrated into the MR system. Thus, prescanning and shimming are performed with the subject at one position and these results are applied for all acquisitions, regardless of the nature of the body part in the scanner. Corrections for field inhomogeneity are again suboptimal in the second and third stations.

> **IMPORTANT POINT:** Even when moving-table technology is not available, bolus chase multistation MRA can be performed, with use of either a patient transfer board or other methods of moving the subject through the MR scanner between consecutive 3D acquisitions.

Bolus Chase Imaging: Automated Moving Table with Phased-Array Coil

State-of-the-art technology for performing multiple-station MRA incorporates moving-table technology with phased-array coil designs that span the entire vascular region of interest. As the table moves to each new position, different coil elements are activated. Prescanning and shimming are performed at each station for optimal image quality. Pre-contrast acquisitions can be performed before the bolus chase and serve as a mask for subtraction. With proper bolus timing, the quality of the bolus chase MRA can match that of dedicated single-station studies.

For peripheral MRA, a multi-element peripheral phased-array coil (Figure II4-15) permits high spatial and contrast resolution imaging of the vessels to the feet. The acquisition times at each station are on the order of 10–20 sec. Table movement time between acquisitions is 5–7 sec. For peripheral MRA, a timing examination or fluoroscopic triggering scheme is used to ensure arterial phase imaging of the first station. The later acquisitions use centric encoding of k-space and are kept short to minimize venous contamination in the last station. The parameters and orientations of each 3D acquisition can be adjusted at each station to optimize visualization of the smaller vessels and to ensure that vessels are not excluded from the field of view.

Contrast doses for multistation imaging vary from institution to institution. In our experience, a double dose of contrast (0.2 mmol/kg, approximately 30–40 mL for adults) is sufficient. The optimal rate of injection for peripheral MRA is unknown, but a two-stage injection protocol is favored to prolong the arterial phase during the full course of the imaging protocol. For example, a typical injection protocol might consist of 20 mL gadolinium contrast injected at 2 mL/sec followed by another 20 mL contrast at 1 mL/sec followed by 20 mL saline flush at 1 mL/sec.

CHALLENGE QUESTION: With multistation MRA, at what location should circulation time be determined with a test bolus timing examination?

Answer: Commonly circulation time at the level of the femoral heads is measured. However, if there is significant discrepancy in disease between the vessels of the legs, it is possible to have delayed enhancement of the arteries on one side relative to the other, particularly at the distal station (trifurcation vessels and feet). Therefore, circulation time at the popliteal arteries may also be useful.

With moving table multistation MRA, the scan delay is defined for the first station. For subsequent stations, the effective scan delay depends on the acquisition times and on the speed the table moves between stations. For example,

$$\text{Scan delay for second station} = \text{Scan delay for first station} + T_{\text{acq for first station}} + T_{\text{moving table}}$$

where T_{acq} is typically 10–20 sec and $T_{\text{moving table}}$ 5–10 sec. For optimal imaging of the second and later stations,

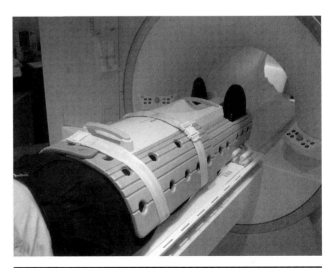

FIGURE II4-15. Peripheral phased-array coil. For imaging of the lower abdomen and pelvic arteries, a torso phased-array coil can be added to this configuration.

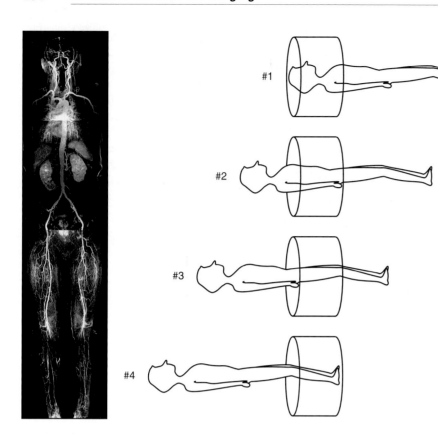

FIGURE II4-16. Whole-body MRA performed in four separate stations over 1 minute following a single bolus of 0.2 mmol/kg gadolinium contrast material. Each station is imaged using dedicated phased-array coils and high-resolution (512 matrix) interpolated 3D spoiled gradient echo sequences with parallel imaging techniques.

these delays must match the bolus transit time from station to station. The bolus transit time depends on the subject's physiology and extent of vascular disease and is difficult to predict a priori without test bolus circulation time measurements at each station. In practice, using a circulation time measured at the femoral heads sometimes results in a mismatch in bolus transit time and scan delay at the third (below the knees) station. Hence, alternative strategies for imaging the third station should be considered to supplement bolus chase peripheral MRA. These include "time-resolved" gadolinium-enhanced MRA (see below) or time-of-flight imaging, both performed prior to the bolus chase acquisitions. A sample protocol is provided at the end of the chapter.

> **IMPORTANT CONCEPTS:** Bolus chase MRA is typically performed with a two-stage injection protocol and with either a bolus detection scheme or a test bolus timing examination at the level of the femoral heads. To supplement imaging at the distal (below the knees) station, time-resolved gadolinium-enhanced MRA or time-of-flight imaging may be performed prior to the bolus chase.

Bolus Chase Imaging: Whole-Body MRA

Provided multiple phased-array coils can be plugged in and selectively activated from station to station, whole-body MR angiography can be performed by chasing a single bolus from the head and neck through to the toes

(Figure II4-16). To achieve a successful bolus chase, imaging times for each station must be kept shorter than 10–12 sec by use of parallel imaging methods. Four-station whole-body imaging, using a combination of phased-array coils, can then be accomplished in under 1 min of acquisition time, allowing for 5 sec moves between each station.

TIME-RESOLVED MRA

In some applications, the kinetics of contrast enhancement may be more important than extended spatial coverage. *Time-resolved MRA* refers to the use of fast imaging techniques to perform multiple MRA acquisitions with sufficiently high temporal resolution to illuminate the dynamics of contrast enhancement during first pass of the bolus and beyond. Examples of useful clinical applications include the evaluation of complex arteriovenous malformations, identification of retrograde filling proximally of occluded vessels (such as in peripheral vascular disease, Figure II4-17), assessment of pulmonary vascular disease, and diagnosis of complex congenital heart disease.

Typically, for time-resolved MRA, the area of interest is limited, and therefore the 3D imaging slab can be designed to be relatively thin with few partitions. Each 3D acquisition should be 5–10 sec or less. To achieve short acquisition times, higher-bandwidth sequences that allow TR times <4 msec are typically needed. Additionally, parallel imaging techniques (SENSE or SMASH, see

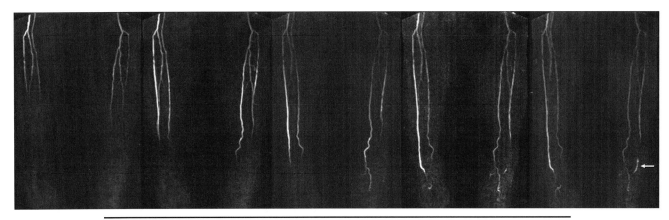

FIGURE II4-17. Time-resolved MRA through calves and feet. Series of sequential 6 sec 3D MR acquisitions in the third station of a peripheral MRA study performed following 7 mL gadolinium contrast material shows retrograde filling of the left dorsalis pedis (arrow) in the setting of an occluded anterior tibial artery. All images are subtracted MIP reconstructions.

Chapter I-8) and view-sharing methods (Chapter I-8) improve the temporal resolution.

To implement time-resolved MRA, the MR system must be capable of generating and reconstructing large amounts of data quickly. Some vendors provide automatic subtraction of unenhanced from enhanced images and automatic MIPs of multiple 3D acquisitions. Such features considerably ease the post-processing demands associated with time-resolved MRA.

Time-resolved MRA is also an alternative solution to the timing challenge of gadolinium-enhanced MRA. With sufficient numbers of short 3D acquisitions, at least one good arterial phase acquisition is expected and the test bolus or bolus detection methods are obviated.

> **IMPORTANT CONCEPT:** Time-resolved MRA requires multiple fast acquisitions, typically on the order of 5–10 sec each, to provide temporal information about contrast enhancement. This is useful for evaluation of pathologies such as arteriovenous malformations, peripheral vascular disease, and pulmonary vascular disease.

MR VENOGRAPHY

The evolution of MR venography has paralleled that of MR angiography. Whereas early approaches relied on 2D time-of-flight imaging, more recent implementations give excellent results using gadolinium-enhanced 3D techniques.

CHALLENGE QUESTION: Why are 3D time-of-flight imaging methods never used for MR venography?

Answer: The slow-flowing blood in venous structures is saturated in 3D time-of-flight imaging. For MR venography, 2D time-of-flight imaging is preferable.

2D MR Venography

Two approaches can be used for non-contrast-enhanced MR venography: time-of-flight and steady-state free precession (True FISP).

Two-dimensional time-of-flight (TOF) imaging is useful for imaging limited portions of the venous system. As discussed in Chapter II-2, with time-of-flight imaging, inflow of fresh, unsaturated protons into a slice will have high signal intensity. Saturation bands are applied on the arterial side of the imaging slice, leaving only signal from veins (Figure II4-18). These saturation bands typically travel with the imaging slice.

There are limitations to 2D time-of-flight for MR venography. Slow flow proximal to a venous thrombosis may mimic thrombosis itself, leading to overestimates of the extent of disease (Figure II4-18). Additionally, flow artifacts at the junctions of veins can be mistaken for thrombus (Figure II4-19).

As a new alternative to 2D time-of-flight imaging, steady-state free precession sequences can be applied for imaging veins. With these balanced gradient sequences, image contrast is based on T2/T1 differences between tissues. Therefore, blood is bright because of its high water content, while thrombus is dark (Figure II4-18). This method, unlike time-of-flight, is not based on flow-sensitivity, and the rate of flow does not influence the detectability of thrombus. However, both arteries and veins have high signal on these images, making image interpretation more difficult.

CHALLENGE QUESTION: Are saturation bands used with steady-state free precession venography?

Answer: No. Because the method is not based on flow-sensitivity, saturation bands are not needed.

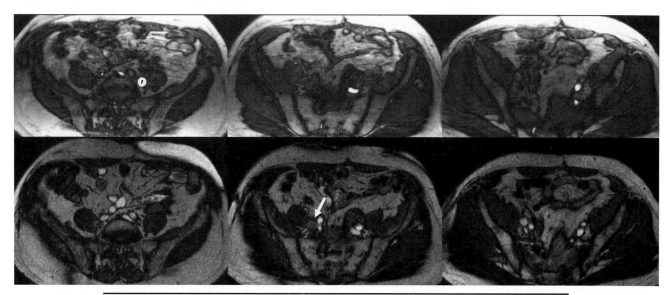

FIGURE II4-18. 2D TOF (top row) and steady-state free precession (bottom row) MR venography in a subject with right common iliac vein thrombus (arrow). Because a saturation band has been applied in the cranial direction on the TOF images, only flow in the veins creates signal. Slow-flow proximal and distal to the thrombus also has low signal and mimics thrombus on TOF images. On steady-state free precession images, blood in both arteries and veins gives rise to high signal intensity. Thrombus in the right common iliac vein (arrow) has lower signal intensity.

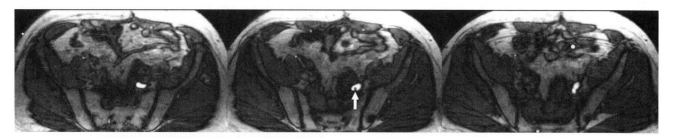

FIGURE II4-19. Time-of-flight image artifact. Flow artifact (arrow) in left common iliac vein at the confluence of the internal and external iliac veins mimics thrombus.

IMPORTANT CONCEPTS: For non-contrast-enhanced MR venography, two strategies can be used: TOF or steady-state free precession (true FISP). When 2D time-of-flight with traveling saturation bands is used, slow flow and flow artifacts at the confluence of vein branches may mimic thrombus. Steady-state free precession sequences are promising for venography based on the intrinsic high signal of blood in arteries and veins.

Direct Gadolinium-Enhanced MR Venography

For an assessment of venous patency, direct venous injection of contrast material for MR venography can be performed, akin to conventional venography. This requires venous access of the limb of interest. Because of the short T2 of concentrated gadolinium contrast (see Chapter I-3,

Figures I3-4 and I3-5), the contrast must be diluted before direct injection. Typically, a ratio of 1:50 works well; for example, 5 mL of gadolinium contrast can be diluted in 250 mL sterile saline.

To perform direct MR venography, a 3D acquisition is positioned to include the entire draining venous system following cannulation of a vein distal to the area of suspected disease. Then, while the contrast is injected slowly into the intravenous catheter, 3D acquisitions can be performed over the area of interest. The resulting images resemble those of a conventional venogram, although data are three-dimensional (Figure II4-20). As with conventional venography, occluded vessels are inferred by the filling of collaterals. To visualize the source of occlusion, a full 3D acquisition can also be performed during recirculation of the contrast to detect thrombus or other extrinsic causes of obstruction (Figure II4-20).

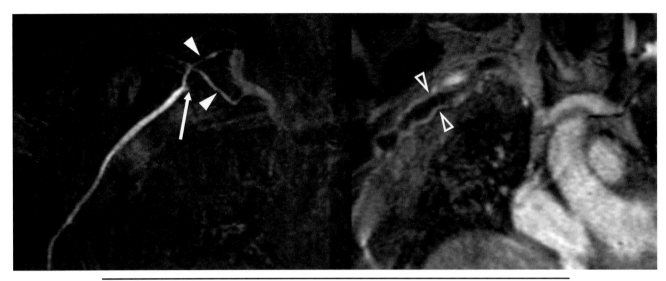

FIGURE II4-20. Direct gadolinium-enhanced MR venography. MIP of a 3D MRA acquisition (left) performed during continuous injection of diluted gadolinium contrast into a right hand vein shows obstruction of the right subclavian vein (arrow) and patent collateral vessels (arrowheads). On a subsequent 3D contrast-enhanced image obtained 2 min after recirculation of the injected contrast (right), the unenhancing thrombus can be seen (open arrowheads).

Indirect, Recirculation Gadolinium-Enhanced MR Venography

Direct gadolinium-enhanced MR venography is limited because the imaging is confined to the venous system draining the injected vein, and venous access on the side of suspected disease may be limited. An alternative gadolinium-enhanced approach is to perform recirculation venography, which enables assessment of the entire venous system in the field of view by means of any venous access.

The concept is straightforward. First, 3D MRA is performed in the area of interest, timed for maximum arterial enhancement. Then, approximately 120 sec later, when the gadolinium contrast has had time to recirculate into the venous system, the same 3D acquisition is repeated. During this delayed phase, both the arterial and venous systems are enhanced. A large-FOV MR venogram can be produced by subtraction (Figure II4-21):

$$\text{Delayed acquisition} - \text{Arterial acquisition}$$
$$= \text{3D MR Venogram}$$
$$(MRA + V) - (MRA) = (MRV)$$

Because the method relies on recirculation of the gadolinium contrast material into the entire venous system, the choice of access vein is inconsequential. This is advantageous in many of the patients referred for MR venography who have had chronic venous access difficulties. Also, the large field of view provides abundant information about patency of alternative sites of venous access.

For MR venography, a double dose of contrast material (0.2 mmol/kg, or about 30 to 40 mL) ensures adequate enhancement of the veins during recirculation. Injection rates and acquisition parameters are otherwise similar to those used for MR arteriography.

> **IMPORTANT CONCEPT:** Contrast-enhanced MR venography enables assessment of venous patency across a large field of view in short study times. Unlike direct venography, or conventional contrast x-ray venography, recirculation techniques can be performed with any venous access, not necessarily distal to the site of suspected venous disease.

PITFALLS

Contrast-enhanced MR angiography is a widely used clinical test that has been validated in innumerable clinical studies. Nevertheless, imaging artifacts can occasionally give rise to diagnostic pitfalls. The most common artifacts and pitfalls are briefly discussed next (refer also to a pictorial essay illustrating many of these findings (5)).

Mistiming of the MR Acquisition

The synchronization of short acquisition times of 20 sec or less and short contrast infusion times of about 10 sec requires precise timing to achieve high-quality angiograms without venous contamination. If the acquisition is too late, venous enhancement can obscure

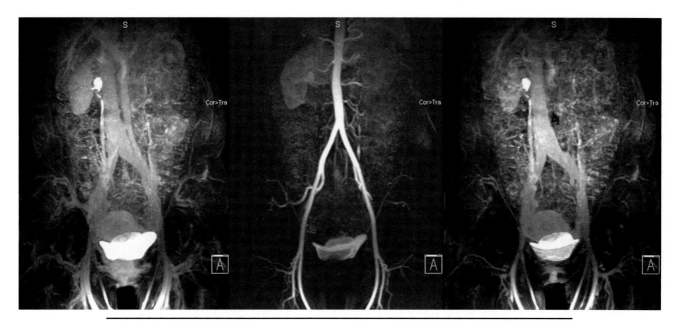

FIGURE II4-21. Indirect gadolinium-enhanced MR venography. Sample recirculation 3D MR venogram (right) obtained from subtracting the arterial phase (middle) from the delayed arterial-venous phase (left).

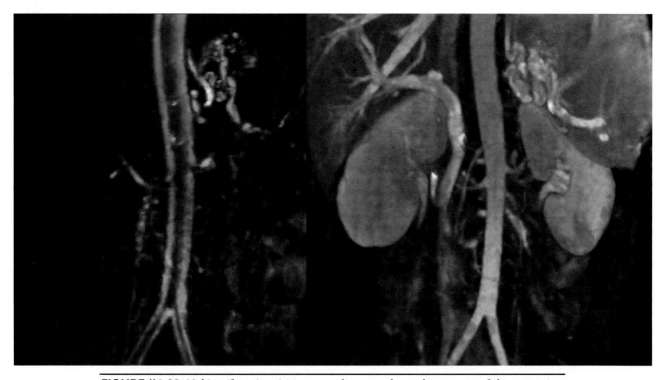

FIGURE II4-22. Maki artifact. Acquisition preceding complete enhancement of the aorta gives rise to an MRA (subvolume MIP) shown to the left. MIP of a 3D acquisition acquired within 10 sec of the first acquisition (right) shows normal appearance of the abdominal aorta. (Modified with permission from Lee VS, et al. Gadolinium-enhanced MR angiography: Artifacts and pitfalls. AJR 2000; 175;197–205.)

visualization of arterial vessels. The source images are usually still diagnostic, although angiographic reconstructions may be degraded. If the acquisition is too early, the arteries may be incompletely opacified in MR images.

When the acquisition is considerably too early, the vessels may have an unusual appearance illustrated in Figure II4-22. The rapid change in contrast enhancement during the filling of central and peripheral lines of k-space can give

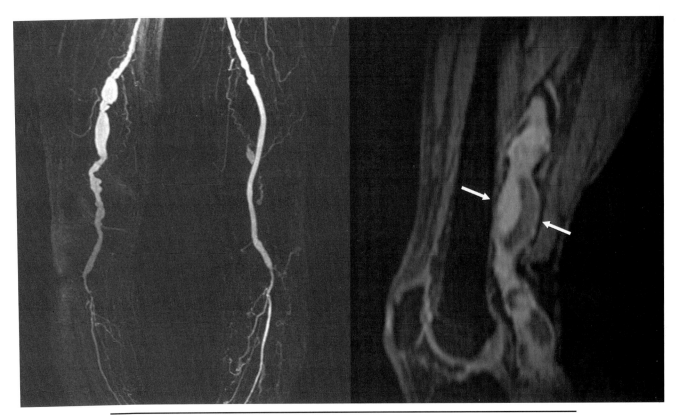

FIGURE II4-23. Nonvisualization of mural thrombus. Subtracted MIP MR angiogram (left) shows extensive aneurysmal dilatation of the right superficial femoral and popliteal artery. Sagittal view of subsequent 3D gradient echo image (right) shows unsuspected mural thrombus in the right leg vessels. The subtracted maximum intensity projection MR angiogram, by depicting only vessel lumen, underestimates the severity of the aneurysmal disease (arrows).

rise to an image in which the walls of a vessel are enhanced while the lumen is unenhanced, referred to as the *Maki artifact* (6). Because of the potential problems with timing, most MRA protocols include a second contrast-enhanced acquisition immediately following the first as part of a routine single station MRA (Table II4-3) and for the last station of a multistation study.

CHALLENGE QUESTION: Can you explain the appearance of the artifact in Figure II4-22 in terms of the filling of k-space?

Answer: During the initial part of the MR acquisition, the contrast bolus was still in transit. The central lines of k-space, defining the low-spatial-resolution components of the image, were collected during the unenhanced phase. The bolus arrived at the end of the acquisition, during the filling of the peripheral lines of k-space. Hence, only the high-spatial-resolution parts of the image, such as the edges of the vessels, appear enhanced.

IMPORTANT CONCEPT: The appearance of the Maki artifact can be understood in terms of the timing relationship between k-space filling and contrast enhancement.

Nonvisualization of Mural or Extraluminal Pathology

The MR angiogram, particularly the post-processed images, depicts gadolinium contrast within the lumen of the vessels. Pathology that involves the vessel wall or that extends outside the vessels is usually not visualized, especially on subtracted post-processed images. Examples include dissection, mural thrombus, particularly in an aneurysm (Figure II4-23), intramural hematoma, vasculitides, and extravascular masses that may compress arterial structures. Imaging protocols should therefore include at least one set of images that includes the vessel wall and extraluminal structures.

IMPORTANT CONCEPT: All MR angiographic studies should include at least one sequence to assess mural and extramural pathology.

Overestimation of Stenosis

All MR angiographic methods tend to overestimate the degree of stenosis when compared with conventional

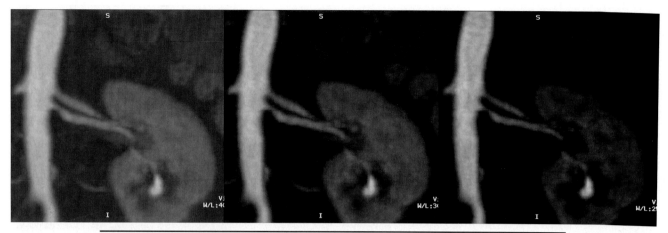

FIGURE II4-24. Variable appearance of left lower renal artery stenoses on MIP images with varying window and level settings.

angiography, in part due to spin dephasing caused by turbulent flow at a stenosis and partial volume effects. The short TE used with contrast-enhanced 3D acquisitions helps to reduce this problem. However, the stenosis is still exaggerated, especially with suboptimal spatial resolution. Angiographic renderings, especially MIP reconstructions, also contribute to overestimation of stenosis severity. Even the conditions under which images are viewed on the workstations, including the window and level settings, can dramatically affect the appearance of moderate stenoses (Figure II4-24). Image analysis should rely on a careful review of source images rather than on post-processed images.

> **IMPORTANT CONCEPT:** MRA tends to overestimate the degree of vascular stenosis. The overestimation is further exaggerated with post-processing techniques such as maximum intensity projection or other 3D renderings. Source images are the most reliable.

Pseudostenosis

Pseudostenoses can be caused by a number of factors (Table II4-5).

Susceptibility artifacts related to adjacent metallic clips or joint prostheses or metallic vascular stents can create the appearance of a vascular stenosis or occlusion (Figure II4-25).

CHALLENGE QUESTION: How can you confirm suspected metallic artifacts with MR imaging?

Answer: By reimaging with sequences that are more sensitive to susceptibility effects, such as gradient echo sequences with long echo times. On these sequences, metallic artifacts become very apparent or "bloom."

▶ **TABLE II4-5**

Pseudostenoses

Metal artifacts
Susceptibility from concentrated gadolinium contrast
Exclusion of vessel from slab
Low spatial resolution/volume averaging

A similar susceptibility artifact can result from other causes of T2* or T2 shortening, such as extremely concentrated gadolinium contrast material. Recall from Chapter I-3 (Figure I3-6) that in its undiluted form, gadolinium contrast material has a very short T2. Because the contrast material is injected intravenously without dilution, the T2 effects of the gadolinium contrast in central veins ipsilateral to the side of injection may cause signal loss in veins and arteries in close proximity, creating the false impression of arterial stenosis (Figure II4-26).

CHALLENGE QUESTION: Into which arm should gadolinium routinely be injected intravenously, right or left, to minimize the undesirable effects of concentrated gadolinium retention in veins causing arterial signal loss?

Answer: Right. A left-sided injection can cause apparent stenosis of not only the left subclavian artery but also the proximal great vessels where the left brachiocephalic vein crosses. Injection of the right arm should be used for most MRA studies of the chest, unless right upper extremity arterial pathology is suspected.

To reduce residual contrast material in the veins, saline flush is used. Venous inflow also helps to dilute and wash out any residual contrast material. Therefore, on repeat

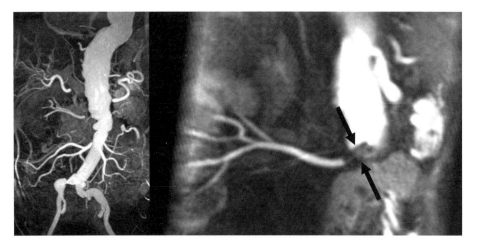

FIGURE II4-25. Pseudostenosis. Maximum intensity projection of abdominal aorta on left shows apparent right renal artery occlusion. Oblique coronal reconstruction of the source data on right reveals a right renal stent (arrow). Patency of the stent is difficult to assess because of the susceptibility artifact caused by the stent.

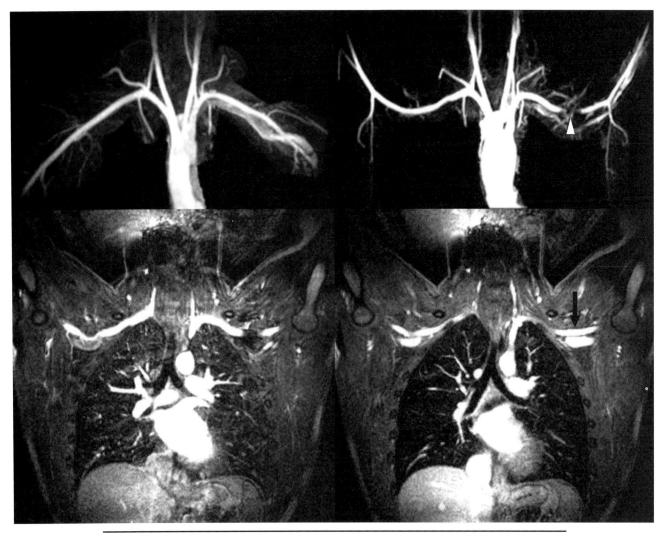

FIGURE II4-26. Pseudo thoracic outlet syndrome. Maximum intensity projections of two separate 3D MRA acquisitions performed with the arms down (top left) and arms elevated (top right) show apparent left subclavian artery stenosis with elevation. Source images (below MIP images) show that the area of signal loss in the left subclavian artery with elevation (arrowhead) extends beyond the expected vessel lumen (lower left), with the appearance of a susceptibility artifact. Delayed acquisition with arms elevated (lower right) confirms left subclavian artery patency (arrow). With arm elevation, venous drainage is impaired and the concentrated gadolinium contrast in the veins creates a pseudostenosis of the left subclavian artery.

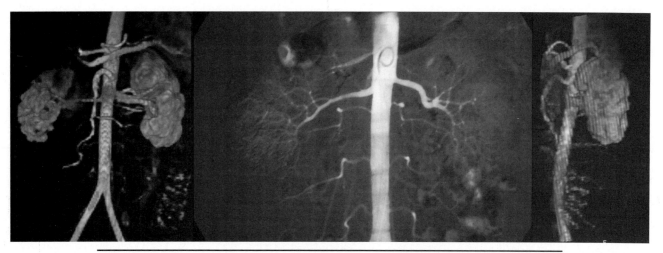

FIGURE II4-27. Pseudo fibromuscular dysplasia of the renal arteries. Maximum intensity projection of a gadolinium-enhanced MRA (left) shows irregular, beaded appearance of the right renal artery, while conventional contrast angiography (middle) shows a normal appearance. The sagittal view of the MRA on the right explains the artifactual appearance. Stair-step artifact resulting from thick (3 mm) partitions in the anterior-posterior direction creates the beaded appearance of the renal artery as it passes anteriorly to posteriorly. (Reproduced with permission from Lee VS, et al. Gadolinium-enhanced MR angiography: Artifacts and pitfalls. AJR 2000; 175;197–205.)

MRA acquisitions done after the arterial phase, the artifact is no longer as severe.

Another cause of pseudostenosis or pseudo-occlusion is exclusion of the vessel from the imaging slab. Areas that are most susceptible to exclusion from the imaging slab include the common and internal iliac arteries posteriorly, the common femoral arteries anteriorly, and the popliteal arteries posteriorly. Careful use of bright-blood scout images for positioning of 3D MRA slabs minimizes these errors.

Low spatial resolution can exaggerate stenosis and can even create pseudostenosis in widely patent vessels. When voxel size is large relative to vessel size, the vessel caliber will be misrepresented and can produce a stair-step artifact that mimics the beaded appearance of fibromuscular dysplasia (Figure II4-27).

> **IMPORTANT CONCEPTS:** Causes of pseudostenoses include susceptibility artifacts such as metal objects in the body and concentrated gadolinium contrast material, low spatial resolution, and exclusion of the vessel from the imaging slab.

Short-T1 Tissues Mimic or Obscure Gadolinium Contrast Enhancement

Contrast-enhanced MRA sequences are T1-weighted sequences. Therefore, tissues such as bone marrow, fat, and bowel contents, which have short T1 relaxation times,

also appear bright on MRA and can obscure visualization of overlying vessels. Other tissues, such as blood products in atherosclerotic plaque, can also have high signal intensity at MR angiography and can interfere with image interpretation (see, for example, Figure II2-Q4). Since these sources of high signal are present on the pre-contrast images, subtraction of the unenhanced from the enhanced images reduces their signal and improves the appearance of angiographic reconstructions (Figure II4-10).

> **IMPORTANT CONCEPT:** Not everything that is bright on a 3D MRA image is gadolinium contrast material. Subtraction images are useful for excluding other sources of high signal intensity on contrast-enhanced MRA.

REVIEW QUESTIONS

1. Many 3D MRA acquisitions use partial Fourier methods, as discussed in Chapter I-8, so that the center of k-space is typically traversed somewhere nearer the beginning of the acquisition time. You know the time to the center of k-space with a 16 sec acquisition is at 6 sec. How should you time the scan delay based on the test bolus, assuming a 20 mL gadolinium contrast bolus injected at 2 mL/sec?

2. Early attempts at using a fluoroscopic bolus detection technique, with axial fluoroscopic images, for timing the acquisition of a thoracic aortic MRA often resulted in an MRA image like that shown in Figure II4-Q2A. Can you explain what happened and why?

3. A patient was referred for evaluation of a right hilar mass seen on chest x-ray. Time-resolved MRA images of the chest are shown in Figure II4-Q3 with a mass again seen (arrow). What is the diagnosis?

4. Referring oncologists have difficulty finding venous access in a patient who requires intravenous access for chemotherapy. A gadolinium-enhanced 3D MR venogram is performed using the recirculation technique (Figure II4-Q4). What is your interpretation of the results?

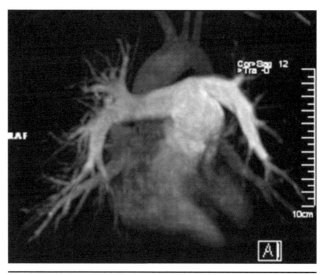

FIGURE II4-Q2A

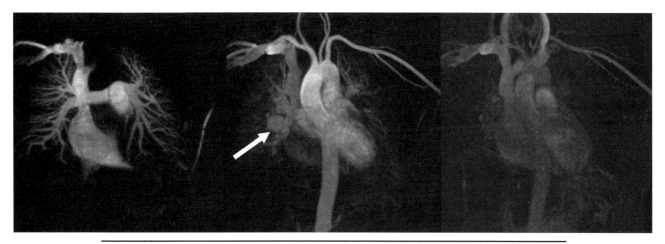

FIGURE II4-Q3. Time-resolved MRA of the chest in the pulmonary arterial phase (left), pulmonary venous phase (middle), and arterial phase (right). Note the hilar mass (arrow) in the pulmonary venous phase.

5. An MRA is performed for right arm symptoms as shown in Figure II4-Q5.
   a. Discuss the differential diagnoses.
   b. To obtain this study, a physician injected gadolinium contrast in the right arm without using a saline flush. With this information, explain the appearance of the MRA shown in Figure II4-Q5. What steps should be taken for correct interpretation of the vasculature?

6. A patient with left thigh claudication has a contrast-enhanced MRA, followed by conventional contrast angiography (Figure II4-Q6). Explain the discrepancy in appearance of the two studies.

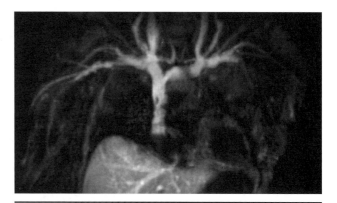

FIGURE II4-Q4. Subtraction 3D MR venogram obtained by subtracting the arterial phase contrast-enhanced 3D MRA from a delayed acquisition.

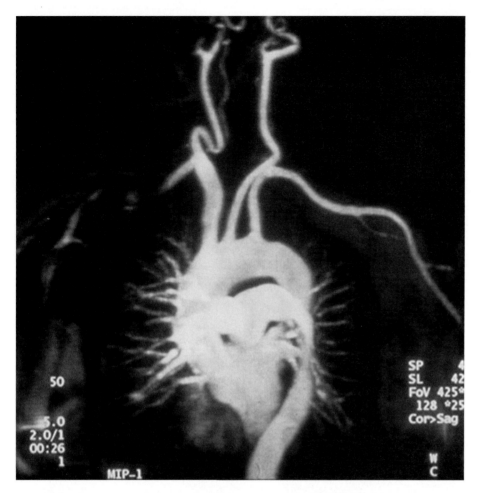

FIGURE II4-Q5

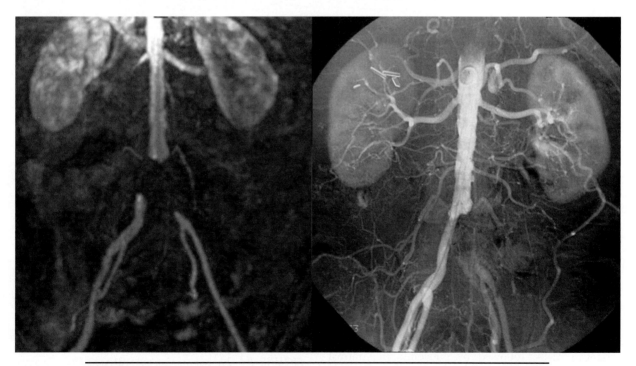

FIGURE II4-Q6. Contrast-enhanced 3D MRA (left) and conventional contrast angiography (right) in a patient with left thigh claudication. (Modified with permission from Lee VS, et al Gadolinium-enhanced MR angiography: Artifacts and pitfalls AJR 2000; 175;197–205.)

REFERENCES

1. Prince MR. Gadolinium-enhanced MR aortography. Radiology 1994; 191:155–164.
2. Earls JP, Rofsky NM, DeCorato DR, Krinsky GA, Weinreb JC. Breath-hold single-dose gadolinium-enhanced three-dimensional MR aortography: usefulness of a timing examination and MR power injector. Radiology 1996; 201:705–710.
3. Ho KY, Leiner T, de Haan MW, Kessels AG, Kitslaar PJ, van Engelshoven JM. Peripheral vascular tree stenoses: evaluation with moving-bed infusion-tracking MR angiography. Radiology 1998; 206:683–692.
4. Pandharipande PV, Lee VS, Reuss PM, et al. Two-station bolus-chase MR angiography with a stationary table: a simple alternative to automated-table techniques. AJR Am J Roentgenol 2002; 179:1583–1589.
5. Lee VS, Martin DJ, Krinsky GA, Rofsky NM. Gadolinium-enhanced MR angiography: artifacts and pitfalls. AJR Am J Roentgenol 2000; 175:197–205.
6. Maki JH, Prince MR, Londy FJ, Chenevert TL. The effects of time varying intravascular signal intensity and k-space acquisition order on three-dimensional MR angiography image quality. J Magn Reson Imaging 1996; 6:642–651.

▶ **PROTOCOL: Carotid Artery MRA with Gadolinium Contrast**[1]

Setup and Preparation	Notes
i.v.	22 G or larger
Gadolinium contrast	0.1 mmol/kg (20 mL)
Coil	Neck phased-array
Positioning tips	Supine, head first
Patient instructions	End-expiratory breath holding

Sequence	Imaging Plane	Parameters
1 Scout (true FISP or spoiled GRE)	Multiplanar	Default
2 2D TOF[1] (optional)	Axial	TR/TE/FA, 25/9/40° Superior saturation band
3 2D TOF[2] (optional)	Axial	4 slices, inferior saturation band
4 T1 SE or TSE[3] (optional)	Axial	Multislice imaging, typically with multiple signal averages and free breathing
5 Pre-contrast 3D MRA sequence	Sagittal	Min TR/TE, FA 25–40°, voxel size ≪ vessel diameter
6 Test bolus (optional)	Axial or sagittal	Images every 1–2 sec 1 mL contrast + 20 mL saline, 2–3 mL/sec
7 Post-contrast 3D MRA sequence 　(a) First acquisition timed using test bolus or bolus detection 　(b) Repeat acquisition a few sec after first acquisition	Sagittal	Same as pre-contrast: 20 mL contrast + saline, 2–3 mL/sec
8 Post-contrast T1-weighted imaging (optional)	Axial	3D interpolated fat-suppressed spoiled GRE Min TR/TE, FA 12°, 2 mm slices, <20 sec breath hold

[1]2D TOF acquisitions are supplemental to the gadolinium-enhanced approach. At the least, a limited set of 4 axial slices spaced over the neck can be useful to determine flow direction in the carotid and vertebral arteries.
[2]A second 2D TOF acquisition is performed using an inferior saturation band to determine flow direction in the vertebral arteries in case of possible subclavian steal. This task requires a limited number of slices.
[3]High-resolution T1 TSE can be helpful in the setting of suspected dissection to evaluate mural pathology in the carotid or vertebral arteries.

▶ PROTOCOL: Thoracic Aorta MRA with Gadolinium Contrast

Setup and Preparation	Notes
i.v.	22 G or larger
Gadolinium contrast	0.1–0.2 mmol/kg (20–30 mL)[1]
ECG leads	Optional for ascending aortic disease or coarctation
Coil	Torso phased-array
Positioning tips	Supine, head first
Subject instructions	End-expiratory breath holding
	Supplemental oxygen by nasal cannula optional

Sequence	Imaging Plane	Parameters
1 Scout (true FISP or spoiled GRE)	Multiplanar	Default
2 Double inversion recovery fast spin echo (single shot optional)	Axial, oblique sagittal	ECG gated if possible 5–8 mm slices
3 STIR[2]	Axial or sagittal	TI = 160 msec, TE >80 msec
4 Cine gradient echo[3]	Oblique coronal, sagittal, or others	Aortic root or coarctation, ECG gated
5 Pre-contrast 3D MRA sequence	Oblique sagittal[4]	Min TR/TE, FA 25–40°, voxel size ≪ vessel diameter
6 Test bolus (optional)	Axial or sagittal	Images every 1–2 sec 1 mL contrast + 20 mL saline, 2–3 mL/sec
7 Post-contrast 3D MRA sequence (a) First acquisition timed using test bolus or bolus detection (b) Repeat acquisition a few sec after first acquisition	Oblique sagittal	Same as pre-contrast 20–30 mL contrast + saline, 2–3 mL/sec
8 Post-contrast T1-weighted imaging (optional)	Axial	3D interpolated fat-suppressed spoiled GRE Min TR/TE, FA 12°, 2 mm slices, <20 sec breath hold
9 2D Cine phase contrast flow quantification[5] (Optional)	Variable	Segmented k-space, view-sharing, Venc 150 cm/sec-maximum, depending on presence of stenosis, retrospective gating for aortic insufficiency TR/TE = 30–60/3–4, FA 30°

[1]Larger doses should be considered for subjects with aneurysmal disease.
[2]STIR images are optional, for use with suspected vasculitis.
[3]Cine images are useful to assess the aortic valve in subjects with ascending aortic aneurysms and also for congenital aortic diseases (Chapter III-4).
[4]Oblique sagittal orientation of the 3D slab should be positioned at the aortic arch (Figure II4-P1).
[5]Cine phase contrast flow quantification can be useful for quantifying aortic valvular stenosis or regurgitation and for assessing aortic coarctation (Figure II3-13, Figure II3-Q3). A segmented k-space sequence with view sharing permits breath-hold acquisitions.

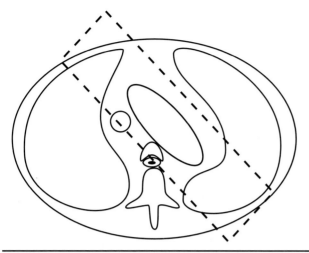

FIGURE II4-P1. Positioning for thoracic aortic MRA 3D slab.

> **PROTOCOL: Abdominal Aorta/Renal Artery MRA with Gadolinium Contrast**

Setup and Preparation	Notes
i.v.	22 G or larger
Gadolinium contrast	0.1–0.2 mmol/kg (20–30 mL)[1]
Coil	Torso phased-array
Positioning tips	Supine, head first Arms propped up at the side or over abdomen[2]
Subject instructions	End-expiratory breath holding Supplemental oxygen by nasal cannula optional

Sequence	Imaging Plane	Parameters
1 Scout (true FISP or spoiled GRE)	Multiplanar	Default
2 T1-weighted gradient echo imaging	Axial	Dual echo (in- and opposed-phase, TE = 2.2 msec, 4.4 msec); include adrenal glands, 5–8 mm slices
3 STIR (optional)[3]	Axial or sagittal	TI 160 msec, TE > 80 msec
4 Pre-contrast 3D fat-suppressed GRE (optional)[4]	Axial	3D interpolated fat-suppressed spoiled GRE Min TR, TE, FA 12°, 2 mm slices, <20 sec breath hold
5 Pre-contrast 3D MRA sequence	Oblique coronal[5]	Min TR/TE, FA 25–40°, voxel size ≪ vessel diameter
6 Test bolus (optional)	Axial	Images every 1–2 sec 1 mL contrast + 20 mL saline, 2–3 mL/sec

7 Post-contrast 3D MRA sequence
  (a) First acquisition timed using test bolus or bolus detection
  (b) Repeat acquisition a few sec after first acquisition
	Oblique coronal	Same as pre-contrast
		  20–30 mL contrast + saline,
		  2–3 mL/sec

8 Post-contrast T1-weighted imaging (optional)	Axial	Repeat 3D interpolated fat-suppressed spoiled GRE

[1]Larger doses should be considered for subjects with aneurysmal disease.
[2]To reduce wraparound artifact from the arms, elevate using cushions so that arms are above the level of the kidneys (Figure II4-P2).
[3]STIR images are optional, for use with suspected vasculitis or retroperitoneal fibrosis.
[4]3D fat-suppressed gradient echo images before and after contrast material are useful for characterizing incidental renal masses found on renal artery studies.
[5]Renal MRA slab can be positioned coronally and tilted parallel the abdominal aorta (Figure II4-P3) to reduce the slab thickness and improve spatial resolution.

FIGURE II4-P2. Patient positioning for renal MRA.

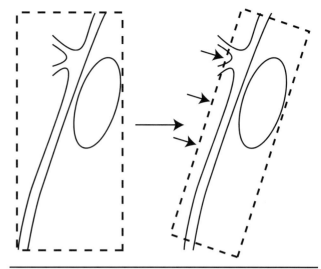

FIGURE II4-P3. Positioning of an oblique coronal slab for renal artery MRA from a sagittal perspective.

▶ **PROTOCOL: Three-Station Peripheral MRA (Renal Arteries to Feet) with Gadolinium Contrast and Moving Table (Option A)**

Setup and Preparation	Notes
i.v.	22 G or larger
Gadolinium contrast	0.2 mmol/kg (40 mL)
Coil	Torso phased-array for lower abdomen/pelvis Peripheral phased-array coil
Positioning tips	Supine, feet first, if possible
Subject instructions	End-expiratory breath holding for first station Supplemental oxygen by nasal cannula optional

Sequence	Imaging Plane	Parameters
1 Scout (true FISP or spoiled GRE)	Multiplanar	Default, three stations: (1) lower abdomen/pelvis (2) thighs (3) calves and feet
2 Test bolus	Axial	Femoral heads Images every 1–2 sec 1 mL contrast + 20 mL saline, 2–3 mL/sec
3 Time-resolved 3D MRA sequence through calves and feet (third station) (optional)[1]	Two sagittal slabs or one coronal slab	Min TR/TE, FA 25–40°, < 1.5 mm slices, < 10 sec each, 8–10 acquisitions 10 mL contrast + 20 mL saline, 2–3 mL/sec
4 Pre-contrast 3D MRA sequence (1st station: abdomen/pelvis)	Coronal	Min TR/TE, FA 25–40°, sequential k-space filling, voxel size ≪ vessel diameter

(continued)

▶ **PROTOCOL: Three-Station Peripheral MRA (Renal Arteries to Feet) with Gadolinium Contrast and Moving Table (Option A)** (Continued)

5 Pre-contrast 3D MRA sequence (2nd station: thighs)	Coronal	Min TR/TE, FA 25–40°, centric k-space filling, voxel size ≪ vessel diameter
6 Pre-contrast 3D MRA sequence (3rd station: calves/feet)	Coronal	Min TR/TE, FA 25–40°, centric k-space filling, voxel size ≪ vessel diameter
7 Post-contrast 3D MRA sequence[2] (1st, 2nd, 3rd stations) First acquisition timed using test bolus or bolus detection (moving table)	Coronal	Same as pre-contrast: 20 mL contrast + saline, 2–3 mL/sec, then 10 mL at 1 mL/sec
8 Post-contrast T1-weighted imaging[3] (optional)	Axial	3D interpolated fat-suppressed spoiled GRE Min TR/TE, FA 12°, 2 mm slices, <20 sec

[1]Time-resolved imaging at distal station provides information about pedal vessel patency, including evaluation of retrograde filling of occluded vessels. The scan delay can be set to the circulation time measured at the level of the femoral heads. Acquisition time for each should be less than 10 sec, using parallel imaging algorithms. If available, automated subtraction and MIP reconstructions should be enabled to reduce image post-processing demands.
[2]With moving-table technology, the acquisitions following contrast injection should be performed in quick succession, with approximately 5 sec or less between each station for table movement.
[3]Contrast-enhanced 3D fat-suppressed images following the MRA can be helpful for evaluation of aneurysmal disease to assess for mural thrombus (Figure II4-23).

▶ **PROTOCOL: Four-Station Peripheral MRA (Renal Arteries to Feet) with Gadolinium Contrast and Manual Patient Move (Option B)**

Setup and Preparation	*Notes*
i.v.	22 G or larger
Gadolinium contrast	0.2 mmol/kg (40 mL)
ECG leads	Improves TOF acquisitions
Coil	Spine coil for calves Head coil for feet Body coil for moving-patient study: two stations (1) pelvis and (2) thighs
Positioning tips	Feet should be secured with toes pointing along the bore of the magnet. For moving-patient portion, legs should be secured with elastic binder and knees and calves slightly elevated so that all peripheral arteries are approximately in the same horizontal plane; subject should be placed on a plastic patient transfer board if table is not movable, and the board marked at 35–40 cm intervals once the subject is centered in the magnet for the first station
Subject instructions	End-expiratory breath holding for 1st station Supplemental oxygen by nasal cannula optional

(*continued*)

▶ **PROTOCOL: Four-Station Peripheral MRA (Renal Arteries to Feet) with Gadolinium Contrast and Manual Patient Move (Option B)** (Continued)

Calves (optional)[1]:

Sequence	Imaging Plane	Parameters
1 Scout (true FISP or spoiled GRE)	Multiplanar	Default
2 2D TOF	Axial	TR/TE/FA: 25/9/30° 3–4 mm slices, 0.5–1 mm overlap ECG triggered

Feet (optional)[1]:

Sequence	Imaging Plane	Parameters
1 Scout (true FISP or spoiled GRE)	Multiplanar	Default
2 2D TOF	Axial	TR/TE/FA: 25/9/30° 2–4 mm slices, 0.5 mm overlap ECG triggered

Abdomen/pelvis:

Sequence	Imaging Plane	Parameters
1 Scout (true FISP or spoiled GRE)	Multiplanar	Default
2 Pre-contrast 3D MRA sequence[2] (1st station)	Coronal	Min TR/TE, FA 25–40°, voxel size ≪ vessel diameter
3 Test bolus (optional)	Axial	Abdominal aorta Images every 1–2 sec 1 mL contrast + 20 mL saline, 2–3 mL/sec
4 Post-contrast 3D MRA sequence[2] (1st, 2nd, optional 3rd stations) First acquisition timed using test bolus or bolus detection (manual patient move)	Coronal	Same as pre-contrast; 2–3 acquisitions with 5 sec delay between each for move 20 mL contrast + saline, 2–3 mL/sec, then 10 mL at 1 mL/sec Allow 5 cm overlap of full of view between acquisitions
5 Post-contrast T1-weighted imaging[3] (optional)	Axial	3D interpolated fat-suppressed spoiled GRE Min TR/TE, FA 12°, 2 mm slices, < 20 sec

[1]Imaging the calves and feet may be unnecessary if the clinical history includes claudication and management options are nonsurgical.
[2]For the 1st and 2nd stations, although phased-array coils are preferable, the body coil may be used when the former are not available. The unenhanced acquisition of the 1st station should be performed first. If the table can be made to float, then an unenhanced acquisition of the 2nd station can also be performed. Otherwise, with the patient transfer board approach, the 2nd station is not imaged without contrast. Careful subject positioning is necessary in the 2nd station to ensure that vessels in the thighs are in the same horizontal plane as in the 1st station, so that the slab positioned for the 1st station correctly applies to the second. For the contrast-enhanced acquisitions, the same 3D acquisition is repeated 2–3 times with a 5 sec delay programmed between each. The subject is moved manually during the delays. Although image quality in the 3rd station (calves and feet) using the body coil is suboptimal, it can be performed as part of the bolus chase.
[3]Contrast-enhanced imaging through the abdomen and pelvis is optional but useful for detecting and characterizing incidental pathology such as renal masses.

▶ **PROTOCOL: Three-Station Peripheral MRA (Renal Arteries to Feet) with Gadolinium Contrast with Separate Stations (Option C)**

Setup and Preparation	Notes
i.v.	22 G or larger
Gadolinium contrast	0.3 mmol/kg (45–60 mL)
Coil	Torso phased-array coil for each station
Positioning tips	Feet should be secured with toes pointing along the bore of the magnet
Subject instructions	End-expiratory breath holding for 1st station Supplemental oxygen by nasal cannula optional

Calves and feet (3rd station)[1]:

Sequence	Imaging Plane	Parameters
1 Scout (true FISP or spoiled GRE)	Multiplanar	Default
2 Pre-contrast 3D MRA sequence	Coronal	Min TR/TE, FA 25–40°, voxel size ≪ vessel diameter
3 Test bolus (optional)	Axial	Popliteal arteries Images every 1–2 sec 2 mL contrast + 20 mL saline, 2–3 mL/sec

4 Post-contrast 3D MRA sequence
  (a) First acquisition timed using test bolus or bolus detection
  (b) Repeat acquisition a few sec after first acquisition
	Coronal	Same as pre-contrast:
		15 mL contrast + saline, 2–3 mL/sec, then 10 mL at 1 mL/sec

5 Post-contrast T1-weighted imaging[2] (optional)	Axial	3D interpolated fat-suppressed spoiled GRE Min TR/TE, FA 12°, 2 mm slices, <20 sec

Thighs (2nd station):

Sequence	Imaging Plane	Parameters
1 Scout (True FISP or spoiled GRE)	Multiplanar	Default
2 Pre-contrast 3D MRA sequence	Coronal	Min TR/TE, FA 25–40°, voxel size ≪ vessel diameter

3 Post-contrast 3D MRA sequence
  (a) First acquisition timed using test bolus (adjusted slightly) or bolus detection
  (b) Repeat acquisition a few sec after first acquisition
	Coronal	Same as pre-contrast:
		18 mL contrast plus saline, 2–3 mL/sec

4 Post-contrast T1-weighted imaging[2] (optional)	Axial	3D interpolated fat-suppressed spoiled GRE Min TR/TE, FA 12°, 2 mm slices, <20 sec

(continued)

▶ **PROTOCOL: Three-Station Peripheral MRA (Renal Arteries to Feet) with Gadolinium Contrast with Separate Stations (Option C)** (Continued)

Abdomen and pelvis (1st station):

Sequence	*Imaging Plane*	*Parameters*
1 Scout (true FISP or spoiled GRE)	Multiplanar	Default
2 Pre-contrast 3D MRA sequence	Coronal	Min TR/TE, FA 25–40°, voxel size ≪ vessel diameter
3 Test bolus (optional)	Axial	Abdominal aorta Images every 1–2 sec 1 mL contrast + 20 mL saline, 2–3 mL/sec
4 Post-contrast 3D MRA sequence (a) First acquisition timed using test bolus or bolus detection (b) Repeat acquisition a few sec after first acquisition	Coronal	Same as pre-contrast: 24 mL contrast plus saline, 2–3 mL/sec
5 Post-contrast T1-weighted imaging[2] (optional)	Axial	3D interpolated fat-suppressed spoiled GRE Min TR/TE, FA 12°, 2 mm slices, <20 sec

[1]The total dose of gadolinium contrast material administered should not exceed 0.3 mmol/kg. Allocation of contrast material should increase from station to station.

[2]Contrast-enhanced 3D fat-suppressed images following the MRA can be helpful for evaluation of aneurysmal disease and to assess for mural thrombus (Figure II4-23). Contrast-enhanced imaging through the abdomen and pelvis is optional but useful for detecting and characterizing incidental pathology such as renal masses.

▶ **PROTOCOL: MR Venography of Chest with Gadolinium Contrast**

Setup and Preparation	Notes
i.v.	22 G or larger; intravenous access contralateral to side of disease
Gadolinium contrast	0.2 mmol/kg (30–40 mL)
Coil	Torso phased-array coil
Positioning tips	Supine, head first
Subject instructions	End-expiratory breath holding Supplemental oxygen by nasal cannula optional

Sequence	Imaging Plane	Parameters
1 Scout (true FISP or spoiled GRE)	Multiplanar	Default
2 SSFP or TOF[1]	Axial and sagittal	5–7 mm slices
3 Pre-contrast 3D MRA sequence	Coronal	Min TR/TE, FA 25–40°, voxel size a vessel diameter

4 Test bolus (optional)	Axial	Thoracic aorta
		  Images every 1–2 sec
		  1 mL contrast + 20 mL
		  saline, 2–3 mL/sec

5 Post-contrast 3D MRA sequence[2]
  (a) First acquisition timed using test bolus or bolus detection
  (b) Repeat acquisition 60 sec after first acquisition
  (c) Repeat acquisition 120 sec after first acquisition
	Coronal	Same as pre-contrast;
		  3 acquisitions;
		  40 mL contrast + saline, 2–3 mL/sec

6 Post-contrast T1-weighted imaging[3] (optional)	Axial	3D interpolated fat-suppressed spoiled GRE Min TR/TE, FA 12°, 2 mm slices, < 20 sec

[1]Vascular scout images are useful for positioning the 3D acquisition and can be performed using SSFP (such as true FISP) or 2D TOF imaging. With TOF, saturation bands on the arterial side of the slices helps clarify venous structures.

[2]Image post-processing can include subtraction of the arterial acquisition from the delayed acquisition to produce an image that depicts veins but not arteries (Figure II4-21).

[3]Contrast-enhanced 3D fat-suppressed images following the MRA can be helpful for evaluation of extraluminal causes of venous obstruction.

Cardiac
MR Imaging

ECG Gating

Section III is devoted to cardiac MR applications. The first two chapters describe some basic principles common to all cardiac MRI: synchronization of acquisitions with cardiac motion (Chapter III-1) and orientations of imaging planes (Chapter III-2). The remainder of the chapters are dedicated to specific types of sequences and applications with sample protocols provided to illustrate their implementation in clinical practice.

One of the most important requirements for successful cardiac MR imaging is the accurate synchronization of data acquisition with respect to motion of the beating heart. The images produced then accurately reflect the state of the heart during its different stages of contraction and relaxation and have minimal motion artifacts. To achieve synchronization, the electrical activity of the heart is used to control timing of the MR acquisition. This technique is called *electrocardiographic (ECG)-gating*. To generate an image, k-space data are typically collected across multiple heart beats. For some sequences, such as spin echo anatomic imaging or contrast-enhanced infarct imaging, echoes are typically collected during the end of the cardiac cycle, when there is minimal motion during diastole. For functional imaging, such as cine gradient echo imaging or phase contrast flow quantification, data are collected throughout the cardiac cycle and then partitioned into separate k-space frames, each correponding to a short segment of the cardiac cycle. Each k-space then reflects a snapshot of the heart during the cardiac cycle. When viewed together in a cinematic loop to produce a "beating heart" video clip, *cine MRI* enables the viewer to assess cardiac motion.

Failure to achieve good gating is the most common and frustrating problem with cardiac MRI. This chapter reviews the specific concepts and terminology associated with ECG synchronization and provides suggestions for troubleshooting.

KEY CONCEPTS

▶ ECG recordings are used to synchronize cardiac MRI data acquisition with specific phases of the cardiac cycle.

▶ The most common sources of poor ECG gating are suboptimal electrode placement, patient arrhythmias, and faulty detection of the R wave. The last is caused by the RF pulse and gradients interfering with the ECG and by blood magnetohydrodynamic effects.

▶ S-T segment changes due to blood magnetohydrodynamic effects can also interfere with ECG gating and impair detection of S-T changes associated with myocardial ischemia.

▶ Peripheral pulse gating is a quick and simple alternative to central gating, although delay of the pulse wave relative to the R wave of the ECG may require parameter adjustment.

▶ Retrospectively gated sequences provide a useful alternative to prospectively triggered sequences. Retrospective gating enables imaging throughout the cardiac cycle.

ELECTROCARDIOGRAM: A REVIEW

The *electrocardiogram (ECG)* tracing depicts the electrical activity of the heart (Figure III1-1). The P wave represents atrial depolarization and the onset of atrial contraction. The QRS complex reflects the electrical activity associated with ventricular depolarization preceding systole. The onset of left ventricular systolic contraction occurs about 50 msec after the R wave, and contraction lasts for about 150–250 msec. The T wave represents repolarization of the ventricle. Until the next QRS, the ventricle remains in diastole.

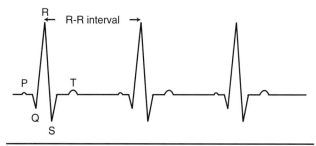

FIGURE III1-1. Schematic diagram of standard electrocardiogram (ECG).

Heart Rate and R-R Interval

The heart rate can be expressed in two ways with ECG-gated sequences: frequency of heartbeats (bpm) or duration of each heartbeat (msec), the latter commonly referred to as the *R-R interval*. Most scanners will provide both values based on the MR ECG tracing. Otherwise, the conversion can be calculated manually:

$$R\text{-}R \text{ interval (msec)} = \frac{60,000}{\text{heart rate (bpm)}}$$

For example, a heart rate of 60 bpm corresponds to an R-R interval of 1000 msec or 1 sec. For a heart rate of 72 bpm, the R-R interval is 60,000/72 or 833 msec. Table III1-1 shows representative heart rates and corresponding R-R intervals.

> **IMPORTANT CONCEPT:** The R-R interval, measured in msec, is the time between consecutive heartbeats. The R-R interval can be calculated as 60,000 divided by the heart rate in beats per minute (bpm).

MR TERMINOLOGY FOR THE ECG TRACING

To synchronize the MR acquisition with the cardiac cycle, conventional *ECG-triggered* sequences rely on detection of the R wave, because it is usually the most prominent feature of the ECG tracing. MR data acquisition usually begins following an R wave. Then, when the data acquisition for a given R-R interval is completed, the scanner waits for the next R wave (Figure III1-2). This pattern of triggering is referred to as *prospective triggering*. Prospective ECG-triggering will be considered standard. There are other types of triggering and gating, which will be discussed later in this chapter.

Terminology specific to ECG-gated MR pulse sequences is reviewed in the following paragraphs. In some cases, the terms may vary across vendors; however, the basic concepts are generally the same.

▶ **TABLE III1-1 Heart Rates (Beats per Minute) and Corresponding R-R Intervals (msec)**

Heart rate (bpm)	R-R interval (msec)	Acquisition Window 85–90% R-R (msec)
50	1200	1020–1080
60	1000	850–900
65	923	785–830
70	857	730–770
75	800	680–720
80	750	640–675
90	667	570–600
100	600	510–540
110	545	460–490
120	500	430–450

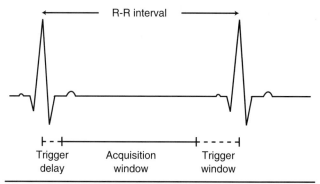

FIGURE III1-2. Nomenclature for ECG-triggered MR acquisitions. For systolic imaging, the trigger delay is zero.

Trigger Delay

For ECG-triggered sequences, the R wave initiates the MR pulse sequence. Imaging that begins immediately after the R wave starts just before the onset of ventricular systole. However, imaging does not have to start immediately after the R wave. For some sequences, such as spin echo imaging, diastolic images may be desired. To obtain diastolic images with R-wave triggering, a delay, called the *trigger delay (TD)*, of at least 150–250 msec is introduced between the detection of the R wave and the start of imaging.

Acquisition Window

Once initiated, the pulse sequence can include a single or multiple RF excitations and echoes. The total duration of data sampling in each heartbeat is called the *acquisition window*. For most prospectively gated cine gradient echo imaging, the acquisition window is about 85–90% of the R-R interval. Sample acquisition window values for subjects with different heart rates are shown in Table III1-1, assuming no trigger delay.

Echoes are typically grouped according to their time interval following the R-wave so that different images correspond to distinct time points of the cardiac cycle.

During each cardiac cycle, usually only a small portion of the data needed to generate each image is collected. Therefore, data acquisition is repeated over many heartbeats.

Trigger Window

If the pulse sequence is designed to acquire data during each heartbeat, then the duration of the acquisition window must fit comfortably within one R-R interval. At the conclusion of each period of data acquisition, the system will ready itself for detection of another R wave to begin the process again. Because subject heart rates are not perfectly constant, it is advisable to leave a reasonable interval between the end of data sampling and the next expected R wave, called the *trigger window (TW)*. In this way, if the QRS is initiated slightly earlier than expected, it will still be detected. Typically the trigger window is defined as 10–15% of the R-R interval (Figure III1-2).

CHALLENGE QUESTION: The trigger window results in exclusion of which portion of the cardiac cycle?

Answer: Assuming no trigger delay, the acquisition window is usually the first 85–90% of the R-R interval. The portion of the cardiac cycle that is excluded usually corresponds to late diastole, just before the QRS complex.

> **IMPORTANT CONCEPTS:** For most ECG-triggered sequences, the imaging parameters should be set up by considering the R-R interval in terms of the following components: trigger delay, acquisition window, and trigger window.

Trigger Frequency

In most of the foregoing discussion, each and every R wave is assumed to initiate data acquisition. However, for some sequences, depending on the desired image contrast, only every other or every third R wave may be used to trigger data acquisition. A parameter called *trigger frequency* determines how frequently an R wave triggers the acquisition.

Acquisition Times

Because subject heart rates vary, acquisition times for different ECG-gated sequences are difficult to predict. Rather than use actual times measured in seconds, it is more practical to think of acquisition times in numbers of heartbeats. Accuracy of predicted acquisition times will depend on how regular the subject's heart rate is and how reliable the gating is. To minimize artifacts associated with respiratory motion, many cardiac MR sequences are performed while the subject suspends respiration. Most

subjects can hold their breath for at least 12–15 heartbeats.

ECG TRACINGS: A HOW-TO

Before the start of every cardiac MRI study, MR-compatible ECG leads should be placed on the subject's chest. It is important to use MR-compatible electrodes and to follow carefully manufacturer's guidelines for their use. To prevent burns, MR electrodes are typically high-impedance electrodes. Three or four electrodes are positioned around the left chest, usually about 4–6 inches apart, either on the anterior chest or on the back (Figure III1-3). It is important to place the electrodes fairly closely together to ensure a high-amplitude signal. For women with large or pendulous breasts, inferior electrodes should be placed immediately under the left breast on the anterior or left chest wall. Good contact between the ECG electrodes and skin is vital and may necessitate shaving of hirsute patients and use of a gentle skin abrasive such as NuPrep (D.O. Weaver and Co, Aurora, CO). MR-compatible lead pads typically have prepackaged conductive gel to improve contact between ECG electrodes and the skin. If the ECG wires are too lengthy, they should be twisted or braided. Loops or circular coil patterns should be avoided.

The MR system usually relies on a high amplitude or steep slope of the R wave to trigger the MR acquisitions. However, the relative amplitude of the R and T waves may vary depending on the subject and the configuration of the leads. Lead polarity typically defaults to a preset configuration, but it is often possible to adjust lead polarity to optimize the ECG triggering (these may be labeled using conventional ECG terms such as I, II, III, aVF, aVR, and aVL). Tracings with desirable features for R wave detection can usually be obtained by toggling through lead polarity options at the console or at the magnet control panel (Figure III1-4).

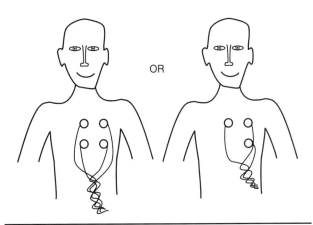

OR

FIGURE III1-3. ECG lead placements vary depending on the type of ECG gating design. Note the twisted or braided configuration of the long wires.

Lead Polarity   ECG Tracing

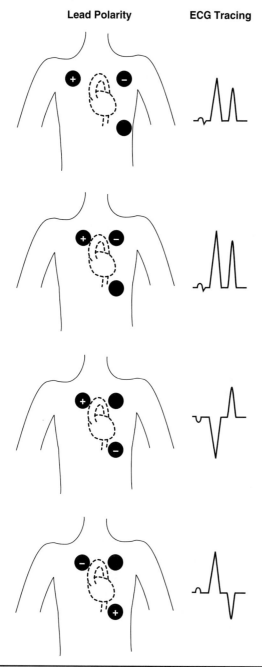

FIGURE III1-4. ECG lead placement and polarity. If the electrodes are placed too far apart, the amplitude of the signal will be attenuated (top). Once the electrodes are repositioned (second), toggling through lead polarity (bottom three) adjusts the appearance of the ECG tracing for improved R wave detection (bottom).

ECG TRACINGS: PROBLEM SOLVING

A summary of common problems encountered with ECG tracings is given in Table III1-2, along with suggestions for possible solutions.

It is common that adequate ECG tracings are obtained while the subject is outside of the bore of the magnet, but

▶ **TABLE III1-2 Basic Troubleshooting Guide**

Problem	Causes	Solutions
Intermittent or absent signal	Poor skin contact	Check electrodes and replace adhesive pads if necessary Shave skin if necessary NuPrep (D.O. Weaver & Co. Aurora, CO) gentle skin abrasive
	Lead cable loose or disconnected	Check lead cable
	Respiratory motion	Consider placing leads on the back
Low amplitude R waves	Signal dampened by tissues	Adjust electrode positions: move closer together and off of breast tissue
	Suboptimal ECG lead selection or polarity	Toggle lead polarity
T waves exceed R waves	Suboptimal ECG lead selection or polarity	Toggle lead polarity
		Vectorcardiograms, if available

once scanning begins, ECG synchronization fails. In some cases the reason for poor synchronization becomes evident right away. A lead may become loose or disconnected and give only intermittent signals. At other times the problem becomes apparent only during scanning. Experienced MR operators listen carefully for the regularity and timing of the sounds emitted by the MR system during ECG-triggered sequences. Poor synchronization can often be heard as irregular MR system sounds ("wahh . . . wahh . . . wahh . . . . wahh . . . wahh-wahh") compared to a subject's regular heart rhythm. It is also important to realize that regular sounds do not necessarily mean perfect gating. For example, triggering off every other heartbeat when every heartbeat is desired will generate regular scanner sounds, although its knocking frequency will be too low.

There are two main reasons why synchronization fails in the scanner: patient arrhythmias and failure of the system to detect the R wave for triggering. These are each discussed next.

Patient Arrhythmias

For ECG-triggered sequences, data acquisition assumes a regular heart rate. Following the R wave, the system begins collecting data, portions of which are assigned to different k-space domains corresponding to different time points in the cardiac cycle. If the heart rate is regular, then all the data collected shortly after the R wave will reflect the left ventricle in systole, while the data toward the end of the R-R interval will image the ventricle in diastole. Figure III1-5 illustrates what happens when the heart rate

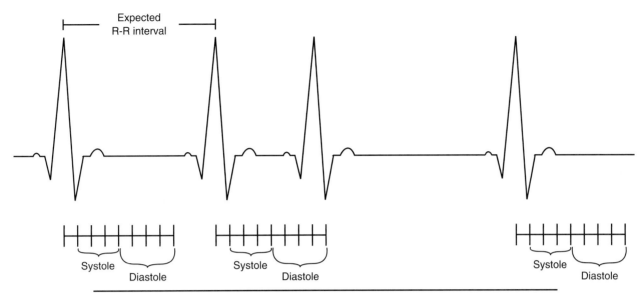

FIGURE III1-5. Irregular heart rate causes irregular triggering, which degrades image quality and lengthens acquisition times.

is irregular. During the second R-R interval, the data collected toward the end of that acquisition window should correspond to diastole, but, because of the premature onset of the third heartbeat, will instead reflect systole. This corrupts the data. The images that should depict diastole will now contain a mix of systolic and diastolic data. To make matters worse, the acquisition time in subjects with irregular heart rates is also longer than expected. In Figure III1-5, for the first three heartbeats, only two sets of data are collected. The third set of data will be collected only after the fourth heartbeat.

Although an occasional irregular beat is tolerable, frequent irregularities cause poor quality and misleading images.

CHALLENGE QUESTION: Heart rates frequently change during breath holding. What is the consequence of a significant heart rate increase above the resting rate during the breath hold acquisition of an ECG-triggered sequence?

Answer: If the heart rate increases significantly, the R-R interval shortens considerably compared to the expected acquisition window. This will cause data to be collected only after every other heartbeat. The acquisition time will be twice as long as expected. If the heart rate is consistent, then the images will still be interpretable although the end diastole images may appear systolic.

IMPORTANT CONCEPTS: With ECG-triggered sequences, arrhythmias can result in erratic triggering and inaccurate depictions of cardiac function. Heart rates that exceed those expected can result in triggering with every other heartbeat and consequently longer acquisition times.

▶ **TABLE III1-3 Fast Imaging Sequences for Subjects with Arrhythmias**

Type of Sequence	Robust to Arrhythmias
Black-blood spin echo	Single-shot double inversion recovery fast spin echo
Bright-blood cine GRE	Real-time cine True FISP
Phase-contrast flow quantification	Real-time phase-contrast (under development)

The imaging of subjects with serious arrhythmias requires special consideration. A general solution is to use faster imaging sequences. Table III1-3 lists specific sequences for imaging subjects with arrhythmias.

A double inversion-recovery single-shot half-Fourier sequence acquires a black-blood image in under a heartbeat (see Chapter III-3). Real-time true FISP sequences acquire all the data for a given frame in less than 100 msec and therefore do not even require cardiac gating (see Chapter III-4). With fast real-time phase-contrast flow quantification sequences, velocities can be sampled in specific regions with real-time or continuous updating. When combined with interactive positioning devices, real-time phase contrast MRI has the potential to function like Doppler ultrasound or echocardiography. Unlike the fast black- and bright-blood methods, real-time phase contrast methods are not yet commercially available.

Faulty Detection of the R Wave

A more pervasive and challenging problem with cardiac MRI is the faulty detection of the R wave for ECG-triggering. This is most commonly due to erroneous triggering due to a prominent T wave. Some of the simplest sources of faulty detection have been discussed above and are listed in Table III1-2. Two more complex sources of error are described next, together with their solutions:

Induced Currents

RF pulses and gradient switching induce currents in the usual carbon fiber ECG wires. These currents can cause spikes that lead to faulty triggering. *Fiber optic cables* transmit the ECG signal by means of light rather than electric current and are more resilient to electromagnetic effects.

Magnetohydrodynamic Effects

The most problematic source of artifactual triggering is due to the magnetohydrodynamic effect of moving blood within the magnetic field. Recall from electromagnetic theory (Chapter I-1) that electrical charges moving through a magnetic field induce a voltage. Blood contains many charged particles (Na^+, Cl^-, HCO_3^-, among others). When these ions move through blood vessels in the setting of a magnetic field, a voltage can be detected, particularly during systole or the ST portion of the ECG tracing. Distortion of the ST portion and peaking or elevation of the T waves (Figure III1-6) results in faulty triggering wherever the T wave is higher than the R wave. Triggering off of the T wave means that much of systole is missed.

New vectorcardiographic approaches (see below) reduce artifactual triggering from the magnetohydrodynamic effect.

> **IMPORTANT CONCEPTS:** Faulty ECG gating can be solved with careful attention to technique, such as better lead contact and testing different lead polarity options. Arrhythmias are more challenging and call for faster imaging sequences that are more resilient in the setting of irregular heart rates. Distorted signals from the blood magnetohydrodynamic effect are harder to solve; more sophisticated solutions, such as vector cardiogram approaches, are preferred.

One important consequence of the magnetohydrodynamic effect is that important ECG changes, such as ST depression or elevation in the setting of ischemia, may be impossible to detect in the magnet bore. As will be discussed in Chapter III-7, changes in ventricular contractility are more sensitive than ECG changes. Fast cine imaging is typically used when imaging subjects with ischemic heart disease, and using dobutamine pharmacologic stress.

> **IMPORTANT CONCEPT:** Distortion of the ST portion of the ECG tracing by the magnetic field limits detection of ST changes in the setting of myocardial ischemia.

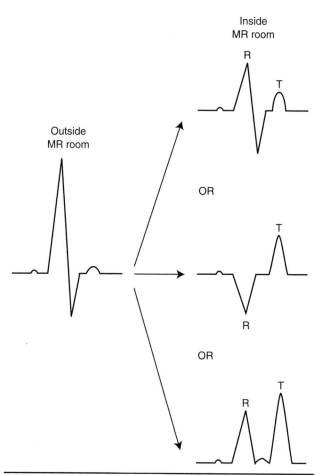

FIGURE III1-6. Distortion of the ECG in the magnetic field due to the magnetohydrodynamic effect.

VECTORCARDIOGRAM TRIGGERING

To overcome magnetohydrodynamic effects, *vectorcardiogram (VCG)*-based triggering systems (1, 2) are commercially available. With vectorcardiography, the electrical activity of the heart is depicted both temporally and spatially, using measured signal from all three leads (Figure III1-7). Because the orientation of the electrical axis of the heart is different from the artifacts associated with the magnetohydrodynamic effect, the vectorcardiogram is more accurate at detecting cardiac activity.

PERIPHERAL PULSE GATING

Occasionally, adequate ECG tracings cannot be obtained, perhaps because of a subject's body habitus or other interference with signal measurement, such as a large pericardial effusion. Peripheral pulse gating is a viable alternative when central gating is not possible. Like plethysmography, peripheral pulse gating detects the pulse wave of

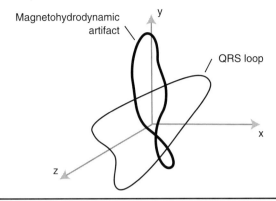

FIGURE III1-7. Vectorcardiogram depicts measured spatial changes in voltages over time. QRS signals follow predictable paths, while the magnetohydrodynamic artifacts give rise to VCG loops that have distinctly different orientations. VCG triggering occurs when the measured signal closely approximates the expected path of the QRS loop.

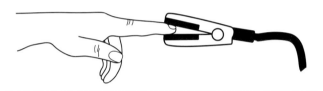

FIGURE III1-8. Peripheral pulse monitor.

blood as it transits through the fingers. Typically peripheral pulse gating monitors are clipped to the fingertips or toes (Figure III1-8). Note that nail polish interferes with the signal measurement. Only MR-compatible peripheral pulse monitors should be used and their operating guidelines followed carefully.

CHALLENGE QUESTION: How would ECG-triggered and peripheral pulse-triggered acquisitions differ in the timing of images relative to the cardiac cycle?

Answer: The R wave typically precedes the onset of systole by about 50 msec. Therefore ECG-triggered sequences (with no trigger delay) start at end diastole and include all of systole. The propagation of the systolic pulse wave in the vascular system requires about 200 msec or more. Imaging that is triggered by the peripheral pulse wave will start after the onset of left ventricular systole (Figure III1-9).

Peripheral pulse monitors are easy to use. However, to ensure imaging during systole (Figure III1-9), prospectively triggered imaging protocols should incorporate a longer trigger delay or double the acquisition window. When available, retrospective gating is well suited for peripheral pulse gating.

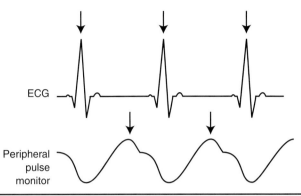

FIGURE III1-9. ECG and peripheral pulse monitor tracings show the temporal relationship between peak R wave and peak peripheral pulse wave (arrows). Peripheral pulse waves occur in early diastole, and so a portion of systole may be missed with prospectively triggered peripheral pulse monitoring.

GATING VERSUS TRIGGERING

The terms *gating* and *triggering* can be confusing. They are often used interchangeably. Generally, gating refers to any means of relating MR data acquisition to the phase of the cardiac cycle during which the data were acquired. Gating can be either prospective or retrospective. Triggering is one form of prospective gating, whereby the MR sequence is initiated with the R wave.

RETROSPECTIVE GATING

Many ECG-gated sequences can also be performed with *retrospective gating* (Figure III1-10). Retrospective gating means that the data are acquired continuously, along with a recording of the ECG tracing. After the acquisition, the imaging data are retrospectively sorted based on the time of the echoes relative to the R-wave. Retrospectively gated sequences provide information about imaging through the entire cardiac cycle, including the full duration of diastole, provided that the patient's heart rhythm is sufficiently regular. Compared to prospectively gated sequences, the image reconstruction of retrospectively-gated sequences is more complex and computationally intensive.

CHALLENGE QUESTION: Why is retrospective gating preferable with peripheral pulse monitoring?

Answer: Prospective gating can be problematic with peripheral pulse monitoring because the peripheral pulse wave may coincide with early diastole, while imaging of systole may be missed during the trigger window (Figure III1-9). Retrospective gating is necessary to include the full duration of systole.

With retrospective gating, the temporal spacing of the frames can be defined by the user, regardless of the true or effective TR of the sequence (Figure III1-11). As illustrated in Figure III1-11, several post-processing steps are necessary to construct images from the data collected. First, all R-R intervals are adjusted to equal a representative R-R interval by expanding or compressing the spacing between echoes. Then, the user-defined temporal resolution is approximated by assigning each echo to the nearest time point desired. For the example in Figure III1-11, to use data from different heartbeats with different R-R intervals, the system stretches or shrinks the time course of each to fit a standard R-R interval, 600 msec in this example. To attain the user-defined temporal resolution, the echoes nearest to the desired time frame contribute to that frame. Two reconstructions are demonstrated: 30 msec and 50 msec temporal resolution.

REAL-TIME IMAGING

Real-time MR imaging consists of the rapid collection and reconstruction of MR images. For cardiac MRI, the aim is to generate images akin to echocardiography. Commercially available sequences include real-time steady-state free precession (true FISP) sequences for imaging cardiac motion, with each frame generated in less than 100 msec. With real time acquisitions, ECG-gating can be obviated. In some cases, however, ECG-triggering may still be advantageous to ensure that acquisitions at multiple slice positions are all initiated at the same time point

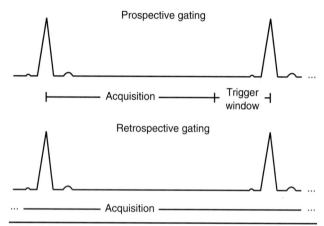

FIGURE III1-10. Prospective versus retrospective gating.

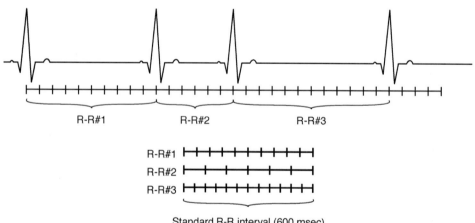

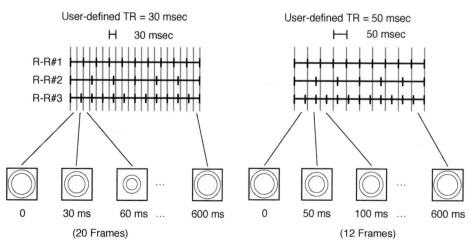

FIGURE III1-11. Retrospective gating with continuous collection of data and ECG tracing.

of the cardiac cycle. For example, a series of short-axis cine true FISP images can be configured to begin immediately after an R wave and then to continue for 1–2 sec at each slice position. In this way, each slice will be imaged starting at the same point in the cardiac cycle. Interactive slice positioning devices are under development. The aim is to allow the user to control the imaging slice plane at the console during the acquisitions. The clinical applications of these new tools are likely to be broad.

REVIEW QUESTIONS

1. A subject has a resting heart rate of 60 bpm. You wish to perform an ECG-gated cine MRI sequence for left ventricular function.
   a. What is the subject's R-R interval? What settings might you choose for a trigger delay, acquisition window, and trigger window?
   b. You ask the subject to hold her breath for this sequence. Her heart rate goes up to 100 bpm. What is the new R-R interval? Having set the parameters in (a) anticipating a heart rate of 60 bpm, what will happen to the acquisition now? How will the acquisition time change?

2. You wish to measure total blood flow through the ascending aorta as an estimate of cardiac output. You have the choice of a prospectively or retrospectively gated phase contrast flow quantification sequence. Which should you choose and why?

3. During an MRA study of the thoracic aorta, you notice a markedly widened aortic root and dilated left ventricle. You suspect aortic valvular disease and wish to perform an ECG-gated cine MRI acquisition. However, the patient does not have central ECG leads on her chest, and because of a tight schedule, you only have a few minutes to acquire more images. You place a peripheral pulse monitor on the subject's index finger and obtain a strong signal.
   a. Your prospectively triggered cine gradient echo sequence has the following ECG settings: trigger delay = 0, acquisition window = 90% R-R interval, and trigger window = 10% R-R interval. How good is your ability to diagnose aortic stenosis versus aortic insufficiency on these images? Assume that the findings of aortic stenosis are seen during systole and aortic insufficiency during diastole.
   b. To image the remainder of the cardiac cycle, how might you modify the sequence parameters?
   c. What alternative sequence might you use to obtain images of the full cardiac cycle more efficiently?

REFERENCES

1. Fischer SE, Wickline SA, Lorenz CH. Novel real-time R-wave detection algorithm based on the vectorcardiogram for accurate gated magnetic resonance acquisitions. Magn Reson Med 1999; 42:361–370.
2. Chia JM, Fischer SE, Wickline SA, Lorenz CH. Performance of QRS detection for cardiac magnetic resonance imaging with a novel vectorcardiographic triggering method. J Magn Reson Imaging 2000; 12:678–688.

Cardiac Imaging Planes

In contrast to most other MRI applications, the imaging planes typically used in cardiac MRI are defined with respect to the orientation of the heart. These planes depict the left ventricle in three orthogonal planes: the *horizontal long axis (four-chamber view), vertical long axis (two-chamber view)*, and *short axis* planes (Figure III2-1). These imaging planes are doubly oblique relative to the conventional axial, sagittal, and coronal axes of imaging, and they differ from subject to subject depending on the particular orientation of the left ventricle, which can vary with respect to the body. In this chapter, a step-by-step guide is presented for positioning slice planes in the desired orientations. Additional views are also discussed.

THE THREE MAIN PLANES

The main planes used for cardiac imaging include two long axis views (the horizontal and vertical long axis) and the short axis view (Figure III2-1). The long axis is defined as the line that passes through the center of the mitral valve orifice and the left ventricular apex. For most studies, a series of short axis views are obtained from the left ventricular base, at the level of the mitral valve, to the apex. The three main planes are called *orthogonal views* because they are each perpendicular to each other. Depending on the orientation of the heart, each of these views is usually oriented obliquely to conventional axial, sagittal, and coronal planes. A systematic method for obtaining images in the correct planes is presented in the following subsections.

The process of obtaining images in the desired doubly oblique planes should take less than 2–3 minutes. For each step, a fast imaging sequence, similar to that used for scout imaging, should be used. This may consist of a fast spoiled gradient echo or balanced steady-state gradient echo (true FISP), or double inversion recovery single-shot fast spin echo sequence. For these sequences, imaging each slice requires 1 sec or less. It is important that the subject's heart be in the same position for each step. Breath holding at end-expiration is generally preferable over breath holding at end-inspiration. If the subject has limited breath-holding capacity, supplemental oxygen via nasal cannula should be provided.

> **IMPORTANT CONCEPT:** To obtain desirable slice positioning, subjects should be instructed to suspend respiration at end-expiration for greater reproducibility. Oxygen via nasal cannula can help improve a subject's ability to suspend respiration.

Step 1: Finding a Transverse Image through the Left Ventricle and Septum

The approach start with routine scout images, which include a standard coronal image of the chest (Figure III2-2). From this coronal view, a series of transaxial images is positioned through the heart. Among the transverse slices, an image that depicts both left and right ventricles and the interventricular septum is selected (Figure III2-3).

Step 2: Defining a Two-Chamber Scout from the Transverse Image

Based on the axial image identified in Step 1, an oblique coronal slice is positioned through the left ventricle that is parallel to the interventricular septum and passes through the left ventricular apex (Figure III2-3). This will produce a long axis view of the heart referred to as a two-chamber scout view.

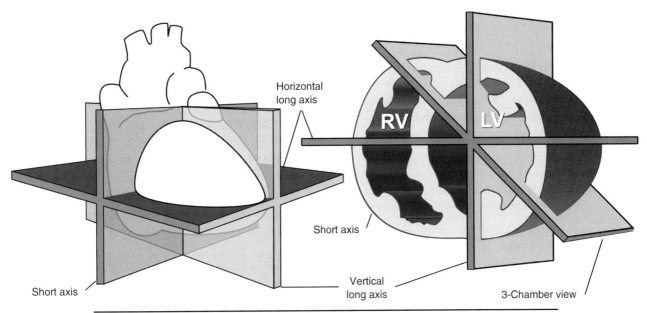

FIGURE III2-1. Conventional imaging planes of the heart. On the left, a whole-heart view depicts the plane defining the short axis view, as shown on the right, together with the planes defining the horizontal, vertical and three-chamber long axis views.

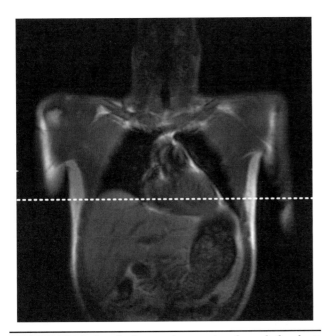

FIGURE III2-2. Standard coronal scout view through the chest. Of a series of axial slices positioned through the left ventricle (Step 1), at least one (dotted line) will depict the left ventricle and the interventricular septum.

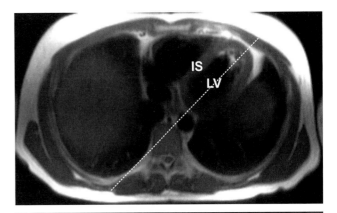

FIGURE III2-3. Axial image through the left ventricle (LV) and interventricular septum (IS) allows positioning of an oblique coronal slice (dashed line, Step 2) parallel to the IS and through the LV apex. The resulting two-chamber scout image is shown in the left panel of Figure III2-4.

Step 3: Obtaining a Short Axis View from the Two-Chamber Scout and a Transverse Image

In subjects whose hearts are vertically oriented, the two chamber scout view (Figure III2-4, left panel) may serve

as a good vertical long axis view. In general, for a true vertical long axis, additional adjustment is needed (see Step 5).

A plane aligned perpendicular to the long axis of the heart on both the two-chamber scout view and the original transverse image (Figure III2-4) gives a short axis view. The resulting short axis plane is a doubly oblique slice plane. The short axis view is used for subsequent positioning of the long axes.

Step 4: Defining a Horizontal Long Axis View from a Short Axis and Two-Chamber Scout

Using the short axis and the two-chamber scout, the horizontal long axis (four-chamber view) can be positioned by bisecting the left ventricle in the horizontal plane. As a guide to the "horizontal" plane, the line should bisect both the left and right ventricles and be parallel to the diaphragm (Figure III2-5).

Step 5: Obtaining a Vertical Long Axis View from the Horizontal Long Axis and Short Axis

Using the horizontal long axis view (four-chamber) and the short axis view, a true vertical long axis view can be defined by bisecting the left ventricle in the vertical plane (Figure III2-6). Note that, in this example, the true vertical

long axis and the two-chamber scout differ only slightly by the off-axis tilt away from a straight vertical line through the short axis. The resulting image through the left ventricle, left atrium, and mitral valve is shown in Figure III2-7.

ADDITIONAL COMMONLY USED IMAGING PLANES

Left Ventricular Outflow Tract/Ascending Aorta

In subjects with ascending aortic pathology, imaging the left ventricle, aortic valve, and ascending aorta can be

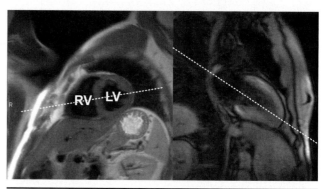

FIGURE III2-5. Positioning of the horizontal long axis view (Step 4) using the short axis view (left) and the two-chamber scout (right). The horizontal long axis plane passes from the midpoint of the mitral valve orifice through the left ventricular apex and usually lies parallel to the diaphragm, bisecting the left ventricle (LV) and right ventricle (RV).

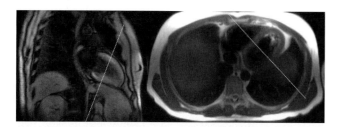

FIGURE III2-4. Positioning of a short axis view (Step 3) using the two-chamber scout (left) and the original axial image (right). The doubly oblique short axis view should be perpendicular to the interventricular septum and perpendicular to the long axis of the left ventricle in both views.

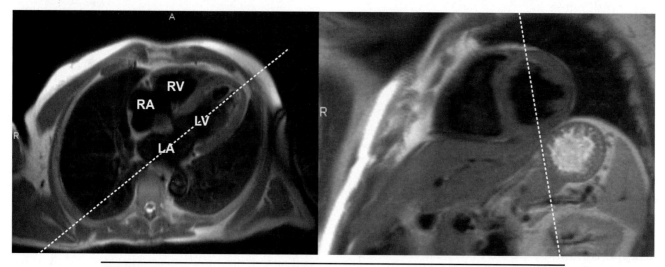

FIGURE III2-6. Positioning of a vertical long axis (two-chamber) view (Step 5) using the horizontal long axis or four-chamber view (left) and the short axis view (right). The plane of the vertical long axis view extends from the center of the mitral valve orifice to the left ventricular apex and bisects the left ventricle (LV). The four-chamber view also shows the right atrium (RA), right ventricle (RV), and left atrium (LA).

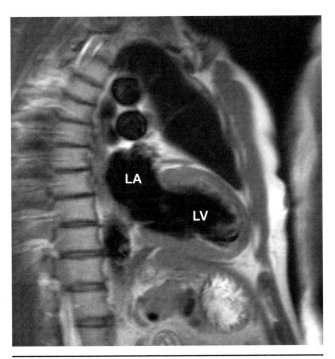

FIGURE III2-7. Vertical long axis or two-chamber view provides another view of the left atrium (LA), left ventricle (LV), and mitral valve.

extremely useful. This view can be obtained by using transverse slices (see Step 1 in the preceding section) to orient a single oblique slice through the aortic root and left ventricle (Figure III2-8).

Left Ventricular Outflow Tract/Three-Chamber View

Because of the close proximity between the aortic and mitral valve annuli, disease processes frequently involve both valves. A three-chamber view can be helpful for evaluation of rheumatic heart disease, endocarditis, hypertrophic cardiomyopathies, and other valvular abnormalities. The three-chamber view is another long axis view of the left ventricle. Figure III2-9 illustrates an efficient approach to constructing a slice in the three-chamber view. Using the left ventricular outflow tract view, a slice can be positioned longitudinally through the left ventricle, aortic valve, and ascending aorta (Figure III2-9, top left).

An alternative method is to position a long axis view orthogonal to the short axis view, similar to the four-chamber view but tilted obliquely through the left ventricular outflow tract (Figure III2-9, bottom left).

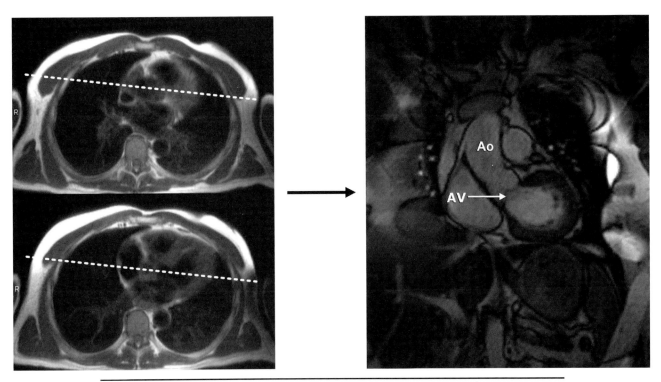

FIGURE III2-8. Left ventricular outflow tract/aortic root view positioned using transverse images through the aortic root and heart (left). An oblique coronal slice (right) permits visualization of the left ventricular outflow tract, aortic valve (AV) leaflets, and ascending aorta (Ao).

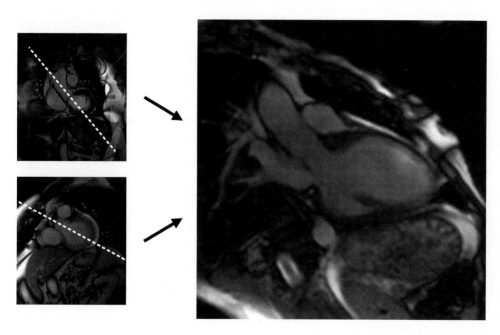

FIGURE III2-9. From either a left ventricular outflow tract view (top left) or short axis view at the left ventricular base (bottom left), a three-chamber view can be obtained.

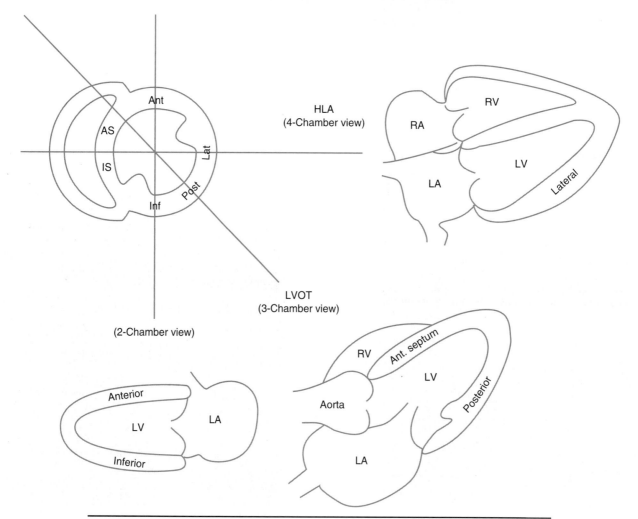

FIGURE III2-10. Left ventricular wall regions identified on the standard imaging views. LA, left atrium; LV, left ventricle; RA, right atrium; RV right ventricle; AS, anterior septum; IS, inferior septum; Inf, inferior; Post, posterior; Lat, lateral; Ant, anterior.

ANATOMIC DEFINITIONS

Left ventricular regions visible on the standard anatomic views are labeled in Figure III2-10. As with all of diagnostic imaging, it is desirable to confirm all abnormalities on two separate views. For example, for the anterior wall, both the short axis and vertical long axis views are useful. For lateral wall disease, the short axis and horizontal long axis views should reveal the pathology. For the apex, the two long axis views are important.

In Figure III2-11, the presumed coronary artery blood supply distributions for the left ventricle are depicted. Recall that the blood supply to the inferior wall is variable. In the majority of individuals, the right coronary artery (RCA) supplies the posterior descending artery. In the remaining population, either the left circumflex (LCx) or both arteries supply the inferior wall.

For purposes of reporting and analysis, the left ventricle may be divided into a number of segments, and different measures of disease or function, such as perfusion, wall motion, and viability, assessed for individual segments. One commonly used classification scheme is shown in Figure III2-12.

A summary of findings for the entire left ventricle can be depicted two-dimensionally by using a compressed bull's eye view or polar map, where the concentric rings that correspond to the basal, mid, and apical portions of the left ventricle are superimposed (Figure III2-13). Bull's eye maps can be used to depict the results of a variety of cardiac parameters—wall motion (thickening, strain, and others), perfusion, and viability, for example.

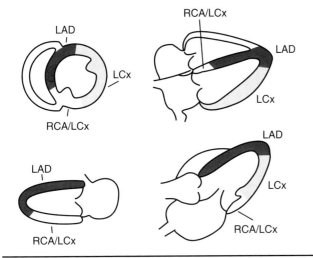

FIGURE III2-11. Presumed coronary artery supply distributions for the left ventricle. The inferior wall of the left ventricle and septum can be supplied by either the right coronary artery (most commonly), the left circumflex artery, or both arteries (1). LAD (dark gray): left anterior descending artery, LCx (light gray): left circumflex artery, and RCA (white): right coronary artery.

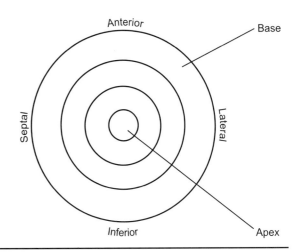

FIGURE III2-13. Schematic of a bull's eye or polar map of the left ventricle that is convenient for summarizing findings for the entire left ventricle on a single image. Each concentric ring represents a short axis slice from base toward the apex, where the apex is represented in the center.

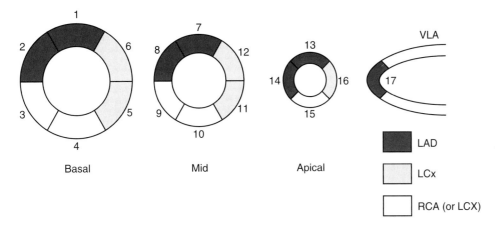

FIGURE III2-12. Seventeen-segment classification system on basal, mid, and apical short axis views and a vertical long axis (VLA) view (1).

REVIEW QUESTIONS

1. An alternative approach to arriving at images in the orthogonal planes of the heart starts with conventional three-plane scout images that include coronal, transverse, and sagittal images through the left ventricle, as shown in Figure III2-Q1. This approach directly generates a short axis view from the scout images. On Figure III2-Q1, draw the slice position guides to indicate how a short axis slice would be defined.

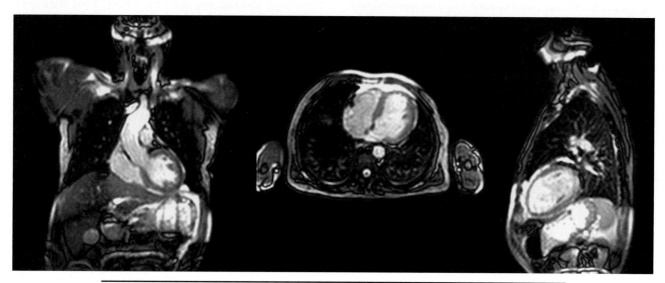

FIGURE III2-Q1(A–C). Conventional orthogonal scout views of heart.

2. You attempt to obtain a horizontal long axis view of the left ventricle using different pulse sequences, each performed after the subject is instructed to take in a deep breath and hold it. The resulting images are shown in Figure III2-Q2. How do you explain these findings, and can you propose a solution?

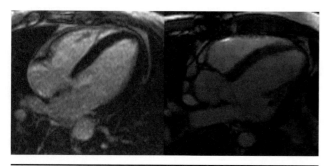

FIGURE III2-Q2

3. Which of the following regions are best depicted on each of the views listed in Table III2-3A?

▶ **TABLE III2-3A**

Region	Short Axis	Horizontal Long Axis (4-Chamber)	Vertical Long Axis (2-Chamber)	LV Outflow Tract (3-Chamber)
Anterior LV wall				
Interventricular septum				
Inferior LV wall				
LV apex				
Mitral valve				
Aortic valve				

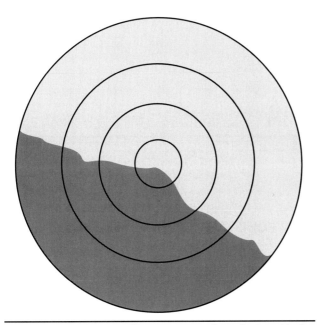

FIGURE III2-Q4A. Bull's eye map of perfusion (darker corresponds to more perfusion).

4. A bull's eye map of left ventricular perfusion is depicted in Figure III2-Q4A, where darker shades of gray reflect normal perfusion. Which coronary artery or arteries is/are most likely diseased based on this map?

REFERENCE

1. Cerqueira MD, Weissman NJ, Dilsizian V, Jacobs AK, Kaul S, Laskey WK, Pennell DJ, Rumberger JA, Ryan T, Verani MS. Standardized myocardial segmentation and nomenclature for tomographic imaging of the heart: A statement for healthcare professionals from the Cardiac Imaging Committee of the Council on Clinical Cardiology of the American Heart Association. Circulation 2002; 105(4):539–42.

Black-Blood Imaging

Black-blood images are produced with MR pulse sequences that to null signal from flowing blood for better visualization of cardiac and mediastinal anatomy and vascular wall pathology. Techniques include conventional spin echo imaging, fast spin echo or turbo spin echo, and ultrafast single-shot turbo spin echo methods, all of which are performed with ECG gating. Preparation pulses are commonly implemented to improve image contrast. This chapter reviews implementations of conventional spin echo and faster echo train sequences, emphasizing methods for optimum blood nulling.

KEY CONCEPTS

▶ For cardiac spin echo sequences, TR is usually equal to one R-R interval for T1- or proton density-weighted images or two R-R intervals for T2-weighted images.

▶ Spin echo sequences achieve blood nulling because moving protons do not experience both the 90° excitation and 180° refocusing pulses and therefore do not contribute to the echo.

▶ When an acquisition time for a spin echo sequence exceeds a breath hold, multiple signal averages can be used to minimize respiratory motion artifacts.

▶ Fast spin echo cardiac MR images can be used for multislice imaging or for high-resolution single-slice images.

▶ Fast spin echo sequences rely on double inversion recovery pulses to null signal from flowing blood during imaging.

▶ Half-Fourier single-shot fast spin echo sequences can produce black-blood images in less than one heartbeat but require double inversion recovery pulses to null blood signal.

▶ Triple inversion recovery fast spin echo sequences generate fat-suppressed, black-blood, T2-weighted images of the cardiovascular system.

SPIN ECHO CARDIAC MR IMAGING

The principles of spin echo imaging have been presented in Chapter I-4. Recall that essential components of the spin echo pulse sequence are the 90° excitation pulse and a 180° refocusing pulse. The parameters that determine image contrast are the repetition time, TR, and the echo time, TE. For T1-weighted imaging, the TR and TE are typically 500–800 msec and <50 msec, respectively, while for T2-weighted imaging, they are ≥1200 msec and ≥80 msec.

Spin Echo: ECG Gating

To minimize motion artifacts due to the beating heart, data for each image must be acquired during the same temporal phase of the cardiac cycle. The acquisition is synchronized to cardiac motion by using ECG gating. The TR is usually set to be equal to the R-R interval. For example, for a subject with a heart rate of 72 bpm, the R-R interval = (60 sec/min)/(72 beats/min) = 0.833 sec, and consequently, the TR would be 833 msec.

In most subjects, defining the TR as equal to one R-R interval will result in T1-weighted imaging, provided a short TE is used. For subjects with slower heart rates, the contrast may be closer to proton density-weighted.

CHALLENGE QUESTION: How can ECG-gated spin echo sequences be used to obtain T2-weighted images?

Answer: By triggering off every other R wave, instead of every R wave, a longer TR can be achieved. For a subject with heart rate of 72 bpm, the TR would be 833 msec × 2 = 1666 msec. The TE also needs to be lengthened to at least 80–100 msec. Because the TR is two times the R-R interval, the T2-weighted sequence will require an acquisition time that is twice as long as that of a T1-weighted sequence.

Spin Echo: Image Contrast

For most routine black blood imaging of the heart, the TR is equal to one R-R interval. It usually does not matter whether the image contrast is strongly T1-weighted or closer to being proton density-weighted. The main function of these images is to provide anatomic assessment of cardiac and vascular structures in the absence of signal from flowing blood.

T2-weighted sequences triggered off every other R wave may be important in certain settings such as evaluation of masses or vasculitis. To enhance conspicuity of pathology, fat suppression is often used.

> **IMPORTANT CONCEPT:** With ECG-gated spin echo images, the TR is usually a multiple of the R-R interval. Typically T1-weighted or proton density-weighted images are used for anatomic imaging (TR = R-R interval), while T2-weighted images may be important for the assessment of certain types of pathology (TR = 2 R-R intervals).

Multislice ECG-Gated Spin Echo Imaging

As described in Chapter I-4, because the TE is short relative to the TR, there is ample time to collect data from multiple slice positions when performing an ECG-gated spin echo sequence (Figure III3-1).

The number of slices that can be acquired during one acquisition depends on the acquisition window and on the total number of 90°–180°-echoes that can fit into the acquisition time. The acquisition window usually corresponds to about 85% of the R-R interval (Chapter III-1).

For the subject with a heart rate of 72 bpm, the R-R interval is 833 msec, and the acquisition window is about 700 msec. If the total time from start of the 90° RF pulse to the end of the echo is 35 msec, then the number of slices that could be imaged in the same time as needed for a single slice would be 700/35 or 20 (Figure III3-1).

With an ECG-triggered spin echo sequence, the first slice position is imaged immediately after the R wave, while the last is acquired toward the end of the R-R interval. Hence, each slice will reflect the heart at a different phase of the cardiac cycle (Figure III3-1). On a series of transaxial images, the more cephalad images may be acquired during systole, and the more caudal slices may be acquired during diastole. Alternatively, the slices could be acquired in reverse order. It is important to recognize that motion artifacts are most likely to affect images collected during peak systole. while signal in the blood pools most likely.

> **IMPORTANT CONCEPT:** With multislice ECG-gated spin echo sequences, each slice position corresponds to a different time point in the cardiac cycle.

Acquisition Times for ECG-Gated Spin Echo Imaging

As with all spin echo imaging, acquisition times are dependent on TR. For cardiac applications, because TR

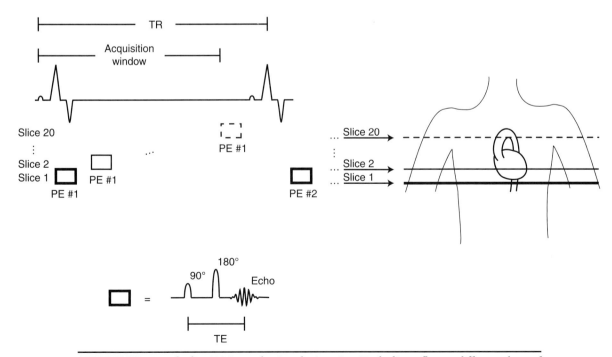

FIGURE III3-1. Multislice ECG-gated spin echo imaging. Each slice reflects a different phase of the cardiac cycle. With conventional spin echo sequences, each R-R interval contributes one echo or one phase-encoding (PE) step to each image at different slice positions.

depends on heart rate or R-R interval, the total acquisition time can be expressed as:

$$\text{Acquisition Time} = \frac{(\text{R-R interval}) \times N_{PE} \times N_{Acq}}{\text{ETL}} \text{ or}$$

$$= \frac{2(\text{R-R interval}) \times N_{PE} \times N_{Acq}}{\text{ETL}}$$

depending on whether triggering occurs with every heartbeat or every other heartbeat. With conventional spin echo imaging, a single line of k-space is acquired during each heartbeat, so that the echo train length, ETL, is equal to 1. If there are 128 phase-encoding lines, then the acquisition time for one set of data (N_{Acq} = 1) will be 128 heartbeats. For a subject with heart rate 72 bpm, and R-R interval = TR = 833 msec, the acquisition time will be 128 × 0.833 sec = 106 sec, or nearly 2 min. If a more T2-weighted sequence is desired, then a TR equal to two R-R intervals will double the acquisition time (212 sec) to nearly 4 min.

CHALLENGE QUESTION: Acquisition times for spin echo sequences exceed the time frame for a breath hold. How can respiratory artifacts be minimized for these acquisitions?

Answer: Averaging multiple signals, say three to four signal averages (N_{Acq}), will minimize respiratory artifacts. Consequently, acquisition times increase proportionately by a factor of 3–4.

Spin Echo: Multiple Signals Averaged

Because acquisition times with spin echo images exceed breath holding times, subjects are usually instructed to breathe normally while multiple signals, typically three or four, are acquired and averaged. If each acquisition requires 2–4 min, then total acquisition time for multiple N_{Acq} ranges from 6 to 16 min. For most subjects, a set of conventional spin echo images through the chest requires about 10 min.

Despite the use of signal averaging, respiratory motion still frequently causes artifacts on conventional spin echo images. Most commonly, these artifacts arise from ghosting from the subcutaneous fat of the anterior chest or abdominal wall (Figure III3-2). Saturation bands placed over the ghosting source are used to reduce these artifacts (Chapter I-9).

Spin Echo Black-Blood Effects

To generate a spin echo, protons must experience both the 90° excitation pulse and the 180° refocusing pulse. If the RF pulses are slice selective and if the protons in the blood are not present within the slice long enough to experience both RF pulses, then no echo is generated, resulting in a signal void. For this reason, flowing blood is typically black with conventional spin echo imaging. As discussed in chapter II-1, to minimize the signal from flowing blood, several strategies can be employed: using a longer TE, thinner slices, and slice positioning orthogonal to the direction of flow. Moreover, acquisitions during systole, when flow is fastest, have more complete nulling of flowing blood.

CHALLENGE QUESTION: Consider routine axial images of the heart using spin echo imaging. How does the order of acquisitions (cranial to caudal or caudal to cranial) affect the image quality and degree of blood nulling on the images?

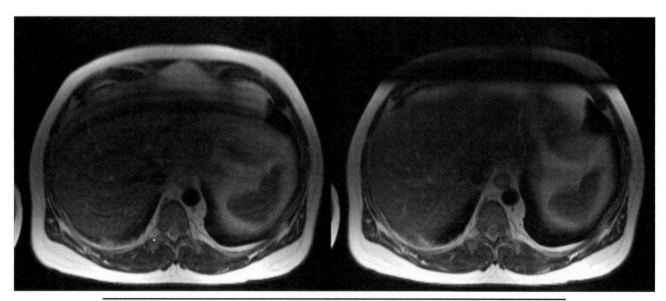

FIGURE III3-2. Spin echo images performed with multiple averages show ghosting artifacts (left) resulting from the high signal of the subcutaneous fat near the surface coils. Artifacts are reduced by placing saturation bands over the anterior abdominal wall (right).

Answer: The images acquired immediately after the R wave will be in systole and have best blood nulling on spin echo images. When visibility of the myocardium (and distinction from blood pool) is important, consider ordering the acquisition from caudal to cranial (Figure III 3-1) so that the heart is imaged during systole, while images of the aorta and great vessels are acquired during diastole.

When is the blood not black on spin echo images? When blood flow is slow or stagnant, blood protons may experience both the 90° and 180° pulses and create measurable signal. In healthy subjects, this occurs during diastole. In disease, blood flow may be relatively stagnant even in systole, for example, in dilated cardiomyopathies or in ventricular aneurysms. Alternatively, if imaging is in the plane of flow, protons, despite their motion, may experience both pulses and consequently generate signal (Figure III3-3).

> **IMPORTANT CONCEPT:** Conventional spin echo images achieve blood nulling because blood moving through the imaging slice does not experience both the 90° and 180° pulses. Blood nulling is helped by use of longer TE, thinner slices, slice positioning orthogonal to flow direction, and acquisition during systole.

TURBO OR FAST SPIN ECHO CARDIAC MR IMAGING

Fast spin echo (FSE) or turbo spin echo imaging, also referred to as rapid acquisition relaxation enhancement (RARE), is a valuable alternative to conventional spin

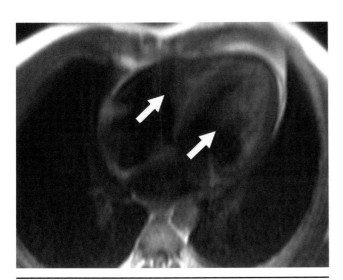

FIGURE III3-3. High signal (arrows) on spin echo-type image may be generated by in-plane flow during diastole.

echo imaging for black-blood cardiovascular MR imaging. (For a detailed discussion of fast spin echo sequences, refer to Chapter I-4.) The acquisition of multiple echoes per RF excitation makes these sequences more efficient. Because fat appears bright on FSE images, fat suppression techniques are frequently used in conjunction with FSE images to enhance the conspicuity of pathology. Frequency-selective fat suppression pulses and inversion recovery methods can be used (Chapter I-9).

Imaging Efficiency with FSE

Compared to conventional spin echo imaging, the acquisition time with FSE is reduced directly in proportion to the ETL. For example, if the ETL is 16, the acquisition time is reduced by a factor of 16. Consider a typical sequence with TR = 2 R-R intervals ≈ 1600 msec. If the imaging matrix is 256 × 128, then the acquisition time with ER = 16 for a single slice is

$$\text{Acquisition Time (sec)} = \frac{1.6 \times 128}{16} = 12.8 \text{ sec}$$

Because 12.8 sec is comfortably within the time frame of a single breath hold for most subjects, the imaging can be performed with one acquisition. Multiple signal averages are no longer needed.

As with all fast spin echo sequences, the TE that controls image contrast is the effective TE (TE_{eff}) (Chapter I-4). Recall that TE_{eff} is defined as the TE associated with the echo used to fill the central line of k-space.

> **IMPORTANT CONCEPT:** Depending on the echo train length, ECG-gated fast spin echo imaging can be performed in one breath hold.

Fast Spin Echo: Imaging in Diastole

With fast spin echo imaging, acquisition of an echo train of, say, 16, might require about 160–200 msec. These relatively long sampling durations have important consequences in cardiac imaging. First, the long echo train duration causes the image to be sensitive to cardiac motion. As discussed in Chapter I-4, intrinsic blurring is associated with echo train imaging. This blurring is exacerbated by motion associated with systole. Consequently, fast spin echo images are best acquired during diastole. This can be achieved by using a trigger delay of at least 150–200 msec. Second, the efficiencies of multislice acquisitions with spin echo imaging have to be reconsidered. For example, for a subject with a R-R interval of less than 700 msec, only about 3–4 slices can be acquired with the multislice method.

Fast Spin Echo: Adding Inversion Recovery Pulses

Conventional spin echo sequences rely on the flow of blood through the slice to suppress its signal. Because fast spin echo acquisitions are sensitive to cardiac motion and are generally performed in diastole, additional measures must be taken to ensure blood nulling.

As introduced in Chapter I-9, a pair of inversion recovery pulses can be added to an FSE sequence to null blood (Figure I9-16).

CHALLENGE QUESTION: Given that the T1 relaxation time of blood is about 1200 msec at 1.5 T, what should the inversion time be for blood nulling?

Answer: This is a tricky question. Following the first inversion pulse, the inversion time (TI) can be calculated based on the equations for exponential recovery (Chapter I-2) to be equal to 0.693 × 1200 or 832 msec. What happens after the second inversion pulse? Because there is incomplete recovery of longitudinal magnetization, M_z, following the first inversion pulse, the starting magnitude of M_z is lower than expected. This means that the time to cross the null point is shorter than 832 msec. The exact time depends on the T1 of blood and on the heart rate and is typically between 400 and 600 msec. Fortuitously, such a long TI ensures that imaging is performed in diastole, thereby minimizing potential motion artifacts associated with imaging in systole.

> **IMPORTANT CONCEPT:** Because diastolic imaging is desired for fast spin echo imaging, a double inversion recovery technique with inversion time of 400–600 msec is commonly used to null blood.

Fast Spin Echo: High-Resolution Single-Slice Imaging

Fast spin echo imaging methods produce high-resolution single-slice images in a single breath hold, or multislice acquisitions with free breathing and multiple signal averaging. The single-slice technique, combined with double inversion recovery prepulses to null blood, is used more commonly.

The imaging efficiency of fast spin echo imaging is exploited by use of a large number of phase-encoding steps. For example, for an image with 192 phase-encoding steps and an echo train length of 24, the acquisition time is 8 (192/24) heartbeats. If the subject can tolerate a 16-heartbeat breath hold (about 15 sec), 384 phase-encoding steps can be performed! How does this translate into spatial resolution? For a typical field of view of 35 cm with 75% rectangular field of view (35 cm × 26.3 cm) and a 512 × 384 matrix (Figure III3-4), the voxel size would be 0.7 mm × 0.7 mm. The in-plane resolution is improved

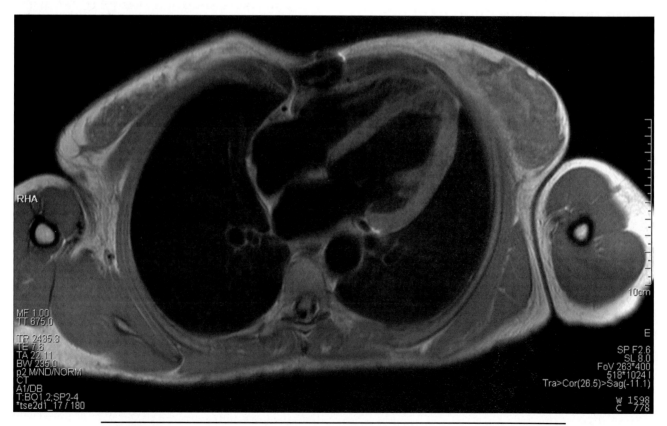

FIGURE III3-4. Example of a high-resolution image of the heart.

▶ **TABLE III3-1**

Sequence Parameters	Imaging Matrix	Spin Echo Acq Time	FSE Acquisition Time		
			ETL 16	ETL 24	ETL 32
TR = 800 msec (T1-weighted)	256 × 128	102 sec	6.4 sec	8.5 sec	3.2 sec
	256 × 192	154 sec	9.6 sec	6.4 sec	4.8 sec
	256 × 256	205 sec	12.8 sec	8.5 sec	6.4 sec
	512 × 384	307 sec	19.2 sec	12.8 sec	9.6 sec
TR = 1600 msec (T2-weighted)	256 × 128	205 sec	12.8 sec	8.5 sec	6.4 sec
	256 × 192	307 sec	19.2 sec	12.8 sec	9.6 sec
	256 × 256	410 sec	25.6 sec	17.1 sec	12.8 sec

twofold in each direction as compared with 1.4 mm × 1.4 mm voxels and 256 × 192 matrix used for an 8-heartbeat acquisition.

Sample acquisition times for spin echo and fast spin echo implementations are shown in Table III3-1 for a subject with an R-R interval of 800 msec.

CHALLENGE QUESTION: What is the drawback of longer echo train lengths in fast spin echo imaging?

Answer: The higher the ETL, the more susceptible is the sequence to blurring caused by cardiac motion during the echo train. For example, for typical interecho spacings of 7–10 msec, an ETL = 16 would require sampling over about 150 msec, while an ETL of 32 would require sampling over 300 msec. Shortening the interecho spacing by means of a higher receiver bandwidth may help, but at the expense of lower signal-to-noise ratios.

For a typical single-slice fast spin echo sequence, the acquisition window is about 85% of the R-R interval. For a subject with a heart rate of 72 bpm and an acquisition window of about 700 msec, an inversion time of 400–500 msec is used with double inversion recovery pre-pulses. This leaves about 200–300 msec for the acquisition of each echo train. The number of echoes that can be obtained depends on the interecho spacing.

High-resolution single-slice fast spin echo images are commonly used for evaluation of right ventricular dysplasia and for assessment of cardiac masses (Figure III3-5).

Multislice Fast Spin Echo

An alternative to breath-hold high-spatial-resolution fast spin echo is multislice fast spin echo imaging. These sequences are very similar to conventional spin echo sequences except for relatively short echo train lengths of 3 to 4 to improve efficiency. Short echo train lengths minimize sensitivity to motion, allowing data acquisition to continue throughout the cardiac cycle. The degree of blood nulling on these images is similar to that of conventional spin echo imaging. When compared with conventional spin echo methods acquisition times are shortened by a factor of 3 to 4. For example, if the subject's heart rate is 72 bpm, the R-R interval = TR = 833 msec and

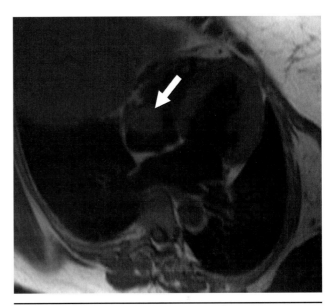

FIGURE III3-5. Fast spin echo imaging demonstrates a right atrial mass (arrow).

ETL = 3, then the acquisition time for a 256 × 128 matrix will be (128/3) × 0.833 sec = 35 sec. Three- to four-signal averages would require about 2 min. For more T2-weighted imaging, the acquisition times would double, given that the TR would consist of two R-R intervals.

HALF-FOURIER SINGLE-SHOT FAST SPIN ECHO

With faster gradient switching and more efficient data sampling, it is possible to sample rapidly a large number of echoes for a long echo train. With half-Fourier single-shot fast spin echo techniques, all the data needed to make each image can be acquired within one heartbeat. As discussed in Chapter I-4, the technique takes advantage of the Hermitian symmetry of k-space. As a reminder, with an ETL of 68, the MR system computes the remaining 60 lines of data to generate a full 256 × 128 matrix for k-space. In less than 500 msec, a single image is generated.

Although all the data needed to generate an image can be obtained in single heartbeat, images are usually acquired only every other heartbeat. This serves two functions: (a) built-in "downtime" reduces the overall specific absorption rate (SAR) associated with the repeated 180° pulses in quick succession and (b) the longitudinal magnetization is more recovered, particularly when fully inversion recovery prepulses are used.

Single-Shot Black-Blood Imaging with Double Inversion Recovery Pulses

Even with interecho spacing times as short as 5 msec, an ETL of 68 would require over 300 msec. To minimize cardiac motion during echo sampling, diastolic imaging is desired. To ensure nulling of signal from flowing blood, these sequences are implemented with double inversion recovery prepulses (Figures I9-16 and I9-17).

The single-shot fast spin echo sequences are routinely used to evaluate cardiac and great vessel anatomy. Because they are half-Fourier techniques, spatial resolution and signal-to-noise ratio are inferior compared to FSE methods. On the other hand, the speed of single-shot acquisitions reduces cardiac and respiratory motion arti-

facts. If high-resolution images are desired, then single-slice fast spin echo or multislice FSE sequences should be performed (Figure III3-6).

FAT SUPPRESSION WITH TRIPLE INVERSION RECOVERY FAST SPIN ECHO

Addition of a third slice-selective inversion recovery pulse to the double inversion recovery fast spin echo sequence achieves both fat and blood nulling for FSE sequences (Figure III3-7). The third 180° pulse is applied around the time of the nulling of blood (TI_1). Following this pulse, an inversion time (TI_2) of approximately 160 msec, is selected for nulling of fat signal. The third 180° pulse has no effect on already nulled blood. Because the left ventricle is in diastole after application of the third 180° pulse, the blood remains within the imaging slice until the readout. This implementation can accompany a single-shot fast spin echo sequence and achieves the same kind of tissue contrast as would be expected with a conventional inversion-recovery fast spin echo sequence. Tissues with short T1, such as fat, are nulled. Additionally, T1 and T2 contrast effects are additive, making

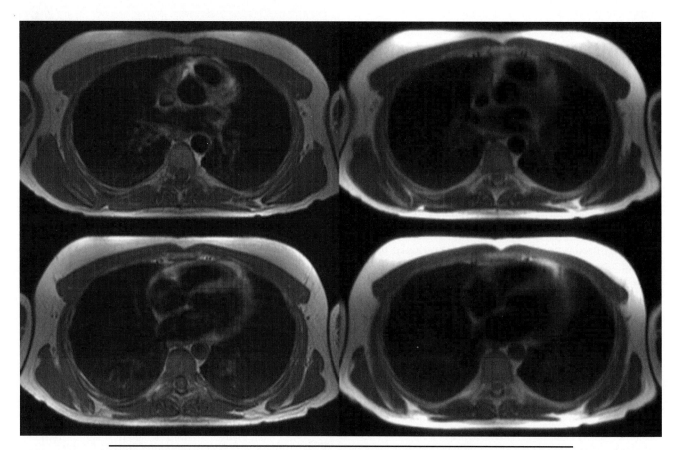

FIGURE III3-6. Comparison of fast spin echo (left) and single-shot half-Fourier fast spin echo (right) images in the same healthy subject. Higher image signal and spatial resolution in fast spin echo images come at the expense of significantly longer acquisition times (8 min versus 25 sec for 15–20 images through the chest).

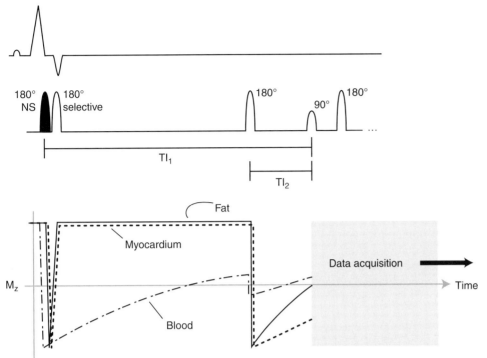

FIGURE III3-7. Triple IR pulse sequence results in nulling of blood as well as fat. The first two IR pulses, one nonselective (NS) and the other slice-selective, null blood signal. The third IR pulse is slice-selective and achieves fat suppression.

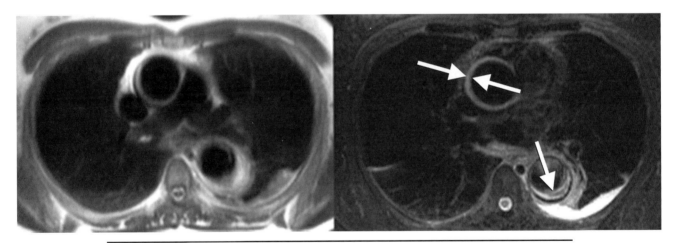

FIGURE III3-8. Intramural hematoma. High-signal-intensity material in the wall of the ascending and descending aorta on single-shot half-Fourier fast spin echo images (left) can be confused with mediastinal fat. Fat suppression with a triple inversion recovery sequence (right) confirms the presence of hemorrhage in the wall of the aorta (arrows).

pathology particularly conspicuous on these sequences (Chapter I, Figure I9-14).

Examples of clinical applications of this fast cardiac triple IR sequence include the detection of acute myocardial infarction and the evaluation of mural vascular pathologies such as vasculitis and intramural hematoma (Figure III3-8).

BLACK-BLOOD IMAGING OPTIONS

The range of black-blood imaging options varies from MR system to MR system. Regardless of the scanner, black-blood imaging should always be possible using ECG-gated spin echo imaging.

When available, ultrafast spin echo methods such as single-shot double-inversion recovery half-Fourier techniques can provide a quick anatomic overview for routine cardiac imaging. The single-shot version usually results in lower spatial resolution and lower signal-to-noise ratios than fast spin echo methods. If higher-resolution images are needed, targeted fast spin echo single slice imaging can then be performed, with one slice per breath hold. For most fast imaging, double inversion recovery prepulses should be used to ensure blood nulling.

REVIEW QUESTIONS

1. Consider the tradeoffs with T1-weighted fast spin echo imaging versus spin echo imaging when 15-slice positions are desired.

   a. For spin echo imaging, how many slices can be imaged in a single acquisition if the TR = R-R = 800 msec, the trigger window is 15%, and the time from the start of the 90° RF pulse to the end of the echo is 40 msec? What is the acquisition time if the imaging matrix is 256 × 100 (N_{PE} = 100)? What will the acquisition time be if three signal averages are used?

   b. For fast spin echo imaging, consider an echo train length of 4. Assume that the heart rate and trigger window are the same as in (a). Given that time from the start of the 90° RF pulse to the end of the echo train is 80 msec, how many slices can be obtained in a single acquisition, assuming that a trigger delay of 200 msec is needed to avoid systole? How long will this acquisition be? To acquire the desired 15 slice positions, how many separate acquisitions are required, assuming that breath-hold acquisitions are favored?

   c. Use the results obtained in (a) and (b) to summarize considerations in deciding between using spin echo and FSE sequences for a T1-weighted acquisition.

2. As will be discussed further in Chapter III-5, for the evaluation of patients with suspected arrhythmic right ventricular dysplasia, high-spatial-resolution images of the right ventricular wall and outflow tract are desired. One method for increasing the spatial resolution requires that the posterior elements of the phased-array coil be turned off during the acquisition (Figure III3-Q2). How can spatial resolution be improved with this approach? What are the advantages and disadvantages of this technique?

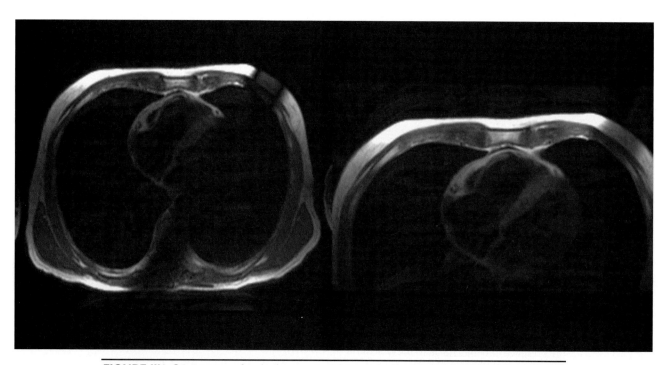

FIGURE III3-Q2. Imaging of arrhythmogenic right ventricular dysplasia with both anterior and posterior phased-array coils (left) and with only the anterior coil (right). In both cases a saturation band is applied over the left ventricle to minimize left ventricular motion artifacts.

Cine Gradient Echo Imaging

Spin echo imaging is the "meat and potatoes" of most cardiac MRI, and used for evaluation of anatomy. Cine gradient recalled echo (GRE) imaging adds the spice of functional imaging. With cine GRE, the same slice is imaged at multiple time points in the cardiac cycle. The multiple frames are viewed in a cinematic loop (hence, the term *cine*). The movie gives the viewer an appreciation for flow and function in the heart and vessels. For example, whereas a routine MR angiogram may depict ascending aortic pathology, cine imaging provides the functional assessment of the aorta and aortic valve. In emergency cases, cine GRE may help distinguish between aortic dissection and intramural hematoma by demonstrating flow in the false lumen.

Like ECG-gated spin echo imaging, cine GRE is performed using ECG-gating Data for each image are acquired across several heartbeats. Compared to spin echo methods, cine GRE pulse sequences are more complex, because they require that several additional parameters be adapted to the subject's heart rate and breath-holding capabilities. The aim of this chapter is to clarify the challenges of optimizing cine GRE.

KEY CONCEPTS

▶ Cine gradient echo acquisitions rely on robust and consistent ECG gating.

▶ Acquisition times are usually defined in terms of number of heartbeats (rather than in absolute units of time).

▶ Temporal resolution and spatial resolution must be balanced against acquisition time.

▶ Retrospective gating allows reconstruction of images throughout the cardiac cycle, whereas prospective gating typically excludes late diastole.

▶ Image contrast depends on whether spoiled gradient echo or steady-state free precession gradient echo sequences are performed.

▶ Segmented k-space sequences allow the user to vary temporal resolution of images; increased temporal

resolution comes at the expense of either decreased spatial resolution or increased acquisition time.

▶ View sharing increases the apparent temporal resolution of a cine gradient echo sequence without increasing acquisition time.

▶ Steady-state free precession sequences have sufficient signal-to-noise ratio to warrant routine implementation with parallel imaging methods.

▶ Accurate quantification of functional parameters such as left ventricular ejection fraction requires careful attention to the demarcation of blood pool at end systole and end diastole.

▶ Pitfalls of cine gradient echo imaging may relate to inaccurate ECG gating, poor image contrast, and flow-related signal loss, among others.

▶ Clinical Protocol:
  ▶ Left ventricular function

PRINCIPLES OF CINE GRE

Before delving into the details of specific types of cine GRE sequences, it is necessary to review some themes common to all cine GRE techniques. These include the definition of temporal resolution, segmented k-space methods, partitioning of MR data into frames, and image contrast.

Cine GRE relies on ECG-gating for an accurate representation of cardiac motion. It may be helpful for the reader to review Chapter III-1 on the electrocardiogram (ECG) and the basics of ECG gating. An understanding of the concepts of trigger delay, acquisition window, trigger window, R-R interval, and prospective versus retrospective gating (Figure III1-2 and III1-10) is assumed.

IMPORTANT CONCEPT: As with all ECG-gated sequences, the most critical step for successful imaging is placement of ECG leads and confirming a good ECG tracing for gated sequences (see Chapter III-1).

Number of Frames and Temporal Resolution

With cine GRE, multiple images at the same slice position are generated to capture different time points in the cardiac cycle. The terminology to describe these images can be confusing. For clarity, the individual images are referred to as *frames*, rather than "cardiac phases" (Figure III4-1).

The multiple frames of a cine GRE sequence are played in a cinematic loop to show a video of the beating heart. The temporal resolution and number of frames define how smooth or jerky the cine loop appears. The temporal

resolution of the cine GRE acquisition is usually defined as the duration of the cardiac cycle that each frame represents. For example, if each frame is acquired in 50 msec intervals after the R wave, then the temporal resolution is 50 msec. If MR data are acquired for 700 msec of each heart beat, then the number of frames will be 14. Higher-temporal-resolution images are needed for more accurate assessment of cardiac motion and function, particularly during systole. As will be discussed later in this chapter, some images can be generated by interpolation (view sharing or echo sharing in k-space). The true temporal resolution of interpolated data is more complicated to determine.

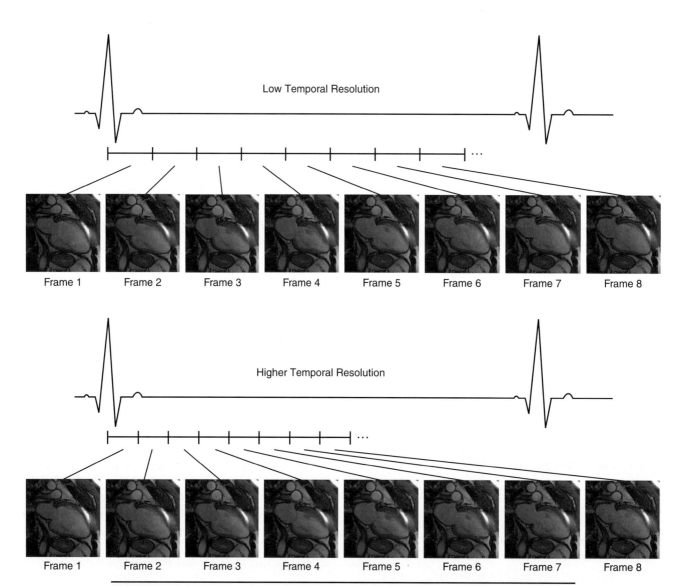

FIGURE III4-1. Lower- versus higher-temporal-resolution prospectively gated cine gradient echo acquisition. The eight low-temporal-resolution images sample fewer time points across the cardiac cycle. The first eight frames of the higher-temporal-resolution images better reflect cardiac motion during systole, when dyskinesis of the thinned apex can be seen. Recall that with prospectively triggered sequences, images of the heart immediately preceding the R wave are not obtained.

ECG-Gated Data: Sorting into k-Space Frames

ECG-gated sequences acquire gradient echoes repeatedly after each R wave for the entire duration of the acquisition window. The manner in which the echoes are partitioned or segmented into different k-spaces determines the temporal resolution of the images and also the total acquisition time. Each k-space corresponds on a one-to-one basis to a specific frame (Figure III4-2). Generally, only a small proportion of the data needed to fill each k-space is collected in a single heartbeat. The amount of data needed to fill each k-space determines the spatial resolution of the images (the number of phase-encoding steps). The number of heartbeats needed to fill a given k-space determines the total acquisition time for the sequence.

Because the k-space data for each frame are collected across a number of heartbeats, the image quality is strongly dependent on the consistency of cardiac motion and gating from beat to beat.

CHALLENGE QUESTION: You run a prospectively triggered sequence and listen to the sounds of the system. The rhythm is irregular. At first there is a run of three bursts at about one every second, but then there is a pause, a couple more bursts, and then more pauses. What is happening, and how can you solve this problem?

Answer: While a prospectively ECG-triggered sequence is running, the noises emanating from the scanner should be rhythmic, one burst per heartbeat. If the noises are erratic, then either the subject's heart rate is irregular or the triggering is not working properly. If it seems that the machine is skipping beats,

the problem may lie in the acquisition window being too long relative to the R-R interval (Figure III4-3). Reducing the acquisition window to 80% of the R-R interval (or increasing the trigger window to 20%) may solve the problem. Another important factor to check is whether the heart rate of the subject is changing during a breath-hold acquisition. The acquisition window should be based on the R-R interval during breath holding.

The quality of ECG-gated images, particularly cine GRE images, relies not only on having a reasonable temporal resolution, but also, importantly, on the consistency of data acquisition with respect to the ECG. For example, the MR system assumes that the cardiac position immediately after the R-wave is the same for all heartbeats. Therefore, when echoes are acquired at this time point over multiple beats, the resulting image should be a perfect representation of the heart at that point in time. The system similarly assumes that the heart position at, for example, 240 msec and 560 msec after the R wave is the same from beat to beat as well. However, with irregular rates or premature beats, this may not be true (Figure III4-3). Combining data that reflects the heart in different states of contraction will degrade image quality substantially.

CHALLENGE QUESTION: What other consequences of poor ECG gating could lead to image degradation?

Answer: Poor ECG gating may also result in many heartbeats where no data is collected (Figure III4-3, fourth heartbeat). An occasional missed R-wave will not degrade image quality substantially. But if this happens often, then the total acquisition time will exceed the breath hold, causing motion artifacts and further reducing image quality.

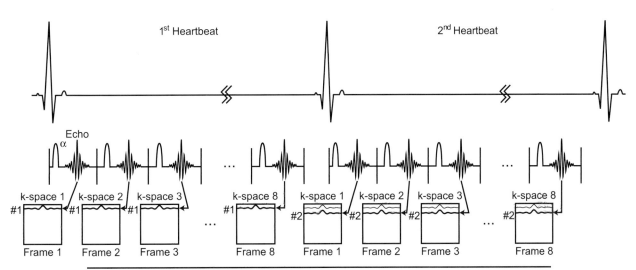

FIGURE III4-2. k-space filling for the multiple frames of an ECG-gated cine gradient echo sequence. In this example, with each heartbeat, one line of k-space is collected for each frame. The total number of heartbeats needed to fill all k-spaces equals the number of phase-encoding steps for each image. For example, if $N_{PE}=100$, then the acquisits time will be 100 heartbeats.

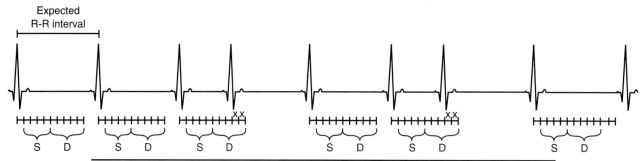

FIGURE III4-3. Effect of irregular heart rate on acquisitions when R-R intervals are shorter than expected. The "x" labels denote data that are presumed to reflect diastole (D) but that in fact correspond to early systole (S).

> **IMPORTANT CONCEPT:** Reliable ECG-gating and regular heart rates are necessary for images to reflect cardiac motion accurately.

Acquisition Time

For cardiac MR pulse sequences, acquisition times are usually a multiple of heartbeats rather than of seconds. The acquisition times therefore depend on a subject's heart rate. Because most cardiac MR examinations require cine acquisitions in multiple planes of the heart, it is vital that cine gradient echo acquisition times be short enough for a comfortable breath hold. A subject's breath-holding capacity is usually thought of in seconds (and not heartbeats!). Most healthy individuals can suspend respiration for 20 sec. Those with moderate cardiac or respiratory ailments are usually still able to hold their breath for 10 sec, particularly if supplemented with oxygen via nasal cannula. If acquisition times exceed the breath-holding capacity of subjects, then the ECG-gated images should be performed during free breathing with 3–4 signals averaged, thereby lengthening the acquisition times by a factor of 3–4.

> **IMPORTANT CONCEPT:** With ECG-gated cine GRE sequences, acquisition times are better thought of in terms of number of heart beats rather than in absolute time (seconds). Sequences with acquisition times that exceed a subject's capacity for breath holding (despite supplementary oxygen) may need to be performed with multiple signal averages during free breathing.

Tradeoffs: Temporal Resolution vs Spatial Resolution vs Acquisition Time

For all cine GRE images, acquisition parameters can be modified to balance the tradeoffs between temporal resolution, spatial resolution, and acquisition times (Figure III4-4). Fundamentally, the parameter that constrains all three is the minimum time needed to generate each gradient echo, reflected in the minimum TR, and this

varies depending on the MR system and the pulse sequence used.

In general, ideal temporal resolution of sequences performed for assessment of cardiac function should be 50–60 msec or less, depending on the subject's heart rate. The faster the heart rate, the better the temporal resolution needed to resolve the motion of the heart during systole. If temporal resolution is inadequate, the cine images are likely to underestimate left ventricular contractility.

The spatial resolution of cine GRE images depends on the structures that need to be resolved. For studies of overall cardiac function, an in-plane spatial resolution of 2–2.5 mm is probably sufficient. Higher spatial resolution, such as 1–2 mm, helps to define finer structures such as cardiac valves, a patent foramen ovale, or smaller vessels such as coronary arteries or bypass grafts. Typical imaging fields of view are about 250 mm × 350 mm (allowing for rectangular field of view for short axis views). Thus for a standard 100–128 × 256 matrix, the in-plane spatial resolution is usually approximately 2–2.5 mm × 1.4 mm. A 192 × 256 matrix provides superior resolution of 1.3 × 1.4 mm.

CHALLENGE QUESTION: What are the drawbacks of setting TR to a minimum?

Answer: Recall from Chapter I-8 that one of the main ways to reduce TR is by using a higher receiver bandwidth. Higher-bandwidth sequences result in lower signal-to-noise ratios. Therefore, there are limits to how low TR can go without sacrificing image signal. Also, as will be discussed subsequently, with spoiled gradient echo sequences, short TRs will reduce the contrast between blood pool and myocardium.

Most vendors preset sequences with a minimum TR based on the desired image quality and contrast of a sequence. After TR is fixed, the next consideration in setting up a cine GRE sequence is usually the acquisition time, constrained by the subject's breath-holding capacity. For a given TR and acquisition time, parameters of a cine GRE sequence are selected based on the desired balance between spatial and temporal resolution (Figure III4-4).

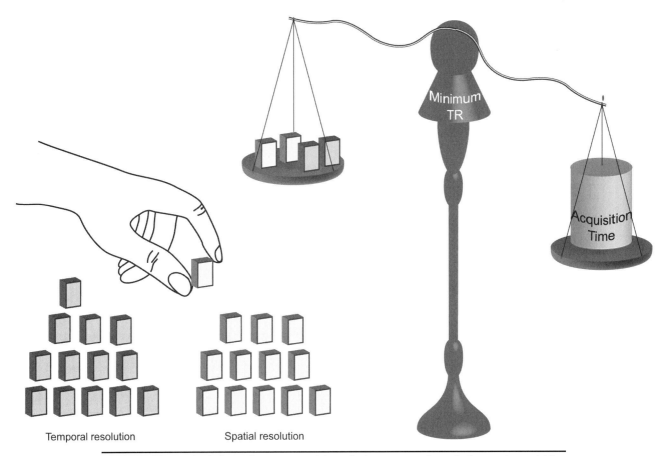

FIGURE III4-4. The balance between spatial resolution, temporal resolution, and acquisition time. For a given minimum TR, acquisition time depends on the spatial and temporal resolution. To keep acquisition time constant (with a given minimum TR), there must be a proper compromise between spatial and temporal resolution.

Temporal resolution

Spatial resolution

IMPORTANT CONCEPTS: Image acquisition parameters, guided by the minimum TR for the sequence, are based on the trade-offs between temporal resolution, spatial resolution, and acquisition times. Ideally, acquisition times should be less than 15–20 sec to accommodate breath holding. Temporal resolution should be 50–60 msec or less. Spatial resolution should be 2–2.5 mm or less.

Image Contrast

Cine GRE sequences are designed to evaluate flow and function of the myocardium and vessels. They are typically referred to as bright-blood sequences, because the signal intensity of the blood is bright relative the myocardium and vessel wall. How this image contrast is achieved varies with the type of pulse sequence. With standard spoiled gradient echo sequences, the image contrast is based on the time-of-flight phenomenon, similar to that discussed in Chapter II-2. Repeated RF pulses

cause saturation of the stationary tissues, while the inflow of fresh, unsaturated protons in moving blood leads to its relatively high signal intensity. To allow time for the inflow of moving blood, the TR of these gradient sequences is on the order of 8 msec or more. Even with a TR of 8 msec, if blood flow is slow, signal of the blood pool can become saturated and the contrast between myocardium and blood pool reduced.

Because of the need to allow time for inflow, these sequences are not able to take advantage of the ultrashort TRs possible with newer MR systems. Steady-state free precession sequences, as described in Chapter I-4, produce images with high contrast between blood and myocardium based on their T2 (and T1) differences (Figure I4-19), independent of flow. These sequences benefit from shorter TRs and TEs, which in turn translate into shorter acquisition times or higher-spatial-resolution images in equivalent acquisition times.

More details about the different methods used to produce cine GRE images are outlined in the following sections and summarized in Table III4-1.

▶ **TABLE III4-1** Cine Gradient Echo Pulse Sequence Options

Sequence	True TR (msec)	TE (msec)	Flip Angle	Views per Segment	Typical matrix	Acquisition time	N_{Acq}	Total time/slice
Standard cine GRE	30–60	3–4	15–20	1	100–150 × 256	100–150 sec	3–4	5–8 min
Segmented k-space cine GRE	7–10	3–4	15–20	3–7	100–150 × 256	15–20 sec	1	15–20 sec
SSFP cine GRE	2–4	1	60–80	10 +	100–150 × 256	7–10 sec	1	7–10 sec
Real-time SSFP cine GRE	2	.8	60–80	n/a	50–55 × 128	50–70 msec (parallel × 2) per frame	1	1–2 sec (depends on user)

SSFP, steady state free precession; GRE, gradient recalled echo.

Note: True TR is the time between RF pulses. Without view-sharing, temporal resolution is equal to true TR × views per segment (sometimes labeled as "TR" on the MR console).

CONVENTIONAL ECG-GATED CINE GRE: BASIC VERSION

A standard ECG-gated cine GRE sequence is available for cardiac imaging on almost all 1.5–3 T MR systems. With the standard spoiled gradient echo sequence, only one echo is collected for each k-space during a given heartbeat (Figure III4-2). Depending on the number of phase-encoding steps, the total acquisition time is between 100 and 128 heartbeats, or about 2 min. Because 2 min is too long for a breath hold, respiratory motion will degrade these acquisitions unless multiple signal averages are performed. With 3–4 signal averages, about 5–8 min are required for one cine loop of a single slice position.

Choosing Parameters for Imaging

With conventional cine GRE, the temporal resolution is equal to the TR for the sequence. TR is usually about 50–60 msec, so that 12–18 frames are produced. The flip angle is selected based on image contrast and the TR. A typical flip angle of 15–20° gives a good balance between the amount of signal in the image and the image contrast between blood and myocardium. Because the image acquisition time is directly proportional to the number of phase-encoding steps, rectangular field of view is valuable for reducing acquisition times without sacrificing spatial resolution.

> **IMPORTANT CONCEPT:** Using the basic cine GRE sequence, the minimum TR and TE should be used with a flip angle of about 20°. To reduce motion artifacts, 3–4 signal averages result in a total acquisition time of approximately 5–8 min per slice position.

SEGMENTED k-SPACE CINE GRE

With stronger gradients and faster slew rates, gradient echoes can be generated in 10 msec or less. Then, in the

same time that a conventional cine GRE sequence takes to acquire one line of k-space, the faster sequence can acquire say, 5. Each consecutive set of 5 echoes is used to fill the k-space of the corresponding frame (Figure III4-5). To fill each k-space completely, the number of heart beats required is reduced by a factor of 5. For example, for images with a matrix of 100 × 256, the acquisition time would be reduced from 100 heartbeats (for each signal or excitation) to 20 heartbeats. This difference is critical, because now the acquisition time is short enough for a single breath hold; multiple signal averaging is no longer necessary.

The acquisition of multiple lines of k-space in a given heartbeat is referred to as segmented k-space cine gradient echo imaging.

The terminology for the TR of segmented k-space sequences can be confusing. For clarity, the following terms and definitions will be used in the remainder of this book:

- *TR*: Although, strictly speaking, the TR should be defined as the time between consecutive RF pulses, with cine GRE imaging the TR is usually used to refer to the temporal resolution. In the foregoing example, the "TR" would be 50 msec.
- *True TR*: This separate term will be used to specify the actual time between consecutive RF pulses. In the example, the "true TR" would be 10 msec.
- *Views per segment (vps)* or *Lines per segment*: The number of gradient echoes acquired for each frame during a single heartbeat. In the example, the views per segment would be 5. The TR is equal to the true TR multiplied by the vps. Examples of different numbers of views per segment are illustrated in Figure III4-5.

Choosing Parameters for Cine GRE

The choice of views per segment offers an additional flexibility in planning a cine GRE acquisition. It is selected based on the desired relationship between spatial

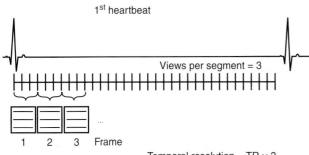

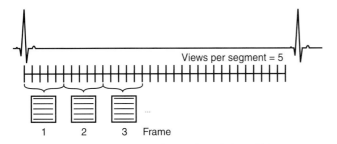

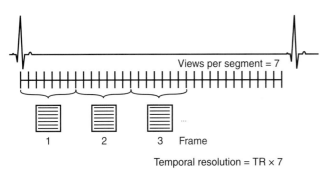

FIGURE III4-5. Segmented k-space cine gradient echo sequences shown with 3, 5, and 7 views per segment. The more views per segment, the shorter the acquisition time at the cost of lowering temporal resolution.

resolution, temporal resolution, and acquisition time. Typically, a temporal resolution of 50–60 msec is desired, corresponding to about 12–18 frames. If temporal resolution is too low (for example, if only 8–10 frames are acquired at 100 msec intervals), then the information about the heart's motion might be inadequate for interpretation. To show fine detail such as cardiac valves, ideally, the spatial resolution should be less than 2 mm. Finally, acquisition time is usually kept less than 20 sec for breath holding. With ECG-gated sequences, acquisition time depends on number of heartbeats, and so the actual acquisition time depends on the subject's heart rate.

Given the interplay of these parameters, how should a sequence be set up based on a subject's heart rate and breath-holding capacity?

Consider the following two sample subjects: one with a heart rate of 60 beats per minute (A) and another with a heart rate of 90 beats per minute (B). In both cases, the same sequence is used—a prospectively gated segmented k-space cine GRE sequence with true TR = 10 msec. The desired imaging matrix for an axial view is 100×256 (assuming recFOV is used). What is the relationship between temporal resolution and acquisition time in these two cases when views per segment is varied?

Case A: Heart Rate of 60 Beats per Minute

In this subject, the R-R interval is 1 sec or 1000 msec. The use of prospective gating means that the usable period of the R-R interval for data acquisition is reduced to about 85% of the R-R interval, or 850 msec. Within this time, for a TR of 10 msec, a total of up to about 85 echoes can be generated. How these echoes are allocated to different k-spaces depends on the vps (Figure III4-6).

Scenario A-1 (Figure III4-6, Case A): vps = 5

If each consecutive set of 5 echoes is assigned to a separate k-space frame, then the temporal resolution of the cine images will be 50 msec. With this temporal resolution, a total of 17 frames (850/50) will be generated. Twenty heartbeats will be needed to fill each k-space with 100 echoes (100 phase-encoding steps). With a heart rate of 60 beats per minute, the acquisition time will be 20 sec, assuming perfect triggering.

Scenario A-2 (Figure III4-6, Case A): vps = 7

If each consecutive set of 7 echoes is assigned to a separate k-space frame, then the temporal resolution of the cine images will be 70 msec, which is still within the acceptable range for detection of most pathology. A total of 12 frames will be generated. Because more echoes are sampled with each heart beat, the total duration of acquisition will be shorter than in Scenario A-1. To fill each k-space with 100 echoes, at a rate of 7 echoes per heart beat, the duration of acquisition will be about 15 heartbeats (the number of phase-encoding steps will default to 105 rather than 100). With a heart rate of 60 beats per minute the acquisition time will be 15 sec, assuming perfect triggering.

The optimal vps depends on the subject's breath-holding capacity. If the subject can tolerate a 20 sec breath-hold, then 5 views per segment will provide an acquisition with excellent temporal resolution of 50 msec. If the subject can only hold his/her breath for 15 sec, then the vps should be increased to 7, with a slight deterioration in temporal resolution.

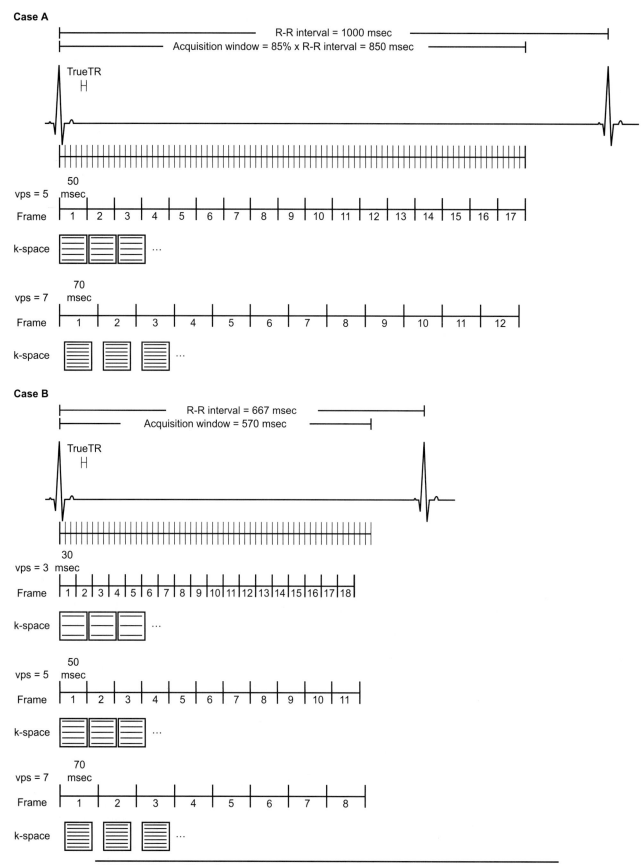

FIGURE III4-6. Effect of varying views per segment (vps) in a subject with a slow heart rate of 60 beats per minute (Case A, above) and a subject with a fast heart rate of 90 beats per minute (Case B, below).

Case 2: Heart Rate of 90 Beats per Minute

In a subject with a much faster heart rate, the R-R interval is shorter (667 msec). Assuming an acquisition window that is 85% of the R-R interval, the usable period of the R-R interval for data acquisition will be about 570 msec. During each heartbeat, a total of up to about 57 echoes can be generated if the true TR is 10 msec. Again, consider scenarios with different assignment of views per segment (Figure III4-6) and evaluate how these affect temporal resolution and acquisition time.

Scenario B-1 (Figure III4-6, Case B): vps = 5

As in Scenario A-1, the temporal resolution of the cine images will be 50 msec. With this temporal resolution, a total of 11 frames (570/50) will be generated from this acquisition. To fill each k-space with 100 echoes, the duration of acquisition will be 20 heartbeats. In this subject with a heart rate of 90 beats per minute, assuming perfect triggering, the acquisition time will be 13.3 sec.

Scenario B-2 (Figure III4-6, Case B): vps = 7

With 7 views per segment, the temporal resolution of the cine images will be 70 msec. For a subject with a fast heart rate, this may be barely enough to resolve motion during peak systole. With a higher number of views per segment, the total duration of acquisition will be shorter than in Scenario B-1. To fill each k-space with 100 echoes, at 7 echoes per heart beat, the duration of acquisition will be about 15 heartbeats (the number of phase-encoding steps will default to 105 rather than 100). With a heart rate of 90 beats per minute, the acquisition time will be only 10 sec.

Scenario B-3 (Figure III4-6, Case B): vps = 3

Instead of using a higher number of views per segment in this case, consider what happens with a lower number of views per segment. With three views per segment, the temporal resolution will improve to 30 msec. For an acquisition time of 33 heartbeats, the acquisition time will be 22 sec.

CHALLENGE QUESTION: Apply the experience from the examples to calculate the acquisition times and temporal resolution for the same sequence using 3, 5, and 7 views per segment in a subject with a heart rate of 72 beats per minute.

Answer: Temporal resolution would be 30, 50, and 70 msec respectively. Acquisition times would be 27.5 sec, 16.7 sec, and 12.5 sec, respectively.

For the example in the preceding Challenge Question,

$$R\text{-}R \text{ interval} = 60/72 = 0.833 \text{ sec} = 833 \text{ msec}$$
$$\text{Acquisition window} = 85\% \text{ R-R interval} = 720 \text{ msec}$$

At 3 views per segment,

$$\text{Temporal resolution} = 10 \times 3 = 30 \text{ msec}$$
$$\text{Number of frames} = 720/30 = 24$$
$$\text{Acquisition time} = 100/3 \text{ heart beats} = 33 \text{ heart beats}$$
$$= 33 \times 0.833 \text{ sec} = 27.5 \text{ sec}$$

At 5 views per segment,

$$\text{Temporal resolution} = 10 \times 5 = 50 \text{ msec}$$
$$\text{Number of frames} = 720/50 = 14$$
$$\text{Acquisition time} = 100/5 \text{ heart beats} = 20 \text{ heart beats}$$
$$= 20 \times 0.833 \text{ sec} = 16.7 \text{ sec}$$

At 7 views per segment,

$$\text{Temporal resolution} = 10 \times 7 = 70 \text{ msec}$$
$$\text{Number of frames} = 720/70 = 10$$
$$\text{Acquisition time} = 100/7 \text{ heart beats} = 15 \text{ heart beats}$$
$$= 15 \times 0.833 = 12.5 \text{ sec}$$

IMPORTANT CONCEPTS: To calculate acquisition times and temporal resolution for a given segmented k-space cine GRE sequence without view sharing, the following steps should be performed:

- Determine the R-R interval based on the subject's heart rate (in beats per minute).
  - □ R-R interval (sec) = 60/heart rate
  - □ R-R interval (msec) = (60/heart rate) × 1000
- Determine the acquisition window (assuming prospective triggering).
  - □ Acquisition window (msec) = 0.85 × R-R interval (msec)
- Calculate the temporal resolution based on the views per segment.
  - □ Temporal resolution = True TR × views per segment
  - □ Number of frames = Acquisition window/temporal resolution
- Compute the acquisition time in heartbeats and in seconds for a given number of phase-encoding steps (N_{PE}).
  - □ Acquisition time (heart beats) = N_{PE}/views per segment
  - □ Acquisition time (sec) = (N_{PE}/views per segment) × R-R interval (sec)

For any given true TR, calculations of temporal resolution and acquisition time for a given number of phase-encoding steps can be performed to optimize the sequence parameters for a given subject. For example, a more thorough set of calculations is given in Table III4-2 for the case of a true TR of 10 msec and an imaging matrix of 100×256. In the table, assuming that the subject can hold his/her breath for around 20 sec, the "optimal" choice is shown in **bold**.

Optimizing Segmented k-Space Cine GRE

For any particular true TR and imaging matrix, a table like Table III4-2 can be constructed to help choose optimal imaging parameters. A blank table (Table III4-3) is provided at the end of this chapter and may be photocopied and completed for posting at the MR console for reference. Short of using such a table, the following general pointers may be helpful when using default scanner parameters.

Tip # 1: Heart Rate Determines Views per Segment

For slower heart rates, use more views per segment. For faster heart rates, use fewer views per segment. With slower heart rates, R-R intervals are longer, and so more views per segment can fit into the acquisition window. By using more views per segment, the total acquisition time will take fewer heartbeats, which is important if the subject's heart rate is slow. The limit of how high the views per segment can go depends on the temporal resolution desired.

▶ **TABLE III4-2** Calculating Acquisition Times for Varying Heart Rates and Views per Segment ($N_{PE} = 100$)

Heart Rate	R-R Interval (msec)	Acq Window (msec)	True TR (msec)	Views per segment (vps)*	"TR" (temporal resolution)	Number of frames	Acq Time in heartbeats	Acq Time (in sec)
(beats per min)	(60/HR) × 1000	R-R × 0.85	Scanner dependent	User defined	True TR × vps	Acq Win/ "TR"	N_{PE}/vps	(N_{PE}/vps) R-R (sec)
Slow								
60 bpm	1000	850	10	10	100	8	10	10
				8	80	10	13	13
				6	**60**	**14**	**17**	**17**
				5	50	17	20	20
				4	40	21	25	25
68 bpm	880	750	10	100	100	7	10	8.8
				8	80	9	13	11.4
				6	60	12	17	15
				5	**50**	**15**	**20**	**17.6**
				4	40	18	25	22
Medium								
75 bpm	800	680	10	10	100	6	10	8
				8	80	8	13	10.4
				6	60	11	17	13.6
				5	**50**	**13**	**20**	**16**
				4	40	17	25	20
80 bpm	750	640	10	10	100	6	10	7.5
				8	80	7	13	9.8
				6	60	10	17	12.8
				5	50	12	20	15
				4	**40**	**16**	**25**	**18.8**
				3	30	21	33	24.8
Fast								
90 bpm	667	570	10	10	100	5	10	6.7
				8	80	7	13	8.6
				6	60	9	17	11.4
				5	50	11	20	13.3
				4	**40**	**14**	**25**	**16.7**
				3	30	19	33	22

*Note that vendors vary the range and selection of views per segment values. Some prefer even numbers and others prefer odd numbers. Similar calculations can be performed regardless.

Tip #2: Temporal Resolution

Aim for a temporal resolution in the range of 30–60 msec. On some systems, the TR shown on the MR console is the true TR; on others, the TR gives the temporal resolution (true TR × views per segment). It is important to realize that the number of frames is not as important as the temporal resolution. The temporal resolution determines how well abnormal wall motion, particularly systolic dysfunction, can be detected on images. Higher heart rates require better temporal resolution for accurate estimates of function.

Tip #3: Poor Breath Holders

For subjects who are poor breath holders, use a higher number of views per segment combined with a lower number of phase-encoding steps. Recall that supplemental oxygen via nasal cannula can be extremely helpful in increasing the breath-holding capacity of subjects. The acquisition time can be reduced with use of higher views per segment. Again the caveat about maintaining reasonable temporal resolution holds. If necessary, the acquisition time can be reduced further by decreasing N_{PE}. One way to achieve this without a loss in spatial resolution is to use rectangular field of view.

Tip #4: Faster Heart Rate During Breath Hold

Beware of changes in heart rate when the subject suspends respiration. The heart rate frequently increases with suspended respiration. If the R-R interval becomes shorter than the prescribed acquisition window, the triggering will occur for every other heartbeat rather than every heartbeat. The acquisition time will double. To have a reasonable estimate of heart rate for sequence parameter optimization, it may be worth having the subject perform a trial breath hold to assess heart rate changes.

> **IMPORTANT CONCEPTS:** Use a higher number of views per segment in subjects with slower heart rates and a lower number in subjects with faster heart rates. Poor breath holders may require a higher number of views per segment as well as a reduced number of phase-encoding steps to shorten acquisition times. Assumptions about heart rates used to determine sequence parameters should be made based on observations during suspended respiration to better reflect what happens during breath-hold cine GRE acquisitions.

VIEW SHARING OR ECHO SHARING

The goal of view sharing, as introduced in Chapter I-8 (Figure I8-20), is to increase the apparent temporal resolution without much increase in acquisition time. In its typical implementation, view sharing roughly doubles the number of frames. However, a twofold improvement in temporal resolution is not actually achieved. The sharing of data across consecutive k-spaces makes the temporal resolution difficult to determine—it lies somewhere between the original value and the apparent value.

Consider, for example, the case of subject with a heart rate of 72 beats per minute (Figure III4-7). As just discussed, the acquisition window will be 720 msec. If 9 views per segment are used (without view sharing), then the acquisition time for a 100 × 256 image will be about 11 heartbeats, and the temporal resolution will be 90 msec, assuming the true TR is 10 msec. There will be 8 frames in the cine acquisition. By using view sharing, the acquisition duration will still be 11 heartbeats, but instead of 8 frames, 15 frames will be generated, and the apparent temporal resolution will nearly double (Figure III4-7). What is the true temporal resolution of this view-shared acquisition? It is difficult to define, because the interpolated frames contain some echoes acquired at the desired time point and other echoes copied from adjacent time points (Chapter I-8). The true temporal resolution lies somewhere between 45 and 90 msec and is probably closer to 45 msec.

> **IMPORTANT CONCEPT:** View sharing increases the apparent temporal resolution of a cine GRE sequence without increasing the acquisition time. When combined with view sharing, higher numbers of views per segment can be used to decrease acquisition times without a loss in apparent temporal resolution.

STEADY-STATE FREE PRECESSION CINE GRE

As introduced in Chapter I-4, steady-state free precession (SSFP) sequences are a valuable alternative to spoiled gradient echo sequences. There are particular advantages in cardiac applications. First, in the absence of artifacts, the image contrast and signal-to-noise ratios are superior to those of spoiled gradient echo cine GRE images. Consequently, these sequences are well suited for parallel imaging (discussed below), which decreases acquisition times at the price of reduced signal-to-noise ratio. Second, because these sequences rely on intrinsic T2 differences between tissues (rather than on inflow) for image contrast, the TR times can be as short as possible, depending on the capabilities of the scanner. Shorter TR times can translate into higher temporal resolution, higher spatial resolution, decreased acquisition time, or some combination of all three.

Steady-state gradient echo sequences require magnetization to be in steady state, so the RF pulses are applied throughout the acquisition. With ECG-triggered sequences, the R waves initiate data acquisition, but during the trigger window, the RF pulses continue to be applied for

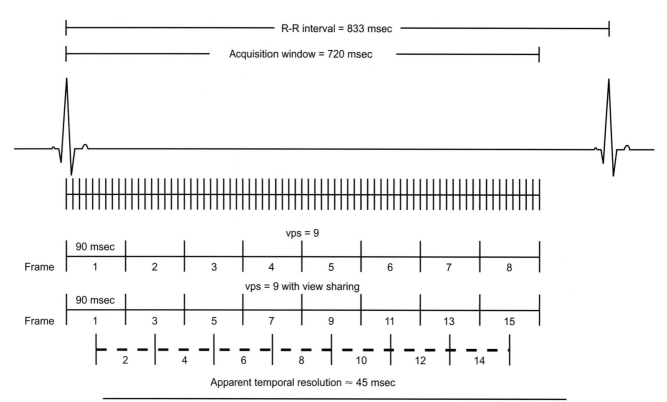

FIGURE III4-7. View sharing or echo sharing using nine views per segment. Without view sharing, the temporal resolution is about 90 msec. With view sharing (dashed lines), 15 frames span the acquisition window, so the apparent temporal resolution is about 45 msec.

the purposes of maintaining steady-state magnetization, although echoes are not recorded.

Choosing Parameters

To maintain steady-state free precession, the repetition times associated with these sequences are always short, typically less than 4–5 msec with TE less than 2 msec. A flip angle of 40–60° is commonly used. Because the true TR is so short, these sequences are always implemented with segmented k-space filling. For example, if the TR = 3.6 msec, and the number of views per segment is 15, then the temporal resolution would be a comfortable 54 msec. Compared to spoiled gradient echo techniques, the steady-state sequences provide images with higher spatial resolution in the same acquisition times as spoiled gradient echo sequences. For example, with 15 views per segment, even an image with N_{PE} = 240 would require only 16 heartbeats.

The most common implementation of steady-state free precession cine GRE sequences uses the shorter TR for faster acquisitions. In fact, if the acquisitions are very short, then multiple slice positions can be imaged per breath hold. For example, with 15 views per segment, a standard image with 100 × 256 might take only 7 heartbeats. If the subject has low cardiorespiratory reserve, the corresponding 5–7 sec breath hold may be the most he or she can tolerate.

But, if the subject can suspend respiration for closer to 20 sec, then 2 or 3 slice positions could be imaged in a single (14 or 21 heartbeat) breath hold acquisition.

The approach to calculating optimal parameters for steady-state free precession sequences are the same as described earlier for spoiled gradient echo sequences. View sharing can also be implemented to increase the apparent temporal resolution for a given sequence. For example, in the preceding scenario, if the number of views per segment is increased from 15 to 25, then the acquisition time for an image with matrix of 100 × 256 would be reduced to 4 heart beats. The temporal resolution without view sharing would be 90 msec (25 × 3.6 msec). With view sharing, however, the effective temporal resolution would be acceptable at about 45 msec, and three separate slice positions could be imaged in a 12-heartbeat acquisition.

Limitations of Steady-State Free Precession Gradient Echo Imaging

While SSFP GRE sequences have desirable speed, contrast, and signal-to-noise properties, they suffer from several limitations. Because of the strict requirements for steady state, these sequences are extremely sensitive to field inhomogeneities. If the field is not sufficiently shimmed or the subject has metallic artifacts near the area of interest, these sequences may have serious artifacts (Figure III4-8). Local shimming or frequency adjustments may be necessary to improve the image quality of these sequences, particularly at 3 T. Also, because the steady-state free precession sequences rely on T2/T1 differences rather than time-of-flight effects, they may demonstrate less sensitivity to turbulent flow, such as occurs with stenotic or regurgitant valves or stenotic vessels. Although steady-state free precession sequences have replaced conventional cine GRE sequences in most centers, spoiled GRE sequences should still be maintained in the repertory for detection of subtle flow abnormalities in valvular disease or when field inhomogeneity leads to insurmountable artifacts with the SSFP sequences.

With steady state free precession sequences, the TE times are typically <2 msec. At 1.5 T, gradient echo imaging at such TEs is associated with chemical shift artifact of the second kind (India ink artifact; see Chapter I-9, Figure I9-3). This artifact may be problematic in certain clinical settings, such as the evaluation of arrhythmogenic right ventricular dysplasia (see Chapter III-5); under those circumstances spoiled gradient echo cine sequences may be preferable.

One other potential limitation is the energy deposition associated with the continuous application of RF pulses to maintain steady state. Depending on subject size and body habitus, SAR limits may be reached, particulary at higher flip angles.

RETROSPECTIVE GATING AND ARRHYTHMIA REJECTION

As described in Chapter III-1, with retrospective gating, data acquisition is continuous and echoes are sorted in k-space according to their timing relative to the R wave. Continuous acquisition is well suited to the requirements of steady-state free precession sequences. With retrospective gating, the entire cardiac cycle is imaged, including end diastole. This method is compatible with peripheral pulse gating. Computationally, image reconstruction is more complex and may result in noticeable delays in appearance of images.

Retrospective gating is useful in patients with arrhythmias, because data can be selected depending on the ECG pattern. For example, if an irregular heartbeat causes some R-R intervals to be shorter than expected, data from these shorter heartbeats can be rejected, and the resulting images are more faithful to cardiac motion during normal heartbeats. Several commercial systems provide such *arrhythmia rejection* software tools.

PARALLEL IMAGING

The high signal-to-noise ratios and high contrast-to-noise ratios of steady-state free precession cine GRE sequences are advantageous for parallel imaging applications (Chapter I-8).

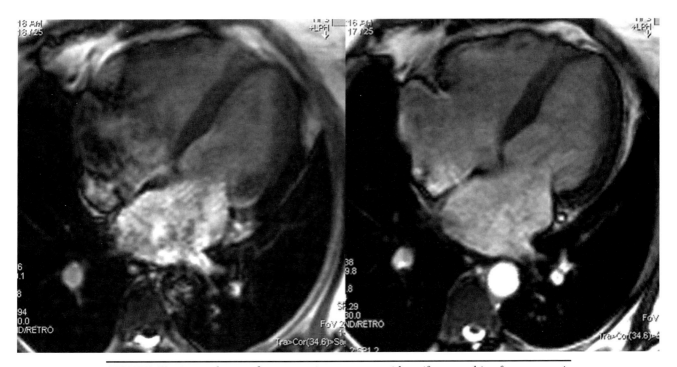

FIGURE III4-8. Steady-state free precession sequence with artifacts resulting from magnetic field inhomogeneity and flow effects (left). Following frequency adjustment, image quality improves substantially (right).

As discussed in Chapter I-8, parallel imaging techniques allow k-space to be undersampled and therefore result in substantial time savings. The degree to which k-space can be undersampled depends on the number of independent coil elements that have separate receiver channels in the phase-encoding direction. A twofold reduction in phase-encoding steps is readily achievable. The development of new cardiac receiver coils and algorithms for parallel imaging is of great research and commercial interest.

Reduction in imaging time with parallel imaging is not proportional to the number of receiver channels because the information from channels is not totally independent. Coil sensitivity mapping is needed for image reconstruction. Depending on the implementation, the coil sensitivity map may require a separate acquisition. Alternatively, it may be embedded within the imaging sequence with the acquisition of additional reference lines of data, typically about 24. For example, for a 128 × 256 image, a parallel factor of 2 would still require collection of about 64 + 24 or 88 lines of k-space. Additionally, parallel imaging methods are generally not tolerant of any phase wrapping due to conventional rectangular field of view. Therefore, some of the gains in time are offset by additional time needed to

imagane increased FOV. Nonetheless, parallel imaging methods are of clear value for cardiac imaging.

REAL-TIME STEADY-STATE FREE PRECESSION CINE GRE

Most cine GRE sequences require data collection across multiple heartbeats. With steady-state free precession sequences, it is possible to perform real-time imaging, similar to echocardiography or fluoroscopy, where the data needed to acquire each frame are collected during a single short portion of a single heartbeat and reconstructed "on the fly" for real-time viewing. Real-time cine GRE requires the fastest MRI systems, ultrashort TRs, high numbers of views per segment, view sharing, and parallel imaging. Even with the use of many time-saving tricks, real-time cine GRE can achieve only modest spatial resolution.

Consider the scenarios in Figure III4-9. On some commercial systems, it is possible to achieve a true TR of about 2.5 msec or less. A large number of views per segment can be selected depending on the desired balance between temporal and spatial resolution.

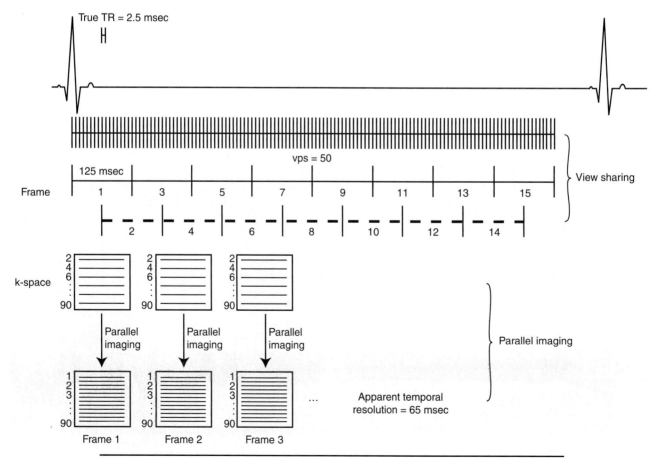

FIGURE III4-9. Real-time steady-state free precession gradient echo sequence implemented with parallel imaging and view sharing to achieve an apparent temporal resolution of 65 msec.

Scenario 1: 70 Views per Segment/Frame

This number equals the number of phase-encoding steps needed to fill the k-space for a single frame. Without parallel imaging techniques, the spatial resolution would be low (because the imaging matrix would be 70 × 128 or 70 × 256), but with parallel imaging it could easily be possible to achieve an imaging matrix of 100 × 256. Assuming a field of view of 250 × 350 mm, the in-plane spatial resolution would be 2.5 × 1.4 mm. The temporal resolution without view sharing would be 175 msec (70 × 2.5 msec), which would be too large for definition of systole, but with view sharing the effective temporal resolution could be as low as 90 msec.

Scenario 2 (Figure III4-9): 50 Views per Segment/Frame

Spatial resolution would be low without parallel imaging (50 × 256 matrix), but with parallel imaging the matrix could be closer to 90 × 256. Assuming a field of view of 250 × 350 mm, the in-plane spatial resolution would be less than 3 mm. In this scenario, the temporal resolution without view sharing would be 125 msec (50 × 2.5 msec), and with view sharing the apparent temporal resolution would be about 65 msec.

TAGGED CINE GRE IMAGES

For a more sophisticated method to evaluate contractility, cine MR with tagging can be performed in conjunction with segmented k-space cine gradient echo imaging, referred to as *spatial modulation of magnetization* *(SPAMM)*. The tagging is achieved by RF prepulses that are spatially selective and cause striped or grid patterns of saturation oriented perpendicular to the imaging plane (Figure III4-10). The tags have low signal intensity because they reflect local saturation. Over time, they fade because of T1 relaxation and so are less apparent on late diastolic images. The tags serve as markers of the position of the underlying myocardium and enable the viewer to appreciate patterns of deformation better than is possible with plain cine MRI. If diastolic function is of interest, the tagging pulse can be applied in late systole and imaging carried out throughout diastole.

Beyond serving as a visual tool, tagging can be used to quantify wall motion and myocordial strain. Quantitative interpretations of strain can be determined from tagged data based on displacement of the tagged regions. Quantitative SPAMM requires special software and expertise that to date have been confined to the research setting.

APPLICATION TIPS WITH CINE GRE SEQUENCES

A complete evaluation of left ventricular function requires a series of short axis cine gradient echo images from base to the apex, typically in 8–10 mm intervals, and at least two to three long axis views (see the protocol at the end of this chapter). Image processing techniques to determine parameters such as left ventricular end diastolic and end systolic volumes, stroke volume, ejection fraction, left ventricular mass, and contractility are reviewed in this section.

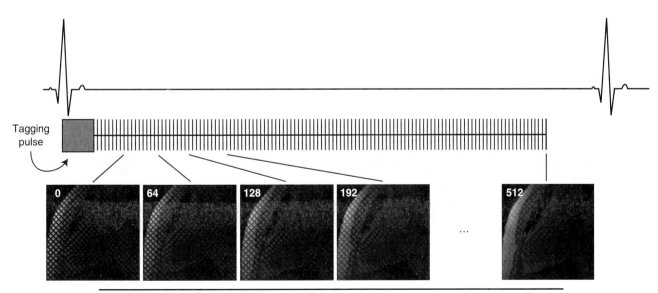

FIGURE III4-10. Tagged cine gradient echo imaging with images starting immediately after the tagging pulse. Note the progressive fading of the tags during each heartbeat due to T1 relaxation of saturated protons.

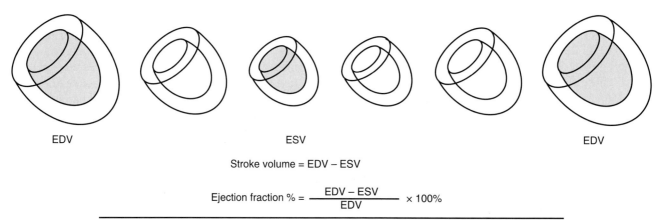

EDV   ESV   EDV

Stroke volume = EDV − ESV

$$\text{Ejection fraction \%} = \frac{\text{EDV} - \text{ESV}}{\text{EDV}} \times 100\%$$

FIGURE III4-11. End diastolic volume (EDV) and end systolic volume (ESV) (shaded) correspond to the largest and smallest volumes of the left ventricular chamber. These volumes are needed for the measurement of ejection fraction (EF).

Left Ventricular Volumes and Ejection Fraction

Quantification of left ventricular function includes measurement of ejection fraction, together with the end diastolic and end systolic volumes. How these values are determined from the cine GRE images is described in this section, following a review of definitions (Figure III4-11).

The *end systolic volume (ESV)* of the left ventricle is defined as the intracavitary volume of the left ventricle when the ventricle has fully contracted. Typically, the ESV is considered equivalent to the minimum volume of the left ventricle. The *end diastolic volume (EDV)* is the volume prior to the onset of systole and is typically considered equivalent to the maximum intracavitary volume. The *stroke volume (SV)* is the difference between EDV and ESV. *Ejection fraction (EF)* is defined as the ratio of the stroke volume to the EDV:

Ejection fraction (EF, %)
$$= \frac{\text{EDV} - \text{ESV}}{\text{EDV}} \times 100 = \frac{\text{SV}}{\text{EDV}} \times 100$$

From these volumetric measurements, calculations of other standard parameters of cardiac function can also be performed. For example, *cardiac output (CO, mL/min)* provides a measure of the net forward flow of blood over time (mL/min) and can be calculated by multiplying the stroke volume and heart rate (HR):

Cardiac output (mL/min)
$$= \text{SV (ml/beat)} \times \text{HR (beats/min)}$$

More commonly, cardiac output is normalized to patient body surface area (BSA) to generate a *cardiac index (CI, mL/min/m²)*.

Cardiac index (mL/min/m²) = CO/BSA

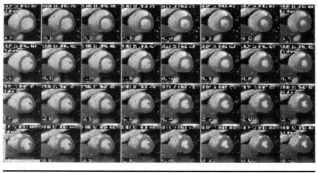

FIGURE III4-12. Short axis cine gradient echo images from the base to mid-left ventricle (top row base, bottom row mid) across the cardiac cycle (left column immediately after the R wave, right column peak systole).

There are several formulas to estimate body surface area (BSA) using body weight and height. Most MRI cardiac software programs will provide estimates of CI.

EDV and ESV can be approximated in a number of ways from the MR images. The most commonly used method relies on a series of short axis images from the base of the left ventricle to the apex. The images are viewed in a matrix layout (Figure III4-12) where slice positions vary from top to bottom while the time point in the cardiac cycle varies from left to right. For any given column or time point in the cardiac cycle, a stack of images in that column would represent the entire left ventricle. For example, in Figure III4-12, the 8th column corresponds to end systole, while the 1st column corresponds to end diastole.

To compute a left ventricular volume from a series of short axis images, Simpson's rule is applied. In its simplest form, the rule estimates the volume as the sum of cross-sectional areas, A, of each slice, multiplied by t, the

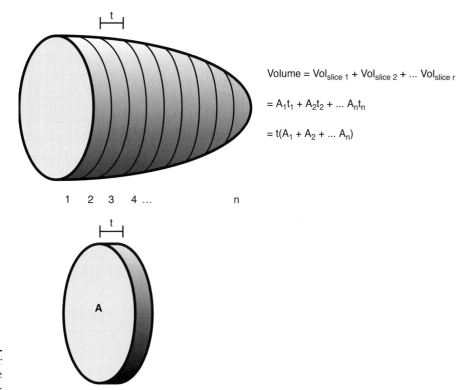

$$Volume = Vol_{slice\ 1} + Vol_{slice\ 2} + ... Vol_{slice\ r}$$

$$= A_1t_1 + A_2t_2 + ... A_nt_n$$

$$= t(A_1 + A_2 + ... A_n)$$

Volume of slice = A x t

FIGURE III4-13. Simpson's rule for computing left ventricular volume based on summing the volumes of individual slices (treated as disks).

distance between slices (Figure III4-13) (or the slice thickness plus interslice gaps):

$$Volume\ (cm^3) = A_1(cm^2) \times t_1\ (cm) + A_2\ (cm^2) \times t_2\ (cm)$$
$$+ \cdots + A_N\ (cm^2) \times t_N\ (cm)$$
$$= (A_1 + A_2 + \cdots + A_N) \times t$$

assuming distance between slices is the same, t, for the entire volume.

A simple way to implement this rule is to image short axis slices at 1 cm intervals (for example, 7 mm slices with 3 mm gap or 8 mm slices with 2 mm gap). With t=1 the sum of the cross sectional areas of each slice (in cm²) will numerically equal the total volume of the left ventricle (in cm³).

To determine ESV, the intracavitary cross-sectional areas of the left ventricle must be calculated for all the images at end systole, while EDV is calculated from the sum of areas for all the images at end diastole.

Cross-sectional areas can be manually defined by drawing regions of interest along the endocardial border on each end diastolic and end systolic image. Alternatively, post-processing software packages provided by MR vendors and others can be used to perform the analysis in a semi-automated fashion.

There are several challenges in performing EF calculations. First, it should be decided whether the papillary muscles and trabeculae are included in the intracavitary volumes. If papillary muscles and trabeculae are excluded from the blood pool at diastole, they must also be excluded on all systolic images. In general, it is easier to draw relatively circular regions of interest around the blood pool, thus including papillary muscles in the chamber volumes (Figure III4-14). On the other hand, the coalescence of papillary muscles on systole may make it difficult to separate them from the myocardial wall. The key is consistency. The same papillary muscles should be included in the intracavitary volume at systole as are included at diastole.

A second challenge is to decide which slices at the left ventricular base to include in the volumetric calculations. The contractile motion of the left ventricle during systole can cause the basal short axis slice to depict left atrium during systole and left ventricle during diastole. Additionally, a slice thickness of 6–8 mm contributes to volume averaging that makes precise definition of boundaries difficult. One guiding principle is to use only images that depict a complete circumferential rim of left ventricular muscle for volume calculations (Figure III4-15). EDV usually includes one or two more short axis slices than ESV.

CHALLENGE QUESTION: For measurements of ejection fraction, what are the expected consequences of low-temporal-resolution cine GRE images on the accuracy of calculation?

Include
papillary muscles
in LV volume

Exclude
papillary muscles
in LV volume

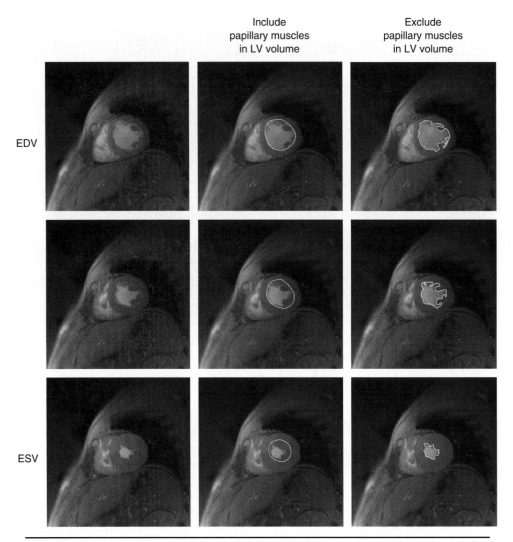

EDV

ESV

FIGURE III4-14. Consistency in defining the left ventricular intracavitary volumes is critical to obtaining accurate estimates of ejection fraction. For the particular short axis slice shown at end diastole, early diastole, and end systole, two approaches are illustrated, indicated by bright outlines around the regions of interest—inclusion of papillary muscles in the left ventricular volumes (middle column) and exclusion (right column).

Answer: End-diastolic volumes are usually accurately measured provided gating is adequate. With inadequate temporal resolution, end-systole may be missed, resulting in misleadingly high end-systolic volumes and, consequently, underestimations of ejection fraction.

Left Ventricular Mass

Left ventricular mass can also be accurately estimated with the standard short axis cine images. By drawing regions of interest around the outer, or *epicardial*, contour of the left ventricle, together with the *endocardial* contour, the area of left ventricular myocardium for a given slice position can be determined (Figure III4-16). The total LV myocardial volume can be calculated by summing the areas for each slice position. Again, this calculation is

simplest if the interval between adjacent slices is 1 cm. Images at end diastole are often used. Assuming that the density of myocardium is 1.05 g/mL, the left ventricular mass can be calculated as

$$\text{LV myocardial mass (g)} = \text{LV myocardial volume} \\ \text{(mL)} \times 1.05 \text{ g/mL}.$$

Assessment of Wall Motion and Thickening

While left ventricular contractility is typically assessed by viewing images in cine loops, software packages are available that provide quantitative measures of wall motion and thickening. Typical algorithms rely on the definition of left ventricle boundaries along endo- and epicardial

EDV   ESV

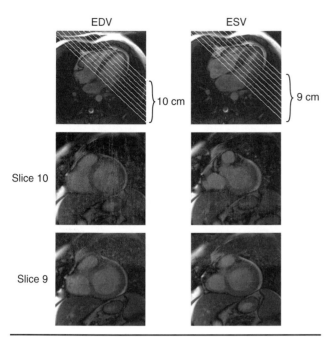

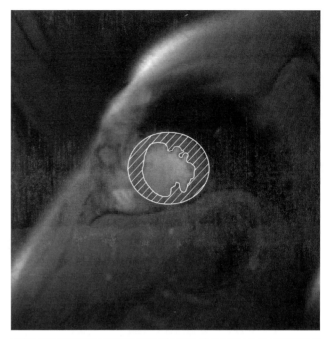

Slice 10

Slice 9

FIGURE III4-15. Calculations of left ventricular volume using short axis images at the base. The long axis dimension of the left ventricle is shorter at end systole (ESV) than at end diastole (EDV). The inclusion of slice 10 for end diastolic volumes is justified by the appearance of a circumferential rim of myocardium, whereas at end systole the same slice position is predominantly in the left atrium and therefore not included in ESV calculations.

surfaces, which are propagated across all the images of all the slices. Motion and thickening of each segment of the wall are assessed for the entire cardiac cycle. These values are quantified and can usually be depicted as a color-coded bull's eye or polar map (similar to those described in Chapter III-2, Figure III2-13). Useful parameters include wall thickness or percent wall thickening (Figure III4-17), defined as

$$\text{Percent thickening (\%)} = (\text{Thickness}_{sys} - \text{Thickness}_{dias})/ (\text{Thickness}_{dias}) \times 100\%$$

Evaluation of Cardiac Valves

Cine gradient echo images can be useful for evaluating cardiac valvular dysfunction. Aortic stenosis is associated with turbulent flow patterns that cause signal loss on images during systole; aortic insufficiency jets are seen during diastole (Figure III4-18). It is important to realize that the turbulent jets may be eccentrically positioned with respect to the valve orifice, so that multiple cine images across the valve are needed to assess fully for disease.

A qualitative assessment of the severity of stenosis or insufficiency may be possible based on the extent of signal loss, but more accurate measures can be determined using cine phase contrast flow quantification methods, described in Chapter III-6.

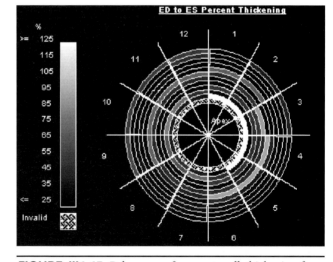

FIGURE III4-16. Left ventricular mass is computed by summing its cross-sectional areas on short axis images, from the base to the apex. Each cross-sectional area requires defining two regions of interest, the epicardial and endocardial regions.

FIGURE III4-17. Polar map of percent wall thickening from end diastole to end systole showing diffuse hypokinesis of the entire left ventricle.

POTENTIAL PITFALLS WITH CINE GRE SEQUENCES

A variety of pitfalls are associated with cine GRE imaging, as reviewed in this section.

Right Atrial Pseudomass

A small filling defect in the right atrial wall is commonly seen on bright-blood sequences and can be mistaken for a mass or thrombus (Figure III4-19). In fact, this projection is present on almost all cardiac MR examinations and represents the confluence of normal anatomic structures— part of the Chiari network, crista terminalis, and remnants from embryonic valves of the coronary sinus and inferior vena cava. The apparent lesion is referred to as a right atrial pseudomass and should be recognized as a normal finding.

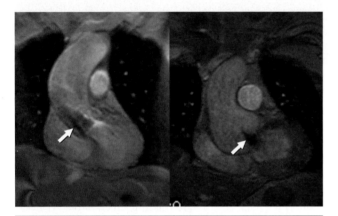

FIGURE III4-18. Oblique coronal cine frames depict systolic jet of aortic stenosis (left, arrow) extending to the ascending aorta and diastolic regurgitant jet of aortic insufficiency (right, arrow) directed toward the left ventricle in two different subjects.

Gating off the T Wave

Because of the magnetohydrodynamic effect described in Chapter III-1, ECG-triggered sequences can inadvertently be triggered by a peaked T wave rather than the desired R wave. Images then span late systole through diastole and exclude systole. The ECG leads should be adjusted or lead polarity changed so that the R wave is more pronounced than the T wave. Alternatively, if available, vectorcardiogram-based triggering mechanisms could be used.

Arrhythmias and Poor Gating

The two manifestations of a poorly triggered sequences are an irregularity in the noises of the MR system during image acquisition and acquisition times that exceed expected directions. It may be difficult to recognize from the images alone that the sequence was acquired with poor gating. Frames that are supposed to reflect systole and diastole may depict these periods less accurately. The images can be misleading and result in inaccurate interpretations, include grossly underestimating left ventrical function. Careful attention at the time of acquisition is criticial to avoid this pitfall.

Stasis

In the setting of relative stasis of the blood pool in the left ventricle, saturation of the signal can produce poor image contrast between the blood pool and the myocardium, resulting in blurring of the endocardial borders and false values of measured parameters.

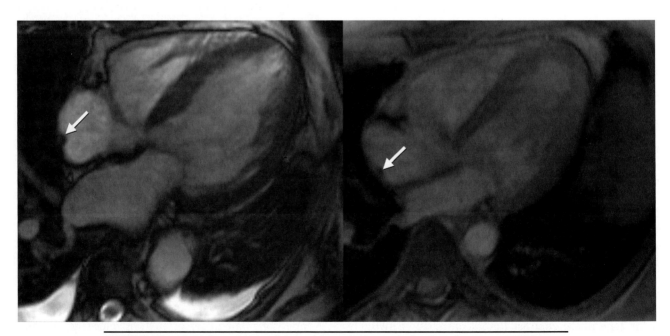

FIGURE III4-19. Right atrial pseudomass (arrows), two examples (see also Figure I4-19).

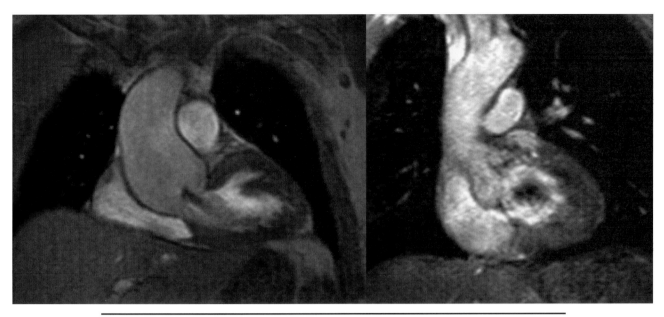

FIGURE III4-20. Real (left) and pseudo (right) aortic insufficiency.

Pseudoaortic Insufficiency

Rapidly moving blood causes dephasing and loss of signal. This phenomenon is the basis for the diagnosis of valvular stenosis and insufficiency. However, normally flowing blood can also cause signal changes. One common pitfall is the appearance of signal loss in the left ventricular chamber as a result of inflow through the mitral valve orifice. Appearing in diastole, this signal loss can be misinterpreted as aortic insufficiency (Figure III4-20). Unlike the regurgitant jet in true aortic insufficiency, however, this region of signal loss is generally diffuse and central within the left ventricle, rather than emanating from the level of the aortic valve leaflets.

REVIEW QUESTIONS

1. You set up a prospectively gated GRE sequence for a subject with a resting heart rate of 60 beats per minute, yielding an acquisition window of 850 msec. However, once the subject holds her breath, her heart rate increases to a regular rate of 75 beats per minute (R-R interval of 800 msec). What will happen to the acquisition time and image quality?

2. In the preceding scenario, with an acquisition window of 850 msec, the number of views per segment was selected so that the acquisition time was near the limits of the subject's breath-holding capacity.
   a. With the increase in heart rate that accompanies her breath holding, how should the number of views per segment be modified to restore the original acquisition time? Should vps be increased or decreased?
   b. If the acquisition window is decreased to 700 msec and the views per segment is kept the same, how will the acquisition time be affected?
   c. With the faster heart rate during breath holding, you are concerned about missing end systole with the temporal resolution of your basic sequence setting. How should the number of views per segment be changed to improve the temporal resolution of the sequence to represent systole accurately?

3. A cine GRE cardiac MR study has a temporal resolution of 100 msec, and the views per segment is 12 for a total acquisition time of about 8 sec (10 heartbeats). If the purpose of the study is to measure left ventricular function, including ejection fraction, what steps can you take to improve the temporal resolution to 50 msec? What will be the effect on acquisition time?

4. In the above case, the subject is only able to suspend respiration for the acquisition time needed to attain 50 msec temporal resolution. What can you do to solve this problem, while still achieving reasonable image quality and temporal resolution?

5. A retrospectively gated cine acquisition is being used for a cardiac MR study. The steady-state free precession sequence has a true TR of 3 msec and is set up with 15 views per segment so that each frame corresponds to 45 msec of the cardiac cycle. The imaging matrix is 105×256, and therefore you expect the entire acquisition to take 7 heartbeats. The subject's heart rate is 72 beats per minute (R-R interval 833 msec) when you set up the sequence parameters, and you define the threshold for arrhythmia rejection

to be heartbeats that are less than 750 msec. Once you start the breath hold acquisition, the systems emits a continuous hum.

a. Why is the hum continuous and not periodic with every beat?

b. After about 10 sec, the system is still acquiring data, but the subject can no longer hold her breath. What has happened? How can you solve the problem?

6. You are asked to evaluate the thoracic aorta in a subject who has a systolic murmur. A cine gradient echo image in systole through the left ventricular outflow tract/ascending aorta is shown in Figure III4-Q6A.

a. What are the findings?

b. How would you position the slice plane to evaluate the possibility of a bicuspid aortic valve?

7. For a cardiac MR study, you wish to administer gadolinium contrast material. You also wish to used tagged cine GRE acquisitions to assess left ventricular wall motion. Should you perform the tagged studies before or after gadolinium contrast injection?

8. As part of an evaluation of left ventricular function, you measure EDV and ESV and calculate stroke volume as the difference. What MR method can you use to verify the accuracy of this calculation independently? (*Hint:* Consider Chapter II-3.)

9. The regions of interest in Figure III4-Q9A were drawn for a calculation of EDV and ESV. Are the regions drawn correctly?

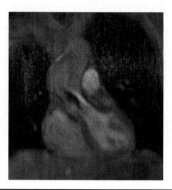

FIGURE III4-Q6A

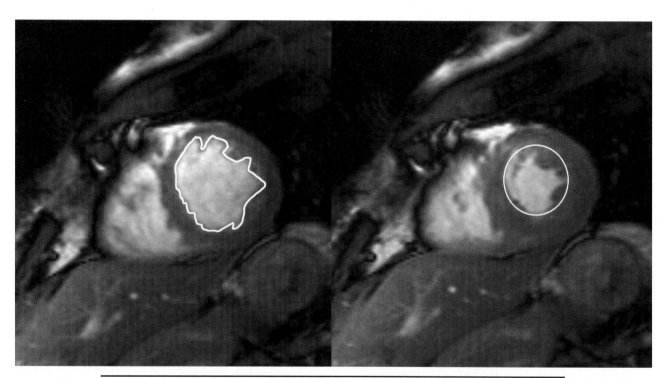

FIGURE III4-Q9A. ROIs drawn for (left) EDV and (right) ESV.

▶ **TABLE III4-3** Table for Determining Views Per Segment Based on Heart Rate and Desired Acquisition Time

Heart Rate (beats per min)	R-R Interval (msec) $(60/HR) \times 1000$	Acq Window (msec) $R\text{-}R \times 0.85$	True TR (msec) Scanner dependent	Views per segment (vps)* User defined	"TR" (temporal resolution) True TR $\times$ vps	Number of phase encoding steps User defined	Number of frames Acq Win/ Win/TR	Acq Time in heartbeats N_{PE}/vps
Slow								
60 bpm	1000	850						
68 bpm	880	750						
Medium								
75 bpm	800	680						
80 bpm	750	640						
Fast								
90 bpm	667	570						

▶ **PROTOCOL: Left Ventricular Function Study**

Setup and Preparation	Notes
ECG Leads	Necessary
Coil	Torso phased-array
Positioning tips	Supine, head first
Subject instructions	End-expiratory breathholding Supplemental oxygen by nasal cannula optional

Sequence	Imaging Plane	Parameters
1 Scout (true FISP or spoiled GRE)	Multiplanar	Default
2 Fast spin echo imaging of the chest (double IR single-shot half-Fourier FSE, if available)	Axial	Single-shot or FSE with TR = R-R interval 8–10 mm slices
3 Single-slice scouts	Obliques to get short axis and long axis views	1 slice/breath-hold
4 Cine GRE (spoiled gradient echo or steady-state gradient echo, segmented k space)	Short axes	8 mm slices with 2 mm gaps Parameters (incl views per segment) defined for temporal resolution <60 msec, and acquisition time within a breath hold, LV base to apex, 8–12 slices
5 Cine GRE (spoiled gradient echo or steady state gradient echo, segmented k-space)	Long axes	8 mm slices Same parameters as above Less rectangular FOV for VLA view[1]
6 Cine phase contrast flow quantification (optional)	Oblique axial through ascending aorta	Temporal resolution <60 msec, retrospective gating, view-sharing for breath hold acquisition

[1]For most acquisitions 75% rectangular FOV can be used. Typically, for the vertical long axis (two-chamber) view, a larger FOV is needed or less rectangular FOV (85%).

Tissue Characterization in the Heart

An important application of cardiac MRI is to characterize tissues using special pulse sequences. Tissue characterization can be useful for subjects with cardiac masses and pericardial disease, as well as intrinsic myocardial diseases such as ischemic heart disease and cardiomyopathies. The most widely used tools are T1- and T2-weighted imaging, fat suppression, and gadolinium contrast enhancement in both the early (less than 5 min) and delayed (greater than 10–15 min) phases. Each of these tools is reviewed in this chapter. Examples of how different tissue characterization methods can be used to assess cardiac masses, myocardial viability, and arrhythmogenic right ventricular displasia are then considered (with full protocols provided at the end of the chapter). The assessment of ischemic myocardium is discussed in more detail in Chapter III-7.

KEY CONCEPTS

▶ T1-weighted imaging can be achieved with spin echo or spoiled gradient echo imaging.

▶ T2-weighted imaging can be achieved with spin echo imaging; T2-like weighting is produced with steady-state free precession gradient echo imaging.

▶ T2*-weighted imaging can be achieved with spoiled gradient echo imaging with relatively long TE.

▶ Fat suppression using frequency-selective saturation pulses is more specific for characterizing fat than inversion recovery techniques.

▶ Cystic masses and bland thrombus are diagnosed based on the absence of gadolinium enhancement.

▶ Delayed enhancement with gadolinium contrast is associated with infarcted myocardium. Other cardiomyopathies can also have delayed enhancement.

▶ Nulling of uninfarcted myocardium with an inversion recovery sequence provides optimal conspicuity of infarcted tissue.

▶ Clinical Protocols:
▶ Cardiac mass
▶ Cardiac viability
▶ Arrhythmogenic right ventricular dysplasia

T1-WEIGHTED IMAGING

T1-weighted images provide anatomic assessment of the myocardium and great vessels, help characterize lesions with short T1 relaxation times, and assess contrast enhancement. T1 weighting can be achieved using spin echo or spoiled gradient echo sequences. To improve conspicuity of myocardial and pericardial anatomy and pathology, black-blood images are often desired. Consequently, spin echo or fast spin echo (FSE) sequences with blood-nulling pulses are usually preferred over bright blood spoiled gradient echo sequences (Figure III5-1).

In addition to providing anatomic images of the heart and chest, T1-weighted sequences may also help to characterize some tissues, particularly those that have short T1 relaxation times and are therefore hyperintense on T1-weighted images. Tissues with short T1 times are listed in Table III5-1. With respect to detecting cardiac masses, the most common sources of confounding signal are fat and hemorrhage. It is important to recall that time-of-flight effects can also give rise to high signal on T1-weighted imaging and can result in a potential pitfall of interpretation.

For cardiac diagnoses, T1-weighted spin echo or fast spin echo sequences are ECG-gated. Since the TR must be set to one R-R interval, image contrast depends on the subject's heart rate. If the heart rate is slow, the TR may approach or exceed 1000 msec, reducing T1 weighting. The TE should be as short as possible for T1 weighting, typically under 50 msec.

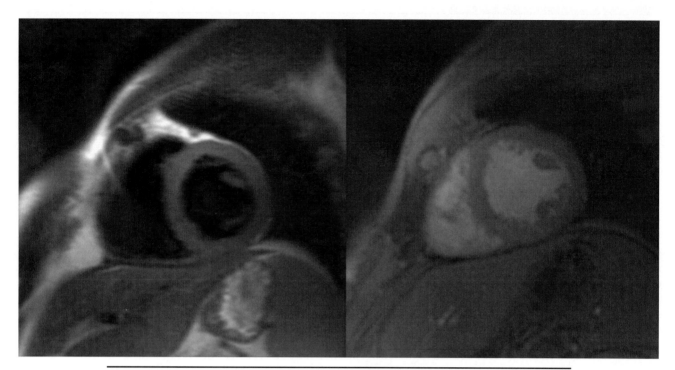

FIGURE III5-1. Short axis T1-weighted (a) fast spin echo and (b) spoiled gradient echo imaging.

▶ **TABLE III5-1**

Tissues Bright on T1-Weighted Images

Lipid (fat and sebaceous material)
Hemorrhagic products
Proteinaceous fluid
Melanin
Some forms of hydrated calcification calcium
Gadolinium, manganese, magnesium, copper, and certain other metals
  (Low or time-of-flight effects) (pitfall)

IMPORTANT CONCEPTS: T1-weighting with spin echo imaging is reduced if the subject's heart rate is slow and the TR exceeds 800–1000 msec. Spoiled gradient echo sequences provide alternative methods for T1-weighted imaging but have the disadvantage of high signal intensity of the blood pool.

T2-WEIGHTED AND T2*-WEIGHTED IMAGING

T2-weighted images of the heart are valuable in the detection and characterization of pathology with long T2 times, which yields high signal intensity on these images. They are generally performed with spin echo or fast spin echo sequences. Depending on the subject's heart rate, the TR is usually defined to be at least 2 R-R intervals with a TE of 80–100 msec. To defect high signal intensity pathology, blood nulling is desirable. With fast spin echo sequences,

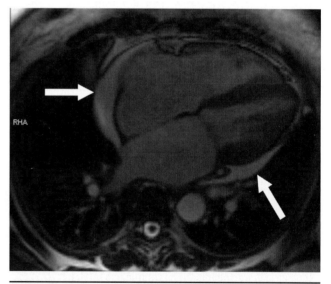

FIGURE III5-2. Pericardial effusion (arrows) is high in signal intensity on a steady-state free precession gradient echo sequence because of its high T2/T1 ratio.

fat is high in signal intensity, so fat suppression will improve lesion conspicuity.

For steady-state free precession gradient echo sequences, as discussed in Chapter III-4, image contrast is T2/T1 weighted, which means that both tissues with high water content and fatty tissue are high in signal intensity (Figure III5-2).

Occasionally, it may be desirable to obtain T2*-weighted images that are sensitive to susceptibility effects.

For example, for the diagnosis of hemochromatosis, a long-TE spoiled gradient echo sequence will demonstrate decreased signal intensity because of the susceptibility effects of iron in the myocardium (Figure III5-3).

> **IMPORTANT CONCEPT:** T2-weighting or T2-like-weighting can be achieved with black-blood spin echo methods or with bright-blood steady-state free precession gradient echo imaging. T2*-weighted imaging is particularly useful as an iron-sensitive sequence for the evaluation of hemochromatosis.

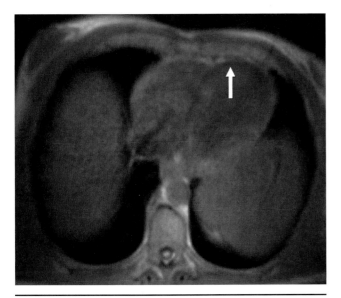

FIGURE III5-3. Low signal intensity in the myocardium on spoiled gradient echo imaging, caused by iron deposition that is due to primary hemochromatosis.

FAT SUPPRESSION

Fat suppression may be useful in cardiac MRI to help distinguish whether lesions that are high in signal intensity on T1-weighted images contain fat. It is also used to improve lesion conspicuity on T2-weighted fast spin echo images, where fat has high signal intensity (Chapter I-4).

Two approaches can be employed to achieve fat suppression: a frequency-selective fat suppression prepulse or an inversion recovery prepulse with short inversion time set to null tissues with short T1, such as fat (Figure III5-4). For tissue characterization, the frequency-selective method is more specific.

CHALLENGE QUESTION: Why is frequency-selective fat suppression preferred over short-inversion-time inversion recovery (STIR) imaging for characterizing tissues with high signal on T1-weighted images?

Answer: STIR imaging nulls signal with short T1, regardless of whether the signal is due to fat, hemorrhage, or melanin. With frequency-selective fat suppression, only fatty tissue will lose signal; blood and melanin will not.

When fat suppression is needed to enhance lesion conspicuity with T2-weighted images, inversion recovery sequences are frequently used. To ensure blood nulling as well as fat suppression on T2-weighted FSE images, triple inversion recovery sequences may be used, as described in Chapter III-3.

CHALLENGE QUESTION: Why is STIR imaging often preferred for suppressing fat on T2-weighted FSE sequences?

Answer: The STIR approach is a more robust method for suppressing fat, particularly in the chest, where field

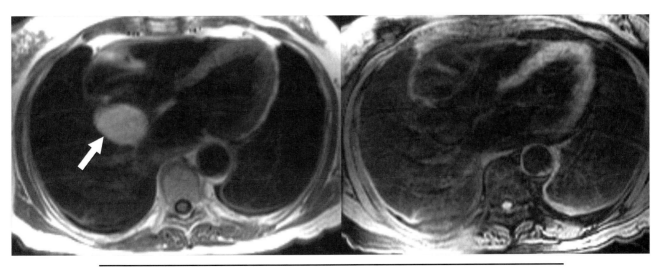

FIGURE III5-4. A mass in the interatrial septum has high signal intensity on T1-weighted imaging (left, arrow). With a frequency-selective fat-suppression pulse (right), the mass becomes uniformly hypointense, indicating that the lesion is a lipoma.

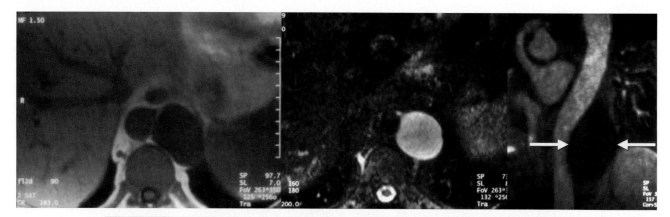

FIGURE III5-5. Periaortic cystic lymphangioma in the retroperitoneum shows uniform low signal intensity on T1-weighted gradient echo image (left) and high signal intensity on T2-weighted fast spin echo image (middle). Following contrast administration, no enhancement is seen in the cyst on a coronal fat-suppressed T1-weighted gradient echo image (arrows, right).

inhomogeneities can result in suboptimal frequency-selective fat suppression (see discussion in Chapter I-9). Field inhomogeneities have no significant effect on T1 relaxation times, and hence fat is reliably suppressed with STIR.

> **IMPORTANT CONCEPTS:** Frequency-selective fat suppression provides more specific characterization of fat-containing lesions, whereas STIR imaging suppresses tissues based only on their short T1 relaxation times. However, frequency-selective fat suppression requires good field homogeneity, which may be difficult to achieve in the chest.

CONTRAST ENHANCEMENT

Contrast-enhanced T1-weighted imaging can also help to characterize pathology in the heart and pericardium. Most commonly, contrast material is useful to differentiate enhancing masses, such as cardiac tumors, from nonenhancing pathology, such as cysts (Figure III5-5) and thrombi. To assess the vascularity of a lesion, the delay time between injection and imaging is typically less than 5 minutes.

Contrast enhancement is assessed with black-blood ECG-gated T1-weighted spin echo sequences. Alternatively, fat-suppressed T1-weighted spoiled gradient echo imaging can be used (Figure III5-5).

DELAYED CONTRAST ENHANCEMENT

One of the most active and still growing areas of cardiac MRI is the use of delayed contrast-enhanced MRI to characterize myocardial infarction or, alternatively, to assess myocardial viability. Following intravenous injection of extracellular contrast agents such as gadolinium chelates, areas of infarct and fibrosis in subacute and chronic

▶ **TABLE III5-2**

Causes of Delayed Contrast Enhancement

Subacute or chronic myocardial infarct
Acute myocardial infarct
Sarcoidosis
Hypertrophic cardiomyopathy
Acute myocarditis
Arrhythmogenic right ventricular dysplasia

infarcts demonstrate delayed enhancement and delayed washout relative to viable myocardium. Delayed enhancement has also been demonstrated in acute infarcts and other diseases listed in Table III5-2, although its patterns of distribution vary for different etiologies.

About 10–30 min after injection, delayed washout of contrast material from infarcted myocardium will cause it to appear slightly hyperintense relative to uninfarcted myocardium. However, this difference may be difficult to detect on routine T1-weighted imaging (and with other modalities such as contrast-enhanced computed tomography, CT). To enhance the conspicuity of infarcted tissue, an inversion-recovery gradient echo sequence is used whereby the inversion time is selected to null signal from uninfarcted myocardium (Figure III5-6). When the uninfarcted myocardium is nulled, hyperintense signal from the infarcted or abnormal myocardium becomes dramatically more obvious.

The pulse sequence is illustrated in Figure III5-7. With this ECG-triggered inversion recovery sequence, the 180° inversion pulse is applied about 150–200 msec after the R wave so that imaging occurs during diastole. Then after an appropriate inversion time, when the uninfarcted myocardium is crossing its null point, the gradient echo acquisition is performed. Either a spoiled gradient echo sequence or a steady-state free precession sequence can

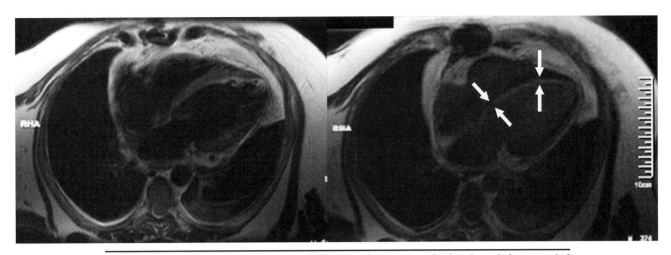

FIGURE III5-6. Improved conspicuity of delayed enhancement of subendocardial myocardial infarct (arrows) with inversion recovery methods (right) compared with T1-weighted fast spin imaging (left). Both images were obtained 10 min following intravenous contrast material, but the inversion recovery sequence was performed using an inversion time selected to null uninfarcted myocardium.

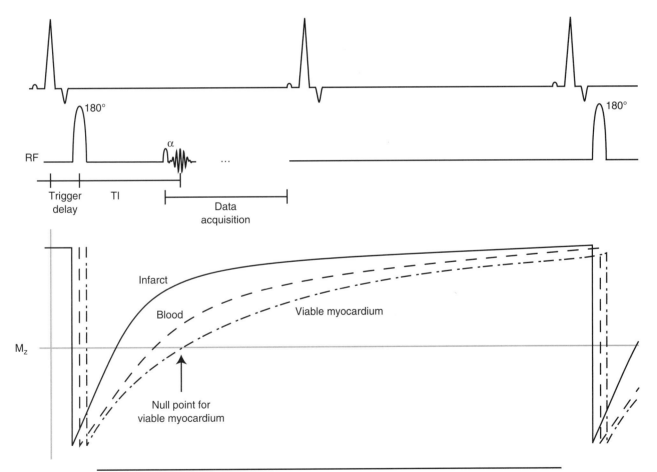

FIGURE III5-7. Inversion recovery sequence achieves nulling of viable myocardium by careful selection of the inversion time centric filling of k-space ensures optimal supperssion. Data are acquired every other heartbeat to allow recovery of longitudinal magnetization.

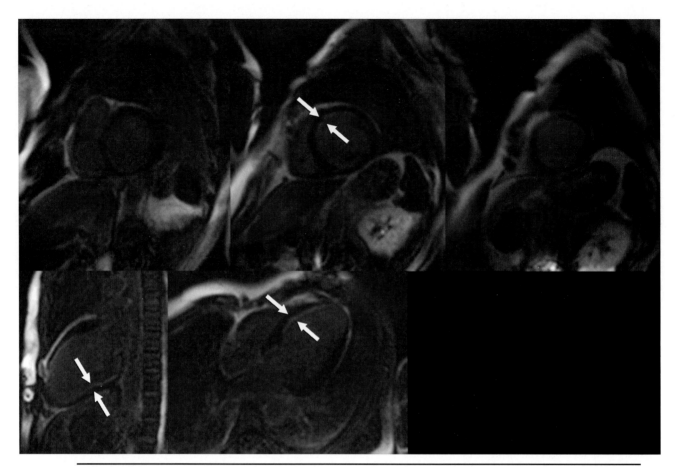

FIGURE III5-8. Selected short (top row) and long axis (bottom row) views of the left ventricle to assess myocardial viability show extensive subendocardial infarction. Some, but not all regions are marked with arrows.

be used with k-space segmentation. The inversion time varies across subjects and also depends on factors such as contrast agent dose and time after injection. Selection of the optimal inversion time is critical to image quality.

To assess left ventricular viability or infarct, the inversion recovery sequence is performed for a series of short axis images from the left ventricular base to the apex. Horizontal and vertical long axis planes confirm short axis findings (Figure III5-8).

> **IMPORTANT CONCEPT:** Myocardial infarcts and other cardiomyopathies can demonstrate delayed contrast enhancement and washout. To enhance conspicuity of areas of abnormal enhancement, inversion recovery sequences are applied with inversion times selected to null normal myocardium.

Choosing an Inversion Time

The selection of inversion time to null the uninfarcted myocardium can critically affect the diagnostic value of the infarct images. To understand why, recall from Chapter I-7 (Figure I9-11) that most MR images are magnitude images. Magnitude images do not distinguish

between signal from protons that are flipped below the xy plane and signal from protons that have recovered above the xy plane. By relying on magnitude data alone, patterns of tissue contrast vary dramatically with different inversion times (Figure III5-9). For example, at the null point of viable myocardium, infarct will have signal intensity that

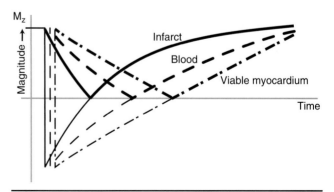

FIGURE III5-9. Signal intensity of cardiac tissues following an inversion pulse, with darker lines depicting the magnitude or absolute value of the magnetization. Image contrast at time points preceding the null point can be confusing.

is higher than that of blood. However, at the inversion time of the infarcted myocardium, image contrast will be inverted, and the viable myocardium will have the greatest signal intensity.

Selection of the inversion time that nulls normal myocardium is commonly performed by successive approximations. Inversion times range from 200 to 350 msec for most subjects when imaged 10–20 minutes after administration of about 0.1 to 0.2 mmol per kg of body weight of gadolinium chelate. It is common for the nulling inversion time to change slightly over the course of the examination.

CHALLENGE QUESTION: Why does inversion time change during the examination? Would it become shorter or longer with time?

Answer: Over time, more of the gadolinium contrast material washes out of the uninfarcted myocardium. With less gadolinium contrast, the T1 time lengthens, and consequently the inversion time is also longer (Figure III5-10). During the 10–15 min of viability imaging, the TI time usually increases by about 25–50 msec.

Inversion Time Mapping Sequence

The inversion time for nulling uninfarcted myocardium can be customized to each subject with an *inversion time mapping* sequence, which is available on some commercial systems. The sequence is an inversion recovery segmented-k-space cine gradient echo sequence that produces images at multiple inversion times (Figure III5-11). Following an electrocardiographic trigger, an inversion pulse (180°) is applied. Then a segmented gradient echo readout is implemented, where each segment corresponds to a different inversion time. The acquired cine images trace the longitudinal relaxation of the tissues imaged (Figure III5-11). With centric reordering of the segments, the central lines of k-space are collected for all phases (all TIs) in the first heartbeat. This reduces the effect of variability of heart rate on image contrast due to differences in longitudinal recovery following the inversion pulse. Data are collected during every other heartbeat to allow for adequate longitudinal relaxation between inversion pulses.

A typical implementation uses a steady-state gradient echo approach with short TR (<3 msec) and flip angle of 50–60°. At least 12–15 lines of k-space are collected per frame per heartbeat, so that for frames with image matrix of about 100 × 192, the acquisition time is about 7–10 heartbeats. The images can be analyzed qualitatively; the optimal inversion time corresponds to that of the image that shows uninfarcted myocardium as darkest intensity.

The temporal resolution of the acquisition determines the precision of the nulling inversion time. For example, if the TR is 3 msec, and the number of views per segment is 12, then the temporal resolution is 36 msec, whereas if the number of views per segment is 33, then the temporal resolution becomes 99 msec. How much precision is necessary? For good discrimination of normal from infarcted myocardium, resolution of at least 40–50 msec is needed.

CHALLENGE QUESTION: Why do the inversion time mapping images show the heart in different states of contraction?

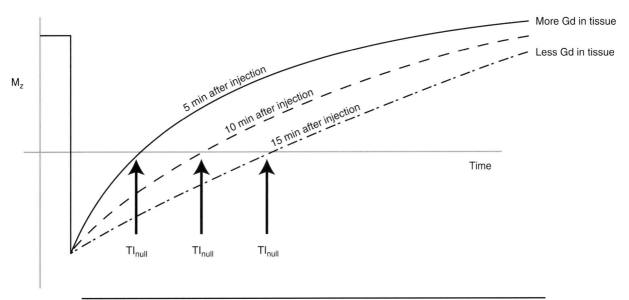

FIGURE III5-10. Evolution of T1 relaxation in uninfarcted myocardium after gadolinium injection. With progressive washout of the contrast material, T1 times lengthen, and consequently the inversion time for nulling increases.

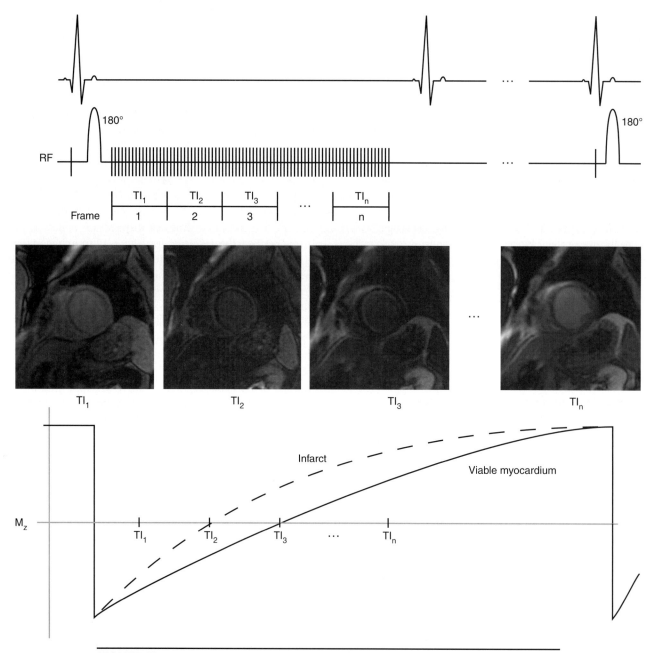

FIGURE III5-11. Inversion time mapping sequence. TI_3 is the optimal inversion time for nulling of uninfarcted myocardium.

Answer: Images are gated to the electrocardiogram. Thus, images at short inversion times show the heart in systole, while later images depict the heart in diastole.

Phase Sensitive Reconstructions

An alternative approach to ensuring good image contrast between infarcted and normal myocardium is to use phase-sensitive reconstructions of inversion recovery sequences, also available on some commercial systems. With phase-sensitive imaging, signal intensity varies with longitudinal magnetization across its full spectrum, from $-M$ to $+M$ in Figure III5-9. Consequently, the infarcted tissue is always higher in signal intensity than the viable myocardium, regardless of the inversion time. Identifying the null point for viable myocardium is no longer critical. Acquisitions are performed for every other heartbeat to allow for recovery of longitudinal magnetization. To correct for field inhomogeneity and its effects on phase, a separate reference image is acquired, usually during the second heartbeat, after nearly complete recovery of the longitudinal magnetization (Figure III5-12).

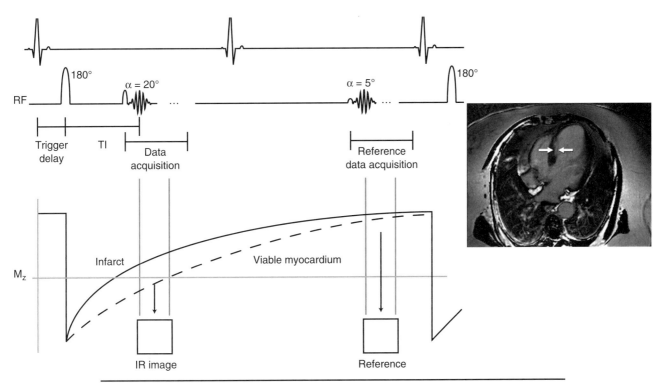

FIGURE III5-12. Phase-sensitive inversion recovery (IR) sequence (left) shows that image data acquisition occurs during diastole of the first heartbeat, while the reference image data is collected toward the end of the second heartbeat, when there is nearly complete recovery of longitudinal magnetization. With phase-sensitive IR imaging (right), signal intensity of the infarct (arrows) is greater than uninfarcted myocardium at virtually all inversion times.

IMPORTANT CONCEPTS: To achieve good contrast between myocardial infarct and viable myocardium, a magnitude-reconstructed inversion recovery sequence requires selection of optimal inversion time to achieve nulling of viable myocardium. Phase-sensitive reconstructions are more forgiving in the selection of TI, but they require acquisition of a reference image and phase correction.

CLINICAL APPLICATIONS: CARDIAC MASSES

This and the following two sections focus on application of tissue characterization pulse sequences to three common clinical problems: cardiac masses, myocardial infarct imaging, and arrhythmogenic right ventricular dysplasia. Representative protocols are provided at the end of the chapter.

For characterization of cardiac masses, a spectrum of MR pulse sequences can be implemented to localize and characterize tumors.

T1- and T2-Weighted Spin Echo Imaging

T1- and T2-weighted spin echo or fast spin echo imaging should be performed with ECG gating. Initially, an ultrafast half-Fourier single-shot black-blood fast spin echo sequence can be used to obtain T2-weighted imaging of the entire chest. Once the mass is localized, higher-resolution T2-weighted spin echo or fast spin echo imaging is needed through the mass. Where metastatic disease is suspected, assessment of the entire chest can yield information about additional lesions in the lungs or mediastinum (Figure III5-13).

Fat-Suppressed Imaging

To characterize fat-containing tumors such as the relatively common lipoma or lipomatous hypertrophy of the interatrial septum, conventional imaging should be supplemented with fat-suppressed imaging, preferably using a frequency-selective fat suppression sequence (Figure III5-4). Additionally, some masses may be more conspicuous on fat-suppressed imaging (Figure III5-13, for example).

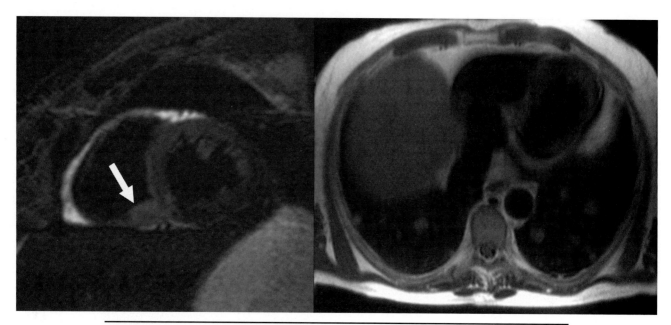

FIGURE III5-13. Fat-suppressed T2-weighted fast spin echo image (left, arrow) shows a right ventricular mass and a small pericardial effusion in a subject with a history of melanoma. On an axial single-shot fast spin echo image through the heart (right), multiple lung masses confirm the diagnosis of metastatic melanoma.

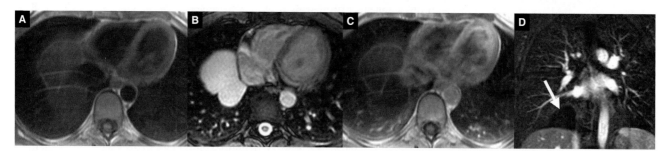

FIGURE III5-14. Pericardial cyst on (**A**) T1-weighted imaging, (**B**) T2-weighted imaging, and (**C**) axial and (**D**) coronal contrast-enhanced T1-weighted images showing a lack of enhancement (arrow), consistent with a cyst.

Gadolinium-Enhanced Imaging

To diagnose cystic lesions in the heart and surrounding structures, intravenous gadolinium contrast material can be administered and T1-weighted imaging performed before and after injection (Figure III5-14). A single dose (0.1 mmol/kg or about 15–20 mL) of gadolinium chelate is sufficient. The time between injection and imaging should be less than 5 minutes. Contrast administration can also be helpful to distinguish tumors from thrombus or to delineate adherent thrombus from ventricular myocardium (particularly in the setting of a ventricular aneurysm or pseudoaneurysm).

Cine Gradient Echo Imaging

Cine gradient echo imaging can provide valuable additional information about the physiologic significance of cardiac masses. For example, an atrial myxoma may prolapse across the mitral valve and cause symptoms mimicking mitral stenosis. To assess the motion of an atrial myxoma, two-chamber or four-chamber cine gradient echo acquisitions can be performed in a single breath hold or two. The physiologic effects of cardiac masses can be well evaluated on cine gradient echo images (Figure III5-15).

Sometimes, vascular lesions can mimic masses in and around the heart. For example, aneurysms of the sinus of

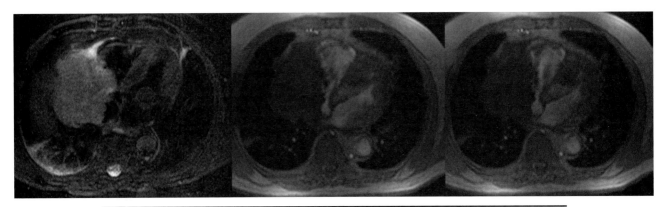

FIGURE III5-15. Lymphoma on (left) T2-weighted (STIR) imaging, and cine gradient echo imaging at (middle) systole and (right) early diastole show a large mass invading the heart, but with preserved motion of the mitral valve.

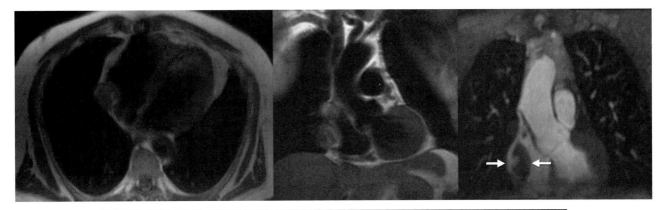

FIGURE III5-16. Apparent cardiac mass in the right atrium on (left) axial and (middle) coronal single-shot fast spin echo images in a patient who has undergone median sternotomy for coronary artery bypass grafting. On a coronal contrast-enhanced image (right), the mass corresponds to an aneurysmal coronary artery bypass graft (arrows) filled with nonenhancing thrombus.

Valsalva or coronary arteries can appear masslike. Cine gradient echo imaging can help demonstrate flow through the vessel. Alternatively, first-pass contrast enhancement can be persuasive (Figure III5-16).

> **IMPORTANT CONCEPTS:** A wide spectrum of MR tools is available for evaluation of cardiac masses: conventional T1- and T2-weighted (fast) spin echo imaging, fat-suppression sequences, contrast enhancement, and cine gradient echo imaging. A suitable protocol depends on the nature of the mass and on the clinical issues at hand—characterization, localization, and assessment of physiologic effects.

A typical cardiac mass protocol is provided at the end of this chapter.

MYOCARDIAL INFARCT IMAGING

Cardiac viability or infarct imaging is commonly used in the clinical setting to determine the likelihood of recovery of left ventricular function following revascularization. Distinction between infarcted and hibernating myocardium may be difficult with conventional imaging methods, as shown in Table III5-3. The high spatial resolution of delayed contrast-enhanced imaging enables precise measures of the extent of myocardial infarct.

For the assessment of myocardial viability, most protocols (see end of chapter) consist of three main parts—cine gradient echo for wall motion imaging, first-pass contrast-enhanced studies for resting perfusion (optional), and delayed contrast-enhanced inversion recovery imaging for infarct imaging. As will be discussed in Chapter III-7, stress perfusion can also be performed as part of a more general protocol for coronary artery disease. If performed without pharmacologic stress, the gadolinium-enhanced perfusion images provide information only about resting perfusion and not inducible ischemia.

Cine gradient echo imaging and delayed contrast-enhanced imaging are performed in the short axis plane from the left ventricular base to apex, typically at intervals of 8–10 mm (6–8 mm slices with 2 mm gaps), with at least

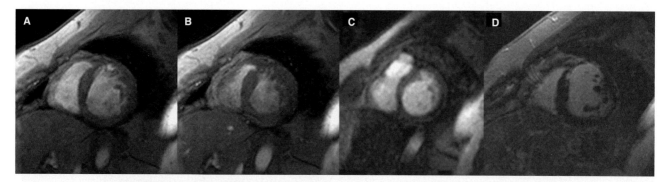

FIGURE III5-17. Case study (**A**) Diastolic and (**B**) systolic short axis cine gradient echo images, (**C**) first-pass resting perfusion, and (**D**) delayed contrast-enhanced short axis images from an inversion recovery viability acquisition.

▶ **TABLE III5-3 Resting Cardiac MR Examinations without Pharmacologic Stress**

Pathologic State	Wall Motion and Thickening	Wall Thickness	First-Pass Perfusion (rest)	Delayed Enhancement
Resting ischemia	↓	±	↓	None
Acute infarct/ unstable angina	↓	Normal	↓	↑
Hibernating myocardium	↓	±	±	None
Chronic/subacute infarct	↓	↓	↓	↑

two long axis views. Cine and viability images are matched in slice positions to allow direct comparison of wall motion and thickness against delayed contrast enhancement (Table III5-3).

Experience with delayed contrast-enhanced MR imaging for evaluation of subacute or chronic infarct is quite extensive. The transmural extent of delayed contrast enhancement appears to predict response to revascularization; infarcts that span less than 50% of the wall thickness have the greatest likelihood of recovery of function following angioplasty or bypass grafting, regardless of the degree of wall motion impairment. Therefore, viability studies can help identify which subjects with diminished contractility will benefit from revascularization.

Case Study: Myocardial Infarct Imaging

Clinical History: A 52-year-old diabetic woman with a history of a prior myocardial infarction complained of four days of nausea and other nonspecific gastrointestinal symptoms. In the emergency room, nonspecific ST changes were detected on the electrocardiogram.

MR Findings: Selected short axis cine gradient echo images are shown in Figure III5-17. The cine images show a global decrease in contractility with wall thinning in the anterior wall. First-pass perfusion studies were performed without pharmacologic stress (Figure III5-17) and revealed hypoperfusion of the thinned anterior wall as well as in the subendocardial region of the inferolateral wall. The hypoperfusion reflects either resting ischemia or infarct. Delayed contrast-enhanced imaging with inversion time selected to null uninfarcted myocardium shows hyperenhancement in the anterior wall as well as in the inferolateral wall. The anterior wall changes, given the thinned appearance of the myocardium, likely reflect prior (chronic) infarct. A new subendocardial infarct in the inferolateral wall is most likely caused by left circumflex artery or right coronary artery disease and explain the subject's nonspecific gastrointestinal symptoms.

Interpretation: Chronic anterior wall infarct (LAD territory) with new subacute infarct (RCA/LCx territory) in the inferolateral wall.

For patients with acute chest pain and acute myocardial infarction, the experience with delayed contrast-enhanced MR imaging is growing. As with subacute and chronic infarcts, the transmural extent of delayed hyperenhancement in acute infarcts is a good predictor of reduced recovery despite revascularization. To date, MR has been shown to be very sensitive in the acute setting for detection of myocardial infarction. One notable finding that is sometimes observed in the setting of acute infarction is the presence of *microvascular obstruction*. Within areas of infarct, there can be regions that are markedly hypovascular in the early minutes after contrast administration. The subsequent rate of enhancement depends in part on the degree of vascular obstruction and may also reflect diffusion of contrast material from adjacent perfused areas. These focal areas of low signal intensity surrounded by hyperintense infarcted myocardium have very poor prognosis for recovery following revascularization (Figure III5-18).

Cardiac MR has several advantages in the assessment of viability compared with existing techniques, including higher spatial resolution and no need for ionizing radiation. Additionally, in contrast to other techniques such as dobutamine echocardiography or ECG-gated scintigraphy, the assessment of viability by delayed contrast-enhanced MRI does not rely on changes in wall motion.

Consequently, subjects who have preserved wall motion in the setting of subendocardial infarcts can be accurately diagnosed with delayed contrast enhancement.

> **IMPORTANT CONCEPTS:** Delayed contrast enhancement, when performed in conjunction with cine gradient echo assessment of wall motion, can diagnose and differentiate between infarcted and hibernating myocardium. Therefore, it can identify which patients with left ventricular dysfunction are most likely to benefit from revascularization. In the acute setting, delayed contrast enhancement is also very sensitive for the detection of infarction.

ARRHYTHMOGENIC RIGHT VENTRICULAR DYSPLASIA

Arrhythmogenic right ventricular dysplasia (ARVD), which is part of a spectrum of causes of arrhythmogenic diseases of the heart that can cause sudden death in otherwise healthy young adults, can be a challenge for MRI. Often individuals have arrhythmias that limit the quality of ECG-gated images. Subjects with gross abnormalities are frequently diagnosed by other imaging methods, leaving only the more subtle cases for MR referral. Nevertheless, given advances in MR methods, MRI often plays a critical role in diagnosing this life threatening diseases. About one-third of cases are familial, and therefore screening of relatives of affected individuals is also often performed with MRI.

Classic MR findings include fibrofatty replacement of the right ventricular myocardium (Figure III5-19). Associated with these structural abnormalities are global or segmental RV dilatation or at least hypokinesis. The

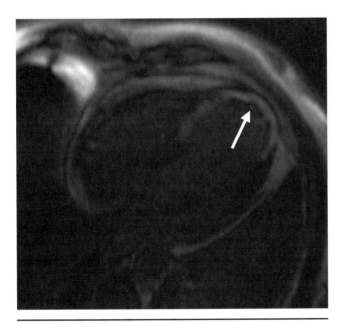

FIGURE III5-18. Apical and septal infarct with hypointense region (arrow) in the apex corresponding to area of microvascular obstruction.

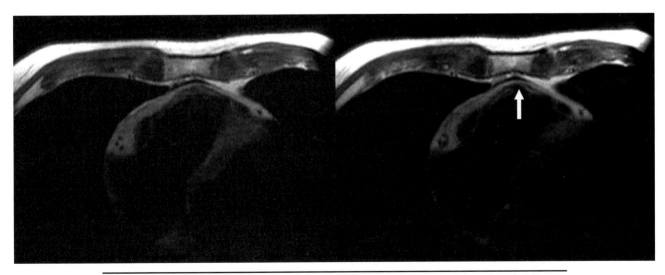

FIGURE III5-19. T1-weighted FSE image through the right ventricle shows normal right ventricular wall (left) adjacent to an area of focal fibrous replacement of the free wall (right, arrow). The focal abnormality also demonstrated dyskinesis on cine images (not shown). Signal loss centrally in the thorax reflects the use of only anterior coil elements for image acquisition. A saturation band was also placed over the left ventricle to minimize ghosting artifacts.

▶ **TABLE III5-4** Diagnostic Criteria for ARVD

Criteria	Major	Minor
Family history	Familial disease confirmed at autopsy or surgery	Family history of premature sudden death (<35 yrs) due to suspected ARVD
ECG depolarization/ conduction abnormalities	Epsilon waves or localized prolongation (>100 ms) of QRS complex in right precordial lead	Late potentials on signal-averaged ECG
ECG repolarization abnormalities		Inverted T waves in V2, V3, >12 yrs old without RBBB
Arrhythmias		Sustained or nonsustained LBBB; frequent (>1000/24 hr) ventricular extrasystoles
Global or regional dysfunction or structural alterations	Severe dilatation and reduction of RVEF (without or mild LV involvement); RV aneurysms; RV segmental dilatation	Mild global RV dilatation or decreased EF with normal LV; mild segmental RV dilatation; regional RV hypokinesia
Tissue characteristics	Fibrofatty replacement of myocardium on endomyocardial biopsy	

LBBB, left bundle branch block; LV, left ventricle
RBBB, right bundle branch block; RV, right ventricle; RVEF, right ventricle ejection fraction

imaging protocol (see end of chapter) therefore requires high-spatial-resolution imaging of the right ventricle in at least two planes and corresponding cine gradient echo imaging to assess for associated wall motion abnormalities. Because many individuals, as they age, develop fatty infiltration of the right ventricular wall, the wall motion abnormalities are generally considered a requirement for considering the diagnosis of ARVD.

For high-resolution images of the right ventricle, T1-weighted fast spin echo methods are usually obtained, one slice per breath hold. Two imaging planes orthogonal to the free wall of the right ventricle are useful, for example a conventional transverse plane and an oblique sagittal view. To improve the spatial resolution, the posterior coil elements of the torso phased-array coil can be turned off, relying only on the anterior coils. This allows the field of view to be reduced substantially without fear of wraparound artifact from the back (Figure III5-19). If motion artifacts from the anterior chest wall or left ventricle are troublesome, spatially selective saturation bands can be applied to minimize ghosting.

It is critical to perform cine gradient echo acquisitions matched in position to the FSE images. While steady-state free precession (true FISP) methods are faster, chemical shift artifacts of the second kind (India ink artifact, Chapter I-9) can limit evaluation of the thin right ventricular wall, and therefore spoiled gradient echo sequences may be preferred. In some cases, right ventricular abnormalities can be associated with abnormal patterns of delayed contrast enhancement. Therefore, gadolinium enhancement should be considered a useful supplementary technique for this difficult diagnosis.

It is worth emphasizing that an diagnosis of ARVD requires more than just MR imaging findings. Of the abnormalities listed in Table III5-4, (a) two major criteria, (b) one major and two minor criteria, or (c) four minor criteria are necessary.

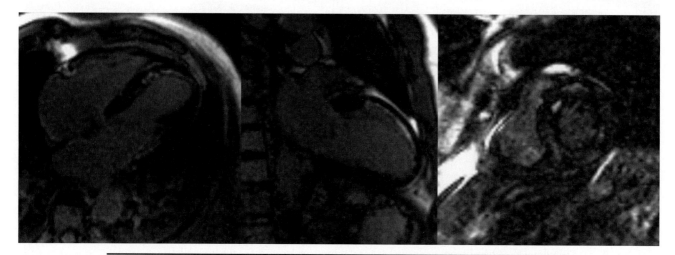

FIGURE III5-Q2. Long axis viability images (**A, B**) show superb suppression of the uninfarcted myocardium at inversion time = 275 msec. Subsequent short axis image (**C**) with the same inversion time suffers from a lack of contrast as a result of poor suppression of uninfarcted myocardium.

REVIEW QUESTIONS

1. In the evaluation of a cardiac mass, an imaging protocol is performed with T2-weighted fast spin echo imaging and contrast enhanced T1-weighted imaging of the mass. Your colleague concludes from the imaging study that the mass is vascular because it is high in signal intensity on the contrast-enhanced images. Is she correct?

2. As part of a myocardial viability study, the first set of inversion recovery images were performed using an inversion time of 275 msec, yielding excellent suppression of uninfarcted myocardium (Figure III5 -Q2A and Q2B). However, by the time the last acquisition was performed (Figure III5-Q2C), the image quality deteriorated. What happened, and what could be done to correct this problem?

3. Consider diseases such as acute myocarditis and sarcoidosis (Table III5-2) that cause hyperintensity on delayed contrast-enhanced imaging. How can these entities be differentiated from myocardial infarction by imaging?

4. Interpret the systolic cine image in Figure III5-Q4, obtained in a subject referred for possible arrhythmogenic right ventricular dysplasia, with particular attention to the right ventricular apex.

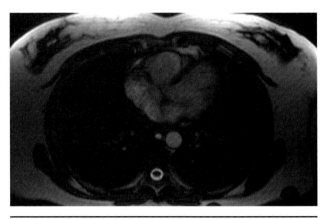

FIGURE III5-Q4

▶ **PROTOCOL: Cardiac Mass Study**

Setup and Preparation	Notes
i.v.	22 G or larger[1]
Gadolinium contrast	0.1 mmol/kg (20 mL)[1]
ECG leads	Necessary
Coil	Torso phased-array
Positioning tips	Supine, head first
Subject instructions	End-expiratory breath holding Supplemental oxygen by nasal cannula optional

Sequence	Imaging Plane	Parameters
1 Scout (true FISP or spoiled GRE)	Multiplanar	Default
2 T2-weighted fast spin echo imaging of the chest (double IR single shot half-Fourier FSE, if available)	Axial	Single shot or FSE with TR = one R-R interval 8–10 mm slices
3 Single-slice high-resolution T1-weighted FSE	Axial and other views through mass	5–6 mm slice; repeated for full coverage of mass, TR = one R-R interval
4 Frequency-selective fat suppressed FSE[1]	Matched to (3)	5–6 mm slice
5 Cine GRE (spoiled gradient echo or steady-state gradient echo, segmented k-space)	Variable[2]	5–6 mm slices with 2 mm gaps Parameters (incl views per segment) defined for temporal resolution < 60 msec, and acquisition time within a breath hold
Gadolinium contrast injection		
6 Single-slice high-resolution T1-weighted FSE[3]	Same as (3)	Same as (3)

[1]Gadolinium contrast material is optional in some cases. For example, for characterization of lipomas, a frequency selective fat-suppressed sequence is usually sufficient, and gadolinium contrast administration is unnecessary.
[2]Cine gradient echo imaging can be performed in positions that match the T1-weighted images. Additionally, depending on the nature of the mass, conventional short or long axis views may be helpful to assess the relationship between masses and cardiac valves.
[3]Alternatively, fat-suppressed 2D or 3D gradient echo imaging (as used in MR angiography) can be performed for the evaluation of enhancement in masses outside the heart (such as some pericardial masses) where cardiac motion has less of an impact on image quality. For evaluation of thrombus adjacent to infarcted myocardium, delayed contrast enhancement sequences can be used (see the cardiac Viability protocol).

▶ **PROTOCOL: Cardiac Viability**

Setup and Preparation	Notes
i.v.	22 G or larger
Gadolinium contrast	0.1–0.2 mmol/kg (20–40 mL)
ECG leads	Necessary
Coil	Torso phased-array
Positioning tips	Supine, head first
Subject instructions	End-expiratory breath holding Supplemental oxygen by nasal cannula optional

Sequence	Imaging Plane	Parameters
1 Scout (true FISP or spoiled GRE)	Multiplanar	Default
2 T2-weighted fast spin echo imaging of the chest (double IR single-shot half-Fourier FSE, if available)	Axial	Single shot or FSE with TR = one R-R interval 8–10 mm slices
3 Single-slice scouts Gadolinium contrast injection[1]	Obliques to get short axis and long axis views	1 slice/breathhold
4 Cine GRE (spoiled gradient echo or steady state gradient echo, segmented k-space)	Short axes	8 mm slices with 2 mm gaps Parameters (incl views per segment) defined for temporal resolution <60 msec, and acquisition time within a breath hold, LV base to apex, 8–12 slices
5 Cine GRE (spoiled gradient echo or steady state gradient echo, segmented k-space)	Long axes	8 mm slices Same parameters as above Less rectangular FOV for VLA view[2]
6 Inversion time mapping	Short axis (through infarct, if possible)	Single slice. Parameters defined to achieve temporal resolution of < 60 msec to determine inversion time for nulling of uninfarcted myocardium
7 Inversion recovery segmented k-space gradient echo imaging[3]	Short and long axes (match cine GRE)	Set inversion time according to Step 6

[1]During contrast administration, first-pass perfusion imaging can be performed (refer to protocol in Chapter III-7), or alternatively, a gadolinium-enhanced thoracic MR angiogram can be acquired (refer to protocol in Chapter II-4).

[2]For most acquisitions 75% rectangular FOV can be used. Typically, for the vertical long axis (two-chamber) view, a larger FOV is needed or less rectangular FOV (85%).

[3]2D and 3D spoiled and steady-state gradient echo sequences are available. For conventional magnitude images, selection of the appropriate inversion time to null uninfarcted myocardium is important. An inversion time mapping sequence can be helpful. Alternatively, a phase-sensitive reconstruction can be performed.

▶ **PROTOCOL:** **Arrhythmogenic Right Ventricular Dysplasia**[1]

Diagnostic criteria for ARVD are given in Table III5–4.

Setup and Preparation	Notes
i.v.	22 G or larger[1]
Gadolinium contrast	0.1 mmol/kg (20 mL)[1]
ECG leads	Necessary
Coil	Torso phased-array
Positioning tips	Supine, head first
Subject instructions	End-expiratory breath holding Supplemental oxygen by nasal cannula optional

Sequence	Imaging Plane	Parameters
1 Scout (true FISP or spoiled GRE)	Multiplanar	Default
2 T2-weighted fast spin echo imaging of the chest (double IR single-shot half-Fourier FSE, if available)	Axial	Single shot or FSE with TR = one R-R interval 8–10 mm slices
3 Single-slice high-resolution T1-weighted FSE[2]	Axial and oblique sagittal through RV wall	4–6 mm slices; repeated for full coverage of the right ventricle through pulmonary infundibulum, TR = one R-R interval
4 Frequency-selective fat suppressed FSE[3]	Matched to Step 3	Selected slices, depending on findings from Step 3
5 Cine GRE (spoiled gradient echo, segmented k-space)	Matched to Step 3	4–6 mm slices Parameters (incl views per segment) defined for temporal resolution < 60 msec, and acquisition time within a breath hold
Gadolinium contrast injection[1] (optional)		
6 Inversion time mapping[1](optional)	Axial, including RV	Single slice. Parameters defined to achieve temporal resolution of <60 msec to determine inversion time for nulling of normal myocardium
7 Inversion recovery segmented k-space gradient echo imaging[1] (optional)	Matched to Steps 3 and 5	Set inversion time according to Step 6.

[1]Gadolinium contrast material is optional. In some cases, delayed contrast enhancement reveals abnormalities of the right ventricular wall.

[2]To improve the spatial resolution of anatomic imaging, use only anterior coil elements for signal reception. Small fields-of-view, 250 mm or less, can then be used without wraparound artifact from the back. If ghosting artifacts from the chest wall or left ventricle are problematic, spatially selective saturation bands can also be used.

[3]If fatty replacement of the right ventricular myocardium is suspected, a frequency-selective fat-suppressed sequence can help confirm the presence of fat.

Chapter 6

Phase Contrast Flow Quantification in the Heart

Many of the physical principles of phase contrast MRI have been presented already in Chapter II-3, and the reader is encouraged to review that chapter. Here, the emphasis turns to cardiac applications, where phase contrast MRI can be viewed as the equivalent to Doppler echocardiography for assessment of flow. A review of the specific physical concepts that relate to cardiac applications is covered first, followed by discussions of applications to the cardiac patient.

PHASE CONTRAST MRI OR "DOPPLER MRI"

MR cine phase contrast provides information very similar to Doppler ultrasonography or echocardiography. On phase images, signal intensity is velocity encoded, so that the images are velocity maps. Unlike Doppler images, phase contrast images are in black and white, where the gradations of signal intensity reflect velocity. On phase contrast images, no flow (velocity = 0) has the appearance of a middling shade of gray (Figure III6-1). Darker signal corresponds to flow in one direction, while brighter signal reflects flow in the opposite direction.

The pulse sequences can be designed to measure in-plane flow (two-dimensional velocity encoding) or through-plane flow (one-dimensional velocity encoding). The serial application of flow-encoding gradients in mutually orthogonal directions makes in-plane and three-dimensional phase contrast flow quantification measurements time consuming. Most examples in this chapter are through-plane measurements. Phase contrast sequences are usually gated to the cardiac cycle and generate multiple magnitude and phase images at different time points throughout the cardiac cycle.

CHALLENGE QUESTION: In Figure III6-1, what does the black signal during diastole in the ascending aorta signify?

Answer: The black signal indicates normal flow reversal in the ascending aorta during diastolic filling of coronary arteries. In aortia insufficiency which will also have this appearance, the diastolic reversal is present regardless of whether the slice plane is positioned above or below the coronary artery ostia and can be confirmed on cine gradient echo images in the left ventricular outflow tract view as a regurgitant jet of low signal (Figure III4-18 and Figure III4-20).

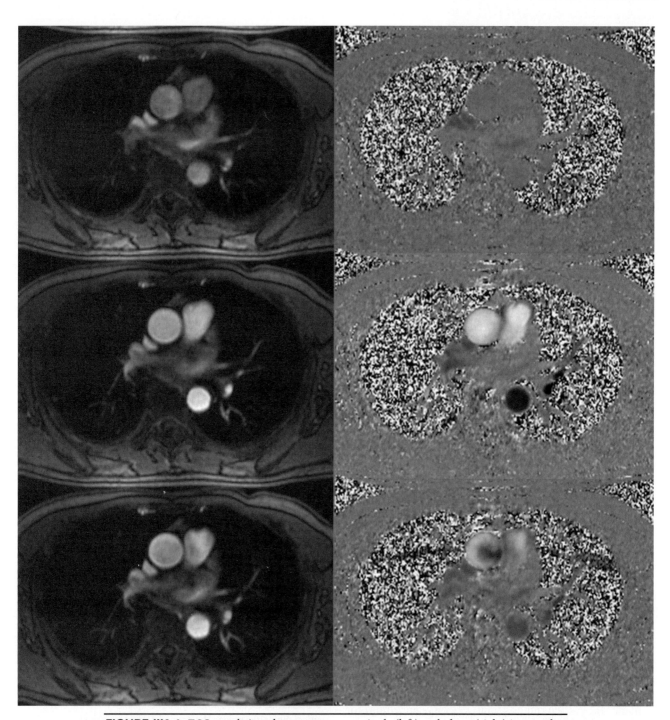

FIGURE III6-1. ECG-gated cine phase contrast magnitude (left) and phase (right) images during end diastole (top), peak systole (middle), and early diastole (bottom). On phase images, bright signal intensity corresponds to cephalad flow, while black signal corresponds to caudal flow. The gray signal intensity of the chest wall reflects stationary tissue, and the mottled appearance of the lungs and air outside the chest is primarily image noise.

The magnitude images of phase contrast acquisitions (Figure III6-1) are identical to the standard cine gradient echo images that have been discussed in Chapter III-4. By defining anatomy, these images help localize signal on phase contrast velocity maps.

IMPORTANT CONCEPT: MR phase contrast flow quantification should be used in cardiac MR studies just as Doppler echocardiography is used in cardiac ultrasound.

CARDIAC CINE PHASE CONTRAST MR: THE PULSE SEQUENCE

The principles of cardiac cine phase contrast MR sequences are identical to those described for vascular applications in Chapter II-3. Fundamental concepts are reviewed next, with an emphasis on considerations specific to cardiac applications.

Flow-Encoding Gradients

The basic principle of phase contrast flow quantification is that protons that move at a constant velocity and are exposed to a flow-encoding gradient (such as a standard bipolar gradient) will accumulate a phase shift that is proportional to their velocity. To correct for phase errors that are introduced by magnetic field inhomogeneities, all phase contrast sequences require two separate acquisitions, each with a different set of flow-encoding gradients (Chapter II-3).

Before considering the details of cine phase contrast MRI, it is important to discuss the assumption about constant velocity. During the systolic portion of the cardiac cycle, blood flow is rarely constant—it accelerates and decelerates. How valid are velocity measurements? The assumptions about constant velocity hold true, provided the temporal resolution of the acquisition is high compared with the time frame of velocity changes. In the setting of normal pulsatile flow, blood can be approximated as having a constant velocity within a given sampling interval. If blood acceleration is too high, such as in the setting of stenoses, then the error in velocity using phase contrast flow quantification will be greater. Note that a similar assumption is needed for Doppler ultrasound measurements of flow. Doppler shifts are assumed to reflect constant velocity of blood, and higher-order flows are neglected.

CHALLENGE QUESTION: In what clinical setting does flow have higher-order components, such as jerk, and what are the implications for phase contrast measurements?

Answer: Stenotic valves and vessels cause turbulent blood flow. Associated with turbulence are high rates of acceleration and also jerk. Conventional velocity-encoded phase contrast measurements will underestimate the velocities of blood. Intravoxel dephasing causes further signal loss with these complex patterns of flow.

> **IMPORTANT CONCEPT:** Conventional phase contrast flow quantification MR sequences assume constant velocity within a voxel during each frame.

Venc

The relationship between phase shift and velocity depends on the strength and duration of the flow-encoding gradients.

Recall that the Venc, or encoding velocity, is the velocity associated with a phase shift of +180°. The range of measurable velocities is ±Venc or from −Venc to +Venc. On the phase contrast images, protons moving away from the viewer at a velocity equal to the Venc will have the highest signal intensity. Protons moving in the opposite direction, at a velocity that approaches −Venc, will be shown with the darkest signal intensity (Figure II3-5).

> **IMPORTANT CONCEPT:** The encoding velocity, Venc, allows the user to define the range of measurable velocities with a phase contrast acquisition, typically ±Venc.

ECG Gating for Cine Acquisitions

For quantification of flow in cardiac applications, measurements are performed either through the great vessels or through the pulmonary arteries or veins; intracardiac measurements are also possible. Segmented k-space sequences are routinely used. The higher the number of segments, the shorter the overall acquisition time. With a higher number of segments, however, the temporal resolution is reduced. As discussed in Chapter II-3, for accurate measurements of peak systolic velocity, the acquisition must have sufficient temporal resolution, preferably less than 50–60 msec.

One important consideration in cardiac phase contrast applications is the effect of motion of the heart during the cardiac cycle. With commercial implementations of phase contrast sequences, the slice position is stationary over the acquisition, but in a beating heart the slice position may image a different slice of the heart across the acquisition period (Figure III6-2). For example, at the aortic root, measurements of flow above the coronary artery orifices differ from those below. Acquisitions at the aortic root should be positioned so that cardiac motion does not result in acquisition slices varying considerably during the cardiac cycle, particularly with reference to the coronary ostia. Flow across the mitral or tricuspid valve orifice can be similarly difficult to measure because of cardiac motion. When accuracy in positioning is critical, scout positions and acquisitions must be obtained in the same phase of suspended respiration, recognizing that scout images are typically obtained with the heart in diastole.

> **IMPORTANT CONCEPT:** Through-plane movement associated with cardiac motion introduces errors in flow measurements with phase contrast MRI.

View Sharing

Using a sufficiently high number views per segment ensures a short acquisition time (<20 sec) and yields an

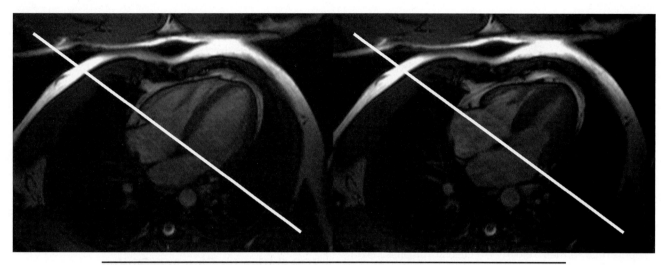

FIGURE III6-2. Motion of the mitral valve during a cardiac cycle (diastole on left and systole on right) relative to a fixed imaging plane (line). During diastole, the slice plane intersects the mitral valve, while in systole, the slice plane is contained in the right atrium.

approximately 100 msec temporal resolution of a conventional phase contrast cine MR.

CHALLENGE QUESTION: Why is the temporal resolution so much worse for phase contrast images than for conventional segmented ECG-gated cine gradient echo imaging?

Answer: To correct for phase errors, phase contrast acquisitions require two separate acquisitions with different flow-encoding gradients, for example two opposite bipolar gradients or gradients with and without flow compensation. Consequently, the acquisition times are usually twice as long as a corresponding segmented cine gradient echo imaging.

A commonly used tool for increasing the apparent temporal resolution of phase contrast acquisitions is view sharing (Figure I8-20). As discussed in Chapters I-8, II-3, and III-4 (Figure III4-7), the apparent temporal resolution can be increased by a factor of two with view sharing. With an apparent temporal resolution of 50 msec or less, reasonably accurate measurements of peak systolic velocity and flow rates can be achieved.

> **IMPORTANT CONCEPT:** Cardiac phase contrast applications should be performed using view sharing for an apparent temporal resolution of about 50 msec or better and acquistion times within a breathhold.

New Research Developments

Some current areas of research with phase contrast acquisitions include the development of real-time phase contrast velocity maps that permit sampling of velocities using an interactive positioning device. Color maps are also being developed that generate images similar to Doppler flow maps.

CINE PHASE CONTRAST IMAGE PROCESSING

All commercial systems that offer phase contrast acquisitions also provide a range of image-processing software for analysis of the results. Calculations of phase contrast velocities require phase difference computations. Complex difference methods are used for phase contrast MR angiographic reconstructions (Chapter II-3). Magnitude images generated from phase contrast acquisitions can serve as anatomic references for comparison with velocity-encoded maps (Figure III6-1).

Measuring Velocities and Flows

To analyze velocity maps, regions of interest (ROIs) are drawn around the vessels or within intracardiac regions. Adjustments to the ROIs across the cardiac cycle may be needed to accommodate change in vessel caliber. Additional ROIs for background correction may be necessary.

The results that are automatically generated include maximum velocity in the ROI, the average velocity in the ROI, and the mean flow in the ROI. All of these values can be plotted versus time points sampled in the cardiac cycle (Figure III6-3).

Some software programs depict the voxel of maximum velocity in the region of interest. For normal laminar flow, the location of the maximum velocity is in the center of the vessel.

Alias Correction

In the presence of aliasing, most vendor-provided software programs allow for modest corrections, typically to correct for velocities up to twice the Venc (Figure III6-4).

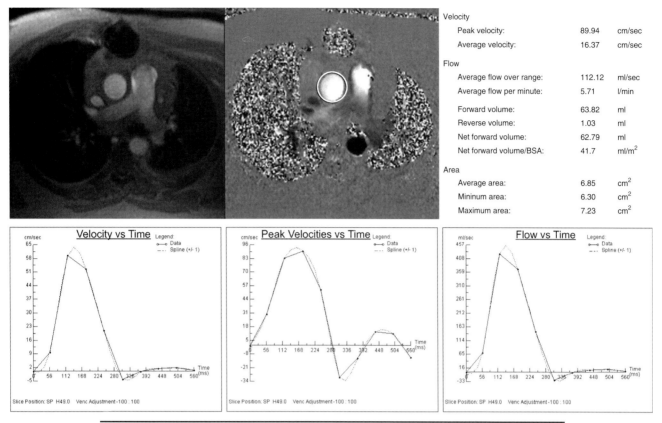

FIGURE III6-3. Magnitude and phase images with summary of results for phase contrast acquisition. Plots of average velocity, maximum velocity, and mean flow in the ascending aorta (ROI drawn on phase image) are shown in the bottom row.

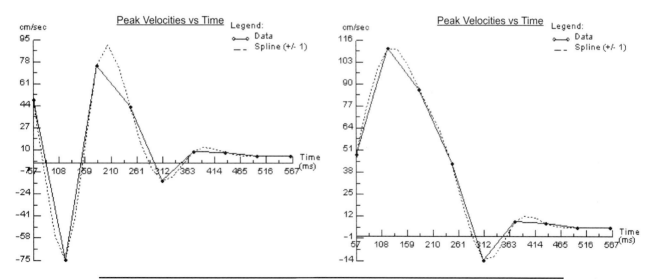

FIGURE III6-4. Aliasing of the peak velocity occurs with a Venc of 75 cm/sec. Alias correction software applied to the data corrects the problem (right).

IMPORTANT CONCEPT: Careful image processing of phase contrast data is essential to extracting accurate quantitative results from images.

CINE PHASE CONTRAST APPLICATIONS: ESTIMATING PRESSURE GRADIENTS WITH v_{max}

As described in Chapter II-3, the peak pressure gradient across a stenosis can be measured by knowing the maximum peak systolic velocity (v_{max}) and by using the modified Bernoulli equation:

$$\text{Pressure gradient (mm Hg)} = 4 \times v_{max}^2$$

where v_{max} is measured in units of meters/sec (m/sec).

Clinical Applications

In cardiac applications, measurements of peak systolic velocity across stenoses are usually confined to stenotic valves, most commonly, aortic stenosis in the adult population. Congenital heart applications are broader. Any region of stenosis for which a pressure gradient should be estimated can be studied with phase contrast MRI. For greater confidence in the accuracy of pressure gradient values, repeated phase contrast acquisitions in different positions may be needed to approximate the peak systolic velocity best.

■ Case Study: AORTIC STENOSIS

Clinical History: An older patient with a heart murmur undergoes a cardiac MR examination.

MR Findings: A cine gradient echo image through the left ventricular outflow tract and ascending aorta is shown in Figure III6-5.

To measure the maximum velocity, the phase contrast acquisition could be performed in the plane of flow to measure in-plane velocities. For an in-plane acquisition, a slice position identical to Figure III6-5a would be used. Alternatively, if the slice is positioned perpendicular to the direction of flow, through-plane velocities can be measured. For this method, the slice was positioned at a level where maximum velocity was expected (Figure III6-5A, dotted line).

Interpretation: Stenotic tricospid aortic valve with peak systolic velocity 2.4m/sec. ■

CHALLENGE QUESTION: What is the pressure gradient across the stenotic aortic valve?

Answer: The peak systolic velocity, as shown in Figure III6-5, is 240 cm/sec or 2.4 m/sec. Using the modified Bernoulli equation, this velocity corresponds to a pressure gradient of

$$\text{Pressure gradient (mm Hg)} = 4 \times 2.4^2 = 23 \text{ mm Hg}$$

To visualize the stenotic aortic valve, a cine gradient echo acquisition at the level of the valve leaflets was performed (Figure III6-5C).

Limitations of Phase Contrast Pressure Gradient Estimates

Clearly the accuracy of pressure gradient measurements with phase contrast MR depends in large part on the

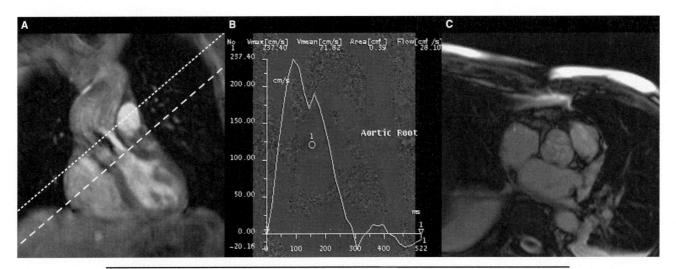

FIGURE III6-5. Case study (**A**) Systolic image through the left ventricular outflow tract shows turbulent jet emanating from the level of the aortic valve leaflets. (**B**) Through-plane velocity map in the ascending aorta (dotted line in (A)). (**C**) Cine gradient echo image through valve plane (dashed line in (A)) at peak systole shows a tricuspid aortic valve, but diminished motion of the valve leaflets, resulting in stenosis.

accuracy of the peak systolic velocity. Velocities can be under- or overestimated for a number of reasons:

- Suboptimal slice positioning
- Higher-order flow patterns and turbulence causing signal loss with simple velocity encoding that may mimic aliasing
- Intravoxel dephasing (becomes more pronounced with larger voxels)
- Inadequate temporal resolution for sampling peak systolic velocity

> **IMPORTANT CONCEPT:** Errors in phase contrast MR measurements of peak velocity can be minimized by careful slice positioning and by acquiring images with high spatial and temporal resolution.

CINE PHASE CONTRAST APPLICATIONS: VOLUME FLOW MEASUREMENTS

As discussed in Chapter II-3, the total flow through vessels can be measured with cine phase contrast MRI by calculating the average flow at each time point in the cardiac cycle. Flow is typically described in terms of mL/sec or mL/min. Summing the values across the cardiac cycle provides a measure of total forward flow (mL/heart beat). In vessels where reverse flow takes place, the forward and reverse flows can be separately calculated.

Retrospective Gating

For many applications that require measurement of volume flow rates, accurate values are needed throughout the entire cardiac cycle. If flow during diastole is negligible, then prospectively gated sequences using a trigger window of 10–15% of the cardiac cycle provide reasonably accurate measurements of flow. However, if flow during diastole contributes significantly to the total flow, then measurements must be performed with retrospective gating.

Clinical Applications

The most common clinical uses of phase contrast flow measurements are estimates of *regurgitant fractions* across valves, *pulmonary/systemic flow ratios (Q_P/Q_S)* in the setting of pulmonary-systemic shunts, and independent estimates of stroke volume. Coronary artery flow with pharmacologic stress, for both native vessels and grafts, has also been used in the research setting to assess coronary flow reserve.

Regurgitant fraction is defined as the regurgitant flow (mL/beat) divided by the forward flow (mL/beat) and is often expressed as a percentage:

$$\text{Regurgitant fraction} = \frac{\text{Regurgitant flow}}{\text{Forward flow}} \times 100\%$$

Pulmonary/systemic flow ratios (Q_P/Q_S) are defined as the total forward flow through the pulmonary artery compared with the total forward flow through the aorta:

$$Q_P/Q_S = (\text{Pulmonary forward flow}/\text{Aortic forward flow})$$

Stroke volume can be calculated based on EDV and ESV calculations as described in Chapter III-4. The forward flow of blood through the ascending aorta is an alternative measure of stroke volume, illustrated in Example 1.

■ EXAMPLE 1: STROKE VOLUME, CARDIAC OUTPUT, AND CARDIAC INDEX

Stroke volume (SV) is defined as the volume of blood per heartbeat that is ejected from the left ventricle during systole. For conventional measurements of stroke volume (Chapter III-4), EDV and ESV are determined from a contiguous series of short axis cine gradient echo slices from the base to apex of the left ventricle. Stroke volume is defined as the difference between the two volumes.

An alternative method for estimating stroke volume uses phase contrast velocity mapping to measure forward flow through the aorta. It is accurate, *provided* that all of the blood leaving the left ventricle during systole passes through the aorta. That is, there must be no mitral regurgitation or ventricular septal defect.

A through-plane phase contrast acquisition is positioned in the ascending aorta. For stroke volume, measures of forward flow can be positioned above or below the coronary ostia. Either prospective or retrospective gating can be used. Using a Venc of about 150 cm/sec, results are shown in Figure III6-6.

The total forward flow during systole is computed by the software. The reverse flow during diastole is ignored. In the example above, the total forward flow is 65 mL. This value should correspond well to the stroke volume computed using the short axis images.

Recall that with the stroke volume and heart rate, an estimate of cardiac output can be derived (Chapter III-4). ■

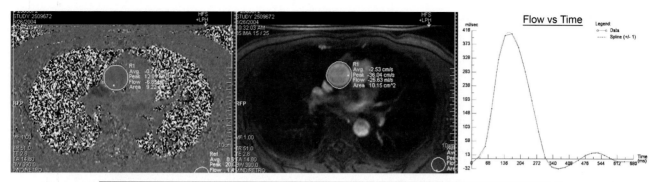

FIGURE III6-6. For stroke volume determination, flow is measured within a region of interest defined around the ascending aorta. The software automatically computes the flow to be 65 mL/heartbeat based on the mean velocity and cross-sectional area of the vessel.

CHALLENGE QUESTION: What is the cardiac output and cardiac index for this subject, given that the heart rate is 70 bpm and body surface area is 2.0 m²?

Answer: The cardiac output (CO) is defined as

$$CO \text{ (mL/min)} = SV \text{ (mL)} \times HR \text{ (beats per minute)}$$

For this example, CO = 65 mL/beat × 70 beats/min = 4550 mL/min or 4.55 L/min. The cardiac index is the cardiac output normalized to BSA, or 4.55 L/min/2 m² = 2.27 L/min/m².

The right ventricular stroke volume can be similarly calculated by determining the forward flow through the pulmonary artery, assuming no tricuspid regurgitation.

■ EXAMPLE 2: PULMONARY-SYSTEMIC SHUNT FRACTION OR Q_P/Q_S

A middle-aged subject has a known atrial septal defect (Figure III6-7). To measure the shunt fraction, two through-plane cine phase contrast acquisitions are positioned, one through the ascending aorta and another through the pulmonary artery. Flow versus time curves are determined for each great vessel and the total forward flow calculated: aortic forward flow = 82 mL/sec and pulmonary forward flow 95 mL/sec.

The pulmonary-systemic blood flow ratio is calculated as:

$$Q_p/Q_s = 95 \text{ mL/sec} / 82 \text{ mL/sec} = 1.2$$

A value greater than 1 is consistent with a left-to-right shunt. As seen on the cine phase-contrast image in Figure III6-7, the flow through the atrial septal defect is as expected, left to right. ■

■ EXAMPLE 3: REGURGITANT FRACTION

A teenager with pulmonic stenosis that had been treated with pulmonic valvulotomy returned for suspected pulmonic valvular regurgitation. Cine gradient echo imaging through the right ventricular outflow tract and pulmonic valve and an oblique axial phase contrast slice across the pulmonic valve are shown in Figure III6-8.

The forward flow during systole is calculated to be 120 mL, while the reverse flow during diastole is 50 mL. The regurgitant fraction is the ratio of the two:

$$\text{Regurgitant fraction} = \frac{\text{Regurgitant flow}}{\text{Forward flow}}$$

$$= \frac{50 \text{ mL}}{120 \text{ mL}} = 0.42 \text{ or } 42\% \blacksquare$$

Limitations of Blood Flow Measurements

Many of the caveats about estimating peak systolic velocity apply to flow rate estimates but have less serious implications on the accuracy of values. Probably the most important factor that reduces measurement accuracy is the spatial resolution. If voxels are large relative to the lumen, then the proportion of voxels that contain both tissue inside and outside the lumen becomes high and leads to inaccuracies in flow measurements (Figure III6-9).

> **IMPORTANT CONCEPTS:** Phase contrast flow measurements can be used to determine stroke volume, shunt fractions, regurgitant volumes, and other quantities. Depending on the application, retrospective gating may be desirable to ensure that measurements reflect the entire cardiac cycle. Spatial resolution is the most important determinant of the accuracy of flow measurements.

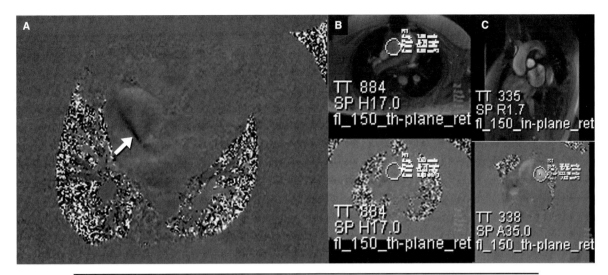

FIGURE III6-7. Atrial septal defect. (**A**) Cine phase-contrast image in the horizontal long axis view, with in-plane flow sensitivity, demonstrates a jet of blood (arrow) flowing from the left atrium to the right atrium through the ASD. Cine phase contrast magnitude (top) and phase (bottom) images measuring through-plane flow through the ascending aorta (**B**) and pulmonary artery (**C**).

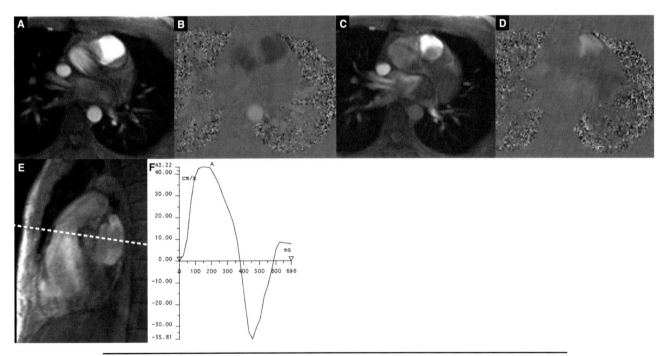

FIGURE III6-8. Pulmonic regurgitation. (**A–D**) Axial magnitude (**A**, **C**) and phase (**B**, **D**) images during systole (**A**, **B**) and diastole (**C**, **D**). (**E**) Sagittal cine gradient echo image through the right ventricular outflow tract and pulmonary artery show the slice positioning for the phase contrast images. (**F**) Corresponding plots of velocity vs. time for the pulmonary artery shows significant flow reversal during diastole, indicative of pulmonic insufficiency.

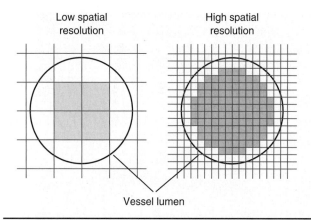

Low spatial resolution   High spatial resolution

Vessel lumen

FIGURE III6-9. Effect of spatial resolution on accuracy in MR phase contrast flow measurements. With low spatial resolution, only four voxels are completely contained within the vessel, the boundary voxels have partial volume of blood and stationary tissue outside the vessel. High-resolution imaging produces more accurate estimates of velocities and flow rates.

REVIEW QUESTIONS

1. To calculate stroke volume, two phase contrast acquisitions were performed (peak systolic magnitude and phase images are shown in Figure III6-Q1). Comment on the appearance of each study. What might be done to improve each acquisition?

2. A subject is referred for evaluation of cystic medial necrosis of the aorta. Cine gradient echo images demonstrate aortic insufficiency. How can you quantify the regurgitant fraction? (Specifically, how can abnormal regurgitant flow be calculated independent of diastolic filling of the coronary arteries?)

3. A subject with mitral regurgitation needs quantitative assessment of the degree of regurgitation. The regurgitant fraction for the mitral valve is calculated using an equation similar to that used for aortic regurgitation.

   Positioning of a phase contrast slice through the mitral valve orifice produces uninterpretable results because of the through-plane motion of the heart during the acquisition. What other techniques can be used to calculate the mitral regurgitant fraction using MRI?

4. A child is referred for evaluation of the differential blood flow between the right and left pulmonary arteries. Phase contrast results for acquisitions through the two sides are shown in Figure III6-Q4. Interpret the results. Are they consistent with the findings seen on the gadolinium-enhanced MR pulmonary angiogram?

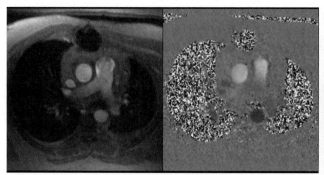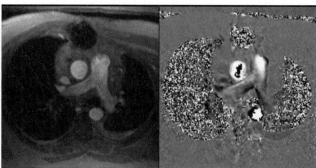

FIGURE III6-Q1. First acquisition (**A**, **B**) and second acquisition (**C**, **D**).

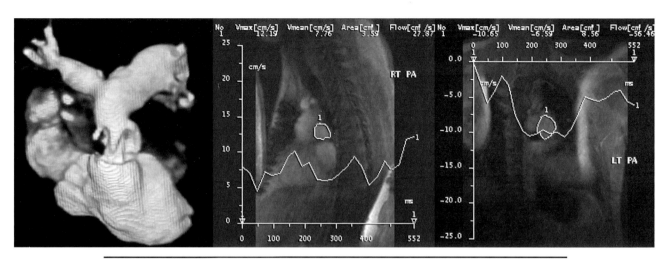

FIGURE III6-Q4. Gadolinium-enhanced MR angiogram of the pulmonary arteries. Separate phase contrast acquisitions through the right (RT PA) and left main pulmonary arteries (LT PA) are shown. The total flow through the right pulmonary artery is 28 mL/sec, and the flow through the left is 56 mL/sec.

▶ **PROTOCOL: Aortic Valve Disease**

Setup and Preparation	Notes
ECG leads	Necessary
Coil	Torso phased-array
Positioning tips	Supine, head first
Subject instructions	End-expiratory breath holding Supplemental oxygen by nasal cannula optional

Sequence	Imaging Plane	Parameters
1 Scout (true FISP or spoiled GRE)	Multiplanar	Default
2 Fast spin echo imaging of the chest (double IR single-shot half-Fourier FSE, if available)	Axial	Single shot or FSE with TR = R-R interval 8–10 mm slices
3 Single-slice scouts	3-chamber view, LVOT view	1 slice/breathhold
4 Cine GRE (spoiled gradient echo or steady-state gradient echo, segmented k-space)	3-chamber view, LVOT view, in-plane valve view[1]	Parameters (incl views per segment) defined for temporal resolution <60 msec, and acquisition time within a breathhold
5 Cine phase contrast flow quantification	Oblique axial through ascending aorta, above and below the coronary sinuses	Temporal resolution <60 msec, retrospective gating, view sharing for breathhold acquisition, through-plane

[1]A cine acquisition in the plane of the valve is helpful for viewing valvular morphology as depicted in Figure III6-5C.
[2]Flow quantification to estimate peak pressure gradient requires acquisition above the valve planes. For quantification of regurgitant fraction, two separate acquisition as listed, may be necessary.

▶ **PROTOCOL: Shunt Fraction Quantification**

Setup and Preparation	Notes
ECG leads	Necessary
Coil	Torso phased-array
Positioning tips	Supine, head first
Subject instructions	End-expiratory breath holding Supplemental oxygen by nasal cannula optional

Sequence	Imaging Plane	Parameters
1 Scout (true FISP or spoiled GRE)	Multiplanar	Default
2 Fast spin echo imaging of the chest (double IR single-shot half-Fourier FSE, if available)	Axial	Single-shot or FSE with TR = R-R interval 8–10 mm slices
3 Cine GRE[1] (spoiled gradient echo or steady-state gradient echo, segmented k-space)	Short and long axes	Parameters (incl views per segment) defined for temporal resolution <60 msec and acquisition time within a breath hold
4 Cine phase contrast flow quantification	Perpendicular to aortic and pulmonary outflow	Temporal resolution <60 msec, retrospective gating, view sharing for breathhold acquisition, through plane

[1]Cine images may be helpful for diagnosing abnormal shunts, including intracardiac defects.

Ischemic Cardiac Disease

Cardiac MRI for the evaluation of ischemic heart disease has tremendous potential because of its high spatial resolution and image contrast. In considering the different diagnostic strategies that can be used, it is helpful to review the progression of detectable abnormalities in ischemic heart disease, shown in Figure III7-1. The two main diagnostic strategies measure changes in either perfusion or ventricular wall motion under pharmacologic stress compared with rest. Although qualitative perfusion imaging is more sensitive for early ischemic change, it is also less specific than wall motion studies and may be less accurate in patients with global ischemia.

The MR imaging techniques and methods for pharmacologic stress vary considerably across various laboratories. Validation studies of both MR approaches are still being performed, and, in the context of alternative techniques such as stress ECG, SPECT, echocardiography, and PET, the role of MR in the evaluation of patients with

ischemic heart disease remains to be defined fully. Some basic principles of stress perfusion and wall motion studies are outlined in this chapter, with the caveat that these methods are continuing to be refined.

KEY CONCEPTS

▶ Pharmacologic stress improves the accuracy of diagnosis of ischemic heart disease and can be performed with catecholamines (dobutamine) for increased contractility and oxygen consumption or with vasodilators (adenosine/dipyridamole) for differential hyperemia.

▶ Performance of stress-rest MRI requires careful monitoring of subjects, ready access to antidotes to stress agents, and the presence of a physician experienced in cardiac resuscitation.

▶ Perfusion imaging sequences are not standardized but generally consist of a magnetization-prepared fast gradient echo or a multishot echo planar sequence following a low-dose bolus of gadolinium contrast material.

▶ Stress contractility examinations require fast cine gradient echo acquisitions with sufficient temporal resolution to detect changes in end-systole, and near-real time reconstruction and display.

▶ Clinical Protocols:
   ▶ Ischemic heart disease: adenosine/dipyridamole perfusion imaging
   ▶ Ischemic heart disease: dobutamine contractility imaging

Perfusion defect - subendocardial

Perfusion defect - transmural

Diastolic dysfunction

Systolic dysfunction

ECG changes

Symptoms (angina)

FIGURE III7-1. Diagnostic studies for ischemic heart disease.

PHARMACOLOGIC STRESS IN THE MRI SETTING

For the evaluation of ischemic heart disease, all diagnostic techniques are performed with cardiac stress. Stress can be achieved with exercise or with pharmacologic agents. In general, for exercise and sympathomimetic stress, the goal is to achieve a submaximal *target heart rate* that depends on age:

$$\text{Target heart rate} = 0.85 \times (220 - \text{Age (yrs)})$$

While ergonomic stress is the most physiologic, exercising in the magnet bore is not generally practical. Therefore, cardiac MR studies typically are performed with pharmacologic agents using one of two approaches: (a) *dobutamine*, a catecholamine that causes increased contractility and oxygen consumption, or (b) either *adenosine* or *dipyridamole*, both vasodilators that cause hyperemia. In both cases, changes that are observed are different for regions of myocardium that are supplied by diseased coronary arteries compared with those supplied by normal coronary arteries.

For all stress testing, careful monitoring of patients in the MR setting is vital. A physician experienced in cardiac resuscitation should be present for all examinations. There must be a continuous communication between the subject and operators to ensure prompt attention to symptoms. Monitoring should include frequent blood pressure measurements, continuous pulse oximetry, and continous single-lead ECG tracings for heart rate and rhythm. Although the detection of ST segment changes is problematic in the MR scanner because of the magnetohydrodynamic effect (see Chapter III-1), wall motion abnormalities generally precede ECG changes. With real-time cine MRI early detection of ischemia is possible.

Dobutamine

Dobutamine is a synthetic catecholamine with potent β_1-receptor and mild α_1- and β_2-receptor agonist activity. The effect of dobutamine depends on the dose administered. At low doses ($\leq$10 μg/kg body weight/min), dobutamine causes increased contractility. The recovery of wall motion with low-dose dobutamine is one technique for assessing cardiac viability in the setting of resting hypokinesis or akinesis. At high doses of dobutamine, increased heart rate and contractility cause an increase in oxygen consumption. Areas supplied by significantly diseased coronaries develop wall motion abnormalities under these conditions. The stress protocol is based on that used for dobutamine echocardiography (Table III7-1).

Beta-blockers reduce the effects of dobutamine and generally are withheld for 24–48 hours prior to the examination. Similarly, calcium antagonists and nitrates are discontinued for 24 hours prior to the study.

Contraindications for the administration of dobutamine include acute coronary syndrome, severe aortic stenosis, hypertrophic obstructive cardiomyopathy, uncontrolled hypertension, uncontrolled atrial fibrillation,

▶ **TABLE III7-1**

Dobutamine Dose	Duration Until Target Heart Rate Is Reached (or Other Criteria, Table III7-2)
10 μg/min/kg body weight	3 min
20 μg/min/kg body weight	3 min
30 μg/min/kg body weight	3 min
40 μg/min/kg body weight	3 min
Optional atropine 0.25 mg × 4 (1–2 mg total)	

▶ **TABLE III7-2**

Criteria for Stopping Dobutamine Infusion

Target heart rate achieved
Systolic blood pressure decrease more than 40 mm Hg
Blood pressure increase greater than 240/120 mm Hg
Intractable symptoms
New or worsening wall motion abnormalities in at least two adjacent left ventricular segments
Complex cardiac arrhythmias

uncontrolled heart failure, and known severe ventricular arrhythmias.

As shown in Table III7-1, the conventional protocol involves incremental increases in dobutamine doses in steps of 10 μg/min/kg body weight, up to a maximum dose of 40 (or even 50) μg/min/kg. If target heart rate is not reached, additional atropine can be administered at doses of 0.25 mg, up to 1–2 mg total, during the ongoing infusion of dobutamine. Criteria for termination of the study are shown in Table III7-2 and include the development of signs and symptoms of ischemia—including wall motion abnormalities in at least two adjacent ventricular segments or anginal symptoms.

Side effects of the dobutamine can be reversed with a β-blocker such as intravenous esmolol or metoprolol if signs and symptoms do not resolve after infusion is stopped. The half-life of dobutamine is short—approximately 2 min. In patients who develop angina, sublingual nitroglycerin can also be used.

Dipyridamole and Adenosine

Dipyridamole (Persantine) and adenosine have almost identical vasodilatory effects. Adenosine is a naturally occuring vasodilator. Dipyridamole blocks the cellular uptake and metabolism of adenosine and consequently also causes vasodilation. With both agents, a four- to five-fold hyperemia is seen in normal myocardial territories but not in regions subtended by stenotic coronary arteries. With significant coronary artery disease, dipyridamole

> **TABLE III7-3** Doses of Adenosine and Dipyridamole

Pharmacologic Agent	Dose	Duration
Adenosine	140 μg/kg body weight/min	6 min (start imaging after 3 min)
Dipyridamole	0.56 mg/kg body weight total	4 min (start imaging after 2 min)

and adenosine cause a steal phenomenon, and the differential perfusion changes with vasodilation are used to diagnose ischemic heart disease.

Contraindications include asthma, high-grade atroventricular block, sinus arrhythmia, aortic or mitral valvular stenosis, and carotid artery stenosis. Medications that contain aminophylline, theophylline, and other xanthines (such as caffeinated products) are withheld for 12–24 hours before the study.

Assessment of perfusion is performed using first-pass gadolinium-enhanced perfusion. The standard dosing regimens for the two vasodilatory agents are shown in Table III7-3.

Reasons for stopping the infusion of these agents include bronchospasm, ventricular arrhythmias, and the onset of second- or third-degree atrioventricular block and bradycardia. Low-workload exercise (such as handgripping exercises) have been shown to reduce the side effects associated with the vasodilators. Intravenous aminophylline is an antidote to both adenosine and dipyridamole and should be available for immediate administration. The plasma half-life of adenosine is less than 10 sec. For intravenous dipyridamole, it is 5 min.

Pharmacologic Stress in the Diagnosis of Ischemic Heart Disease

Both categories of pharmacologic agents—sympathomimetics such as dobutamine or vasodilators such as adenosine or dipyridamole—improve the diagnosis of ischemic heart disease by accentuating differences between territories supplied by normal coronary arteries and those that receive inadequate blood supply. In the clinical setting, the most common imaging strategies for detecting these differences are stress radionuclide perfusion examination and stress echocardiography. The MR tools recapitulate these approaches. MRI can be used either to measure perfusion, typically with first-pass gadolinium-enhanced T1-weighted imaging, or to detect changes in wall motion with fast cine gradient echo imaging. Each class of stressor agent can be used with either MRI approach. However, most commonly, perfusion imaging is performed with vasodilators and contractility studies are performed with dobutamine. Whether to use perfusion or contractility methods remains the subject of active research. Some considerations include the extent of coronary disease, tradeoffs

between sensitivity and specificity, tolerance by patients, cost, and ease of administration.

PERFUSION IMAGING

The controversies in cardiac perfusion imaging span virtually the entire range of protocol options: from the imaging sequence to the rate and amount of contrast injection to the post-processing analysis of the images. This section begins with a brief discussion of the desired features of perfusion imaging sequences. Characteristics of different commonly used imaging methods are described in the remainder of this section.

Desired Features of MR Perfusion Imaging

The underlying principle of first-pass myocardial perfusion MR imaging is that differences in blood flow to the myocardium can be tracked by the direct visualization of enhancement with rate of uptake, directly visualized by gadolinium contrast agents. The diagnosis of myocardial ischemia or infarction is based on its lower blood flow, recognized by slower rates of both uptake and washout of contrast material during the first pass through the myocardial circulation (Figure III7-2). To maximize detection of ischemia, particularly subendocardial ischemia, several features of the imaging technique are necessary (Table III7-4).

Most cardiac perfusion sequences are T1-weighted fast gradient echo sequences or echo planar sequences performed with magnetization preparation to improve image contrast. Considerations in optimizing MR perfusion sequences include the design of the magnetization preparation prepulse (Chapter I-9), selection of a fast gradient echo readout, gadolinium contrast material injection protocol, and image analysis, each of which is discussed next.

Magnetization Preparation Prepulses

The goal is to differentiate areas of normal perfusion and hypoperfusion during first-pass contrast-enhanced MR imaging using gadolinium contrast agents. Magnetization preparation prepulses are used to accentuate T1 differences. Typically either a 90° saturation prepulse, referred to as *saturation recovery*, or a 180° inversion recovery prepulse is used (Figure III7-3). The prepulse is nonslice-selective to minimize in-flow effects and is typically applied at a fixed time after the R wave. After a selected inversion time, data acquisition is performed with either a gradient echo or an echo planar readout.

The higher the flip angle of the prepulse, the greater the T1 contrast. However, high flip angles require a longer time for recovery between prepulse the and data acquisition,

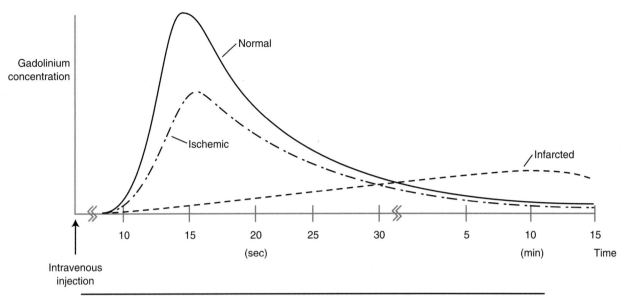

FIGURE III7-2. Schematic of first-pass tracer kinetics in coronary artery disease. Ischemic myocardium demonstrates a lower rate of enhancement and a lower peak compared with nonischemic myocardium. Enhancement of infarcted myocardium is significantly slower than that of ischemic tissue.

▶ **TABLE III7-4** **Desired Features of First-Pass MR Perfusion**

Features	Desired Attributes
Spatial coverage	Entire left ventricular myocardium
Temporal resolution	High resolution to detect differences during first-pass (<1–2 sec)
Spatial resolution	High resolution to detect subendocardial ischemia (<2 mm)
Signal-to-noise ratios	High SNR to differentiate normal and ischemic myocardium
Image contrast	High contrast to differentiate normal and ischemic myocardium
Motion artifact	Minimum
Gadolinium contrast concentration vs. SI	A known and quantifiable relationship between gadolinium contrast concentration and signal intensity

called the inversion time. Ideally, the inversion time is selected so that the unenhanced myocardium is relatively low in signal, or nearly nulled, compared to the enhancing myocardium. The time required for recovery of longitudinal magnetization restricts the number of slices that can be imaged. Additionally, because this sequence is an ECG-gated sequence, recovery of longitudinal magnetization depends on the heart rate, and therefore arrhythmias are detrimental to good image contrast.

An *interleaved notched saturation perfusion* method builds in a longer inversion time between the prepulse and the readout without lengthening the acquisition time. The magnetization prepulse is designed to have a notched slice

profile so that all but a central notch is saturated (Figure III7-4). As shown in Figure III7-4, rather than performing the readout shortly after the saturation pulse, the readout is delayed until the subsequent slice, which allows for a longer inversion time and consequently better image contrast.

Readout Sequences

Following the prepulse, data are acquired. For sufficient spatial coverage and temporal resolution, three slices are acquired per heartbeat, or 6–7 slices every two heartbeats. The readout for each image is therefore constrained to less than 200 msec. This can be achieved by fast gradient echo, multishot echo planar imaging, or, more recently, steady-state free precession gradient echo imaging. In all cases, for maximal T1 weighting, the TE must be kept short.

One of the most commonly used sequences is a saturation or inversion recovery fast low-flip-angle gradient echo sequence (also referred to as turbo fast low-angle shot or turboFLASH sequence, Figure III7-5, see also Chapter I-4).

Following each R wave and a short trigger delay (100 msec) to minimize motion effects during systole, a saturation (or inversion recovery) prepulse is applied. Immediately thereafter, a series of low-flip-angle gradient echoes are generated. To minimize the effects of residual transverse magnetization on subsequent imaging, gradient crusher pulses are typically applied following the readout. With TR less than 2 msec, acquisition of a

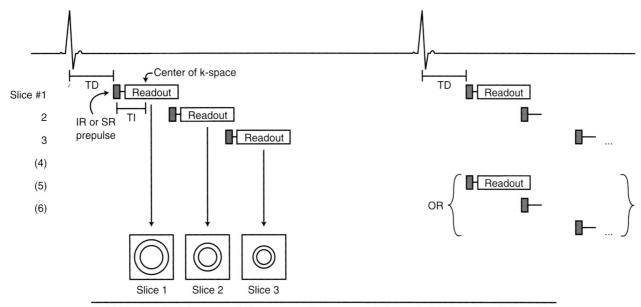

FIGURE III7-3. Schematic of IR or saturation recovery (SR) perfusion imaging of three slice positions every heartbeat (or six slice positions every other heartbeat). TD represents the trigger delay and TI the inversion time between the IR or SR prepulse and the center of k-space during the readout period.

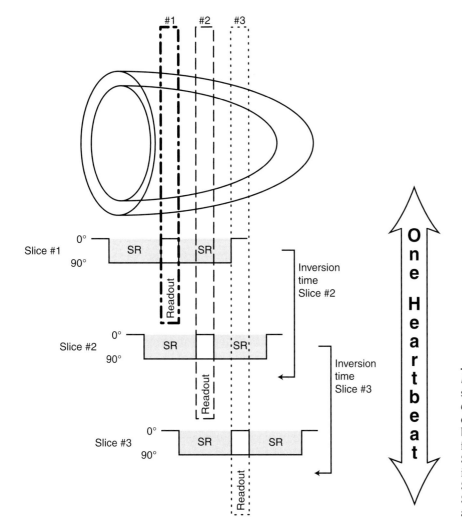

FIGURE III7-4. Notched saturation perfusion method. Time is reflected in the vertical direction. The initial step is application of a notched SR pulse that "spares" Slice #1 but affects Slice #2. Then, after the interval for readout for Slice #1, the notched SR pulse is applied again, this time sparing Slice #2. Then readout is performed for Slice #2. The longer inversion time for Slice #2 means better T1 image contrast is achieved.

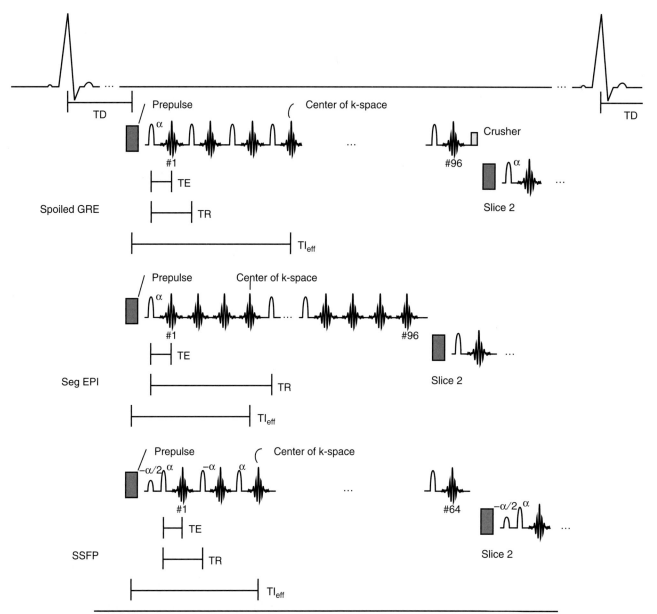

FIGURE III7-5. Fast readout sequences used for first-pass perfusion MR imaging include fast low-angle snapshot imaging ("Spoiled GRE"), segmented EPI ("Seg EPI"), and steady-state free precession ("SSFP") methods.

complete image with matrix of 64–96 × 128 can be achieved in less than 150–200 msec.

CHALLENGE QUESTION: What determines the effective inversion time for this sequence when segmented k-space methods are used?

Answer: The echo that is used to fill the central line of k-space determines image contrast and is acquired at a time called the effective inversion time.

One challenge of fast gradient echo imaging is the maintenance of sufficient T1-weighted image contrast

despite repeated application of the RF pulses needed to generate the gradient echoes. As discussed in Chapter I-4, low flip angles are necessary to minimize disturbance of the T1 recovery during readout.

Although single-shot echo planar imaging is frequently used in brain perfusion studies, the long echo train and, consequently, relatively long TE make this sequence sensitive to susceptibility and other artifacts when imaging the heart. More successful has been multishot echo planar imaging, where the the echo train length can be significantly shorter, such as 4, and repeated 16–24 times for acquisition of each image. With a TR of less than

8 msec, an ETL of 4, each 64–96 × 128 image requires less than 150–200 msec (Figure III7-5).

Recently developed versions of steady-state free precession sequences (Figure III7-5) use a single-shot readout to provide improved signal-to-noise and contrast-to-noise ratios compared with conventional fast gradient echo imaging. While conventional steady-state free precession sequences have T2/T1 weighting, use of a saturation pulse can increase T1 weighting. Despite the improved signal resulting from the refocused transverse magnetization, the TR for these sequences is longer than for other fast methods because of the requirement for balanced gradients. Parallel imaging allows one to acquire the same number of slices per heartbeat (typically 3) as fast low-flip-angle gradient echo approaches.

Alternative fast readout techniques, such as radial k-space trajectories for both 2D and 3D perfusion, are the focus of current investigations.

Gadolinium Contrast Administration

There is no consensus as to the optimal strategy for administering gadolinium contrast material for first-pass perfusion imaging. Important considerations include the need for two injections (one each for stress and rest imaging) and high image contrast. Equally important may be the need for preservation of the monotonic relationship between signal intensity and gadolinium contrast concentration, particularly in the blood pool. The importance of the latter depends on the image analysis approach taken.

The implicit assumption in first-pass perfusion imaging is that the signal intensity of voxels directly relates to the amount of gadolinium contrast in the tissue, and therefore on the amout of blood flow to the myocardium. To have the greatest image contrast between tissues that have different rates of coronary perfusion, higher concentrations of gadolinium contrast seem to be most advantageous. However, as discussed in Chapter I-3, gadolinium chelates shorten both T1 and T2 relaxation times. The T2 effects become significant at higher concentrations of gadolinium contrast, although the exact relationship depends on pulse sequence parameters.

CHALLENGE QUESTION: How does TE affect the relationship between image signal intensity and gadolinium contrast concentration?

Answer: The longer the TE, the more T2-weighted an image is. Sequences with longer TEs will see the effect of T2 shortening on image signal intensity at lower concentrations of gadolinium contrast than sequences with shorter TEs.

Weighing up these considerations, typical contrast material doses for first pass perfusion images range from 0.025 to 0.1 mmol/kg, most commonly 0.05 mmol/kg (approximately 10 mL). Higher doses are generally considered acceptable for analysis by visual inspection, while for quantitative measures of perfusion, lower doses are preferred to avoid T2 effects. Typically stress images are performed first, followed by a delay of 3–15 min depending on the stress agent used, and then repeated at rest with the same, or slightly higher gadolinium dose. To ensure a tight bolus and minimal dispersion of the bolus at the level of the coronary arteries, rates of injection are typically 3–5 mL/sec followed by a saline flush of 20 mL injected at the same rate.

Image Analysis

For analysis of first-pass myocardial perfusion images, the left ventricle can be divided into the standard 17-segment model (Figure III2-12). Interpretation is based on the expected coronary artery distributions for the segments. Analysis can be qualitative, semiquantitative, and fully quantitative.

The simplest form of analysis is a visual assessment of perfusion defects. Localized coronary artery disease first manifests as subendocardial hypoperfusion, as shown in Figure III7-6.

It is important to realize that because surface coils are used for imaging, the signal intensity of the image may

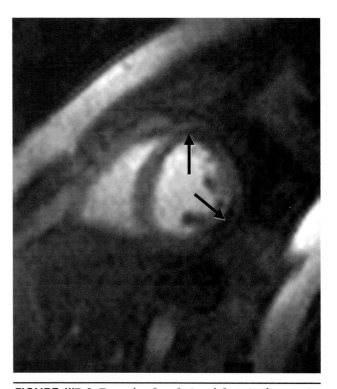

FIGURE III7-6. Example of perfusion defects in the anterior wall and inferolateral wall (arrows).

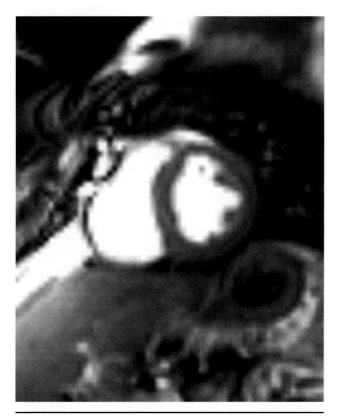

FIGURE III7-7. Low signal along the subendocardial layer circumferentially mimics diffuse subendocardial hypoperfusion. These patterns most likely represent susceptibility artifact due to the arrival of highly concentrated contrast material. They can also be due to cardiac motion.

vary spatially because of nonuniform coil sensitivity. As a result, the inferior and inferolateral wall may appear artifactually less perfused than the anterior wall. Additionally, transient hypointense artifacts are frequently seen along the myocardial-blood pool interface, mimicking subendocardial perfusion defects (Figure III7-7). These are likely either susceptibility effects of the highly concentrated contrast agent in the blood pool, or artifacts due to cardiac motion. Typically the artifacts precede peak myocardial enhancement.

Most commercial vendors offer semi-quantitative methods for analysis of perfusion data. These programs generate time-signal intensity curves for each voxel in the image (Figure III7-8). The curves can then be analyzed in terms of various parameters that characterize the curves and differentiate regions of normal and hypoperfusion (Table III7-5). To facilitate interpretation, commercial software can display parametric maps of the images using these parameters.

The most commonly used parameter is the *upslope* value. An accurate estimate of upslope requires sufficiently high temporal resolution to ensure that multiple frames are acquired before the peak. An important limitation of this index is that it is influenced by the subject's cardiac output.

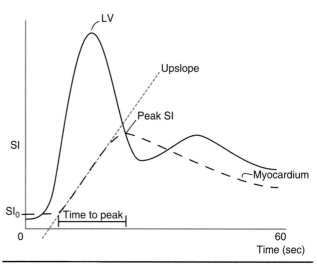

FIGURE III7-8. Typical left ventricular blood pool (LV) and myocardium time-signal intensity curves with selected semi-quantitative parameters depicted. The precontrast myocardial signal intensity (SI) is denoted SI_0.

▶ **TABLE III7-5 Semiquantitative Parameters**

Parameter	Calculation
Peak signal intensity	Peak SI/precontrast SI
Peak contrast enhancement	(Peak SI-precontrast SI)/precontrast SI
Time to peak	Time to peak enhancement from the onset of enhancement
Upslope	Slope of initial rise in myocardium
Upslope ratio	Upslope myocardium/Upslope blood pool
Mean transit time	Average time to pass through the voxel
Area under SI curve	Area under the curve, typically from onset to peak

Because the injection of the contrast material is intravenous, the profile of the bolus at the time of transit through the coronary arteries depends on the hemodynamics of the subject (Figure III7-9). These hemodynamics can change during stress and rest. Consequently, the upslope of signal in the myocardium at stress and rest may vary because of changes in hemodynamics and/or changes in coronary perfusion. To help control for differences in cardiac output, the ratio of left ventricular and myocardial upslopes, called the *upslope ratio* (Table III7-5), is more informative. By normalizing against the upslope of the signal intensity curve in the left ventricular blood pool, the upslope ratio is more likely to reflect changes in perfusion that are attributable to coronary disease.

Qualitative and semi-quantitative methods of interpretation rely on the differentiation of normally perfused areas from hypoperfused regions to diagnose ischemic heart disease. More complex methods have been developed by research laboratories to derive absolute, quantitative

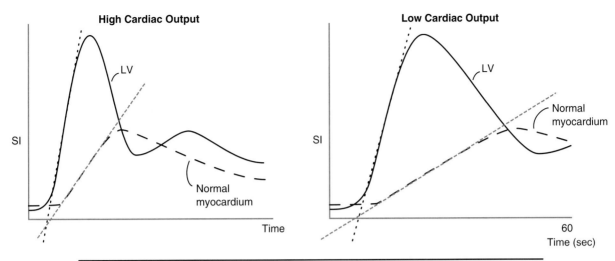

FIGURE III7-9. Effect of different cardiac output on the input function or left ventricular blood pool signal intensity curve (LV). With a lower cardiac output, a more dispersed input function or bolus leads to a broader pattern of enhancement of the normal myocardium, and consequently a lower upslope, which could be mistakenly interpreted as diminished perfusion. Taking the ratio of myocardium upslope (dashed lines) to LV upslope (dotted lines) helps correct for variability due to global cardiac function.

measures of perfusion (in units mL/min/g tissue). These are based on compartmental models and established tracer kinetic techniques. Challenges to these approaches include the derivation of gadolinium contrast concentrations from signal intensity measurements and the stability of computational algorithms such as deconvolution. Nonetheless, quantitative measurements have the potential of improved sensitivity for the detection of changes in perfusion, particularly in the setting of global hypoperfusion. Quantitative perfusion measurements may prove useful markers for studying the effects of therapeutic interventions.

CONTRACTILITY STUDIES

Stress-contractility studies of the heart require very high temporal resolution with multislice cine imaging. It is also important to permit viewing in real time or near-real time, because the detection of wall motion abnormalities is a criterion for termination of the examination, as it reflects underlying myocardial ischemia (Figure III7-1). Rapid detection of these abnormalities is essential. During these examinations, short and long axis images are acquired at rest and then at each dose increment of dobutamine. The more extensive the imaging coverage, the more sensitive is the examination to focal abnormalities.

Modifying Acquisitions for Increased Heart Rate

The required temporal resolution depends on heart rate. For resting studies, a temporal resolution of about 40 msec or less is desirable. Dobutamine increases not only contractility but also heart rate. Therefore, at high doses, high subject heart rates necessitate adjustment of cine gradient echo sequence parameters—reducing the number of lines per segment or views per segment with an associated increase in the number of heartbeats to generate each image. For a review of these concepts, the reader is referred to Chapter III-4, in particular Table III4-2.

CHALLENGE QUESTION: Why is improved temporal resolution important at higher heart rates?

Answer: To assess left ventricular contractility, it is important to image the heart at end systole. If end systole is not imaged, left ventricular contractility will be underestimated. At high doses of dobutamine, this underestimation could lead to false positive interpretations of ischemia. The narrow window of peak systole becomes even more narrow when the heart is beating quickly. To increase the likelihood of imaging at peak systole, higher-temporal-resolution images are needed.

A reduction in the number of lines per segment will improve the temporal resolution, because the temporal resolution is equal to the true TR × the number of lines per segment. With fewer lines acquired in each heartbeat, the number of heartbeats needed per acquisition will increase. However, since the subject's heart rate is higher, the time of acquisition may actually decrease.

CHALLENGE QUESTION: For a particular cine gradient echo sequence, the true TR is 10 msec and the number of phase-encoding steps necessary to generate an image is 100. A subject starts with a heart rate of 60 beats per min (R-R interval of 1000 msec), and the number of views per segment is selected to be 6. With pharmacologic stress, the heart rate increases to

90 beats per minute (R-R interval of 667 msec). The views per segment is reduced to 4. What are the temporal resolution and acquisition time under the two circumstances?

Answer: Based on a review of Table III4-2, the temporal resolution at rest will be 60 msec, and the total acquisition time will be 100/6 heartbeats, or about 17 heartbeats, which is equal to 17 sec. Under stress, the faster heart rate necessitates a higher-temporal-resolution acquisition to evaluate systolic motion accurately. The lower number of views per segment translates into a temporal

resolution of 40 msec. The acquisition time will be 100/4 or 25 heart beats, which is equal to about 17 sec, the same as at rest.

Pulse Sequences

Original reports of stress-contractility exams used single-slice breath-hold segmented k-space fast gradient echo sequences. However, the requirement for multiple breath holds—typically at least 3 short axis and 2 long axis—makes

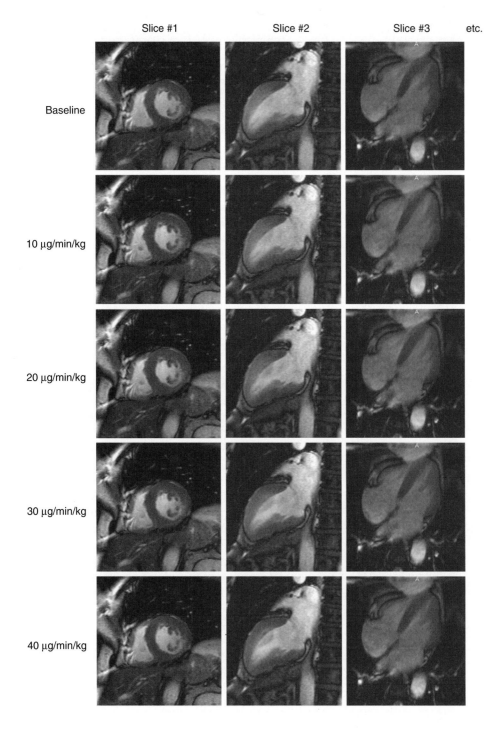

FIGURE III7-10. Selected cine images during a stress contractility study with increasing dose of dobutamine in lower rows and each slice position in a separate column (three shown here).

this approach challenging for some subjects. Faster imaging sequences are preferred.

Steady-state free precession imaging can be used to acquire multiple slice positions in a single breath hold. For example, a series of short axis slices can be obtained in one breath hold and several long axis images in a second breath hold (Chapter III-4). Ideally, spatial resolution should be 2 mm (with slice thickness of 6–10 mm), and temporal resolution as just discussed.

Real-time steady-state free precession sequences, as described in Chapter III-4, are well suited for stress imaging, with the advantage of real-time viewing of the effects of pharmacologic stress agents on contractility, akin to echocardiography. However, the high temporal and spatial resolution demands of stress contractility studies present technical challenges. Further development of parallel imaging and new cardiac coils has the potential to overcome these challenges.

Real-Time Viewing

Regardless of the sequence performed, a common requirement for all stress contractility studies is rapid image reconstruction and simultaneous display of cine loops of multiple imaging slices at different levels of stress. To detect the onset of abnormal wall motion due to ischemia, it is very important to be able to view all the images as they are reconstructed, and also to compare them against baseline and lower stress levels (Figure III7-10).

Interpretation and Analysis

Ventricular contractility at each stress level is analyzed using the standard 17-segment model (Chapter III-2).

▶ **TABLE III7-6** Grading Left Ventricular Contractility

Wall Motion	Definition
1	Normal
2	Hypokinetic
3	Akinetic
4	Dyskinetic

Contractility is typically graded on a score of 1–4 (Table III7-6) based on systolic wall thickening and extent of wall motion.

Segments that develop wall motion abnormalities or show worsening contractility with high-dose dobutamine are considered ischemic. Wall motion abnormalities that are present at rest and worsen at high doses of dobutamine (with possible improvement at low dose) are considered to reflect inducible ischemia. Each segment is assigned to a specific coronary artery territory (Figure III2-12), although coronary distributions, particularly in the setting of collateral vessels, vary considerably across subjects.

Most vendors provide imaging software that relies on the segmentation of the left ventricular endo- and epicardial borders to perform quantitative analysis of left ventricular wall thickening and motion (Figure III4-17).

REVIEW QUESTIONS

1. On first-pass perfusion images, you observe hypoperfusion throughout the inferior wall. How would you differentiate between coronary artery disease and an artifact of coil sensitivity?

2. Interpret the bull's eye maps of perfusion under conditions of stress and rest shown in Figure III7-Q2. (Darker shades of gray represent lower perfusion.)

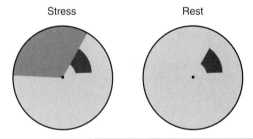

FIGURE III7-Q2. Bull's eye map of perfusion; darker areas correspond to relative hypoperfusion.

3. Interpret the bulls'eye maps of percent wall segmental thickening under conditions of high- and low-dose dobutamine and at rest shown in Figure III7-Q3.

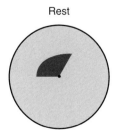

FIGURE III7-Q3

▶ **PROTOCOL: Ischemic Heart Disease: Adenosine/Dipyridamole Perfusion Imaging**

Setup and Preparation	Notes
i.v.	22 G or larger
Gadolinium contrast	0.1–0.2 mmol/kg (20–40 mL)
ECG leads	Necessary
Coil	Torso phased-array
Positioning tips	Supine, head first
Subject instructions	End-expiratory breath holding Supplemental oxygen by nasal cannula suggested
MR-compatible infusion pump	For adenosine infusion
Monitoring/safety checklist	Blood pressure, pulse oximetry, ECG monitoring for heart rate and rhythm; intravenous aminophylline on hand Close monitoring for symptoms; 12-lead ECG before and after examination

Sequence	Imaging Plane	Parameters
1 Scout (true FISP or spoiled GRE)	Multiplanar	Default
2 T2-weighted fast spin echo imaging of the chest (double IR single-shot half-Fourier FSE, if available)	Axial	Single-shot or FSE with TR = one R-R interval 8–10 mm slices
3 Single-slice scouts	Obliques to get short axis and long axis views	1 slice/breath hold
4 Perfusion GRE with adenosine or dipyridamole[1]	Short axes and long axes	6 slices every other heartbeat, 8 mm slice, 0.05 mmol/kg (approx 10 mL) Gadolumine contrast
5 Perfusion GRE at rest (optional)[2]	Same as Step 4	0.05 mmol/kg (approx 10 mL) Gadolumine contrast
6 Cine GRE (spoiled gradient echo or steady-state gradient echo, segmented k-space)	Short axes	8 mm slices with 2 mm gaps Parameters (incl views per segment) defined for temporal resolution <60 msec, and acquisition time within a breath hold, LV base to apex, 8–12 slices
7 Cine GRE (spoiled gradient echo or steady-state gradient echo, segmented k-space)	Long axes	8 mm slices Same parameters as above Less rectangular FOV for VLA view
8 Inversion time mapping (optional)[2]	Short axis (through infarct, if possible)	Single slice. Parameters defined to achieve temporal resolution of < 60 msec to determine optimal inversion time for nulling of uninfarcted myocardium
9 Inversion recovery segmented k-space gradient echo imaging (optional)[2]	Short and long axes (match cine GRE)	Set inversion time according to Step 8.

[1]Perfusion sequence options are detailed in the text. They include a notched saturation perfusion method or saturation recovery True FISP imaging.
[2]Resting perfusion may be optional if delayed contrast-enhanced imaging is performed to distinguish stress perfusion defects due to ischemia or infarct.

▌**PROTOCOL: Ischemic Heart Disease: Dobutamine Contractility Imaging**

Setup and Preparation	Notes
i.v.	22 G or larger
Gadolinium contrast	Optional for delayed contrast-enhanced imaging
ECG leads	Necessary
Coil	Torso phased-array
Positioning tips	Supine, head first
Subject instructions	End-expiratory breath holding Supplemental oxygen by nasal cannula suggested
Monitoring/safety checklist	Blood pressure, pulse oximetry, ECG monitoring for heart rate and rhythm; intravenous esmolol or metoprolol and sublingual nitroglygerin on hand Close monitoring for symptoms; 12-lead ECG before and after examination

Sequence	Imaging Plane	Parameters
1 Scout (true FISP or spoiled GRE)	Multiplanar	Default
2 T2-weighted fast spin echo imaging of the chest (double IR single-shot half-Fourier FSE, if available)	Axial	Single-shot or FSE with TR = one R-R interval 8–10 mm slices
3 Single-slice scouts	Obliques to get short axis and long axis views	1 slice/breath hold
4 Cine GRE (spoiled gradient echo or steady-state gradient echo, segmented k-space) Dobutamine infusion increments until target heart rate (atropine, as needed) or other criteria for stopping infusion met	Short axes and long axes	8 mm slices Parameters (incl views per segment) defined for temporal resolution <40 msec, and acquisition time within a breath hold
5 Repeat cine GRE Limited number of slices at each dobutamine level Gadolinium injection (optional)[1]	Short axes and long axes	0.1–0.2 mmol/kg
6 Inversion time mapping (optional)[1]	Short axis (through infarct, if possible)	Single-slice. Parameters defined to achieve temporal resolution of <60 msec to determine optimal inversion time for nulling of uninfarcted myocardium
7 Inversion recovery segmented k-space gradient echo imaging (optional)[1]	Short and long axes (match cine GRE)	Set inversion time according to Step 6.

[1]Delayed contrast-enhanced imaging is optional for delineation of regions of infarcted myocardium.

Coronary Artery Imaging

Imaging of the coronary arteries is potentially one of the most important applications in cardiac MRI, and, at the same time, one of its most technically challenging areas. Spatial resolution requirements are very high. Coronary vessels are small to begin with, and differences between, say, 60% stenosis and 80% stenosis in a 2 mm vessel can be clinically significant. In addition, respiratory and cardiac motion pose serious obstacles to imaging. With recent advances in multidetector CT angiography, noninvasive coronary imaging is being performed with impressive results. However, in patients who have contraindications to iodinated contrast material, MRI may be a valuable alternative. This chapter reviews the principles of coronary artery MR imaging and discusses the most commonly performed sequences. The information is offered with the caveat that coronary MR angiography is very much an evolving field.

KEY CONCEPTS

▶ The tortuous course of the coronary arteries makes slab positioning challenging. Whole-heart imaging approaches with large 3D volumes simplify positioning.

▶ Spatial resolution of coronary artery MRA must be less than 1 mm, and ideally less than 0.5 mm.

▶ To minimize artifacts related to cardiac motion, data acquisition should be confined to the brief stationary period of diastole, which typically is 120–160 msec long but is highly variable across individuals.

▶ To minimize artifacts related to respiratory motion, data acquisition should either be confined to a breath hold, performed at end expiration, or performed with navigator echoes.

▶ Navigator echo coronary imaging compensates for changes in diaphragm position during the acquisition period. Prospective adaptive motion correction further improves image quality.

▶ Preparation pulses such as fat suppression, T2 preparation pulses, and magnetization transfer are helpful to improve image contrast for bright-blood coronary imaging.

▶ Clinical Protocols:
  ▶ Anomalous coronary arteries
  ▶ Comprehensive examination of coronary artery disease

INTRODUCTION TO CORONARY ARTERY ANATOMY

The normal pattern of coronary artery anatomy is diagrammed in Figure III8-1. The coronary arteries originate from the coronary sinuses just superior to the aortic valve. The left main (LM) coronary artery divides into the left circumflex artery (LCx), which travels in the left atrioventricular groove, and the left anterior descending artery (LAD), which travels in the anterior interventricular groove, typically wrapping around the apex. The right coronary artery (RCA) lies in the right atrioventricular groove and usually becomes the posterior descending artery (PDA) in the posterior interventricular groove. The LAD gives off diagonal artery branches, while the circumflex artery gives rise to marginal arteries. The purpose of most coronary artery imaging is the diagnosis of atherosclerotic stenoses. Other kinds of pathologies include anomalous coronary artery anatomy and coronary artery aneurysms. Occasionally imaging is done to evaluate the patency of coronary artery bypass grafts.

CHALLENGES OF CORONARY ARTERY MRI

Before turning to specific MR sequences that are used for coronary artery imaging, it may be helpful to review the primary challenges of imaging the coronary arteries and some of the general strategies used to overcome each of these.

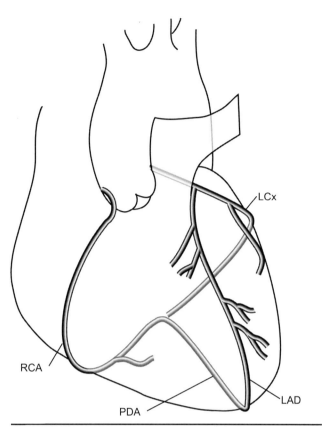

FIGURE III8-1. Main coronary arteries of the heart.

Positioning of the Imaging Slabs

The coronary arteries curve around the epicardial surface of the heart. Their tortuous course makes slice positioning a challenge. One or two oblique thin 3D slabs can be used to image the RCA and LCx. A separate slab is needed to image the LAD. However, even with accurate positioning of slabs, exclusion of large branch vessels may limit the diagnostic accuracy of slab-based coronary MRA studies.

> **IMPORTANT CONCEPT:** The tortuous and variable course of coronary arteries along the epicardial surface of the heart necessitates careful positioning of multiple thin imaging slabs.

Slice or Slab Positioning

Positioning of the 2D imaging slice or 3D slab for each of the coronary arteries requires scout images that facilitate double oblique orientation. A series of scout images through the heart is helpful to position slices or slabs through each of the coronary arteries (Figure III8-2).

The right coronary artery can be best imaged by means of an oblique sagittal slab (Figure III8-2) that is prescribed through the right coronary ostia, mid right coronary artery, and distal coronary artery.

Sometimes, the left circumflex artery is also imaged in the acquisition performed through the right coronary artery (in the plane of the atrioventricular groove), but often a second oblique sagittal acquisition is required.

Typically, for the left coronary artery and proximal left circumflex artery, a separate acquisition is performed using an axial or oblique axial 3D slab (Figure III8-2).

Small Vessel Size

The largest artery is the left main coronary with a typical luminal diameter of 4.5 mm. A series of diagonal branches arise from the LAD, so that the luminal diameter of the distal LAD is reduced to about 2 mm. The RCA and LCx arteries are typically 3–4 mm in diameter proximally and decrease in diameter over their course.

The spatial resolution demands on coronary MR angiography depend on the indication for the examination. As a reference for comparison, conventional contrast angiography, the gold standard diagnostic test for coronary imaging, has a spatial resolution of 0.3 mm or less. In the typical case of coronary atherosclerosis, where coronary artery stenosis needs to be detected and quantified, the spatial resolution of images should be less than 1 mm, ideally closer to 0.5 mm. The high spatial resolution should be isotropic; that is, the voxel resolution should be less than 1 mm in all three dimensions. With most two-dimensional acquisition strategies, this is difficult to achieve; consequently, three-dimensional methods are favored. Imaging of suspected anomalous coronary artery anatomy, on the other hand, does not demand isotropic resolution, and two-dimensional imaging may be sufficient.

> **IMPORTANT CONCEPT:** The small luminal diameters of the main epicardial coronary arteries, between 2 and 5 mm, necessitate spatial resolution of less than 1 mm, and preferably less than 0.5 mm, for accurate depiction of stenoses in the large vessels.

Cardiac Motion

For noncoronary MR imaging of the heart, confining the acquisition window to diastole is one common strategy for minimizing motion artifacts. However, the requirements of coronary artery imaging are even greater. Even during diastole, the coronary arteries move enough to cause artifacts. One study (1) showed that the duration of time during which the coronary arteries undergo less than 1 mm motion is only a short part of middiastole, during isovolumetric relaxation, and varies considerably across individuals. The interval can be as short as 66 msec and as long as 333 msec (averaging 161 msec) for the left coronary artery, while for the right coronary

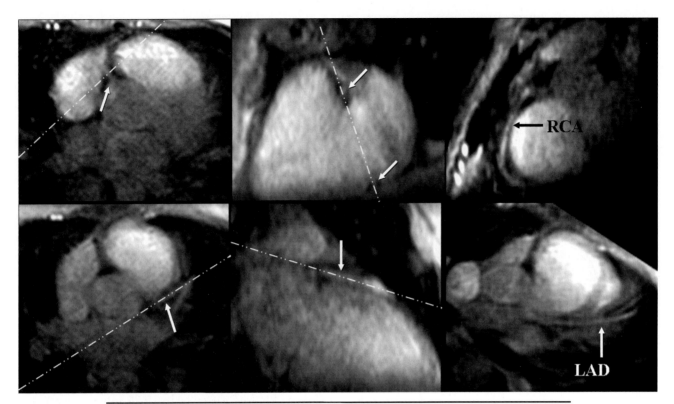

FIGURE III8-2. Slice positioning for the RCA (top row) and LAD (bottom row). Starting from an axial slice, scout images are obtained through the RCA (top, middle) and LAD (bottom, middle). Slices through each vessel are then prescribed along oblique planes, shown as white dashed lines. (Modified with permission from Li D, et al. Coronary arteries: magnetization-prepared, contrast-enhanced, three-dimensional volume-targeted breath-hold MR angiography. Radiology 2001; 219:270–277, 4).

artery the range is 66 to 200 msec (averaging 120 msec). These observations have two important consequences for coronary imaging:

1. Data acquisition is typically constrained to a window of less than 150–200 msec per heartbeat.
2. Because the acquisition window varies across individuals, surveying cardiac motion in each individual may be necessary for coronary acquisitions.

> **IMPORTANT CONCEPT:** To minimize artifacts related to cardiac motion, data acquisition should be confined to the brief stationary period of diastole, which varies across individuals but typically is 120–160 msec.

CHALLENGE QUESTION: How is it possible to determine the stationary period of diastole for a given subject in order to define the trigger delay and acquisition window accordingly?

Answer: A high-temporal-resolution cine acquisition can be performed through the coronary arteries to determine the diastolic window for acquisition.

Respiratory Motion

A major source of motion artifact is related to the motion of the diaphragm in breathing. Two strategies are used to minimize respiratory motion artifacts. One is to perform acquisitions during short breath-hold acquisitions. The other is to use the diaphragm as a reference for cardiac position and to adjust the imaging volume accordingly.

Breath Holding

Studies have shown that the diaphragm is not completely stationary even during breath holding. The drift of the diaphragm is greater when respiration is suspended at end inspiration, where motion varies during the breath hold and has been measured to be as much as 8 mm/sec (typical range 0.1–7.9 mm/sec) (2). At end expiration, when drifts are smaller and more consistent, the diaphragm moves 0.15 mm/sec on average.

> **IMPORTANT CONCEPT:** For breath-hold acquisitions, end-expiratory breath holding results in less diaphragmatic motion than end-inspiratory breath holding.

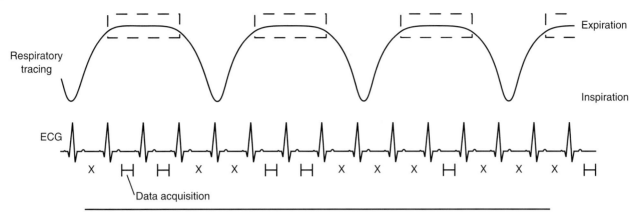

FIGURE III8-3. Combined respiratory and cardiac gating result in limited opportunities to collect data. X's mark heartbeats during which no data are collected.

Navigator Echoes

Navigator echo methods are used to monitor and/or correct for respiratory-related motion by tracking the movement of the diaphragm. Typically the right hemidiaphragm at the lung-liver interface is monitored while the subject breathes freely. Data are acquired only when the interface is positioned within a narrow positional window, usually defined at the end-expiratory phase of breathing.

Generating a Navigator Echo

The purpose of navigator echoes is to track the craniocaudal motion of the diaphragm over time without interfering with imaging of the coronary arteries. Navigators are typically implemented by imaging a thin column of tissue. The excitation is performed by a slice-selective 90° RF pulse and then a separate slice-selective 180° refocusing pulse, positioned to intersect the 90° slice over the dome of the right hemidiaphragm. The intersecting slices are usually positioned to avoid the heart (Figure III8-4).

The navigator echo is effectively a one-dimensional image of the diaphragm-lung interface. When images are acquired continuously, the resulting two-dimensional image (navigator versus time) depicts the motion of the diaphragm (Figure III8-5). This concept is akin to M-mode echocardiographic imaging.

Applications of the Navigator Echo

The navigator echo can be used in a variety of ways. In all applications, a user-defined *acceptance window* or *gating window* must be selected, centered on the interface to be tracked, typically the lung-diaphragm edge. The acceptance window is typically defined as ±1.5–2.5 mm, for a total window of 3–5 mm. The wider the window, the more time during each breath that data can be collected, but this benefit comes at the price of greater motion or misregistration artifacts. Coronary MR imaging with navigator

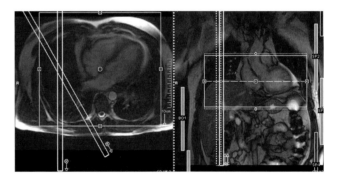

FIGURE III8-4. Navigator echo slab positioning. Two slices are positioned to intersect at the dome of the diaphragm and generate a thin column of signal. This signal is collected throughout the acquisition to track diaphragmatic motion.

approaches are both respiratory and electrocardiographically gated. Within the acceptance window, the data acquisition is further confined to the short periods of diastole during which the coronary arteries are relatively stationary (Figure III8-3).

Navigator efficiency refers to the percentage of heartbeats during which data are acquired. Efficiency depends on the width of the acceptance window and on the subject's breathing pattern. Efficiency should ideally be about 50%, but it often falls to about the 30% level, particularly with drifts in respiratory patterns and narrow acceptance windows.

CHALLENGE QUESTION: For the pattern depicted in Figure III8-3, what would the navigator efficiency be for the duration shown?

Answer: The total number of heartbeats in the interval shown is 15. Of these, data are sampled during 6 beats, for an efficiency of 6/15 or 40%.

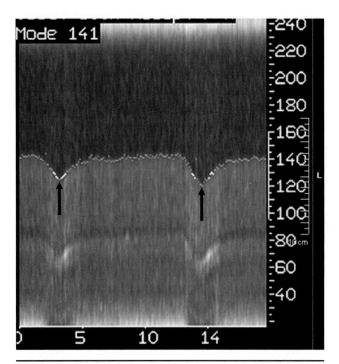

FIGURE III8-5. Tracing of the navigator echo. Columns reflect the lung (dark signal) and the diaphragm (high signal). The tracing is used to depict motion of the diaphragm over time, which is measured along the x axis. Periodic dips (arrow) correspond to inspiration (similar to Figure III8-3). The y axis labels represent distances measured in millimeters. In this case, the position of the diaphragm at end expiration is consistently at position 141 mm (Mode 141).

In its simplest implementation, the navigator echo can be used to gate the acquisition of data, either prospectively or retrospectively, in a manner very similar to electrocardiographic gating. In the prospective setting, data are acquired when the selected interface falls within the acceptance window. In the retrospective setting, data are acquired continuously (interleaved with the navigators), and the selection of data is based on the position of the diaphragm and the ECG.

In a more advanced implementation, the navigator echo is used to refine the position of the imaging volume. *Prospective adaptive motion correction* is based on the observation that there is a relatively constant relationship between diaphragmatic motion and coronary artery motion. For every millimeter of motion of the diaphragm, the right coronary artery moves about 0.6 mm and the left coronary artery moves about 0.7 mm (3). Therefore, if the diaphragm falls within the acceptance window, any motion within the window is corrected for by a slight adjustment in the imaging slice position. With motion correction, wider acceptance windows can be used. The motion correction can be used for prospective free-breathing acquisitions. Alternatively, if data are to be acquired in a series of breath holds, this method can be used to adjust imaging volumes

to compensate for differences in diaphragm position across breath holds.

> **IMPORTANT CONCEPT:** Prospective adaptive motion correction improves the image quality of navigator echo-based coronary imaging by compensating for slight changes in diaphragmatic position during the acquisition period.

Improving Image Contrast

The coronary arteries lie against the epicardial surface of the heart and are surrounded by epicardial fat. Most coronary artery imaging techniques rely on bright-blood approaches. Methods to increase signal from the blood and decrease signal from surrounding fat and myocardium were discussed in Chapters I-9 and II-2. Here, techniques that are useful specifically for improving contrast for coronary artery imaging are reviewed.

Fat Suppression

For bright-blood imaging approaches, suppression of the high signal intensity of fat surrounding the coronary arteries is desirable to improve delineation of the coronary arteries. Most coronary artery imaging sequences include frequency-selective fat suppression pulses. However, because of the lung-tissue interface, field homogeneity around the heart may be suboptimal and fat suppression inadequate. Selective shimming in the volume of interest may be necessary for effective fat suppression.

CHALLENGE QUESTION: Why does field inhomogeneity interfere with fat suppression?

Answer: Frequency-selective fat suppression is based on the premise that the fat protons are precessing approximately 220 Hz more slowly than water protons (at 1.5 T). If the field varies slightly, then water and fat protons no longer precess at the expected frequencies (see Chapters I-1 and I-9). Consequently fat may not be suppressed, and even worse, water may be inadvertently suppressed (Figure I9-9).

Myocardial Suppression

Suppression of myocardial signal also improves conspicuity of the coronary arteries. The most common strategies use *T2 preparation* or *magnetization* transfer.

T2 preparation prepulses are illustrated in Figure III8-6. The purpose of T2 preparation is to accentuate T2 contrast. In the case of coronary artery imaging, the goal is to increase the signal of blood relative to myocardium, based on large differences in their T2 values (250 msec versus

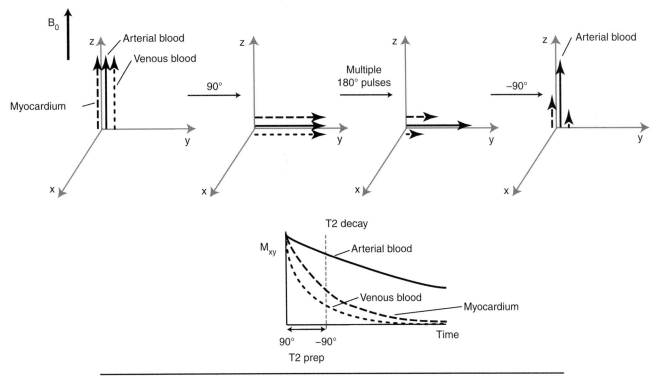

FIGURE III8-6. T2 preparation pulses increase contrast between arterial blood and both myocardium and venous blood.

50 msec, respectively). T2 preparation pulses also exploit the difference between arterial and venous blood T2 times— arterial blood has a T2 of 250 msec, whereas venous blood has a much lower T2 of approximately 35 msec. Consequently, with T2 preparation, the venous blood is also suppressed relative to arterial blood.

With T2 preparation pulses, a 90° pulse is applied first. All protons are tipped into the transverse plane. Left on their own, the differences in decay of the signal would reflect T2* relaxation. However, with a series of 180° refocusing pulses, the decay is based on T2 relaxation. Myocardial signal decays faster than signal from blood, and consequently, after a time period (T2 prep, Figure III8-6), the myocardial and venous blood signal are much lower than that from arterial blood. A −90° pulse that tips the magnetization vectors back into the longitudinal plane concludes the preparation. Following this preparation, arterial blood protons have significantly higher magnetization than venous or myocardial protons. T2 preparation pulses require about 30–50 msec.

An alternative approach to suppressing myocardial signal is the use of magnetization transfer pulses. The concept was illustrated in Chapter I-3. With magnetization transfer, suppression of the myocardium is achieved using off-resonance RF pulses, which cause saturation of protons in myocardium relative to blood.

Minimizing Ghosting Artifacts

In the setting of free-breathing acquisitions using navigator echo approaches, signal from the anterior chest wall can give rise to motion artifacts. Anterior saturation bands and fat suppression can minimize these effects. Prone imaging, although less comfortable for most, has also been advocated as a means of reducing anterior chest wall motion artifacts.

> **IMPORTANT CONCEPTS:** Bright-blood imaging benefits from fat suppression and myocardial suppression methods, such as T2 preparation pulses and magnetization transfer.

CORONARY ARTERY SEQUENCES: OVERVIEW

A staggering number of MR sequences have been used for coronary artery imaging. Bright-blood methods using spoiled gradient echo, echo planar imaging, and steady-state free precession gradient echo sequences have been advocated. Black-blood spin echo-based approaches also have their proponents. Furthermore, conventional gadolinium contrast agents, as well as newer intravascular agents, have been implemented. Both two-dimensional and three-dimensional sequences are available.

Among the broad choices, three of the more commonly used categories of MR pulse sequences are discussed here, beginning with the most standard sequence: two-dimensional segmented k-space gradient echo imaging. Then two different families of three-dimensional MR methods (segmented k-space and steady-state free precession) are considered. These sequences are performed with either breath holding or navigator echoes, with acquisitions limited to the motion-free portion of diastole. A variety of preparation pulses are used to improve image contrast. A template for these pulse sequences is given in Figure III8-7.

Two-Dimensional Segmented k-Space Gradient Echo Imaging

The most widely available coronary MR angiography sequence is a 2D segmented k-space gradient echo acquisition. Data acquisition is usually performed in a single breath hold of fewer than 12 heartbeats (Figure III8-8). Typically 8–16 lines of k-space (one segment) are collected per heartbeat, and a frequency-selective fat suppression pulse is applied. As a 2D approach, thick slices and breath-hold variability can limit the registration of images from slice to slice. However, for applications such as the assessment of anomalous coronary artery anatomy, this sequence may be of sufficient spatial resolution. Compared to the 3D sequences described in the following subsections, this method has the advantage of relative simplicity.

Three-Dimensional Segmented k-Space Methods: GRE, EPI, Spiral

To visualize stenoses in tortuous coronary arteries, 3D imaging methods are usually preferred over 2D methods. Although these sequences can be performed using breath-hold methods, with or without gadolinium-based contrast agents, the most common implementations use navigator echo methods and free breathing with prospective motion correction. These 3D methods are designed to achieve bright-blood images.

The standard format for these sequences is illustrated in Figure III8-7. Incorporated into the navigator-based sequences are fat suppression, either T2-preparation or magnetization transfer pulses for myocardial suppression, and a fast readout. Readout methods include segmented gradient echo techniques, segmented echo planar sequences, and interleaved spiral acquisitions.

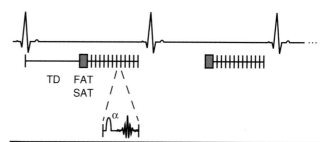

FIGURE III8-8. 2D Segmented k-space gradient echo imaging with 12 lines of k-space acquired per heart beat. For an imaging matrix of 144 × 256, the acquisition time is 12 heartbeats.

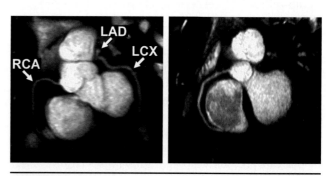

FIGURE III8-9. Contrast-enhanced 3D coronary MRA through the RCA plane in two subjects using an inversion recovery segmented spoiled gradient echo sequence. Sequence parameters are: TR/TE/flip angle 4.0/1.7/25°, 31–35 lines collected per heart beat. Slab thickness of 18 mm was imaged with 6 partitions, interpolated to 12 partitions, interpolated voxel size is 1.8 mm × 0.7 mm × 1.5 mm. (Modified with permission from Bi X and Li D, J Magn Reson Imaging 2005; 21:133–1395, 5.)

FIGURE III8-7. Generic coronary MRA pulse sequence. Data acquisition occurs during a period of less than 150–200 msec during diastole and consists of preparation pulses (such as fat saturation, T2 preparation, and magnetization transfer), motion correction with the navigator echo (NAV), and the 2D or 3D imaging pulse sequence and readout.

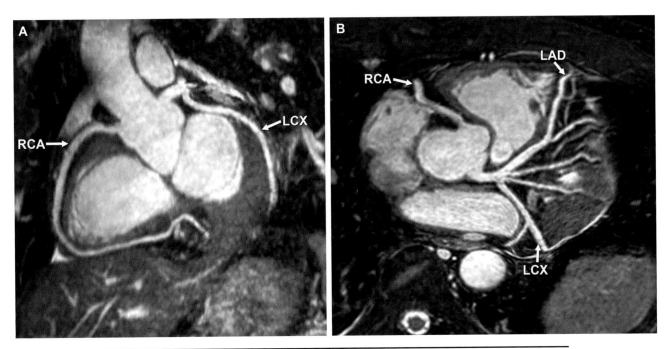

FIGURE III8-10. Reformatted 3D steady-state free precession whole-heart coronary MR angiography in a 42 year-old man with normal coronary arteries. Sequence parameters are 4.6/2.3/90°, navigator gated with fat saturation and T2 preparation. (**A**) Left anterior oblique whole-heart coronary MR angiogram reformatted with curved multiplanar reformatting clearly depicts the right coronary artery (RCA) and left circumflex (LCX) arteries. (**B**) Oblique axial whole-heart coronary MR angiogram reformatted with curved multiplanar reformatting shows the left main coronary artery, left anterior descending (LAD) artery, proximal RCA, and LCX arteries. (Reproduced with permission from Sakuma H et al. Assessment of coronary arteries with total study time of less than 30 minutes by using whole-heart coronary MR angiography. Radiology 2005; 237: 316–321, 6.)

To keep acquisition times short, the coronary arteries are imaged using several 2–3 cm thick slabs (Figure III8-9). When multiple slabs are stacked to visualize one coronary artery, 20–30% overlap in the adjacent slabs is introduced to reduce artifacts at the junctions.

Three-Dimensional Steady-State Free Precession Imaging

Steady-state free precession imaging, unlike contrast enhancement, relies on the intrinsic T2/T1 differences between blood and other tissues. Fast 3D acquisitions can be performed with linear or radial k-space filling. As discussed with cine gradient echo imaging of cardiac function, the independence from inflow for image contrast means that steady-state free precession sequences can benefit from use of ultrashort TR and TE possible with newer MR systems. Additionally, the higher image signal-to-noise ratios accommodate parallel imaging techniques.

Improvements in acquisition efficiency translate into the ability to perform whole-heart evaluation, including the major coronary arteries and branch vessels, in approximately 10 min (Figure III8-16). For best results, the

steady-state free precession approach includes magnetization preparation pulses such as a T2 preparation pulse and frequency selective fat suppression. 3D coronary MRA can be performed without intravenous contrast, taking advantage of the high signal of blood on true FISP sequences. Depending on the diastolic period of minimal motion, approximately 20–50 excitations can be performed per cardiac cycle with TR of 4–5 msec and TE 2 msec. Interpolation of acquisition matrices such as $256 \times 256 \times 80$ to $512 \times 512 \times 160$ results in reconstructed voxels <1 mm in all three dimensions. Acquisition times exceed a breath hold and therefore respiratory gating with motion correction are implemented with an acceptance window of ±2.5 mm or 5 mm.

REVIEW QUESTIONS

1. A middle-aged man underwent a coronary MRA for suspected anomalous coronary artery anatomy. The multiplanar reformatted image in Figure III8-Q1A of a 3D respiratory-triggered steady-state free precession sequence was obtained. Interpret the findings.

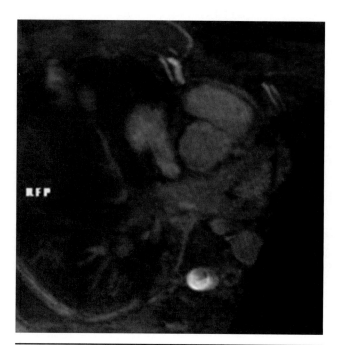

FIGURE III8-Q1A

2. An elderly subject is referred for evaluation the coronary arteries. A curved multiplanar reformat of a 3D whole-heart steady-state free precession acquire through the RCA is shown in Figure III8-Q2A. Interpret the findings.

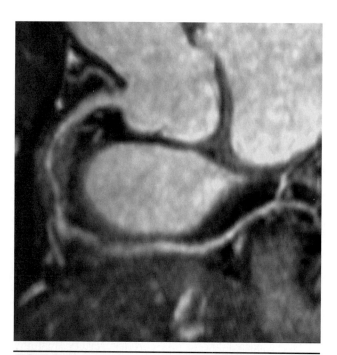

FIGURE III8-Q2A. (Reproduced with permission from Sakuma H et al. Radiology 2005.)

3. A curved multiplanar reformat of the LCx is shown in Figure III8-Q3A. Interpret the findings from this 3D steady state free precession image.

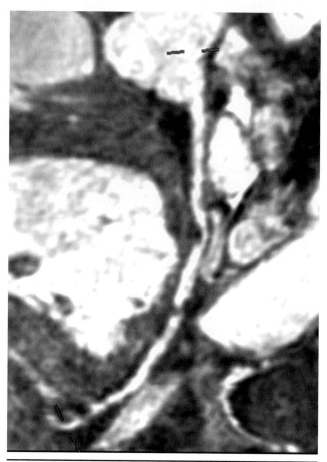

FIGURE III8-Q3A. (Courtesy of H. Sakuma, M.D.)

REFERENCES

1. Wang Y, Vidan E, Bergman GW. Cardiac motion of coronary arteries: variability in the rest period and implications for coronary MR angiography. Radiology 1999; 213:751–758.
2. Holland AE, Goldfarb JW, Edelman RR. Diaphragmatic and cardiac motion during suspended breathing: preliminary experience and implications for breath-hold MR imaging. Radiology 1998; 209: 483–489.
3. Wang Y, Watts R, Mitchell I, et al. Coronary MR angiography: selection of acquisition window of minimal cardiac motion with electrocardiography-triggered navigator cardiac motion prescanning—initial results. Radiology 2001; 218:580–585.
4. Li D, Carr JC, Shea SM, Zheng J, Deshpande VS, Wielopolski PA, Finn JP. Coronary arteries: magnetization-prepared, contrast-enhanced, three-dimensional volume-targeted breath-hold MR angiography. Radiology 2001; 219:270–277.
5. Bi X, Li D. Coronary arteries at 3.0 T: Contrast-enhanced magnetization-prepared three-dimensional breathhold MR angiography. J Magn Reson Imaging 2005; 21: 133–139.
6. Sakuma H, Ichikawa Y, Suzawa N, Hirano T, Makino K, Koyama N, Van Cauteren M, Takeda K. Assessment of coronary arteries with total study time of less than 30 minutes by using whole heart coronary MR angiography. Radiology 2005; 237:316–321.

▶ PROTOCOL: Ischemic Heart Disease: Anomalous Coronary Arteries

Setup and Preparation	Notes
i.v.	Optional/22 G or larger
Gadolinium contrast	Optional
ECG leads	Necessary
Coil	Torso phased-array
Positioning tips	Supine, head first
Subject instructions	End-expiratory breath holding Supplemental oxygen by nasal cannula suggested

Sequence	Imaging Plane	Parameters
1 Scout (true FISP or spoiled GRE)	Multiplanar	Default
2 T2-weighted fast spin echo imaging of the chest (double IR single-shot half-Fourier FSE, if available)	Axial	Single-shot or FSE with TR = one R-R interval 8–10 mm slices
3 Single-slice scouts	Oblique images	1 slice/breath hold to get short axis and long axis views
4 Perfusion GRE with adenosine or dipyridamole (optional)[1]	Short axes and long axes	6 slices every other heart beat, 8 mm slice, gadolinium contrast dose 0.05 mmol/kg (approx 10 mL)
5 Perfusion GRE at rest (optional)[2]	Same as Step 4	Gadolinium contrast dose 0.05 mmol/kg (approx 10 mL)
6 Cine GRE (spoiled gradient echo or steady-state gradient echo, segmented k-space)	Short axes	8 mm slices with 2 mm gaps Parameters (incl views per segment) defined for temporal resolution < 60 msec, and acquisition time within a breath hold LV base to apex, 8–12 slices
7 Cine GRE (spoiled gradient echo or steady-state gradient echo, segmented k-space)	Long axes	8 mm slices Same parameters as above Less rectangular FOV for VLA view[2]
8 Coronary MRA[2]	Whole-heart 3D approach slabs, or 2D slices	Sequence details depend on approach Whole-heart 3D True FISP: navigator (±2.5 mm with perspective motion correction), T2 preparation, fat suppression, number of segments depend on duration of diastole (determine by cine), voxel size < 1mm
9 Inversion time mapping (optional)[3]	Short axis (through infarct, if possible)	Single-slice. Parameters defined to achieve temporal resolution of <60 msec to determine inversion time for nulling of uninfarcted myocardium
10 Inversion recovery segmented k-space gradient echo imaging (optional)[3]	Short and long axes (match cine GRE)	Set inversion time according to Step 9

[1]Depending on the clinical indication, stress and rest perfusion imaging are optional parts of this protocol. If anomalous coronary arteries are suspected to cause myocardial ischemia, stress-rest perfusion imaging may be helpful for diagnosis. Perfusion sequence options are detailed in Chapter III-7 and include a notched saturation perfusion method or saturation recovery true FISP imaging.

[2]Coronary artery MRA sequence options are detailed in this chapter. 3D whole-heart true FISP imaging can be performed without intravenous contrast and require approximately 10 min acquisition time.

[3]Delayed inversion recovery imaging for myocardial viability is optional, depending on the clinical history.

▶ **PROTOCOL:** Ischemic Heart Disease: Comprehensive Examination of Coronary Artery Disease

Setup and Preparation	Notes
i.v.	22 G or larger
Gadolinium contrast	0.1–0.2 mmol/kg (20–40 mL)
ECG leads	Necessary
Coil	Torso phased-array
Positioning tips	Supine, head first
Subject instructions	End-expiratory breath holding Supplemental oxygen by nasal cannula suggested
MR-compatible infusion pump	For adenosine infusion
Monitoring/safety checklist	Blood pressure, pulse oximetry, ECG monitoring for heart rate and rhythm; intravenous aminophylline on hand. Close monitoring for symptoms; 12-lead ECG before and after examination

Sequence	Imaging Plane	Parameters
1 Scout (true FISP or spoiled GRE)	Multiplanar	Default
2 T2-weighted fast spin echo imaging of the chest (double IR single-shot half-Fourier FSE, if available)	Axial	Single-shot or FSE with TR = one R-R interval 8–10 mm slices
3 Single-slice scouts	Oblique images to get short axis	1 slice/breath hold and long axis views
4 Perfusion GRE with adenosine or dipyridamole[1]	Short axes and long axes	6 slices every other heartbeat, 8 mm slice, gadolinium contrast dose 0.05 mmol/kg (approx 10 mL)
5 Perfusion GRE at rest (optional)[2]	Same as Step 4	Gadolinium contrast dose 0.05 mmol/kg (approx 10 mL)
6 Cine GRE (spoiled gradient echo or steady-state gradient echo, segmented k-space)	Short axes Parameters (incl views per segment)	8 mm slices with 2 mm gaps defined for temporal resolution < 60 msec, and acquisition time within a breath hold LV base to apex, 8–12 slices
7 Cine GRE (spoiled gradient echo or steady-state gradient echo, segmented k-space)	Long axes	8 mm slices Same parameters as above Less rectangular FOV for VLA view
8 Inversion time mapping (optional)[2]	Short axis (through infarct, if possible)	Single-slice. Parameters defined to achieve temporal resolution of < 60 msec to determine inversion time for nulling of uninfarcted myocardium
9 Inversion recovery segmented k-space gradient echo imaging (optional)[2]	Short and long axes (match cine GRE)	Set inversion time according to step 8
10 3D whole-heart true FISP[3]	Axial	Navigator (±2.5 mm with prospective motion correction, T2 preparation, fat suppression, number of segments depend on duration of diastole (determined by cine), voxel size < 1 mm

[1]Perfusion sequence options are detailed in Chapter III-7 and include a notched saturation perfusion method or saturation recovery true FISP imaging.
[2]Resting perfusion may be optional if delayed contrast-enhanced imaging is performed to distinguish stress perfusion defects as ischemic vs. infarcted.
[3]Coronary artery MRA sequence options are detailed in this chapter. 3D whole-heart true FISP imaging can be performed without intravenous contrast and requires approximately 10 min acquisition time.

SECTION I: MR PHYSICS

CHAPTER I-1

1. $f = \gamma \times B$
   a. At 1 T, $f = 42.6$ MHz/T $\times$ 1 T $= 42.6$ MHz
   b. At 3 T, $f = 42.6$ MHz/T $\times$ 3 T $= 127.8$ MHz

2. The difference in precessional frequencies is proportional to the magnetic field.
   a. At 1 T, the difference in frequencies is two-thirds that at 1.5 T:

   $$220 \text{ Hz}/1.5 = 147 \text{ Hz}$$

   b. At 3 T, the difference in frequencies is double that at 1.5 T:

   $$220 \text{ Hz} \times 2 = 440 \text{ Hz}$$

   Note that at higher field strengths, there is a greater difference in Lamor frequencies gap between fat and water.

3. $f = 1.49999 \times 42.6$ to 1.50001×42.6 or 63.899575 to 63.900425 MHz. This represents a range of frequencies that differs by .00085 MHz or 0.85 kHz or 850 Hz.

4. For a gradient of 25 mT/m across a 0.5 m field of view, the range of magnetic field strengths will be 25 mT/m $\times$ 0.5 m $= 12.5$ mT (for example, 1.49375 T to 1.50625 T).

   The corresponding Larmor frequencies will be

   $$1.49375 \text{ T} \times 42.6 \text{ MHz/T} = 63.63375 \text{ MHz}$$
   $$1.50625 \times 42.6 \text{ MHz/T} = 64.16625 \text{ MHz}$$

   This represents a range of frequencies that differs by 0.5325 MHz or 532.5 kHz.

5. The signal in in Figure I1-18 represents a sinc function, which is a composite of multiple sinusoidal functions with a range of frequencies. To determine the frequency components that form the sinc function, a 1D Fourier transform should be performed.

6. The distortions at the ends of the image are due to nonlinearity of the gradients. Typically, the range of the field of view across which gradients are nearly linear is at the upper limits of the maximum imaging field. Most systems have correction schemes to minimize these artifacts (Figure I1-Q6B).

7. The corduroy artifact is similar to a superimposed pattern of ripples over the image (Figure I1-29F). This artifact can be attributable to a spike in k-space (upper

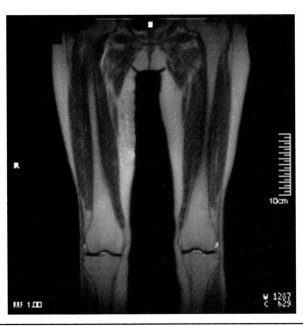

FIGURE I1-Q6B. Large-field-of-view correction eliminates distortion caused by nonlinearity of gradients at the edges of the field.

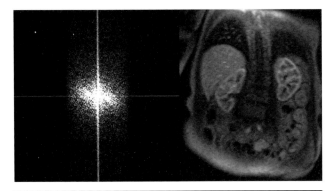

FIGURE I1-Q7B, C. k-space and corrected image (courtesy of N. Oesingmann, Ph.D.).

left quadrant) (Figure I1-Q7B). The image generated without the k-space spike is shown in Figure I1-Q7C.

8. The myocardial SNR is defined by the mean signal of the myocardium (ROI 1) divided by the SD of the signal outside the body (but within the coil), which is ROI 3:

   $$\text{Myocardial SNR} = 85/5 = 17.$$

   The myocardial-to-blood pool CNR is the difference in signal intensities divided by noise:

   $$\text{Myocardial-to-blood pool CNR} = (195 - 85)/5 = 22.$$

   ROI 4 is located outside the image and should not be used.

CHAPTER I-2

1.

   a. The Larmor equation is $f = \gamma B$.

   b. The gyromagnetic ratio is $\gamma = 42.6$ MHz/T.

   c. At 1.5 T, the Larmor frequency is

$$f = \gamma B = 42.6 \text{ MHz/T} \times 1.5 \text{ T} = 63.9 \text{ MHz}$$
$$\text{(approximately 64 MHz)}$$

   d. For a Larmor frequency $\gamma = 128$ MHz, the field strength is

$$B = f/\gamma = 128 \text{ MHz}/42.6 \text{ MHz/T} = 3 \text{ T}$$

2.

   a. To achieve half the flip angle, the B_1 should be on for half of the duration, or 0.3 msec.

   b. To achieve the same flip angle in a third of the time, B_1 would need to be three times as strong, or 30 μT.

   c. At 3 T, the Larmor frequency is 128 MHz, and therefore B_1 would have to rotate around the z axis at 128 MHz instead of 64 MHz in order to resonate with the protons. The frequnecy of the RF excitation pulse would have to change.

   d. The effect of B_1 on flip angle depends only on B_1 and not on B_0. Therefore it would take the same time as at 1.5 T: 0.6 msec.

3. By definition, $M_{xy} = M \sin 30°$ and $M_z = M \cos 30°$. Therefore, the amount of signal following a 30° RF pulse would be $M_{xy} = 0.5$ M, while the residual longitudinal magnetization, $M_z = 0.87$ M.

4.

Tissues	Curve Label
Myocardium: T1 = 800 msec and T2 = 40 msec	C
Blood: T1 = 1200 msec and T2 = 250 msec	A
Fat: T1 = 250 msec and T2 = 90 msec	B

5. Because fat (Curve B) has the shortest T1, it shows the fastest recovery of longitudinal magnetization. Longitudinal magnetization reflects potential signal that translates into measured signal following the next RF pulse. For this reason, fat is often brighter than other tissues on MR images, especially when the RF pulses are applied in relatively close succession.

CHAPTER I-3

1. Free Gd^{3+} is toxic because it binds sites with an affinity for calcium ion (Ca^{2+}).

2. The additivity of relaxivity expresses the T1 value of contrast-enhanced blood in terms of the T1 of blood and T1 of gadolinium chelate. Plugging in the known quantities,

$$\frac{1}{T1_{blood+Gd}} = \frac{1}{T1_{blood}} + \frac{1}{T1_{Gd}} = \frac{1}{T1_{blood}} + (r1 \times C)$$

$$\frac{1}{50 \text{ msec}} = \frac{1}{1200 \text{ msec}} + (4 \times C)$$

$$C = \frac{1}{4}\left(\frac{1}{50} - \frac{1}{1200}\right) = 4.8 \text{ mmol/L}$$

which is less than 1/100 of the originally injected dose of 0.5 mol/L in the vein.

3.

   a. As discussed in the chapter and illustrated in Figure I3-6, a sample of gadopentetate dimeglumine straight from a commercial preparation will have a T1 of 0.5 msec and a T2 of 0.4 msec. The extremely short T2 time means that most signal will have decayed before it can be sampled. For example, if a pulse sequence is designed to measure the signal at 2 msec after the RF pulse (echo time or TE = 2 msec), this will correspond to five T2 time constants. Based on the Background Reading on exponential decay (see Chapter I-2), less than 1% of the original magnetization will be available for measurement.

     The solution to this problem is to dilute the gadolinium contrast material.

   b. If 5 mL of gadopentetate dimeglumine is injected into a 250 mL bag of normal saline, the T1 and T2 values can be calculated knowing that the relaxation time is inversely proportional to the concentration. Expanding on the discussion in part (a), at a 50 : 1 dilution, reducing the concentration by a factor of 50 will increase T1 and T2 values by a corresponding factor of 50. T1 will still be short, at 25 msec, while T2 will have a value of 20 msec. Now there is ample time to sample signal before T2 decay. At an echo time of 2 msec, there will be minimal signal loss from T2 effects.

4. A single dose of gadolinium contrast material having a concentration of 0.5 mol/L is 0.2 mL/kg. For a 10 kg child, the total volume would be 2 mL for a single dose and 4 mL for a double dose. When gadolinium contrast material is required for cardiovascular studies in young children, the contrast doses are frequently diluted 100% with normal saline in order to increase the volume of the injected dose to a more manageable amount.

CHAPTER I-4

1.

	TR	TE or TE_{eff}	ETL	Weighting? (T1, PD, T2)
a.	500	20	1	T1
b.	1200	40	1	PD
c.	1500	80	1	T2
d.	1500	80 (effective)	32	T2
e.	1500	120	1	T2

Most ___e___ ___c___ ___d___ ___b___
___a___ Least

The degree of T2-weighting depends on the TE of the sequence. The fast spin echo sequence with ETL 32 with an effective TE of 80 msec has less T2-weighting than the conventional spin echo sequence with the same TE.

2.

	TR	TE	Flip Angle	Spoiling?	Weighting?
a.	200	2	80	Yes	**T1**
b.	200	4	80	Yes	**T1**
c.	25	10	25	Yes	**T2***
d.	25	4	15	Yes	**PD**
e.	4	1.5	60	No*	**T2/T1**

*Balanced gradients

Sequences with long TR, short TE, and high flip angles (a, b) tend to be T1 weighted. Short TR, long TE sequence are usually T2* weighted (c). To obtain a proton density-weighted sequence, TR should be short to minimize T1 weighting and TE short to minimize T2 weighting (d). A steady-state gradient echo sequence requires that the TR be very short so that transverse magnetization is preserved. The flip angle is usually alternating (in this case, $+60°$, $-60°$, $+60°$, etc). With steady state gradient echo sequences such as in (e), the image contrast is T2/T1.

3.

a. The acquisition time is $TR \times N_{PE} = 700$ msec $\times 100 = 70$ sec for a single acquisition. Since this is longer than the time of a single breath hold, multiple signal averages (3 to 4) would be used, thereby increasing the acquisition time proportionately.

b. The number of slices that can be acquired is 700 msec/35 msec = 20 slices.

c. With the fast spin echo version, the echoes obtained at TE = 30 msec should be used to fill the central lines of k-space to achieve image contrast most comparable to a conventional spin echo sequence with TE = 30 msec. The echoes at TE = 60 msec should be placed furthest away from the center. Despite this action, because the TEs are varying considerably, the image contrast and object sharpness will be less than that of the conventional spin echo sequence. The acquisition time, however, will be reduced by a factor of the echo train length (ETL = 5): 70/5 = 14 sec. The number of slices that can be imaged will be 700/70 = 10 slices.

4.

a. T1-weighted imaging: (1), (2), (4)

b. T2-weighted imaging: (1), (2), (3), (5)

(1) Conventional spin echo

(2) Fast spin echo

c. T2*-weighted imaging: (4)

(3) Half-Fourier single-shot fast spin echo

(4) Spoiled gradient echo

(5) True FISP steady-state gradient echo

All of the sequences except for half-Fourier single-shot fast spin echo and steady-state gradient echo sequences are used for T1-weighted imaging. The spoiled gradient sequences are typically T2* weighted. Although the steady-state gradient echo sequence is T2/T1 weighted, most tissues with long T2 relaxation times also have higher T2/T1 compared with other tissues. Therefore, it is reasonable to consider it a sequence that provides T2-like contrast.

5. With spin echo imaging, there is no residual transverse magnetization at the time of each subsequent RF pulse. This is because the TR times are generally long, much longer than T2 times of most tissues. For example for a TR of 500 msec, all transverse magnetization from tissues with T2 times on the order of 20–100 msec has decayed. Consequently, spin echo imaging is always spoiled.

CHAPTER I-5

1.

a. For a 2-period RF pulse, a suitable slice:interslice gap ratio is 5 : 1. For a 5 mm slice, the smallest reasonable interslice gap would be about 1 mm.

b. See Figure I5-Q1B. With twice the slice gradient strength, the slice thickness can be halved, 2.5 mm, using the same transmitter bandwidth. Since the transmitter bandwidth is the same, the appearance of the RF pulse will be the same. Assuming again that 2 periods are used for the RF pulse, the slice:interslice gap ratio should remain 5 : 1. For a 2.5 mm slice, the interslice gap should then be 0.5 mm.

c. With twice the slice thickness and at the stronger gradient strength, the transmitter bandwidth will be doubled. An RF pulse of 1 msec will correspond to an RF pulse with 4 periods. Hence, the slice profile will be improved, and a smaller interslice gap will be needed.

d. One solution is to acquire two separate sets of images with interleaved slice positions. For example, with 5 mm slices, the first acquisition could consist of a set of 5 mm slices with 1 mm gaps. Then, by repeating the acquisition and shifting all slices by 3 mm, all areas that were in the gap on the first acquisition will be imaged (Figure I5-Q1D).

2.

a. If the gradient strength is 10 mT/m, then the field changes 10 mT over a distance of 100 cm, or 5 mT

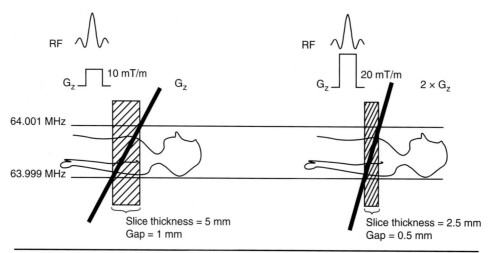

FIGURE I5-Q1B

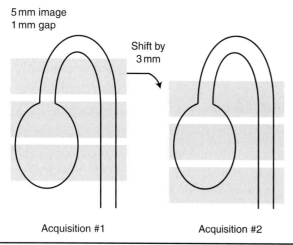

FIGURE I5-Q1D. Separate acquisitions of overlapping slices reduces the problem of missed pathology caused by interslice gaps and poor slice profiles.

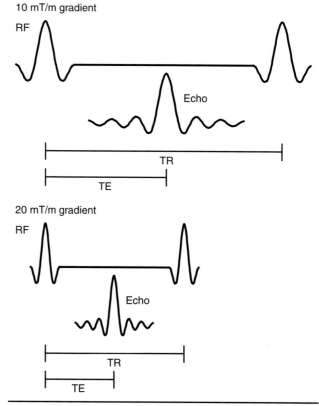

FIGURE I5-Q2

over 50 cm. To convert the range of magnetic field strengths, $\Delta B = 5$ mT, to the range of precessional frequencies, Δf, the Larmor equation is needed.

$$\Delta f = \gamma \times \Delta B$$

That is, the range of frequencies $\Delta f = 42.6$ MHz/T $\times$ 5 mT = 213 kHz.
  b. If the gradient strength is doubled, then the receiver bandwidth will also double, $\Delta f = 426$ kHz.
  c. With double the receiver bandwidth, the sampling frequency will be doubled. This means that the total time to sample the echo, say 256 times, will only be half as long as the original case. Additionally, with the increased gradient strength, the transmitter bandwidth will also be doubled. This can be used to decrease the duration of the RF pulse by one-half. As a result, the TR and TE will

both be reduced considerably. Note that the resulting image quality will not be the same. At higher receiver bandwidths, the decreased sampling time comes at the cost of a decreased signal-to-noise ratio. Therefore, it is usually prudent not to push receiver bandwidths to the maximum possible value (Figure I5-Q2).

3. See Figure I5-Q3B.

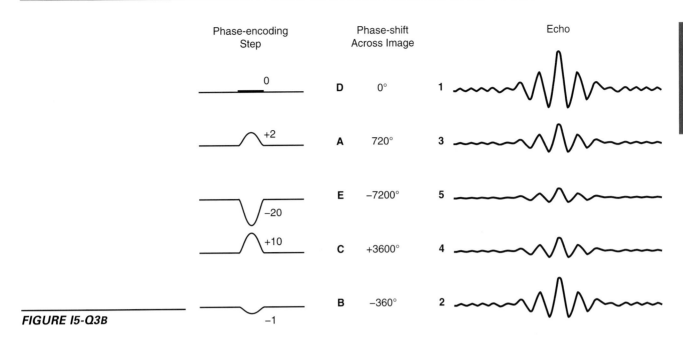

FIGURE I5-Q3B

CHAPTER I-6

1.

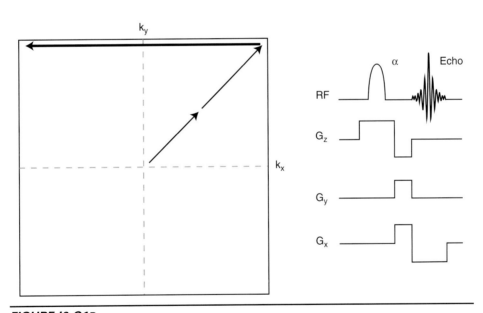

FIGURE I6-Q1B

2.

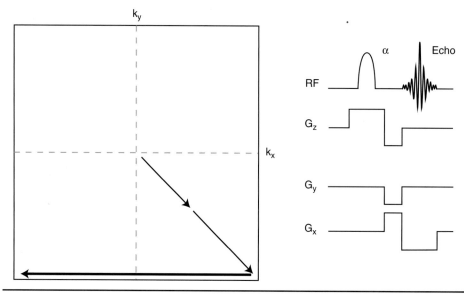

FIGURE I6-Q2B

3.

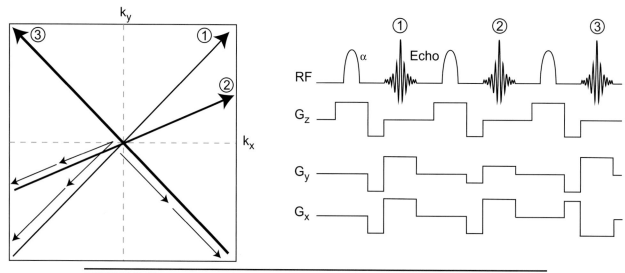

FIGURE I6-Q3B

4.

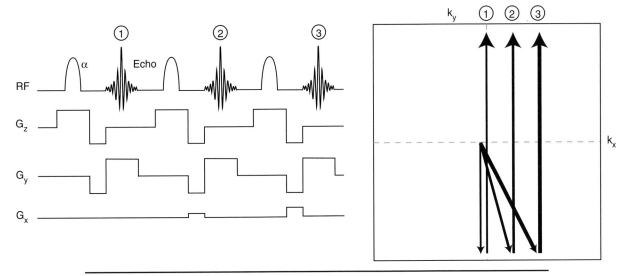

FIGURE I6-Q4B

5. 128×128 matrix

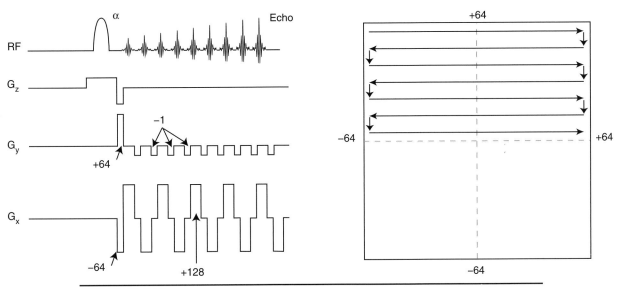

FIGURE I6-Q5B

6.

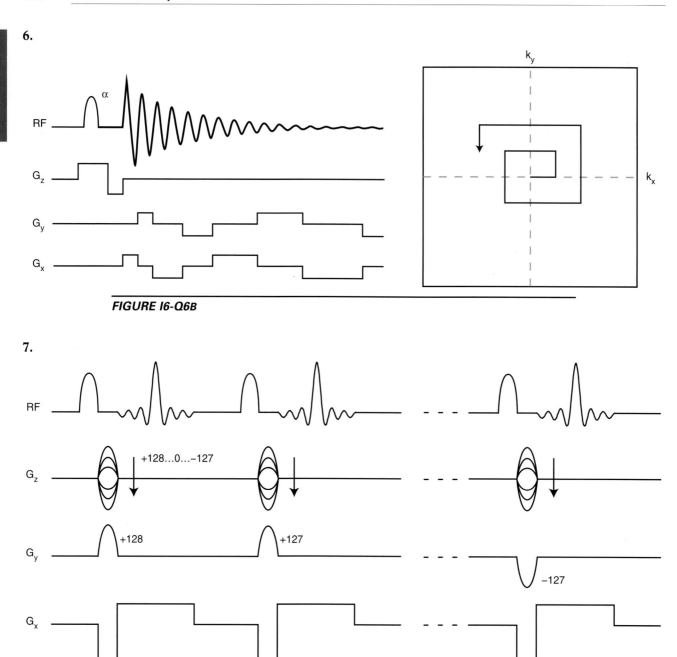

FIGURE I6-Q6B

7.

FIGURE I6-Q7B

CHAPTER I-7

1.

    a. outer 99% Fourier space: (4)

    b. full 100% Fourier space: (1)

    c. center 1% Fourier space: (2)

    d. outer 85% Fourier space: (3)

2.

    a. The central portions of Fourier space describe the overall shade of gray or white in the image, also known as the image contrast.

    b. The abdominal aorta is a larger structure, and therefore the data points that describe it are in the low-spatial-frequency portion—nearer the center of Fourier space.

    c. The lumbar arteries are small, fine structures, and therefore the data points that describe it in Fourier space are further out toward the edges.

3.

    a. 2 mm × 2 mm. The spatial resolution is the FOV divided by the matrix size. 500 mm/256 is approximately 2 mm.

    b. If the FOV is reduced to 300 mm, then the subject's arms may cause wraparound artifact. Frequency oversampling is necessary to avoid this problem, provided the frequency-encoding direction is left-to-right, and phase-encoding is arterior-posterior. The acquisition time will be the same. The spatial resolution will now be 300 mm/256 or 1.2 mm × 1.2 mm.

    c. This subject's body habitus is well suited to using rectangular FOV. With the 225 mm anterior-to-posterior dimension, a 75% rectangular FOV (225/ 300) can be applied, so that the matrix is now 256 × 192. Spatial resolution will not be affected, because the FOV and matrix decrease proportionally (225 mm/192 = 1.2 mm, Figure I7-Q3B). The acquisition time will be reduced to 0.75 × 20 sec, or 15 sec.

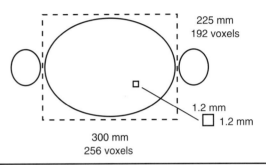

225 mm
192 voxels

1.2 mm
1.2 mm

300 mm
256 voxels

FIGURE I7-Q3B

4.

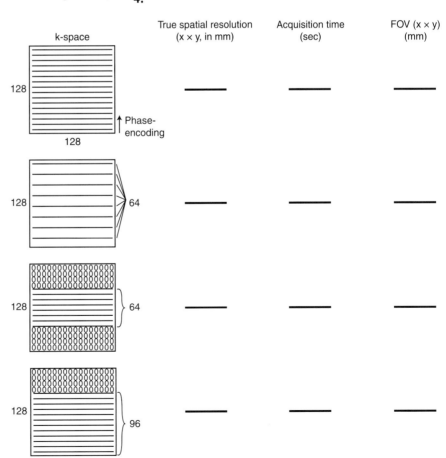

FIGURE I7-Q4

CHAPTER I-8

1.

a. See Table I8-2B. The acquisition time is $TR \times N_{PE1} \times N_{PE2}$ or, in this case. $TR \times 128 \times 32$. Recall that SNR is proportional to the square root of time taken to sample the echo. If time is reduced by a factor of 2, then the SNR will be reduced by $1/\sqrt{2}$ or approximately a factor of 0.7.

b. The reduction in acquisition time when receiver bandwidth is increased from 250 Hz/voxel to 500 Hz/voxel is significant when considering imaging in the torso because most patients can tolerate a breath hold of 16 sec, whereas fewer can tolerate 25 sec. The SNR is reduced by 30% in this transition.

c. The shift to the even higher bandwidth of 1000 Hz/voxel (256 kHz) results in a less significant reduction in acquisition time, from 16 sec to 12 sec, although again the SNR is reduced by 30%. In the clinical setting, the reduction in acquisition time may not be worth the loss in SNR.

2.

a. The number of slices that can be imaged in the same acquisition time as a single slice depends on the number of times the echo train fits into the TR. The echo train duration is measured as the time from the beginning of the RF pulse to the end of the eighth echo. If that interval is 100 msec and the TR is 500 msec, then at most five slices can be imaged.

b. The acquisition time is reduced by a factor equal to the echo train length. The echo train length is 8, and so the acquisition time is 128 sec/8 = 16 sec.

c. The advantage of this short acquisition time is that each acquisition of 5 slices can be performed in a single breathhold. For 20 slices, 4 breathhold acquisitions are needed. In contrast, the spin echo

sequence with an acquisition time of 128 sec is too long for a breathhold, and consequently multiple signal averages are needed to reduce respiratory motion. Allowing for 3–4 averages ($N_{acq} = 3$–4), total acquisition times will be at least about 6–8 min. This is longer than the time needed for four breath holds, and images are likely to suffer from respiratory motion artifacts. The disadvantage of the fast spin echo acquisition is reduced image contrast, because the echo times will span from TE = 20 msec to 90 msec. Image contrast will depend on which echoes are used to fill the central lines of k-space, but inevitably it will not be as good as with conventional spin echo imaging.

3. See Table I8-3B. The spatial resolution in each dimension is FOV/N. Because rectangular FOV is used for the sagittal approach, the time saved from the reduction in N_y can be used to increase N_z, and consequently, spatial resolution is improved with the same (or slightly lower) acquisition time. The actual voxel size will be $0.8 \times 2.5 \times 2$ mm and $0.8 \times 2.5 \times 1$ mm for the coronal and sagittal acquisitions, respectively.

Of the two choices, the sagittal approach is desirable, provided the FOV values are acceptable. Other factors could also play into the decision. For example, if the study requires that the subclavian arteries be assessed, then coronal view would have to be selected.

4. The maximum reduction in phase-encoding steps using parallel imaging techniques depends on the number of independent coil elements in the phase-encoding direction. With the array as shown in Figure I8-Q5, the maximum number is three in the left-to-right direction. Therefore the acquisition with parallel imaging should be performed with phase encoding in the left-to-right direction.

Considering all fast imaging strategies, it may not pay to focus on the optimal R factor with parallel imaging.

▶ TABLE I8-2B

Receiver Bandwidth		Echo sampling duration (msec)	TR (msec)	TE (msec)	Acquisition Time	Relative SNR
125 Hz/voxel	32 kHz	8	10	4	**41 sec**	1
250 Hz/voxel	64 kHz	4	6	2	**25 sec**	0.7
500 Hz/voxel	128 kHz	2	4	1.5	**16 sec**	0.5
1000 Hz/voxel	256 kHz	1	3	1	**12 sec**	0.35

▶ TABLE I8-3B

	FOV_x	FOV_y	FOV_z	N_x	N_y	N_z	x (mm)	y (mm)	z (mm)	Time
Coronal	400	400	128	512	160	32(64)	0.8	2.5	4	20.5 sec
Sagittal	400	400(250)	96	512	160(100)	48(96)	0.8	2.5	2	19.2 sec

Other considerations are important. For example, in 2D imaging of the torso, if phase-encoding is oriented in the left-to-right direction, then rectangular FOV cannot be used, whereas phase encoding in the anterior-to-posterior direction, although resulting in a lower maximum R factor, permits recFOV as well.

For 3D imaging, there are two phase-encoding directions. Parallel imaging techniques can theoretically be applied in one or both of the phase-encoding directions. For the array shown in the figure, the reduction in the left-to-right direction can be a factor of 3. The reduction in either of the other two directions could be 2 (two coil elements in each of those directions). Therefore the maximum reduction in acquisition time with a 3D sequence would be R = 3 × 2 or a factor of 6.

CHAPTER I-9

1.

   a. Inversion recovery fast spin echo imaging using a short inversion time to null fat would be an excellent way to image the vessel wall in the presence of field inhomogeneities. Frequency-selective fat suppression pulses are very sensitive to field inhomogeneity, which is challenging enough in the neck even without metallic hardware. To ensure that signal from blood is also nulled, an inversion recovery sequence can be combined with double inversion recovery prepulses to form a triple inversion recovery sequence, as will be discussed in Chapter III-5 (and illustrated in Figure I9-14B).

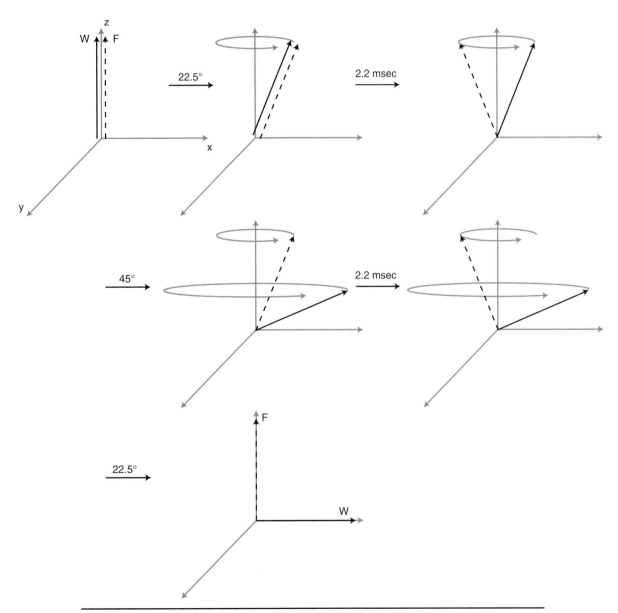

FIGURE I9-Q3B

b. Frequency-selective fat saturation should be implemented with the T1-weighted sequence to test whether the lesion contains fat. Inversion recovery is not a specific method—any tissue with short T1 values will be suppressed on a short-inversion time recovery sequence, and therefore both fat and hemorrhagic material would be suppressed on STIR.

c. A spatially selective saturation band should be applied over the anterior chest wall to reduce this artifact.

2. For the axial slice, frequency-encoding will be left to right while phase-encoding will be anterior to posterior. Because frequency oversampling does not increase the image acquisition time, it is preferable over saturation bands as a method to avoid wraparound artifact from left-to-right. Avoiding wraparound from the anterior and posterior chest wall is more challenging. Saturation bands require less time, but they are also less effective because they are usually not sharply defined. Phase oversampling will definitely decrease aliasing artifact, but at the expense of increased acquisition times, proportional to the degree of phase-oversampling (Chapter I-7). As a compromise, both can be implemented; saturation bands can be used in conjunction with a more limited degree of phase-oversampling.

3. Magnetization vectors for fat and water are illustrated in Figure I9-Q3B for the series of RF pulses:

$22.5° \rightarrow 2.2$ msec $\rightarrow 45° \rightarrow 2.2$ msec $\rightarrow 22.5°$.

4. This sequence produces a fat-suppressed spin echo image (Figure I9-Q4B). The effect of the 45° RF pulse and then the −45° pulse is to cause the fat proton magnetization to be tipped 90°, leaving the water magnetization in the longitudinal direction. With the crusher gradient, the fat magnetization is dephased. This sequence illustrates an alternative technique for fat saturation using binomial RF pulses.

5.

a. The infarct appears nulled, while the uninfarcted myocardium is not. The inversion time used in this sequence is too short. To null the viable myocardium, a longer TI should be used and should give this result as shown in Figure I9-Q5C.

b. Half-Fourier acquisition turbo spin echo (HASTE) imaging of the aorta for assessment of vessel wall pathology: The images show heterogeneous signal in the lumen of the aorta, limiting assessment of wall pathology. The sequence used is a typical HASTE sequence used for biliary imaging. To correct this problem, the double inversion recovery HASTE sequence should be used.

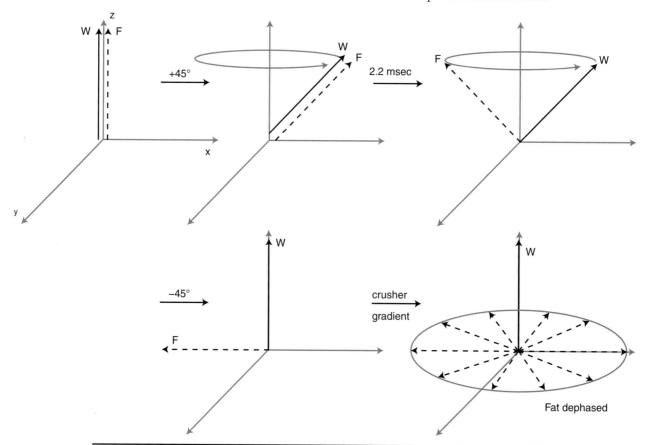

FIGURE I9-Q4B

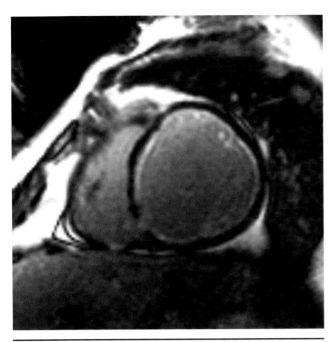

FIGURE I9-Q5C

SECTION II: VASCULAR MR IMAGING

TABLE II1-4B

Proposed Changes	Check Which Apply
a. Electrocardiographic gating to systole	√
b. Electrocardiographic gating to diastole	
c. Change TE to 5 msec	
d. Change TE to 20 msec	√
e. Change slice thickness to 8 mm	√
f. Change slice thickness to 15 mm	
g. Add flow compensation gradients to frequency-encoding gradients	
h. Add double inversion recovery prepulses	√

TABLE II1-5B

Proposed Changes	Check Which Apply
a. Change the slice orientation to axial	√
b. Change the slice orientation to coronal	
c. Electrocardiographic gating to systole	√
d. Electrocardiographic gating to diastole	
e. Change TR to 20 msec	
f. Change TR to 30 msec	√
g. Change TE to 5 msec	√
h. Change TE to 12 msec	
i. Change flip angle to 5°	
j. Change flip angle to 25°	√
k. Add flow compensation gradients to frequency-encoding gradients	√
l. Add double inversion recovery prepulses	

CHAPTER II-1

1. a, d, e, h. (See Table II1-4B.)
For optimal black-blood imaging, the goal is to allow all the protons to flow out of the imaging slice between the RF pulses. To achieve this, gating to systole will synchronize imaging with periods of faster flow. A thinner imaging slice and longer TE also facilitate the flow voids. Flow compensation reduces flow-related dephasing and is not desired. However, double inversion recovery prepulses can be helpful for nulling blood signal.

2. a, c, f, g, j, k. (See Table II1-5B.)
For optimal bright-blood imaging, the goal is to maximize inflow of fresh, unsaturated protons into the imaging slice. This is best achieved by orienting the slice perpendicular to the direction of flow—in this case, an axial slice would be preferable. Additionally, imaging during systole using a longer TR would increase the inflow. A shorter TE would minimize dephasing, as would flow compensation gradients. A higher flip angle suppresses background tissue—in this case the intimal flap—to provide better image contrast between it and the surrounding blood.

3. The signal loss emanating from the aortic valve and extending into the ascending aorta during systole results from dephasing caused by turbulent flow. The turbulence is caused by a stenotic aortic valve. First-order gradient moment nulling or flow compensation will not eliminate this appearance, because the effects are primarily due to higher-order flows. Shortening the TE will reduce the flow-related dephasing and, hence, the extent of the signal void. Unlike the signal voids associated with vascular stenoses, dephasing in this setting is desirable, because it facilitates the diagnosis of valvular stenosis or insufficiency.

4. To minimize ghosting artifacts, signal from flowing blood could be saturated using spatial presaturation pulses. If the saturation band is applied above the imaging slice shown in Figure II1-9, the signal from the flowing aortic blood would be nulled and ghosting minimized (Figure II1-Q4). This approach would be faster than altering the phase-encoding direction or using electrocardiographic gating.

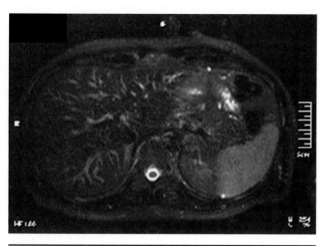

FIGURE II1Q-4

CHAPTER II-2

1.

a Both common carotid arteries and the left vertebral artery are seen as areas of high signal intensity. The right vertebral artery is not visualized. The differential diagnosis includes an absent or atretic right vertebral artery, an occluded right vertebral artery, or flow reversal in the right vertebral artery.

b. Given the clinical history, right subclavian or brachiocephalic steal is suspected. With right subclavian steal, the flow in the right vertebral artery is reversed and is used to supply the right arm, particularly during exertion. To confirm flow reversal, a 2D TOF acquisition could be performed with an inferior saturation band, as shown in Figure II2-Q1B. In the figure, signal can be seen in the jugular veins as well as in the right vertebral artery (circled), indicating retrograde flow.

Alternatively, a contrast-enhanced MR angiogram could be performed (Figure II2-Q1C). The brachiocephalic stenosis explains the subject's right subclavian steal.

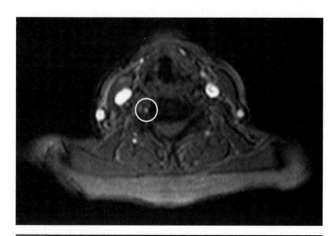

FIGURE II2-Q1B

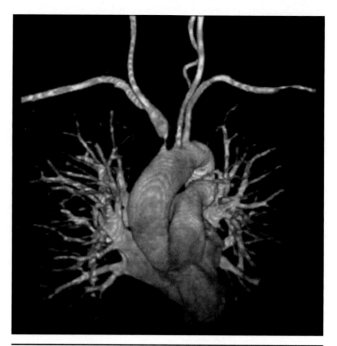

FIGURE II2-Q1C

2.

a. The apparent stenosis of the proximal anterior tibial artery is commonly seen on 2D TOF imaging. The anterior tibial artery has a horizontal course at its origin, which results in in-plane flow on the axial slices. The protons of the moving blood become partially saturated (similar to the stationary tissue), and the resulting signal loss mimics a stenosis. This can be problematic in patients who may also have a stenosis in this region, because the artifact cannot be distinguished from a stenosis.

b. To confirm that the apparent stenosis is an artifact, the TOF sequence can be modified to enhance flow sensitivity. Use of thinner slices, oriented perpendicular to the direction of flow, will improve the visibility of the proximal anterior tibial artery. Alternatively, contrast-enhanced MR angiography can be performed (Figure II2-Q2B).

3. See Table II2-2B. A traveling saturation band superior to the imaging slice will suppress signal from venous structures. More accurate estimations of stenoses are

TABLE II2-2B

Parameter Changes	Check Which Apply
a. Saturation bands superior to the imaging slice	√
b. Decreased voxel size	√
c. Increased TR	
d. Decreased TR	√
e. Increased flip angle	
f. Flow compensation (gradient moment nulling)	√

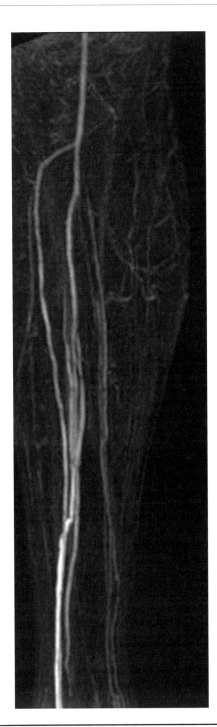

FIGURE II2-Q2B. Gadolinium-enhanced MRA shows patent right anterior tibial artery.

achieved by minimizing flow-related dephasing. This can be achieved with smaller voxel sizes (higher spatial resolution), reduced TE, and flow compensation. Although use of higher flip angles will increase the signal from moving blood, it will cause saturation of more slowly flowing blood. Increased flip angles will also not improve flow-related dephasing associated with turbulent flow at stenoses. Increasing the TR will increase

sensitivity to slow flow, but this is unlikely to improve the depiction of stenotic vessels.

4. The high-signal-intensity material seen adjacent to the proximal internal carotid artery on TOF images, but not seen on the contrast-enhanced images, most likely represents hemorrhagic material in the atherosclerotic plaque. The TOF images are relatively T1-weighted, and consequently tissues that have short T1, such as blood products, may appear bright on these images. These sources of signal can be difficult to differentiate from flow-related enhancement, which is a limitation of TOF imaging.

5. The appearance of venous signal at the caudal portion of the acquisition suggests that the saturation band that is applied to the TOF acquisition is not as effective for the caudal slices. Because the saturation band is too far from the imaging slice, the venous protons have time to recover magnetization and generate signal. To solve this problem, a traveling saturation band should be positioned just cephalad to the imaging slice.

CHAPTER II-3

1. Phase contrast imaging can be used in two ways to assess the severity of an apparent stenosis (1) phase contrast MR angiography and (2) phase contrast flow quantification.

   With phase contrast angiography, a 3D phase contrast acquisition is performed through the proximal renal artery. Because phase contrast is sensitive to turbulent flow, a significant stenosis usually causes marked signal loss on a phase contrast angiographic sequence (Figure II3-7).

   An alternative approach is to position a through-plane 2D phase contrast flow quantification acquisition perpendicular to the left renal artery, just distal to the level of stenosis (see Figure II3-Q1B). If the measured peak systolic velocity exceeds about

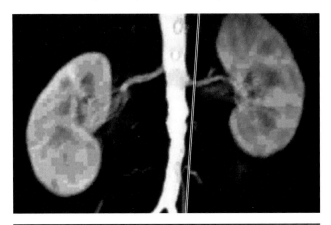

FIGURE II3-Q1B. Slice positioning for 2D through-plane phase contrast flow quantification.

100–150 cm/sec (extrapolating from Doppler ultrasound criteria for main renal artery velocities), then the stenosis is assumed to be flow-disturbing and likely physiologically significant.

2. The peak velocity measurements will be underestimated, although the overall flow volumes (mL/min) will still be correct.

The velocity, v, can be expressed as the vector sum of its two components—the component in the flow direction, $v_{measured}$, and the component perpendicular to the flow direction, v_h (very much similar to breaking down magnetization vectors into longitudinal and transverse components). The terms can be expressed in terms of sine and cosines, relative to the angle, $\theta = 30°$, between the flow-encoding direction and the true direction of flow (Figure II3-Q2B):

$$V_m = \text{Measured velocity component}$$
$$= \text{True velocity} \times \cos \theta = 0.87$$

$$V_h = \text{Unmeasured velocity component}$$
$$= \text{True velocity} \times \sin \theta$$

The measured velocity will equal 87% of the time velocity

Extra challenging question: The volumetric flow rate will not be affected, because, while the velocity component is underestimated by $\cos \theta$, the cross-sectional area will be increased (an oval instead of a circle) by a factor of $\cos \theta$. Therefore the two factors will cancel, and the volume flow rate will be correct.

3. In this application, the total volume of blood flow, measured in volume per time (mL/min, for example) is the measurement of interest. To determine the rate of blood flow in the distal thoracic aorta that originates from the intercostal arteries, one could measure the total blood flow at two levels: in the proximal descending thoracic aorta and in the distal descending thoracic aorta (Figure II3-Q3). The difference in blood flow at the two levels represents flow coming from the intercostal arteries:

Aortic flow (diaphragmatic hiatus)
− Aortic flow (proximal descending aorta)
= intercostal artery inflow

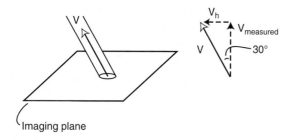

FIGURE II3-Q2B

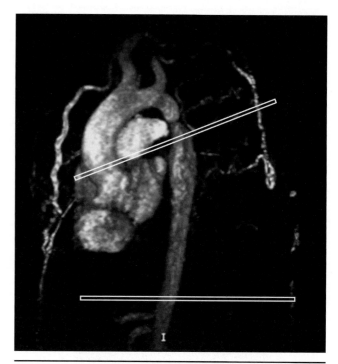

FIGURE II3-Q3. Positioning of two through-plane 2D phase contrast flow quantification slices to measure the total blood flow in the proximal and distal descending thoracic aorta.

Volume flow rates are calculated by multiplying the mean velocity by the cross-sectional area of a vessel lumen, which is typically manually defined by the user for the proximal and distal aortic acquisitions.

4. Setting a high Venc that far exceeds the usual range of measured velocities will prevent most aliasing. However, this is probably not a wise decision in most cases, because with a high Venc the sensitivity and accuracy of low-velocity measurements are poor. For example, with a Venc of 500 cm/sec the ability to differentiate between, say, 80 cm/sec and 120 cm/sec velocities will be not as good as if the Venc were 150 cm/sec. This may be important when assessing the significance of stenoses in the renal or carotid arteries. As a guiding principle, the Venc should be slightly higher than the maximum velocity.

CHAPTER II-4

1. Referring to Figure II4-1, to synchronize the period of maximum contrast enhancement with the acquisition of the central lines of k-space, the midpoint of enhancement, $T_{circulation} + \frac{1}{2}T_{Gd\ injection}$, should coincide with the time to the center of k-space:

$$T_{circulation} + \frac{1}{2}T_{Gd\ injection} = T_{scan\ delay} + T_{center\ of\ k\text{-}space}$$

where $T_{center\ of\ k\text{-}space}$ is the time to the center of k-space or 6 sec in this example. Note that the $T_{center\ of\ k\text{-}space}$

replaces the term, $\frac{1}{2}T_{acquisition}$ for sequential acquisitions. Rearranging this formula,

$$T_{scan\ delay} = T_{circulation} + \tfrac{1}{2}T_{Gd\ injection} - T_{center\ of\ k-space}$$

If the contrast volume is 20 mL and it is injected at 2 mL/sec, then $T_{Gd\ injection} = 10$. The formula reduces to

$$T_{scan\ delay} = T_{circulation} + 5\ sec - 6\ sec$$
$$= T_{circulation} - 1\ sec$$

2. In the excitement of looking for the bolus to arrive in the chest, the operator may not realize that the first region to enhance on axial images is the superior vena cava. If imaging is initiated after bolus detection in the superior vena cava, then a pulmonary angiogram will result. For thoracic aortic MRA, the operator must wait until the bolus first appears in the ascending thoracic aorta before initiating imaging (Figure II4-Q2B).

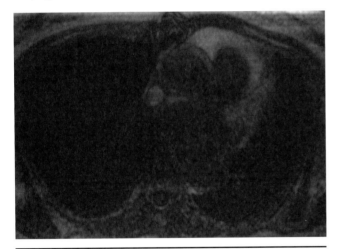

FIGURE II4-Q2B

3. Time-resolved images show that the mass enhances during the pulmonary venous phase and that it communicates directly with the left atrium. The diagnosis is a pulmonary varix (Figure II4-Q3D).

4. The MR venogram shows that the left axillary vein is occluded. However, alternative sites of access, including both jugular veins, both subclavian veins, and the right axillary veins appear patent to the level of the superior vena cava.

5.
   a. The MRA appears to depict complete lack of enhancement of the right arm vasculature from the level of the right subclavian artery, suggesting occlusion at that level. These findings could be due to extrinsic compression (thoracic outlet syndrome), vasculitis, atherosclerotic disease, embolus, or post-traumatic injury such as dissection or occlusion.

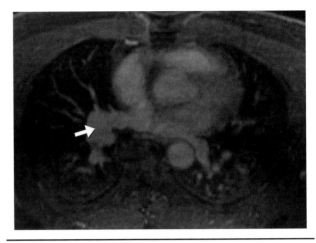

FIGURE II4-Q3D

   b. Concentrated gadolinium contrast material injected in the vein has a very short T2, which causes dephasing of the protons in the blood. When the T2 is sufficiently short (relative to the TE), the signal loss dominates the imaging appearance. By not flushing the concentrated gadolinium contrast in the vein with saline, the concentrated contrast material causes marked signal loss in the veins and adjacent structures such as the arteries. In regions such as the central veins and arteries, where the gadolinium bolus has become relatively dilute by mixing with unenhanced venous blood, the T2 effects are less evident.

   To salvage the case, the second MRA acquisition (refer to the standard protocol in Table II4-3) should be reviewed carefully. Frequently venous inflow will wash out residual concentrated gadolinium and permit evaluation of the arterial structures on the second acquisition. For future studies, a saline flush should be used!

6. There is left common iliac artery occlusion. The right common iliac artery has a metallic stent, which causes signal loss on the MRA, giving the appearance of occlusion. On the source images there is blooming associated with the right common iliac artery (Figure II4-Q6C left), a clue to the presence of the stent. In contrast, the stenotic left common iliac artery (Figure II4-Q6D right) has no associated blooming. Note that because of the susceptibility artifact associated with the stent, the patency of the vessel cannot be assessed on the contrast-enhanced MRA. Other MR techniques, such as phase contrast flow quantification, may detect and quantify flow beyond the stent, whereby patency can be inferred. Note that the appearance of gadolinium contrast in the left common and external iliac arteries does not necessarily indicate vessel patency. When vessels are reconstituted, as in this case, the contrast material can appear distal to an occlusion even on the arterial phase acquisition.

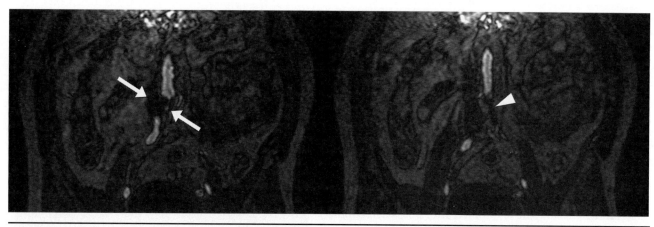

FIGURE II4-Q6C, D. Contrast-enhanced 3D MRA (left) and conventional contrast angiography (right) in a patient with left thigh claudication. (Modified with permission from Lee VS, et al. Gadolinium-enhanced MR angiography: artifacts and pitfalls. AJR 2000; 175: 197–205.)

SECTION III: CARDIAC MR IMAGING

CHAPTER III-1

1.

a. For a heart rate of 60 bpm, the R-R interval will be 1 sec or 1000 msec. The trigger delay should be zero to ensure that systole is included in the imaging. Typically the acquisition window will be 850–900 msec and the trigger window 100–150 msec (or 10–15% of the R-R interval).

b. For a heart rate of 100 bpm, the R-R interval will be 600 msec. The acquisition window or 850–900 msec will now extend beyond one R-R interval, and so the images will include two systolic periods. The acquisition time will be doubled because the triggering will occur only with every other heartbeat rather than with every heart beat. To adjust for the faster heart rate, the acquisition window should be reduced to about 510–540 msec (see Table III1-1) with a trigger window of 60–90 msec.

2. To estimate cardiac output, total blood flow throughout the cardiac cycle must be computed. Retrospective gating is necessary for measurements that include the entire cardiac cycle.

3.

a. With the peripheral pulse triggering, by the time the first images are obtained, the left ventricle is in late systole/early diastole. The trigger window happens to fall during peak systole. Therefore diagnosis of aortic insufficiency should be straightforward, but aortic stenosis may be missed.

b. To image during systole, the acquisition window needs to be shifted or widened. To shift the window, a trigger delay of perhaps 300–400 msec can be used. By keeping the same acquisition window and trigger window durations, the images will now span systole. However, the sequence will trigger off every other heartbeat, and therefore the acquisition time will be twice as long.

Alternatively, rather than using a trigger delay, the acquisition window can be lengthened to about 85–90% of the time of two R-R intervals. For example, if the R-R interval is 1000 msec, and the initial acquisition window was 850 msec, then for the repeat acquisition, the acquisition window can be lengthened to about 1700 msec. In this way, the images will comprise two cardiac cycles, ensuring that systole will be imaged. Note that with this approach, the sequence will again trigger off every other heartbeat, and therefore the acquisition will still be twice as long.

c. Retrospectively-gated cine gradient echo imaging would ensure imaging of the full cardiac cycle.

CHAPTER III-2

1. To obtain a short axis view, a slice should be positioned perpendicular to the long axis of the left ventricle on the three scout views (Figure III2-Q1D–F). From a true short axis view (Figure III2-Q1G), the horizontal and vertical long axis views can be defined as described in the chapter.

2. The position of the heart in each acquisition is shifted because of differences in breath holding. For greater

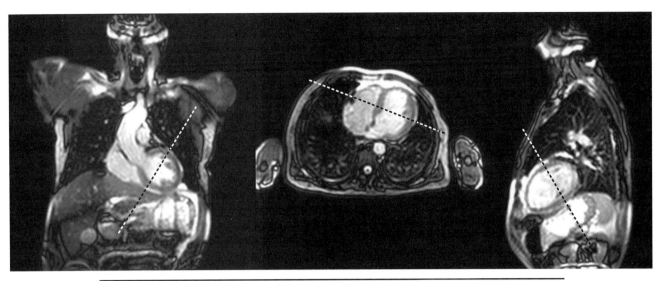

FIGURE III2-Q1D–F. Slice positioning for a short axis view of the left ventricle.

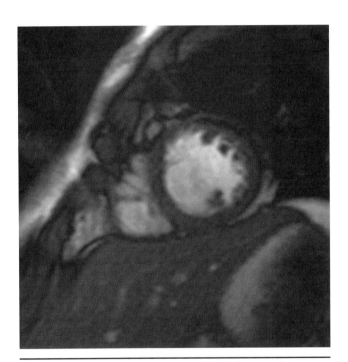

FIGURE III2-Q1G. Short axis view of the left ventricle.

reproducibility, breath holding at end expiration should be used.

3. See Table III2-1B.

4. Both the left coronary artery and left circumflex artery territories show diminished perfusion. Disease of the left main coronary artery could also account for this appearance. A general guide to territories of myocardium supplied by each coronary artery is depicted on the bull's eye or polar map shown in Figure III2-Q4B.

TABLE III2-1B

Region	Short Axis	Horizontal Long Axis (4-Chamber)	Vertical Long Axis (2-Chamber)	LV Outflow Tract (3-Chamber)
Anterior LV wall	√		√	
Interventricular septum	√	√		√
Inferior LV wall	√		√	
LV apex		√	√	√
Mitral valve		√	√	√
Aortic valve				√

*Note that for a full assessment of the aortic value, additional views, including left ventricular outflow tract/ascending aorta view and a slice with the value leaflets en face should be performed.

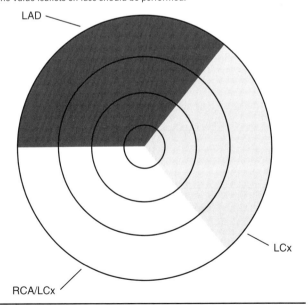

FIGURE III2-Q4B

CHAPTER III-3

1.

a. With an RR = 800 msec and a trigger window of 15%, the acquisition window per heartbeat is 0.85×800 msec = 680 msec. The number of slices that can be imaged is equal to the number of times the 90°–180°-echo can be fitted into this acquisition window. 680 msec/40 msec is approximately 17. Thus, as desired, all 15 slices can be obtained in one acquisition. Assuming that the heart rate is regular and each R wave triggers an acquisition, then the total acquisition time is 100 R-R intervals or 100×0.8 sec = 80 sec. Because this is too long for a breath hold, multiple signal averages must be used. If N_{acq} = 3, then the total acquisition time will be 240 sec or 4 min.

b. The same acquisition window of 680 msec is reduced by 200 msec to 480 msec to ensure diastolic imaging. The number of slices that can be imaged with FSE is 480 msec/80 msec or 6. The acquisition time will be reduced by a factor of the echo train length, so the acquisition will be 80 sec/4 or 20 sec. Multiple signal averaging is not necessary because 20 sec is short enough for one breath hold. To acquire 15 slices, three separate breath holds are needed.

c. With spin echo, a 4 min acquisition is required with the patient freely breathing to obtain the desired 15 slices. With FSE, three separate 20 sec breath holds are required to achieve the same number of slices. Allowing for the time needed to set up the three acquisitions, the total table time for the two approaches is probably comparable. The spin echo sequence will provide superior signal-to-noise ratios and image contrast, when compared with the echo train imaging, but it may be degraded by motion artifact. Repeated breath-hold acquisitions with fast spin echo may result in varying slice positions depending on reproducibility of diaphragmatic position.

2. If the patient is large enough, then most of the signal from the anterior right ventricular wall is detected primarily by the anterior coil elements of the phased-array coil. Turning off the posterior elements will enable the field of view to be reduced dramatically without concern for wraparound artifact in the anterior-posterior direction. The cost of this change is primarily loss of signal that would have been measured from the posterior coil elements.

CHAPTER III-4

1. Because the acquisition window is longer than the subject's R-R interval, the acquisitions will span a full heart beat, but skip every other R wave trigger (Figure III4-Q1). The acquisition time will therefore double, provided the subject's heart rate is regular at 75 beats per minute. The images will cover more than one cardiac cycle.

2.

a. The views per segment should be decreased. The total number of heartbeats needed for the acquisition, which is equal to the N_{PE}/vps, will increase, but because the R-R interval is shorter, the total acquisition time can be maintained.

b. The acquisition time will decrease, since the total number of heartbeats needed for the acquisition will be the same (N_{PE}/vps), but with shorter R-R intervals during breath holding, the overall acquisition time will be shortened.

c. The temporal resolution is equal to the true TR times vps. To improve temporal resolution, vps should be decreased.

3. To improve temporal resolution by a factor of two, the vps should be reduced by one half, to 6. As a consequence, the total acquisition time will double to 20 heartbeats, or about 16 sec.

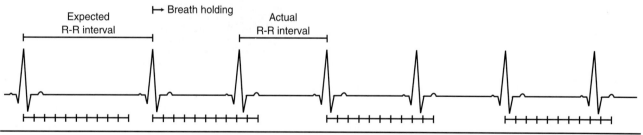

Expected R-R interval   ⟼ Breath holding   Actual R-R interval

FIGURE III4-Q1

4. There are several possibilities, many of which can be tried together:

(1) Provide the patient with supplemental oxygen via nasal cannula to improve breath-holding capacity.

(2) Increase vps slightly. For example, an increase to 7 will result in a slight worsening of temporal resolution, it but may be worthwhile for the concomitant reduction in acquisition time to 17 heartbeats.

(3) Decrease the number of phase-encoding steps slightly. This can be performed using rectangular field of view with no loss in spatial resolution. Further decreases in N_{PE} will cause a a loss in spatial resolution. For example, a reduction in the number of phase-encoding steps from 120 to 98 will reduce the acquisition time by a few more heartbeats to about 14 heartbeats.

(4) Parallel imaging, if available, will reduce acquisition times dramatically. For an R factor of 2, the acquisition time can be reduced by almost a factor of 2. Note that some of these gains are offset by reduced rectangular field of view.

(5) View sharing (or echo sharing) can also be used to increase the apparent temporal resolution. Although it may appear that the temporal resolution is doubled, the actual increase in temporal resolution is not quite that good.

5. a. With retrospectively gated sequences, the acquisition should be continuous. Only after the data are acquired is there partitioning of the echoes into different k-spaces to correspond to different frames.

b. The acquisition time is exceeding the expected time mostly likely because the arrhythmia rejection algorithm is ignoring many heartbeats' worth of data. This is probably because the subject's heart rate has increased with breath holding, so that the R-R interval is frequently less than 750 msec. Before repeating or modifying parameters, check the subject's heart rate with breath holding, and then adjust parameters. For example, if heart rate increases, vps should be reduced.

6. a. On this systolic view, a dark jet is emanating from the aortic valve leaflets, signifying aortic stenosis.

b. Positioning a cine gradient echo slice in the plane of the aortic valve leaflets will show the number of valve leaflets present (Figure III4-Q6B). Images through the aortic valve during systole (Figure III4-Q6C) and diastole (Figure III4-Q6D) show a bicuspid aortic valve (arrows).

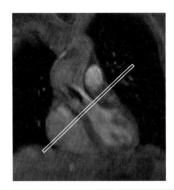

FIGURE III4-Q6B

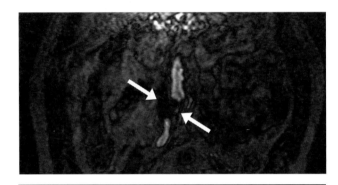

FIGURE III4-Q6C, D. Systolic (left) and diastolic (right) views through the aortic valve show that there are only two aortic valve leaflets, indicating bicuspid aortic valve (arrows).

7. You should perform tagged studies before gadolinium contrast injection. The shortened T1 relaxation following gadolinium contrast injection will cause more rapid fading of the tags, because recovery of the saturated spins will occur more quickly.

8. As will be detailed in Chapter III-6, a phase contrast acquisition through the ascending aorta will provide a measure of forward blood flow in one heartbeat, which is equal to stroke volume, assuming there is no mitral insufficiency.

9. In this example, the papillary muscles are included in the blood pool at end systole but excluded at end diastole. The inclusion or exclusion of papillary muscles should be performed consistently in any given study, from slice to slice and for both EDV and ESV. The ESV region of interest could be modified to Figure III4-Q9B, to be consistent with EDV.

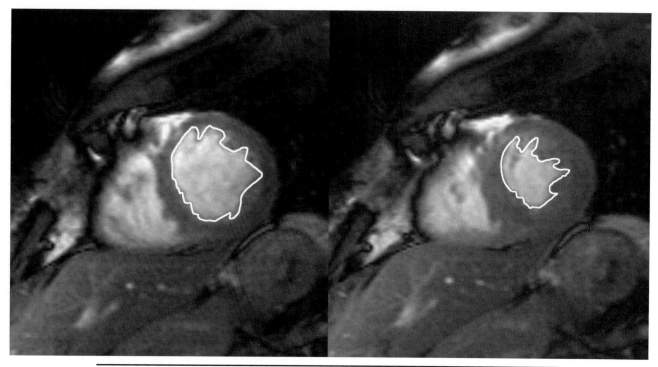

FIGURE III4-Q9B. ROIs drawn for (left) EDV and (right) ESV.

CHAPTER III-5

1. Not necessarily. A mass containing hemorrhagic products, proteinaceous fluid, melanin, or fat (Table III5-1) would appear hyperintense on unenhanced T1-weighted imaging as well as enhanced imaging, regardless of the degree of vascularity. In order to assess vascularity of a mass, both unenhanced and enhanced T1-weighted MR images are needed.

2. Over time, the contrast material in the viable myocardium continues to wash out (Figure III5-10). With less gadolinium contrast material, the T1 of the viable myocardium becomes longer, and consequently, the inversion time to achieve its nulling will also be longer. To solve this problem, the inversion time can be empirically increased at intervals of 25 msec (Figure III5-Q2D). Alternatively, the inversion time mapping sequence can be repeated to determine the new TI more precisely. These issues arise only with magnitude-reconstructed inversion recovery sequences and not the phase-sensitive reconstructions.

3. In addition to clinical history, the spatial distribution of the delayed enhancement is one of the best differentiating features. The regions of the myocardium that are most susceptible to ischemia are the subendocardial layers. Therefore, most infarcts involve at least the subendocardial layer if not the entire wall. The infarcts also tend to follow predictable patterns of distribution

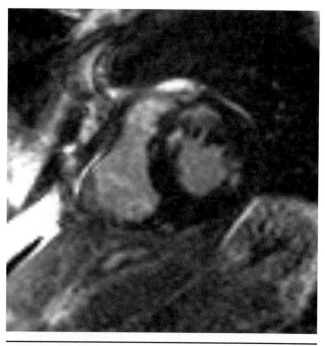

FIGURE III5-Q2D

based on coronary artery territories (see Chapter III-2, Figure III2-11, III2-12). Diseases such as sarcoidosis or hypertrophic cardiomyopathy have a more patchy distribution of hyperintensity and frequently affect subepicardial areas without subendocardial involvement.

4. The axial cine image demonstrates a normal finding. The moderator band inserts into the free wall of the right ventricle and can cause a focal tethering at its insertion that results in a pseudoaneurysmal appearance of the apex. This should not be mistaken for right ventricular dysplasia.

CHAPTER III-6

1. The two acquisitions were performed with suboptimal Venc selection. In images A and B, the peak velocity causes only a mild increase in signal intensity, suggesting that the Venc is much larger than the peak systolic velocity. To improve the accuracy of measurements, the Venc should be decreased to a value that is slightly higher than the expected peak velocity.

In images C and D, the Venc has been set too low. When velocity exceeds the Venc, aliasing is observed. The acquisition should be repeated with higher Venc to avoid aliasing. Alias correction algorithms can be applied in the post-processing phase in order to salvage the data.

For an example of phase contrast imaging at an ideal Venc, refer to Figure III6-Q1.

2. To calculate regurgitant fraction, the volume of regurgitant flow must be calculated together with the volume of forward flow. To avoid calculating the contribution of normal flow reversal due to filling of the coronary arteries during diastole, the slice position should be placed below the level of the coronary sinuses, at the level of the aortic valve leaflets (Figure III6-Q2, bold line). (For ease of calculating the forward flow component, a separate acquisition can be performed above the sinuses of Valsalva for that calculation.) (Figure III6-Q2, Fine line) It is critical that the acquisition be conducted with retrospective gating to ensure that all retrograde diastolic flow is included in the measurement.

3. Several approaches could be used. The stroke volume reflects the total flow of blood out of the left ventricle during each heartbeat. The difference between left ventricular stroke volume and the forward flow out of the aorta can be used to estimate regurgitant flow. Stroke volume (SV) requires separate calculations of EDV and ESV using short axis cine images as described in Chapter III-4. A separate phase contrast acquisition through the ascending aorta would provide a measure of the forward flow through the aorta.

Mitral regurgitant fraction [%] =
[SV − Aortic forward flow]/SV × 100%

The total forward flow out of the heart can also be measured at other points in the cardiovascular system,

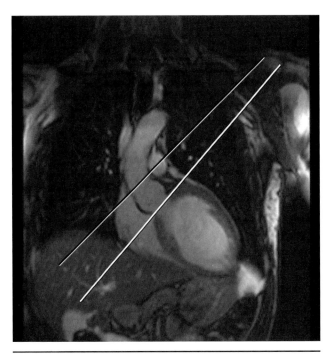

FIGURE III6-Q2

provided there are no other shunts or regurgitant valves. For example, total forward flow through the pulmonary artery should be equal to the aortic forward flow.

Mitral regurgitant fraction =
(SV − Pulmonary forward flow)/SV)

4. The total flow through the left pulmonary artery is twice as great as the flow through the right pulmonary artery. This flow ratio is consistent with what would be expected given the the preponderance of stenoses on the right.

CHAPTER III-7

1. Coil sensitivity effects should be apparent on all images, including unenhanced images, while ischemia should be most obvious only on a few perfusion images. Semiquantitative or quantitative paramitiator analysis may also help.

2. A fixed perfusion abnormality is located in the anterolateral wall of the mid left ventricle. A stress-induced perfusion abnormality is demonstrated throughout the entire anterior wall and anterior septum.

These findings suggest an infarct in the territory of the left circumflex artery, likely a marginal branch, giving rise to the fixed perfusion defect. The stress-induced abnormality implies ischemia in the LAD territory, likely due to a proximal LAD stenosis.

3. At rest, the anterior apex and apical portion of the anterior septum are hypokinetic. Motion recovers with low-dose dobutamine suggesting that this area is viable, though hibernating at rest. The likely culprit is a stenosis in the distal LAD. With high-dose dobutamine, in addition to worsening function in this region, moderate hypokinesis develops along the entire lateral wall, suggesting a significant stenosis of a proximal portion of the left circumflex artery.

CHAPTER III-8

1. The right coronary artery originates anomalously from the left main coronary artery and travels anteriorly to the pulmonary artery toward the right atrioventricular groove (Figure III8-Q1B). This anomaly is usually not clinically significant since there is no abnormal compression of the coronary artery along its course.

2. The MRA demonstrates diffuse atherosclerotic disease. Additionally, in the proximal and mid RCA, significant stenoses are identified. When combined with stress

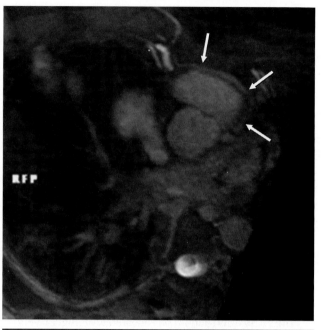

FIGURE III8-Q1B. Anomalous right coronary artery (arrows).

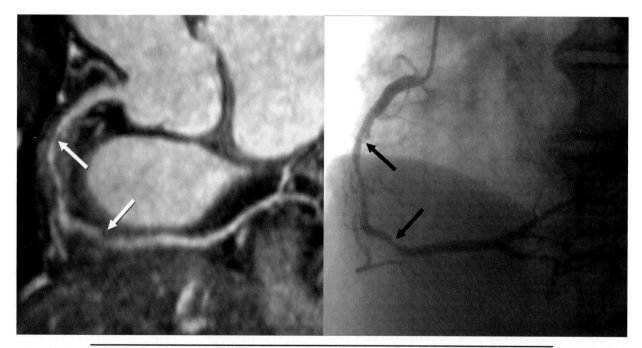

FIGURE III8-Q2B. Correlation between coronary MRA (left) and conventional catheter angiography (right) with multiple areas of stenosis in the RCA (two stenoses labeled with arrows). (Reproduced with permission from Sakuma H et al. Assessment of coronary arteries with total study time of less than 30 minutes by using whole-heart coronary MR angiography. Radiology 2005; 237: 316–321.)

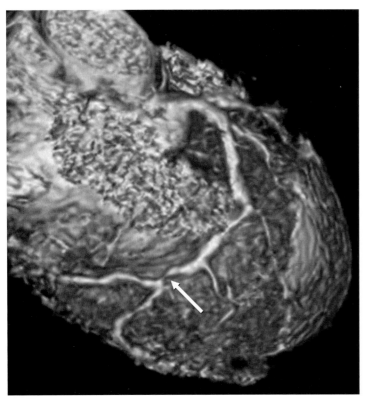 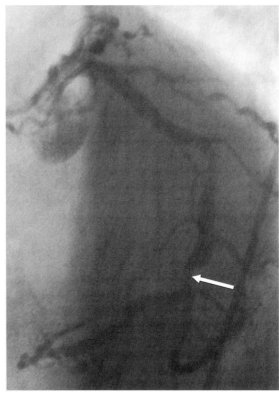

FIGURE III8-Q3B, C. (Courtesy of H. Sakuma, M.D.)

perfusion MR imaging, these lesions were found to be physiologically significant. Conventional coronary artery angiography is shown in Figure III8-Q2B.

3. The coronary MRA depicts significant stenosis in the distal LCx. Figure III8-Q3B demonstrates the same findings (arrows) with a volume-rendered reconstruction of the whole heart MRA. Figure III8-Q3C shows the corresponding conventional contrast angiogram of the LCx.

Acceptance window, or **gating window**: The range of diaphragmatic motion considered acceptable for data acquisition, as shown by navigator echoes.

Acquisition window: The total duration of data sampling during each R-R interval in an ECG-triggered cardiovascular sequence.

Additivity of relaxivity: The principle that the measured relaxivity rate in a heterogeneous tissue can be expressed as the sum of the relaxivities of each component in that tissue. For example, the relaxivity rate of gadolinium-enhanced tissue is equal to the sum of the relaxivity rate of the unenhanced tissue plus the relaxivity rate of the gadolinium contrast. The same concept can also be applied when different factors contribute to relaxivity, such as T2′, T2, and T2*.

Adenosine: A naturally occuring vasodilator, used in stress-cardiac MRI.

Analog-to-digital converter (ADC): An electronic component that samples a continuously varying signal (such as the MR echo) and converts the echo into digital numbers (for storage in k-space, for instance).

Angular frequency: The rate of change of an angle, ϕ, per unit time.

Array: A matrix of numbers.

Arrhythmia rejection: A feature of an ECG-gated MR pulse sequence that allows rejection of data from R-R intervals that fail to meet certain criteria for acceptance.

Asymmetric function: A mathematical function, such as the sine function, that is not symmetric around zero.

Asymmetric sampling of the echo: Measurement of an echo that includes the central peak and more points on one side than the other.

B_0 ("B zero", "B naught"): The main magnetic field of an MR system, which for superconducting magnets is the magnetic field induced by current passing through the superconducting wire (typically 1.5–3.0 T).

B_1 ("B one"): The magnetic field generated by the transmitter coil and used to achieve RF excitation.

Balanced fast field echo (FFE): See **True FISP**.

Band artifct: An image artifact that areas from transverse magnetization interfering with the generation of consistent MR sequences following the RF excitation.

Bandwidth: The range of frequencies used to describe transmitter RF pulses (transmitter bandwidth) and measured signal (receiver bandwidth), usually centered around 0 Hz and described in terms of the maximum frequency minus the minimum frequency.

Binomial pulses: A sequence of RF pulses whose amplitudes follow the pattern of coefficients in an expression for a binomial raised to a power, such as "1–2–1" corresponding to $(a + b)^2 = 1a^2 + 2ab + 1b^2$.

Bipolar gradient: A gradient with a negative lobe and a positive lobe.

Black-blood imaging: Techniques for generating images of the heart and vessels in which signal intensity from moving blood is very low (black on the image), typically spin echo.

Blood flow rate (mL/sec or mL/min): The volume of blood passing through a vessel in a given time.

Blooming artifact: Signal loss around regions such as air-tissue interfaces or metal, which are exaggerated by increased sensitivity to susceptibility or T2* effects.

Bright-blood imaging: Techniques for generating images of the heart and vessels in which signal intensity from moving blood is high (bright on the image), typically gradient echo.

Cardiac index (CI, mL/min/m²): Cardiac output normalized to body surface area.

Cardiac output (CO, mL/min): The net forward flow rate of blood out of the left ventricle over time.

Centric filling of k-space: Use of a k-space trajectory in which central portions of k-space (in 2 or 3 dimensions) are filled first and peripheral portions later.

Chemical shift: The difference in precession rates between protons in different molecular environments, such as between hydrogen protons in fat and hydrogen protons in water.

Chemical shift artifact of the first kind: The mismapping of image signal intensities from fat because of the slower precession of fat protons (about 220 Hz at 1.5 T) compared to water protons. The artifact appears as artifactual white or dark bands at fat-water (fat-organ) interfaces in the frequency-encoding direction.

Chemical shift artifact of the second kind, or **India ink artifact**: Cancellation of signal in voxels that contain nearly equal amounts of fat and water (or nonfatty tissue) on opposed-phase images. The effect causes fat-tissue interfaces to be marked with a black outline and signal loss in organs or masses with intracellular fat.

Cine MRI, or **cinematic MRI**: A series of MR images that depict cardiac motion throughout a heart cycle when viewed in a cinematic or movie loop.

Circulation time: The transit time of a contrast bolus from peripheral venous injection to its appearance in the arteries of interest.

Complex number: A number that has a real and an imaginary component, typically expressed as (a + ib), where i is the imaginary number defined as $\sqrt{-1}$. k-space consists of a matrix of complex numbers whose real and imaginary components are usually considered separately.

Contrast: See **Image contrast**.

Contrast-to-noise ratio: A parameter describing image quality, determined by the ratio of the difference in signal intensities between two tissues (contrast) divided by image noise.

Conventional spin echo imaging: A technique of generating MR images that uses a pulse sequence consisting of a 90° and a 180° radiofrequency pulse and collection of a single echo.

Cross-talk artifact: An artifact of imperfect slice excitation that results from truncated RF pulses and is usually solved by introducing a gap between adjacent imaging slices.

Crusher gradient: See **Spoiler gradient**.

Δk: Dimension of a voxel in k-space.

Dephasing gradient: See **Spoiler gradient**.

Demodulation: The process by which low-frequency signals superimposed on high carrier frequencies are restored by separation from the carrier frequency.

Dipyridamole: A vasodilator that functions by blocking the cellular uptake and metabolism of adenosine, used in stress cardiac MRI.

Distance factor: The slice thickness-to-gap ratio, typically expressed as the fraction of gap per slice thickness. For a slice thickness to gap ratio of 5 : 1 (e.g., 5 mm slices and 1 mm gaps), the distance factor is 0.2.

Dobutamine: A synthetic catecholamine that has potent β_1-receptor and mild α_1- and β_2-receptor agonist activity and whose two main effects depend on the dose administered. At low doses ($\leq$10 μg/kg body weight/ min), dobutamine causes increased contractility; at high doses of dobutamine (30–40 μg/kg body weight/ min), increased heart rate and contractility causes an increase in oxygen consumption, mimicking ergonomic stress.

Double dose: 0.2 mmol/kg subject body weight gadolinium contrast material.

Duality property: A property of a function, whereby f(x) = y, if f(y) = x.

Echo planar imaging (EPI): A fast imaging sequence in which multiple echoes are acquired following each excitation and that can be used to perform single-shot imaging.

Echo time (TE): The time between the RF pulse and the peak of an echo.

Echo train imaging: See **Fast spin echo**.

Echo train length (ETL): The number of echoes generated for every 90° radiofrequency excitation of a fast spin echo sequence; also called the turbo factor.

Effective echo time (TE_{eff}): The echo time (TE) of the echo that is used to fill the center line of k-space in a multiecho sequence.

Ejection fraction (EF, %): The ratio of stroke volume to end diastolic volume (SV/EDV).

Electrocardiogram (ECG): A record of the electrical signals of the heart, which must be measured for cardiovascular MRI to synchronize the acquisitions with cardiac motion.

Electrocardiographic (ECG) gating: Synchronization of cardiac or vascular MR acquisitions with the electrical signal of the heart.

Electrocardiographically triggered (ECG-triggered): The term to describe cardiac or vascular MR acquisitions that are initiated when an ECG signal reaches a predefined threshold.

Electromagnetic induction: A property of electromagnetism in which moving current through a wire induces a magnetic field; conversely, a changing magnetic field across a wire induces a current.

Electromagnetic theory: The field of mathematics and physics that describes the relationship between electricity and magnetism, forming the basis for MR imaging.

Encoding velocity, or **Venc**: The maximum velocity that can be measured using a given phase contrast MR pulse sequence, defined as the velocity that causes a 180° phase shift. The range of velocities that can be measured ranges from −Venc to +Venc.

End diastolic volume (EDV): The intracavitary volume of the left ventricle at end diastole, typically considered equivalent to the maximum volume.

End systolic volume (ESV): The intracavitary volume of the left ventricle at end systole when the ventricle has fully contracted, typically considered the minimum volume of the left ventricle.

Entry slice: The first slice(s) in a series of 2D or 3D images, which depicts most flow-related enhancement.

Ernst angle (α_E): The optimal flip angle in gradient echo imaging for maximizing signal intensity based on pulse sequence TR and tissue T1.

Excitation: The process of pulling the proton magnetic moments away from the axis of the main magnetic field B_0 through the temporary application of a second magnetic field B_1.

Exponential decay: A decline in signal given by the equation, $M_{xy}(t) = Me^{-t/\tau}$, where τ is the time constant of decay; by definition, τ is the time at which the signal declines to 0.37 of its original value.

Exponential recovery: A rise in longitudinal magnetization given by the equation, $M_z(t) = M(1e^{-t/\tau})$, where τ is the time constant of recovery; by definition, τ is the time at which the longitudinal magnetization recovers to 0.63 of its final value.

Fast field echo (FFE): See **Gradient echo, Spoiled gradient echo**.

Fast imaging excitation with steady state acquisition (FIESTA): See **True FISP**.

Fast low angle shot imaging (FLASH): See **Spoiled gradient echo, turboFLASH**.

Fast Spin Echo (FSE): A spin echo sequence that uses multiple 180° refocusing pulses to generate multiple spin echoes per radiofrequency excitation.

Fat saturation or **Fat suppression**: Elimination of signal from fat protons but not from water protons. Fat saturation typically implemented with an RF pulse (a frequency-selective fat suppression pulse) at the precession frequency of fat protons followed by a crusher gradient

Fiber optic cables: Cables that transmit signals in the form of pulses of light rather than electric currents. In cardiovascular MRI, they are used for transmitting ECG signals from the subject to the MR system with minimum interference from RF pulses and gradient switching.

Field of view (FOV): The dimensions of the image (typically described in terms of the x dimension and y dimension and, for 3D imaging, the z dimension).

5 gauss line (5 G line): The minimum distance from an MR scanner at which the static magnetic field strength is 5 gauss or less, considered safe for all individuals (note that 1 tesla = 10,000 gauss).

Flip angle (α): The angle through which the magnetization vector is tipped away from the z axis by an RF pulse.

Flow: A measurement of blood motion in units of volume per time, typically mL/sec or mL/min.

Flow compensation, or **gradient moment nulling**: Application of positive- and negative-lobed gradients that serve to reduce dephasing caused by moving blood with constant velocity.

Flow-related enhancement (FRE): High signal intensity caused by the inflow of unsaturated protons in flowing blood; the basis for time-of-flight imaging methods.

Flow sensitivity direction: The direction(s) in which moving protons generate a phase shift in a phase contrast sequence.

Flow separation: The disturbance of laminar flow at branch points that can give rise to eddies and vortices, such as at the carotid artery bifurcation.

Four-chamber view: See **Horizontal long axis**.

Fourier transformation or **Fourier transform**: Conceptually, a histogram of the distribution of contributions of different frequency components that, when summed, recreate the original function. "Frequency" can refer to the spatial frequency components that are comprised in a function of distance (such as an image) or the temporal frequency components that are comprised in a function of time (such as an MR echo).

Fractional echo: Sampling of an asymmetric echo that serves as a means of reducing image acquisition times by decreasing TE and TR.

Frames: Images from an ECG-gated acquisition that correspond to different time points in the cardiac cycle.

Free induction decay (FID): Decay of transverse magnetization generated from application of an RF pulse, caused by loss of phase coherence of precessing protons.

Frequency: The rate of oscillation of a function that varies in space or in time, such as cosine ωx or cosine ωt, where x is distance and t is time, ω represents the frequency (in radians per second). Frequency can also have units of cycles per second or hertz (Hz), in which case it is usually represented by the symbol f; $\omega = 2\pi f$.

Frequency encoding: The process of spatial localization that relies on gradients to vary precessional frequency linearly with distance.

Frequency-encoding gradient, or **readout gradient**: A magnetic field gradient applied during the sampling of the echo to enable spatial localization in one direction, referred to as the frequency-encoding direction; source of the gradient echo with gradient echo.

Frequency oversampling, or **no frequency wrap**: A technique for reducing wraparound artifact in the frequency-encoding direction by increasing the sampling frequency of the echo.

Fringe field: A magnetic field extending beyond the bore of the magnet.

Gating window: See **Acceptance window**.

Geometric factor, g: The factor by which signal-to-noise ratio calculations are reduced for parallel imaging acquisitions. The parameter reflects the lack of total spatial independence of coil sensitivity profiles used for parallel imaging.

Ghosting artifact: A repetitive appearance of part of an image that is due to any periodic motion caused by breathing, vascular pulsation, or CSF pulsation, typically in the phase-encoding direction.

Gibbs truncation artifact or **Gibbs ringing artifact**: Blurring of edges and signal extending outside of objects as a result of truncation of k-space and incomplete sampling of high-spatial-frequency components in the image.

Gradient: A linear change in a quantity (such as magnetic field strength) across a distance within the bore of the magnet. The gradient can be in any direction (x, y, z, or an oblique direction).

Gradient echo: See **Gradient recalled echo**.

Gradient moment nulling: See **Flow compensation**.

Gradient recalled echo (GRE): An echo produced by application of a single RF pulse and refocusing gradients.

Gyromagnetic ratio, γ: The constant of proportionality that relates the Larmor frequency to the magnetic field. γ = 42.6 MHz/T for protons.

Half-Fourier acquisition single-shot turbo spin echo (HASTE): A single-shot echo train spin echo sequence that uses short interecho spacing to generate enough echoes from a single radiofrequency excitation to fill more than half of k-space. The remainder of k-space is filled numerically using the property of Hermitian conjugate symmetry.

Hermitian conjugate symmetry: The pattern of symmetry in k-space that enables incomplete collection of k-space and computational approximations to substitute for uncollected data.

Hertz (Hz): A unit of frequency, equal to one cycle or sample per second. 1 kilohertz (kHz) is 1000 cycles or samples per second, 1 megahertz (MHz) is 1,000,000 cycles or samples per second.

Horizontal long axis (HLA), or **four-chamber view**: The plane of the heart that is defined by the long axis, which traverses the midpoint of the mitral valve orifice and the left ventricular apex, bisecting the left ventricle horizontally.

Image contrast: The difference in signal intensity between different tissues and between normal and abnormal tissues.

Image noise: Undesirable and meaningless signal contributed by random perturbations from the body and imaging system.

Imaginary component of k-space: The part of the complex numbers represented in k-space that reflects the sine spatial frequency components of an image.

Imaginary image: The Fourier transform of the imaginary component of k-space.

In-phase imaging: Imaging at an echo time at which water and fat protons precess coherently and contribute additively to the signal intensity. At 1.5 T, in-phase gradient echo imaging occurs at echo times that are a multiple of 4.4 msec. See also **Opposed-phase imaging**.

In-plane flow: A term that relies to phase contrast imaging where flow sensitivity is in one or both of the directions of the imaging plane.

India ink artifact: See **Chemical shift artifact of the second kind**.

Interecho spacing: The time between consecutive echoes that are generated after a single radiofrequency pulse.

Interleaved notched saturation perfusion: A perfusion sequence designed with a notched excitation slice profile for the magnetization prepulse that saturates all but the central notch; this approach allows for a longer inversion time between the saturation or inversion prepulse and the readout.

Interpolation: The process of estimating values for data points that lie between measured values.

Interslice gap: The distance between adjacent imaging slices that is left unimaged in order to avoid cross-talk artifacts.

Intravoxel dephasing: Loss of signal as a result of differences in proton velocities leading to phase dispersion within a voxel.

Inversion time (TI): The interval between 180° inversion pulse and RF excitation for an inversion recovery sequence, usually defined to null the signal from a particular tissue.

Inversion time mapping (TI mapping): A sequence performed to determine the inversion time to null signal from a particular tissue, such as viable myocardium.

Isotropic voxels: Voxels that have equal dimensions in all three directions.

k-space: The raw data space that contains all measured signals from an MR pulse sequence; it also represents the Fourier transform of the MR image.

k-space trajectory: The order in which k-space is filled with data, as determined by the pulse sequence diagram.

k_{total}: The overall size of k-space, equal to Δk times the number of voxels in that dimension of k-space.

Keyhole imaging: A rapid imaging approach used when multiple images are acquired over time and repeated images are generated by updating only the central portions of k-space; the periphery of k-space is copied from other time points.

Laminar flow: Flow in a vessel with a parabolic flow profile, where the maximum velocity is twice the average velocity across the vessel.

Larmor equation: The relationship between the precessional frequency of magnetic moments, ω or f, and the magnetic field, B_0, given by the equation, $\omega = \gamma B_0$, where γ is the gyromagnetic ratio.

Larmor frequency: The precessional frequency of magnetic moments in a magnetic field. In this book, the Larmor frequency will have units of hertz (Hz or cycles/sec) or radians/sec .

Left ventricular outflow tract (LVOT)/three-chamber view: The long axis view of the left ventricle that includes visualization of both the mitral and aortic valves.

Left ventricular outflow tract (LVOT)/ascending aorta view: The oblique view of the left ventricle that is orthogonal to the three-chamber view and provides a view of the aortic valve and ascending aorta.

Linear k-space trajectory, or **rectilinear k-space trajectory**: A k-space trajectory that fills k-space one row or column at a time. Linear trajectories can be centric or sequential, depending on whether the filling starts with the central lines of k-space or with the peripheral lines.

Lines per segment: See **Views per segment**.

Longitudinal magnetization: The component of the net magnetization aligned in the same direction as the main magnetic field B_0.

Longitudinal relaxation: See **T1 relaxation**.

Magnetic moment (μ): The magnetization associated with a single object such as a proton.

Magnetic field gradient: See **Gradient**.

Magnetic resonance angiography (MRA): Imaging of blood vessels using magnetic resonance imaging.

Magnetization transfer: Image contrast that relies on the differences in T2 relaxation times between free, unbound water protons and protons that are bound to macromolecules, resulting in suppression of most tissues other than free water and fat.

Magnetization vector (M): Cumulative magnetization from the entire population of visible protons.

Magnetohydrodynamic effect: The consequences of a conductive fluid moving within a magnetic field; magnetohydrodynamic effects on blood during MR procedures generate artifactual signal in the ECG tracings and cause ST elevation and an increase in T wave.

Magnitude image: See **Modulus image**.

Maki artifact: A heterogeneous appearance of a vessel lumen on gadolinium-enhanced MR angiography attributable to a change in enhancement during the filling of k-space.

Matrix: Numbers arranged in an array in rows and columns. The voxels comprised in an MR image form a matrix; "matrix" often means the size of this matrix, expressed as the product of the number of voxels in each dimension, for example 256×192 or $256 \times 128 \times 40$.

Maximum flow-related enhancement velocity (v_{maxFRE}): The velocity of flowing blood associated with maximum flow-related enhancement, above which signal intensity will not increase.

Maximum intensity projection (MIP): An image post-processing reconstruction algorithm commonly used for MR angiography that uses a ray casting algorithm to select the brightest pixels along each ray to generate an angiographic image.

Microvascular obstruction: An especially hypovascular region surrounded by infarcted tissue in a setting of acute myocardial infarction.

Modified Bernoulli equation: The approximate relationship between peak systolic velocity, v (m/sec), through a stenosis and the peak pressure gradient, P (mm Hg) across the stenosis, given by $P = 4v^2$.

Modulation: The process by which low-frequency signals are superimposed on high carrier frequencies.

Modulus image, or **magnitude image**: An image generated by taking the square root of the sum of the squares of real and imaginary data; clinical images are usually modulus images. See also **Phase image**.

Multiple overlapping thin-slab acquisition (MOTSA): A time-of-flight angiographic technique that consists of multiple thin 3D acquisitions that overlap slightly.

Multiplanar reconstruction (MPR): An image post-processing tool that enables datasets to be viewed in any plane regardless of the acquisition.

Navigator echo: A one-dimensional signal acquisition at the level of the lung-liver interface that is used to monitor and correct for respiratory motion for cardiac imaging, particularly of the coronary arteries.

Navigator efficiency: The percentage of heartbeats in a navigator echo acquisition during which data are acquired.

Net phase shift or **phase difference**: The difference in phase shifts between two phase contrast acquisitions, typically one performed using flow-encoding gradients and the other using flow-compensated gradients, used to generate velocity maps.

No frequency wrap: See **Frequency oversampling**.

No phase wrap: See **Phase oversampling**.

Noise: See **Image noise**.

Nonselective RF excitation: An RF excitation pulse that affects all of the protons in the bore of the magnet.

Null point: The point, following inversion with a 180° pulse, at which tissue magnetization has zero longitudinal component.

Number of acquisitions (N_{acq}): The number of times a signal is collected in signal averaging.

Number of excitations (N_{ex}): See Number of acquisitions.

Number of lines per segment: The number of echoes collected per radiofrequency excitation.

Number of phase-encoding steps (N_{PE}): The number of times the phase-encoding gradient is to be applied in generating an image. In general, this number corresponds to the number of pixels in the phase-encoding direction of the image. Number os signal average: see Number acquisting.

Number of signal averages: See **Number of acquisitions**

Nyquist theorem of sampling: The theorem that states that, to detect a signal of a frequency f accurately, the signal must be sampled at a frequency of at least twice the frequency, 2f.

Opposed-phase imaging or **out-of-phase imaging:** Imaging at an echo time at which water and fat protons precess with a phase difference of 180°; voxels that contain equal proportions of fat and water show signal cancellation. At 1.5 T, opposed-phase imaging occurs at echo times of 2.2 msec and 6.6 msec. See also **In-phase imaging**.

Orthogonal views: Views that are perpendicular to each other (the planes are 90° to each other), such as the axial, coronal, and sagittal views.

Out-of-phase imaging: See **Opposed-phase imaging**.

Oversampling: Collection of extra data in k-space that does not manifest directly in the image. See also frequency oversampling and phase oversampling.

Parallel imaging: Technique for undersampling k-space that uses coil sensitivity profiles. See **Sensitivity encoding (SENSE)** and **Simultaneous acquisition of spatial harmonics (SMASH).**

Partial echo: See **Fractional echo**.

Partial flip angle: Flip angle of less than 90°.

Partial Fourier: Incomplete filling of k-space by a reduced number of phase-encoding steps and the use of the symmetry of k-space or zero filling to complete unfilled lines.

Partial number of excitations, or **Partial Nex**: See **Partial Fourier**.

Partition dimension: Term used for the dimension that is orthogonal to the frequency- and phase-encoding directions in a 3D acquisition.

Partition loop: Portion of a 3D pulse sequence that completes the filling of k-space for one position in the partition direction.

Peak amplitude: The maximum gradient strength across the magnet, the range of the field-of-view to which this applies is also important.

Peak systolic velocity: Maximum velocity of flow during systole.

Period: Time for a full oscillation of a sinusoidal or oscillating function, for example, from maximum to minimum to maximum, or from positive to negative to positive peaks.

Phase: Relationship between the direction of a vector and a particular axis or another vector. Phase is typically expressed in terms of degrees (°), where the full range of phase is $-180°$–$+180°$ or 0°–360°. For example, two vectors perpendicular to each other have a phase difference of 90°.

Phase coherence: Degree to which magnetization vectors are precessing together ("in-phase") in the transverse plane.

Phase contrast imaging: Technique that uses pairs of gradients (such as a pair of bipolar gradients) to create velocity-encoded images; protons moving in the direction of the gradients accumulate differences in precessional phase.

Phase difference: See **Net phase shift**.

Phase encoding: Use of differences in phase between precessing protons along a gradient for spatial localization.

Phase-encoding gradient: A magnetic field gradient applied during a pulse sequence other than at the time of the RF pulse and the echo to enable spatial localization in one direction, referred to as the phase-encoding direction. The phase-encoding gradient must be applied in numerous different ways, each referred to as a phase-encoding step, in order to permit localization in this direction.

Phase-encoding steps: See **Number of phase-encoding steps**.

Phase image: An image generated by taking the arc tangent of the imaginary image data divided by the real image data. See also **Modulus image**.

Phase oversampling or **no phase wrap**: A technique for reducing wraparound artifact in the phase-encoding direction; the method is based on increasing the phase-encoding steps and causes an increase in acquisition time.

Phase shift: The relative difference in phase between magnetization vectors, typically refers to vectors in the transverse plane.

Phased-array coil: A coil comprising of several smaller coils that can each receive signal simultaneously and independently, typically used for receiving signal only.

Pixel: A picture element of a two-dimensional image with dimensions in two directions (x and y); because "two-dimensional" MR images correspond to tissue slices with finite thickness, they have a third dimension, and the term **voxel** is more appropriate for describing MR image components.

Plug flow: A flow pattern in a vessel in which velocity is constant across the lumen, typically seen at the orifice of a branch vessel.

Precession: Rotation of magnetic moments about the axis of a magnetic field.

Precessional frequency: See **Larmor frequency**.

Prepulse: An RF excitation pulse performed prior to the echo-producing RF excitation in order to modify image contrast, for example, to suppress signal from particular tissues in the image.

Prospective adaptive motion correction: A method for adjusting the positioning of an acquisition guided by navigator echo data.

Prospective gating, or **prospective triggering**: Initiation of MR data acquisition with the R wave of an electrocardiogram or the pulse wave from a peripheral pulse monitor.

Prospective triggering: See **Prospective gating**.

Proton density-weighted images: Images whose contrast is based on proton density differences with little contrast effect from T1 or T2 relaxation differences.

Pulmonary/systemic flow ratios (Q_P/Q_S): The total forward flow through the pulmonary artery relative to total forward flow through the aorta.

Pulsation artifact: A form of ghosting artifact typically caused by aortic or arterial pulsation.

Pulse sequence: The orchestration of the transmitter coil, three gradient coils, and receiver coil to produce an MR image.

Pulse sequence diagram: A depiction of the RF pulses, gradient behavior, and resulting signal used to generate and MR image.

Quench: The loss of superconductivity with evaporation of cooling agents around the superconducting wire of the magnet.

R factor: A factor of k-space undersampling with parallel imaging.

R-R interval: The time between consecutive R waves of the electrocardiogram, indicating the duration of one heartbeat, typically expressed in milliseconds (msec).

Radial k-space trajectory: Filling of k-space with a series of linear trajectories that all traverse near or through the center of k-space.

Radiofrequency (RF) phase: The orientation of transverse component of magnetization following a radiofrequency pulse relative to the x or y axis.

Radiofrequency (RF) pulse: An energy pulse that can be thought of as a rotating magnetic field, B_1, aligned in the xy plane that pulls the magnetization vector away from the longitudinal direction towards the transverse plane.

Radiofrequency (RF) spoiling: Phase offsets to radiofrequency pulses used to reduce transverse magnetization from excitation to excitation in spoiled gradient echo imaging.

Rapid acquisition with relaxation enhancement (RARE): See **Fast spin echo**.

Readout gradient: See **Frequency-encoding gradient**.

Real component of k-space: The part of the complex numbers represented in k-space that reflects cosine spatial frequency components.

Real image: The Fourier transform of the real component of k-space.

Receiver bandwidth: The range of frequencies detected in a measured MR signal. The receiver bandwidth and sampling frequency are interdependent.

Receiver channels: Separate input channels that relay MR signals from particular receiver coils into the computer for analysis.

Receiver coil: A configuration of wires that are used to record signal from protons.

Rectangular field of view (recFOV): A technique to reduce acquisition times by undersampling k-space in the phase-encoding direction, which causes a proportional reduction in FOV in the phase-encoding direction without a loss of spatial resolution.

Rectilinear k-space trajectory: See **Linear k-space trajectory**.

Refocusing angle: The flip angle of the radiofrequency pulse used with spin echo imaging to cause refocusing, typically 180°.

Refocusing pulse: A radiofrequency (RF) pulse applied after the initial RF excitation to form a spin echo.

Region of interest (ROI): A manually defined area on an image, used to measure signal intensities.

Regurgitant fraction: The ratio of regurgitant flow (mL/beat) to forward flow (mL/beat), often expressed as a percentage.

Relaxation: The return of protons to alignment with the external field B_0 following RF excitation see T1 relaxation and T2 relaxation.

Relaxivity, R1,2: The inverse of the relaxation time T1,2 (i.e., $R_1 = 1/T_1$ and $R_2 = 1/T_2$), which has the units of sec^{-1} and, for a contrast agent, is the product of the relaxivity constant r1, r2 of the agent and the concentration of the agent.

Relaxivity constant, r1,2: The amount of relaxivity produced by a given agent per unit of concentration, which has the units of $(mmol/L\text{-}sec)^{-1}$.

Repetition time (TR): The time between consecutive RF excitations.

Retrospective gating: Continuous acquisition of MR data and simultaneous recording of the electrocardiogram to allow image reconstruction based on the sorting of data relative to time after the R wave.

Rise time: The time needed for a gradient to reach peak amplitude.

Sampling frequency: The rate at which the echo is sampled and digitized. The units of sampling frequency are usually in kHz. See **Hertz**.

Saturation: Suppression of unwanted signal by using RF prepulses to shift the spins of the unwanted protons into the xy plane and dephasing them, then applying the RF pulse for generating the signal echo before the unwanted protons have recovered.

Saturation recovery: An approach that uses a 90° prepulse to improve image contrast, usually applied to fast T1-weighted gradient echo imaging.

Scan delay: The time between start of contrast bolus injection and initiation of imaging acquisition.

Segmented k-space: The acquisition of multiple echoes or lines of k-space per frame per heartbeat in cine gradi-

ent echo imaging, or acquisition of multiple echoes or lines of k-space per radiofrequency excitation in echo planar imaging.

Sequential filling of k-space: Use of a k-space trajectory in which the filling of k-space is performed from one peripheral edge through the center and then finished at the other edge of the periphery, typically refers to linear trajectories.

Sensitivity encoding (SENSE): A parallel imaging technique that uses coil sensitivity information to correct for k-space undersampling in the post-Fourier domain.

Shielding: Methods used to reduce the fringe field, including active and passive shielding.

Shimming: Use of additional coils to improve field homogeneity over the area of imaging.

Short axis: The plane of the heart that is positioned orthogonal to the long axis and depicts the left ventricle as a doughnut shape, usually aquired in a series from the base to the apex of the left ventricle in conjunction with long axis views.

Short tau inversion recovery (STIR): An inversion recovery spin echo sequence, usually used to generate T2-weighted imaging with fat suppression.

Signal averaging: The practice in which a number of signals are averaged to generate an image, usually to improve the signal-to-noise ratio of an image and to reduce the effects of respiratory or abdominal motion; see **Number of signal averages**.

Signal intensity: The brightness of a voxel in an image displayed on the MR monitor, with arbitrary units.

Signal-to-noise ratio: A parameter describing image quality, determined by the ratio of the signal intensity in a region of an image divided by image noise.

Simultaneous acquisition of spatial harmonics (SMASH): A parallel imaging technique that uses coil sensitivity information to correct for k-space undersampling in the pre-Fourier domain.

Sinc function: A function defined as (sin x)/x, and used to describe the sum of sinusoidal functions across a continuous range of frequencies.

Sinc interpolation: See **Zero filling**.

Single dose: 0.1 mmol/kg subject body weight gadolinium contrast material.

Single-shot imaging: MR sequences that generate enough data to produce a single image with only one radiofrequency excitation.

Slab-selective RF excitation: An RF pulse a tissue accompanied by a gradient in the z direction to excite selectively a tissue slab in 3D MR imaging.

Slew rate: The maximum rate of increase of the gradient amplitude to reach its maximum.

Slice profile: The distribution of signal across the thickness of a slice.

Slice-select gradient: A magnetic field gradient applied during RF excitation to ensure that only a thin tissue slice is excited by the RF pulse.

Slice thickness to gap ratio: A relationship between slice thickness and interslice gaps, usually dependent on the nature of the truncated RF excitation pulse; for example, for an RF pulse truncated to 2 periods, the slice thickness to gap ratio would be 5 : 1; See also **Distance factor**.

Spatial localization: The process by which individual contributions to overall MR signal are resolved on a voxel-by-voxel basis.

Spatial modulation of magnetization (SPAMM): A technique for using radiofrequency prepulses to tag myocardium in order to track local myocardial deformation and quantify strain.

Spatial resolution: A parameter of image quality that reflects the size of the smallest lesions that may be depicted and how sharp edges appear.

Specific absorption rate (SAR): The rate at which RF energy is absorbed by a subject being imaged, expressed in watts per kilogram.

Spin echo: A signal generated from application of two RF pulses, usually 90° and 180°.

Spin-lattice relaxation: See **T1 relaxation**.

Spin-spin relaxation: See **T2 relaxation**.

Spiral k-space trajectory: Filling of k-space using a spiral path starting from the center.

Spoiled gradient echo (SPGR) or **fast low angle shot imaging** or **fast field echo**: A type of gradient echo sequence in which the residual transverse magnetization following the gradient echo does not contribute to signal measured from subsequent excitations.

Spoiler gradient or **crusher gradient**: A technique to create spoiled gradient echo images by extended application of a gradient to dephase the residual transverse magnetization following a gradient echo before the next RF pulse.

Steady-state gradient echo: A type of gradient echo sequence in which residual transverse magnetization following the gradient echo is preserved and used to contribute to subsequent gradient echoes.

Steady state free precession (SSFP): See **True FISP**.

Stroke volume (SV): The volume of blood that is ejected from the left ventricle during systole per heartbeat,

computed as the difference between the end diastolic volume and the end systolic volume.

Surface shaded display (SSD): An image post-processing reconstruction algorithm that uses a ray casting algorithm to generate surfaces and frequently implements a simulated light source for shading of surfaces.

Symmetric function: A type of function, such as cosine, that is the mirror image of itself around zero, so that $f(-x) = f(x)$.

T1 recovery: See **T1 relaxation**.

T1 relaxation or **longitudinal relaxation** or **spin-lattice relaxation**: The process in which protons that are perturbed away from the direction of the main magnetic field become realigned and fully recover longitudinal magnetization after the perturbing field is turned off.

T1-weighted images: Images whose contrast is based on differences in T1 relaxation.

T2 decay: See **T2 relaxation**.

T2 Preparation: A technique used to increase T2 weighting by means of +90°, −180°, 180°, ..., 180°, −90° prepulses.

T2 relaxation or **spin-spin relaxation**: Loss of phase coherence of transverse magnetization resulting from the variability in exchange of energy between adjacent protons.

T2* relaxation: Loss of phase coherence of transverse magnetization, due to both intrinsic T2 relaxation and T2′ relaxation.

T2′ relaxation: Loss of phase coherence of transverse magnetization as a result of heterogeneity in the B_0 magnetic field.

T2-weighted images: Images whose contrast is based on differences in T2 relaxation

TE: See **Echo time**.

TR: See **Repetition time**.

Target heart rate: 85% of the age-specific maximum expected heart rate, calculated as $0.85 \times (220 - \text{Age (yrs)})$.

Three-chamber view: See **Left ventricular outflow tract/three-chamber view**.

Through-plane flow: A term that refers to phase contrast imaging where the flow sensitivity is in the direction perpendicular to the imaging plane.

Time-of-flight (TOF): Increased signal from inflow of unsaturated moving protons into a gradient echo image during acquisition.

Time-resolved magnetic resonance angiography (MRA): Repeated MRA acquisitions performed with high temporal resolution to assess contrast enhancement kinetics during the first pass of the contrast bolus.

Transmitting coil: A configuration of wires that are used to cause radiofrequency excitation.

Transmitter bandwidth: The range of frequencies contained an RF excitation pulse. The transmitter bandwidth, coupled with the slice-select gradient, determines the thickness and location of the imaging slice.

Transverse magnetization: The component of the net magnetization aligned in the plane perpendicular to the axis of the main magnetic field.

Trigger delay (TD): The delay time between detection of the R-wave and the start of imaging, used with ECG-triggered sequences.

Trigger frequency: A parameter indicating how frequently an R wave triggers an acquisition; for example, an acquisition might occur every R wave or every other R wave.

Trigger window (TW): The short interval between the end of data sampling and the next expected R wave in prospectively-triggered sequences.

True fast imaging with steady-state precession (true FISP), or **fast imaging excitation with steady-state acquisition** or **balanced fast field echo**: A balanced steady-state gradient echo sequence frequently used in cardiovascular applications in which image contrast depends on the ratio of relaxation times, T2/T1, causing blood to have high signal intensity relative to other soft tissues.

Turbo factor: See **Echo train length**.

Turbo fast low angle shot imaging (turboFLASH): A fast spoiled gradient echo technique that is used for 2D and 3D imaging that typically uses a 180° prepulse for T1-weighted image contrast.

Turbo field echo (TFE): See **Turbo fast low angle shot imaging**.

Turbo spin echo (TSE): See **Fast spin echo**.

Turbulent flow: Flow in a vessel that is nonlaminar, often characterized by eddies and vortices of flow, such as across areas of stenosis.

Two-chamber view: See **Vertical long axis**.

Undersampling: Sampling of a function at less than twice the maximum frequency f; causing misrepresentation of that function. See also **Nyquist theorem of sampling**.

Upslope ratio: A parameter to quantify myocardial perfusion based on the upslope of the myocardial enhancement

curve divided by the upslope of the left ventricular blood enhancement curve.

Upslope: The rate of initial enhancement of the myocardium or left ventricular blood pool in first-pass contrast-enhanced myocardial perfusion imaging.

Vector: A quantity that has magnitude and direction, typically expressed as an arrow.

Vectorcardiograms (VCG): A method for synchronization of MRI with cardiac motion that uses temporal and spatial information about cardiac electrical activity to differentiate better between true signals and artifactual signals resulting from magnetohydrodynamic effect and other noise.

Velocity: Measurement of motion (such as that of blood) in units of distance per time, typically cm/sec or m/sec.

Venc: See **Encoding velocity**.

Vertical long axis, or **two-chamber view**: The plane of the heart that is defined by the long axis, which traverses the midpoint of the mitral valve orifice and the left ventricular apex, bisecting the left ventricle vertically.

View sharing, or **echo sharing**: A technique for increasing apparent temporal resolution by undersampling k-space data for certain time points or frames and utilizing data from adjacent frames to fill in the missing data.

Views per segment, or **lines per segment**: The number of lines of k-space collected per frame per heartbeat in cine gradient echo imaging.

Volume rendering (VR): An image post-processing reconstruction algorithm that can be used for MR angiography whereby the opacity of a voxel is varied to reflect relative positions of structures in the imaging volume.

Voxel: A volume element of an image that has dimensions in three directions (x, y, and z). See also **Pixel**.

Wraparound artifact: The undesired appearance of tissue outside the desired field of view within the image.

Zero filling, or **sinc interpolation**, **zero interpolation**, **zero padding**, or **zip interpolation**: The addition of data points in k-space consisting of zeroes, which have the effect of increasing the matrix size and the apparent spatial resolution, although the true spatial resolution of the image is not increased.

Zero interpolation: See **Zero filling**.

Zero padding: See **Zero filling**.

Zip interpolation: See **Zero filling**.

INDEX